Netter's Obstetrics, Gynecology, and Women's Health

Netter's Obstetrics, Gynecology, and Women's Health

Roger P. Smith, M.D.
University of Missouri–Kansas City

Illustrations by Frank H. Netter, M.D.

Contributing Illustrators

John A. Craig, M.D.
Carlos A. G. Machado, M.D.

Icon Learning Systems • Teterboro, New Jersey

Published by Icon Learning Systems LLC, a subsidiary of MediMedia USA, Inc.
Copyright © 2002 MediMedia, Inc.

FIRST EDITION

ISBN 0-914168-96-7

Library of Congress Catalog No 2002101815

Printed in Canada
First Printing, 2002

NOTICE

Editorial Director: Greg Otis
Managing Editor: Jennifer Surich
Print Production Manager: Jim O'Keeffe
Art Production Managers: Jonna Armstrong and Michelle Jahn
Art Director: Joanie Krupinski

Binding and Printing by Friesens
Color Corrections by Page Imaging
Digital Separations by R. R. Donnelly and Page Imaging
Composition and Layout by Graphic World, Inc.

This work is dedicated to my father,

who taught me the "art" of medicine

and who first introduced me to the art of Dr. Netter.

Preface

No student of medicine, past or present, is unaware of the extraordinary series of medical illustrations created by Dr. Frank Netter; an incredible body of work that has been carried forward since Dr. Netter's passing by the talented John Craig, M.D. Older physicians have looked in envy at these images wishing they had been available when they were learning; established physicians return to them as comfortable sources of information; young physicians seek them out for the wealth of information they contain and their ability to make clear difficult clinical concepts. This spirit of concise reference and resource is the premise of this text.

This text revisits the classic illustrations of Dr. Netter with new and updated material skillfully rendered by Dr. Craig. In addition, we have enlisted the painting talents of two gifted illustrators, Ms. Enid Hatton and Mr. David Mascaro, to paint the new sketches that Dr. Craig has created for this work. We have also included numerous, outstanding paintings created by Carlos Machado, M.D., throughout the book.

The text has been organized to provide a quick, concise resource for the diagnosis and treatment of common conditions encountered by anyone who cares for women. The text material is presented in a consistent format to facilitate rapid access—the same information is in the same location. The topics chosen for inclusion are not meant to be exhaustive of the field of women's care, but rather to address those conditions and challenges that are common and lend themselves to the magic of the visual image. The look, feel, utility, and organization of this work is due in no small part to the vision and talents of Ms. Susan Gay, who has acted as the consulting editor and cheerleader for the project. Bringing the rough draft to final polish has been the task of Jennifer Surich from Icon Learning Systems and Noelle Barrick from Graphic World Publishing Services, who have been more than tolerant of this author's linguistic and typographic failings.

It is our hope that this work will be both a useful resource and celebration of the artistic richness that is clinical medicine.

About the Author

Although Roger P. Smith, M.D., is Vice Chairman, Professor and Director of the Residency Program for the Department of Obstetrics and Gynecology at the University of Missouri–Kansas City, Truman Medical Center, and has a "CV" that is appropriately long, he regards himself as a clinician. Dr. Smith received his undergraduate education at Purdue University, and his medical education, internship (in General Surgery), and residency at Northwestern University in Chicago. He then spent almost ten years in a multi-disciplinary group practice at the Carle Clinic in Urbana, Illinois, before moving to the Medical College of Georgia in 1985, where he was Chief of the Section of General Obstetrics and Gynecology.

Dr. Smith joined the Truman Medical Center in 1999.

Frank H. Netter, M.D.

Frank H. Netter was born in 1906 in New York City. He studied art at the Art Student's League and the National Academy of Design before entering medical school at New York University, where he received his M.D. degree in 1931. During his student years, Dr. Netter's notebook sketches attracted the attention of the medical faculty and other physicians, allowing him to augment his income by illustrating articles and textbooks. He continued illustrating as a sideline after establishing a surgical practice in 1933, but he ultimately opted to give up his practice in favor of a full-time commitment to art. After service in the United States Army during World War II, Dr. Netter began his long collaboration with the CIBA Pharmaceutical Company (now Novartis Pharmaceuticals). This 45-year partnership resulted in the production of the extraordinary collection of medical art so familiar to physicians and other medical professionals worldwide.

Icon Learning Systems acquired the Netter Collection in July 2000 and continues to update Dr. Netter's original paintings and to add newly commissioned paintings by artists trained in the style of Dr. Netter.

Dr. Netter's works are among the finest examples of the use of illustration in the teaching of medical concepts. The 13-book Netter Collection of Medical Illustrations, which includes the greater part of the more than 20,000 paintings created by Dr. Netter, became and remains one of the most famous medical works ever published. The Netter Atlas of Human Anatomy, first published in 1989, presents the anatomical paintings from the Netter Collection. Now translated into 11 languages, it is the anatomy atlas of choice among medical and health professions students the world over.

The Netter illustrations are appreciated not only for their aesthetic qualities, but more importantly, for their intellectual content. As Dr. Netter wrote in 1949, ". . . clarification of a subject is the aim and goal of illustration. No matter how beautifully painted, how delicately and subtly rendered a subject may be, it is of little value as a medical illustration *if it does not serve to make clear some medical point.*" Dr. Netter's planning, conception, point of view, and approach are what inform his paintings and what makes them so intellectually valuable.

Frank H. Netter, M.D., physician and artist, died in 1991.

Contents

SECTION VI
Adnexal Disease 231

SECTION VII
Breast Diseases and Conditions 291

SECTION VIII
Genetic and Endocrine Conditions 335

SECTION IX
Women's Health/Primary Care 395

Vulvar Disease

BARTHOLIN'S GLAND: ABSCESS/INFECTION

INTRODUCTION

Description: An infection in one or both Bartholin's glands resulting in swelling and/or abscess formation. Usually the process is unilateral and marked by pain and swelling. Systemic symptoms are minimal except in advanced cases.

Prevalence: Two percent of adult women develop infection or enlargement of one or both Bartholin's glands.

Predominant Age: Eighty-five percent of Bartholin's gland infections occur during the reproductive years.

Genetics: No genetic pattern.

ETIOLOGY AND PATHOGENESIS

Causes: Infection by *Neisseria gonorrhoeae*, secondary infection by other organisms (eg, *Escherichia coli*).

Risk Factors: Exposure to sexually transmitted disease, trauma.

CLINICAL CHARACTERISTICS

Signs and Symptoms:

- Cystic, painful swelling of the labia in the area of the Bartholin's gland (5 and 7 o'clock on the vulva) developing rapidly over 2–4 days; cysts can range to 8 cm or greater
- Fever and malaise (uncommon)

DIAGNOSTIC APPROACH

Differential Diagnosis:

- Cellulitis
- Necrotizing fasciitis
- Mesonephric cysts of the vagina
- Lipomas
- Fibromas
- Hernias
- Hydrocele
- Epidermal inclusion or sebaceous cyst
- Bartholin's gland malignancy (rare)
- Neurofibroma

Associated Conditions: Dyspareunia

Workup and Evaluation

Laboratory: Because bartholinitis or a Bartholin's gland abscess may be gonococcal in origin, further evaluation for other sexually transmitted disease is prudent. Most often, culture-positive cysts are secondarily infected by coliform organisms or are polymicrobial, limiting the value of routine culture from the cyst.

Imaging: No imaging indicated.
Special Tests: None indicated.
Diagnostic Procedures: Inspection.

Pathologic Findings

Inflammation, dilation of the Bartholin's gland duct, abscess formation.

MANAGEMENT AND THERAPY

Nonpharmacologic

General Measures: Evaluation, perineal hygiene.

Specific Measures: Mild infections may respond to antibiotic or topical therapies. Warm to hot sitz baths provide relief and promote drainage. Spontaneous drainage typically occurs in 1–4 days. Simple drainage is associated with recurrence; therefore, placement of a Word catheter, packing with iodoform gauze, or surgical marsupialization of the gland is desirable.

Diet: No specific dietary changes indicated.

Activity: No restriction.

Patient Education: Reassurance, American College of Obstetricians and Gynecologists Patient Education Pamphlet AP088 (*Diseases of the Vulva*), AP009 (*How to Prevent Sexually Transmitted Diseases*).

Drug(s) of Choice

Ampicillin (500 mg PO qid) or other broad-spectrum antibiotic if cellulitis is present.

Contraindications: Known hypersensitivity or allergy to agent.

Alternative Therapies

Excision of the gland is often difficult and is associated with significant risk of morbidity, including intraoperative hemorrhage, hematoma formation, secondary infection, scar formation, and dyspareunia. For these reasons, excision is not generally recommended.

FOLLOW-UP

Patient Monitoring: Follow up to monitor for spontaneous drainage or the need for surgical intervention.

Prevention/Avoidance: Reduced exposure to sexually transmitted disease and vulvar trauma.

Possible Complications: Chronic cyst formation.

Expected Outcome: Recurrences occur to 5%–10% of patients after marsupialization.

MISCELLANEOUS

Pregnancy Considerations: No effect on pregnancy.
ICD-9-CM Codes: 616.3.

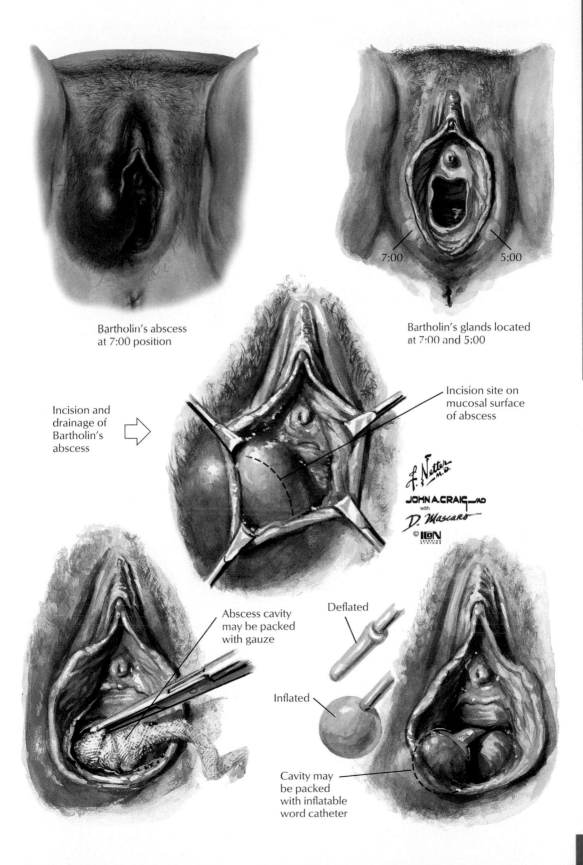

Bartholin's abscess
at 7:00 position

Bartholin's glands located
at 7:00 and 5:00

7:00   5:00

Incision and
drainage of
Bartholin's
abscess

Incision site on
mucosal surface
of abscess

Abscess cavity
may be packed
with gauze

Deflated

Inflated

Cavity may
be packed
with inflatable
word catheter

REFERENCES

Aghajanian A, Bernstein L, Grimes DA. Bartholin's duct abscess and cyst: a case-control study. *South Med J* 1994;87:26.

Cheetham DR. Bartholin's cyst: marsupialization or aspiration? *Am J Obstet Gynecol* 1985;152:569.

Smith RP. *Gynecology in Primary Care*. Baltimore, Md: Williams & Wilkins; 1997:603.

Wells EC. Simple operation of the vulva. In: Sciarra JJ, ed. *Gynecology and Obstetrics*. Vol 1. Philadelphia, Pa: JB Lippincott; 1997;11:6.

BARTHOLIN'S GLAND: CYSTS

INTRODUCTION

Description: A chronic cystic dilation of the Bartholin's gland and duct generally secondary to past infection.

Prevalence: Two percent of adult women develop infection or enlargement of one or both Bartholin's glands.

Predominant Age: Eighty-five percent of Bartholin's gland cysts occur during the reproductive years.

Genetics: No genetic pattern.

ETIOLOGY AND PATHOGENESIS

Causes: Bartholin's gland infection or abscess leading to obstruction of the duct.

Risk Factors: Exposure to sexually transmitted disease, trauma, prior Bartholin's gland abscesses.

CLINICAL CHARACTERISTICS

Signs and Symptoms:
- Smaller, more chronic cysts, caused by obstruction of the Bartholin's duct, may be identified by gentle palpation at the base of the labia majora. These cysts are smooth, firm, and tender with varying degrees of induration and overlying erythema. The cysts may be clear, yellow, or bluish in color.

DIAGNOSTIC APPROACH

Differential Diagnosis:
- Epidermal inclusion or sebaceous cyst
- Mesonephric cysts of the vagina
- Lipomas
- Fibromas
- Hernias
- Hydrocele
- Bartholin's gland malignancy (rare)
- Neurofibroma

Associated Conditions: Dyspareunia.

Workup and Evaluation

Laboratory: No evaluation indicated. (More than 80% of cultures of material from Bartholin's gland cysts are sterile.)

Imaging: No imaging indicated.

Special Tests: None indicated.

Diagnostic Procedures: Inspection.

Pathologic Findings

Cystic dilation of the duct and/or gland, often with chronic induration or inflammation.

MANAGEMENT AND THERAPY

Nonpharmacologic

General Measures: Evaluation, perineal hygiene.

Specific Measures: Asymptomatic small Bartholin's cysts require no therapy. Larger or symptomatic cysts require surgical marsupialization. If surgery is undertaken, it should be reserved for a time when any infection is quiescent.

Diet: No specific dietary changes indicated.

Activity: No restriction.

Patient Education: Reassurance, American College of Obstetricians and Gynecologists Patient Education Pamphlet AP088 (*Diseases of the Vulva*).

Drug(s) of Choice

None indicated.

Alternative Therapies

Excision of the gland is often difficult and is associated with significant risk of morbidity, including intraoperative hemorrhage, hematoma formation, secondary infection, scar formation, and dyspareunia. For these reasons, excision is not generally recommended.

FOLLOW-UP

Patient Monitoring: Normal health maintenance.

Prevention/Avoidance: Reduced exposure to sexually transmitted disease and vulvar trauma.

Possible Complications: Dyspareunia, recurrent inflammation.

Expected Outcome: Recurrences occur to 5%–10% of patients following marsupialization.

MISCELLANEOUS

Pregnancy Considerations: No effect on pregnancy.

ICD-9-CM Codes: 616.2.

REFERENCES

Aghajanian A, Bernstein L, Grimes DA. Bartholin's duct abscess and cyst: a case-control study. *South Med J* 1994;87:26.

Cheetham DR. Bartholin's cyst: marsupialization or aspiration? *Am J Obstet Gynecol* 1985;152:569.

Smith RP. *Gynecology in Primary Care*. Baltimore, Md: Williams & Wilkins; 1997:603.

Wells EC. Simple operation of the vulva. In: Sciarra JJ, ed. *Gynecology and Obstetrics*. Vol 1. Philadelphia, Pa: JB Lippincott; 1997;11:6.

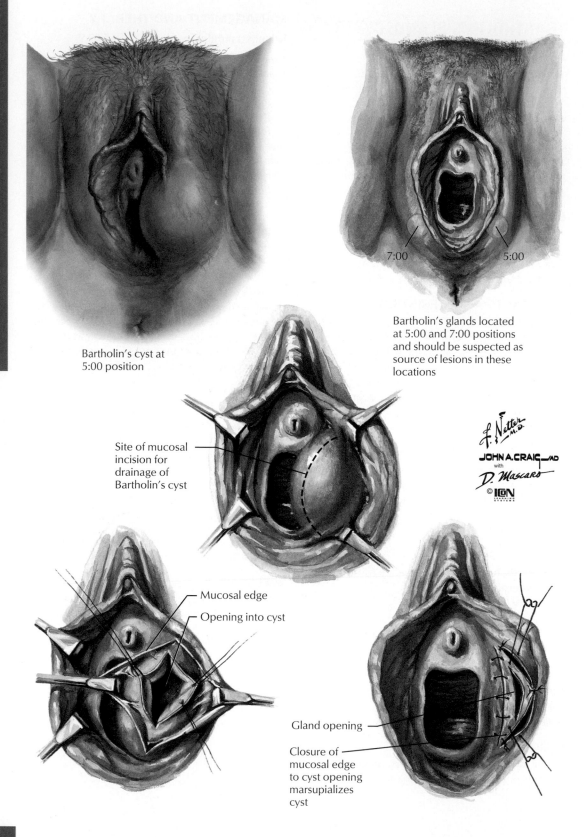

Bartholin's cyst at
5:00 position

7:00   5:00

Bartholin's glands located
at 5:00 and 7:00 positions
and should be suspected as
source of lesions in these
locations

Site of mucosal
incision for
drainage of
Bartholin's cyst

Mucosal edge

Opening into cyst

Gland opening

Closure of
mucosal edge
to cyst opening
marsupializes
cyst

CONTACT VULVITIS

INTRODUCTION

Description: Vulvar irritation caused by contact with an irritant or allergen.

Prevalence: Relatively common.

Predominant Age: Any, but most common in reproductive and menopausal years.

Genetics: No genetic pattern.

ETIOLOGY AND PATHOGENESIS

Causes: Irritants may be primary or immunologic in character. The list of potential irritants can be extensive, including "feminine hygiene" sprays, deodorants and deodorant soaps, tampons or pads (especially those with deodorants or perfumes), tight-fitting or synthetic undergarments, colored or scented toilet paper, and laundry soap or fabric softener residues. Even topical contraceptives, latex condoms, lubricants, "sexual aides," or semen may be the source of irritation. Soiling of the vulva by urine or feces can also create significant symptoms. Severe dermatitis of the vulva resulting from contact with poison ivy or poison oak is occasionally found.

Risk Factors: Exposure to allergen (most often cosmetic or local therapeutic agents), immunosuppression, or diabetes.

CLINICAL CHARACTERISTICS

Signs and Symptoms:

- Diffuse reddening of the vulvar skin accompanied by itching or burning
- Symmetric, red, edematous change in the tissues
- Ulceration with weeping sores and secondary infection possible

DIAGNOSTIC APPROACH

Differential Diagnosis:

- Vaginal infection
- Local *Candida* infection
- Vulvar dermatoses
- Atrophic vulvitis
- Vulvar dystrophy
- Pinworms
- Psoriasis
- Seborrheic dermatitis
- Neurodermatitis
- Impetigo
- Hidradenitis suppurativa

Associated Conditions: Dyspareunia, dysuria.

Workup and Evaluation

Laboratory: Examination of vaginal secretions under saline and 10% KOH to rule out possible vaginal infection.

Imaging: No imaging indicated.

Special Tests: Vulvar biopsy rarely required although it may be diagnostic.

Diagnostic Procedures: A careful history, combined with the withdrawal of the suspected cause, usually both confirms the diagnosis and constitutes the needed therapy.

Pathologic Findings

Vulvar biopsy shows chronic inflammatory change and infiltration by histiocytes.

MANAGEMENT AND THERAPY

Nonpharmacologic

General Measures: Perineal hygiene (keep the perineal area clean and dry; avoid tight or synthetic undergarments), education regarding prevention, encourage completion of the prescribed course of therapy.

Specific Measures: Removal of identified (or possible) allergens, topical therapy.

Diet: No specific dietary changes indicated.

Activity: No restriction.

Patient Education: Reassurance, education about avoidance or risk reduction, American College of Obstetricians and Gynecologists Patient Education Pamphlet AP088 (*Diseases of the Vulva*), AP116 (*Menstrual Hygiene Products*).

Drug(s) of Choice

Wet compresses or soaks using Burow's solution (three to four times daily for 30–60 minutes), followed by air drying or drying with a hair dryer (on cool). (Loose-fitting clothing and the sparing use of a nonmedicated baby powder may facilitate the drying process.)

Steroid creams, (hydrocortisone 0.5%–1%) or fluorinated corticosteroids (Valisone 0.1%, Synalar 0.01%) applied two to three times a day if needed.

Precautions: Further evaluation is warranted (including biopsy) if initial therapy does not produce significant improvement.

Alternative Drugs

Eucerin cream may be used to rehydrate the skin and reduce itching.

VULVAR DISEASE

FOLLOW-UP

Patient Monitoring: Normal health maintenance.
Prevention/Avoidance: Avoidance of possible allergens.
Possible Complications: Excoriation, chronic vulvar change (thickening).
Expected Outcome: With removal of causative agent, complete resolution should be expected.

MISCELLANEOUS

Pregnancy Considerations: No effect on pregnancy.
ICD-9-CM Codes: 616.10.

REFERENCES

American College of Obstetricians and Gynecologists. *Vulvovaginitis.* Washington, DC: ACOG; 1989. ACOG Technical Bulletin 135.

McKay M. Vulvar dermatoses. *Clin Obstet Gynecol* 1991;34:614.

Nanda VS. Common dermatoses. *Am J Obstet Gynecol* 1995;173:488.

Smith RP. *Gynecology in Primary Care.* Baltimore, Md: Williams & Wilkins; 1997:603.

Summers P. Vaginitis in 1993. *Clin Obstet Gynecol* 1993;36:105.

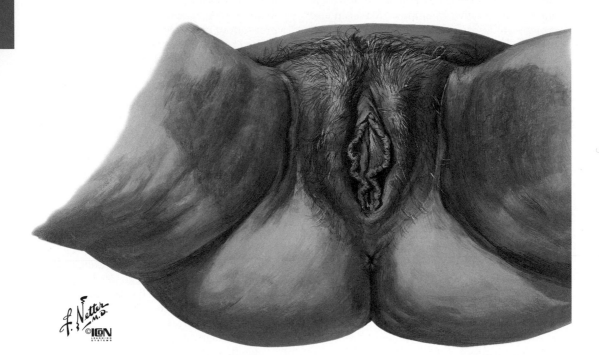

DYSPAREUNIA: INSERTIONAL

INTRODUCTION

Description: Pain that occurs with sexual penetration. This may be in the form of mild discomfort that may be tolerated, pain that completely prevents intromission, or any level of pain in between. In severe cases, pain may lead to severe vaginal spasms that interfere with penetration (vaginismus).

Prevalence: Roughly 15% of women each year (severe—less than 2% of women).

Predominant Age: Reproductive and beyond.

Genetics: No genetic pattern.

ETIOLOGY AND PATHOGENESIS

Causes: Congenital factors (duplication of the vagina, hymenal stenosis, vaginal agenesis, vaginal septum), cystitis (acute or chronic), hemorrhoids, inadequate lubrication (abuse [current or past], arousal disorders, insufficient foreplay, medication, phobias), pelvic (levator) muscle spasm, pelvic scarring (episiotomy, surgical repairs [colporrhaphy]), proctitis trauma (acute or chronic sequelae), urethral diverticula, urethral syndrome, urethritis (bacterial or chlamydial), vaginismus, vulvar (atrophic vulvitis, chancroid, chemical irritation [deodorants, adjuncts, lubricants]), herpes vulvitis, hypertrophic vulvar dystrophy, lichen sclerosis, lymphogranuloma venereum, vestibulitis, vulvitis (infectious), vulvodynia.

Risk Factors: Those associated with causal pathologic conditions.

CLINICAL CHARACTERISTICS

Signs and Symptoms:
- Sharp, burning, or pinching discomfort felt externally (vulva and perineum) during attempts at vaginal penetration (not limited to the penis). The discomfort is generally localized to the vulva, perineum, or outer portion of the vagina. The symptoms may help to localize the cause, but are often generalized and nonspecific.

DIAGNOSTIC APPROACH

Differential Diagnosis:
- Vulvitis (including condyloma)
- Vestibulitis
- Vaginitis
- Bartholin's gland infection, abscess, cyst
- Atrophic change
- Anxiety, depression, phobia
- Sexual or other abuse
- Postherpetic neuralgia
- Hymenal stenosis
- Hymenal caruncle

Associated Conditions: Vaginismus, orgasmic dysfunction.

Workup and Evaluation

Laboratory: No evaluation indicated. Urinalysis, microscopic examination of vaginal secretions, and cultures (cervical and urethral) only for the evaluation of specific processes and clinical suspicion.

Imaging: No imaging indicated.

Special Tests: Colposcopic examination of the vulva and introitus if vestibulitis is suspected.

Diagnostic Procedures: History and pelvic examination.

Pathologic Findings

None.

MANAGEMENT AND THERAPY

Nonpharmacologic

General Measures: Evaluation, reassurance, and relaxation measures. Vaginal lubricants (water-soluble or long-acting agents such as Astro-Glide, Replens, Lubrin, K-Y Jelly, and others), local anesthetics (for vulvar lesions), or pelvic relaxation exercises may be appropriate while more specific therapy is underway. These may be especially useful during the early phase of therapy when arousal may be compromised by the experience of pain.

Specific Measures: Because dyspareunia is ultimately a symptom, the specific therapy for any form of sexual pain is focused on the underlying cause.

Diet: No specific dietary changes indicated.

Activity: No restriction.

Patient Education: Reassurance, relaxation training, progressive desensitization, American College of Obstetricians and Gynecologists Patient Education Pamphlet AP020 (*Pain During Intercourse*), AP042 (*You and Your Sexuality*).

Drug(s) of Choice

The judicious use of anxiolytics or antidepressant medications for selected patients may be appropriate, for short periods of time only.

Alternative Therapies

Modifying the sexual techniques used by the couple may reduce pain with intercourse. Delaying penetration until maximal arousal has been

Self-perpetuating sexual pain

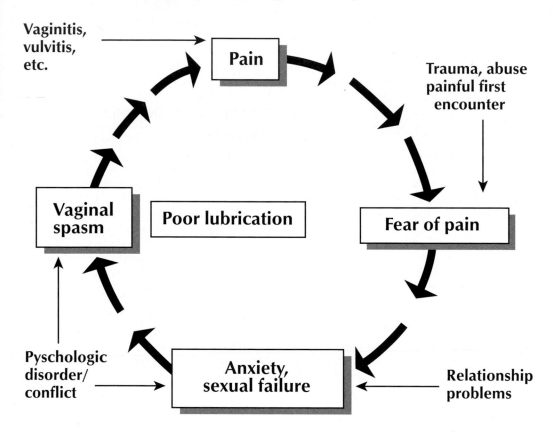

Vaginitis, vulvitis, etc.

Pain

Trauma, abuse painful first encounter

Fear of pain

Vaginal spasm

Poor lubrication

Anxiety, sexual failure

Relationship problems

Pyschologic disorder/ conflict

achieved improves vaginal lubrication, ensures vaginal apex expansion, and provides an element of control for the female partner. Sexual positions that allow the women to control the direction and depth of penetration (such as woman astride) may also be of help.

FOLLOW-UP

Patient Monitoring: Normal health maintenance. Watch for signs of abuse, anxiety, or depression.

Prevention/Avoidance: None.

Possible Complications: Marital discord, orgasmic or libidinal dysfunction.

Expected Outcome: With diagnosis and treatment of the underlying cause, response should be good.

MISCELLANEOUS

Pregnancy Considerations: No effect on pregnancy.

ICD-9-CM Codes: 625.0.

REFERENCES

Bachmann GA. Superficial dyspareunia and vestibulitis. In: Sciarra JJ, ed. *Gynecology and Obstetrics.* Vol 1. Philadelphia, Pa: JB Lippincott; 1998;77:1.

Fink P. Dyspareunia: current concepts. *Med Aspects Hum Sex* 1972;6:28.

Fordney DS. Dyspareunia and vaginismus. *Clin Obstet Gynecol* 1978;21(1):205.

Fullerton W. Dyspareunia. *BMJ* 1971;2:31.

Lamont JA. Dyspareunia and vaginismus. In: Sciarra JJ, ed. *Gynecology and Obstetrics.* Vol 6. Philadelphia, Pa: JB Lippincott; 1998;102:2.

Peckham EM, Maki DG, Patterson JJ, Hafez GR. Focal vulvitis: a characteristic syndrome and cause of dyspareunia. Features, natural history, and management. *Am J Obstet Gynecol* 1986;154:855.

Steege JF. Dyspareunia and vaginismus. *Clin Obstet Gynecol* 1984;27:750.

Steege JF, Ling FW. Dyspareunia. A special type of chronic pelvic pain. *Obstet Gynecol Clin North Am* 1993;20:779.

VULVAR DISEASE

VULVAR DISEASE

FEMALE CIRCUMCISION

INTRODUCTION

Description: Removal of part or all of the external genitalia including the labia majora, labia minora and/or the clitoris. Female circumcision (female genital mutilation, infibulation) is generally performed as a ritual process, often without benefit of anesthesia and frequently under unsterile conditions. The resulting scaring may preclude intromission. The amount and location of tissue removed determine the type of infibulation:

Type I—excision of the prepuce, with or without excision of part or the entire clitoris.

Type II—excision of the clitoris with partial or total excision of the labia minora.

Type III—excision of part or all of the external genitalia and stitching/narrowing of the vaginal opening (infibulation).

Type IV—pricking, piercing, or incising of the clitoris and/or labia; stretching of the clitoris and/or labia; cauterization by burning of the clitoris and surrounding tissue.

Other forms of female genital mutilation include the following:

Scraping of the tissue surrounding the vaginal orifice (angurya cuts) or cutting of the vagina (gishiri cuts).

Introduction of corrosive substances or herbs into the vagina to cause bleeding or for the purpose of tightening or narrowing it.

Any other procedure that falls under the definition given above.

Prevalence: 168,000 women in the United States, up to 96+% of women in some African countries (eg, Somalia).

Predominant Age: Majority performed during early teens (48,000 younger than 18).

Genetics: No genetic pattern.

ETIOLOGY AND PATHOGENESIS

Causes: Electively performed as part of ritual or religious beliefs, generally without the permission and often without the cooperation of the young girl herself.

Risk Factors: Most common in some African and Southeast Asian cultures.

CLINICAL CHARACTERISTICS

Signs and Symptoms:
- Significant scaring and deformity of the external genital structures, often to the point of complete obliteration of vaginal introitus

(varies with the type and extent of the procedure performed)
- Obstruction may be sufficient to result in amenorrhea or dysmenorrhea
- Dyspareunia
- Orgasmic dysfunction
- Libidinal dysfunction

DIAGNOSTIC APPROACH

Differential Diagnosis:
- Childhood burn injuries
- Intersex condition
- Imperforate hymen

Associated Conditions: Dyspareunia, libidinal dysfunction, and orgasmic dysfunction.

Workup and Evaluation

Laboratory: No evaluation indicated.
Imaging: No imaging indicated.
Special Tests: None indicated.
Diagnostic Procedures: History and physical examination.

Pathologic Findings

Absent or grossly scarred and deformed external genital tissues.

MANAGEMENT AND THERAPY

Nonpharmacologic

General Measures: Evaluation, support, and culturally sensitive education.
Specific Measures: Surgical opening of fused or scared genital tissue may be necessary to allow for menstrual hygiene and sexual function. An anterior episiotomy, with or without subsequent repair, may be required at the time of child birth (see the following).
Diet: No specific dietary changes indicated.
Activity: No restriction.
Patient Education: Culturally sensitive discussion of female anatomy, sexuality, and menstrual hygiene.

Drug(s) of Choice

None.

FOLLOW-UP

Patient Monitoring: Normal health maintenance. (Cervical samples for cytologic examination may be difficult to obtain in patients with extensive scarring until or unless surgical revision is performed.)
Prevention/Avoidance: Education of parents of young girls in cultures at risk for the procedure.

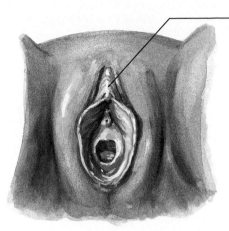

Clitoris
and
prepuce
removed

Type I: Clitoridectomy

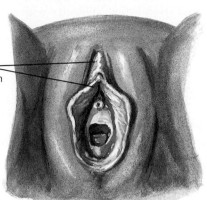

Clitoris
and portion
of labia
minora
excised

**Type II: Clitoridectomy and
partial excision of labia minora**

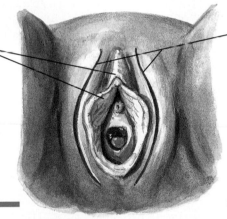

Total excision
of clitoris and
labia minora

Incisions in labia
majora for
approximation
over urethra
and vaginal
entrance
(infibulation)

JOHN A.CRAIG—AD
D. Mascaro
©IGN

Excision of clitoris and labia minora and
incision of labia majora in types III and IV

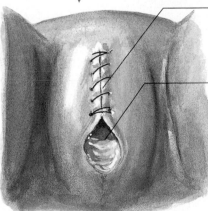

Anterior 2/3
of labia majora
closed over
urethra and
vaginal entrance

Opening

**Type III: Modified (intermediate
infibulation)—allows moderate
posterior opening**

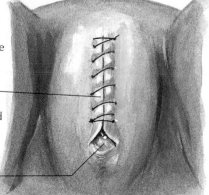

Majority of
labia majora
approximated
over urethra
and vaginal
entrance

Opening

**Type IV: Total infibulation—allows
only small posterior opening for
urine and menstral flow**

VULVAR DISEASE

Possible Complications: Acutely (at the time of the procedure)—bleeding and infection (including tetanus), urinary retention, pain. Long term—sexual dysfunction, difficulty with menstrual hygiene, recurrent vaginal or urinary tract infections, retrograde menstruation, hematocolpos, chronic pelvic inflammatory disease.

Expected Outcome: Sexual sequelae are often lifelong despite surgical revision (especially when clitoridectomy has been performed).

MISCELLANEOUS

Pregnancy Considerations: No effect on pregnancy, but presence may complicate conception and delivery. Delivery may require an anterior episiotomy with attendant increased risk of bleeding. (Subsequent repair of the episiotomy is illegal in some locations such as the United Kingdom and others because this amounts to reinfibulation.)

ICD-9-CM Codes: 624.4 (Old laceration or scarring of the vulva).

REFERENCES

American College of Obstetricians and Gynecologists. *Female Genital Mutilation*. Washington, DC: ACOG; 1995. Committee Opinion 151.

Aziz FA. Gynecologic and obstetric complications of female circumcision. *J Gynaecol Obstet* 1980;17:560.

Baker CA, Gilson GJ, Vill MD, Curet LB. Female circumcision: Obstetric issues. *Am J Obstet Gynecol* 1993;169:1616.

Council on Scientific Affairs, American Medical Association. Female genital mutilation. *JAMA* 1995;274:1714.

Cuntner LP. Female genital mutilation. *Obstet Gynecol Surv* 1985;40:437.

Khaled K, Vause S. Genital mutilation: a continued abuse. *Br J Obstet Gynaecol* 1996;103:86.

Miller L. Female circumcision. In: Sciarra JJ, ed. *Gynecology and Obstetrics*. Vol 1. Philadelphia, Pa: JB Lippincott, 1997;96:1.

Toubia N. Female circumcision as a public health issue. *N Engl J Med* 1994;331:712.

World Health Organization, Estimated prevalence rates for female genital mutilation, updated May 2001. http://www.who.int/frh-whd/FGM/FGM%20prev%20update.html

HIDRADENITIS SUPPURATIVA

INTRODUCTION

Description: A chronic, unrelenting, refractory infection of the skin and subcutaneous tissue initiated by obstruction and subsequent inflammation of apocrine glands, with resultant sinus and abscess formation. This process may involve the axilla, vulva, and perineum.

Prevalence: Uncommon.

Predominant Age: Reproductive (not found before puberty).

Genetics: Suggestions of family pattern but genetic link remains unproved.

ETIOLOGY AND PATHOGENESIS

Causes: Recurrent infections that arise in subcutaneous nodules. Proposed—hypersensitivity to androgens.

Risk Factors: None known.

CLINICAL CHARACTERISTICS

Signs and Symptoms:
- Recurrent and chronic inflammatory and ulcerated portions of labia associated with pain and foul-smelling discharge
- Multiple draining sinuses and abscesses

DIAGNOSTIC APPROACH

Differential Diagnosis:
- Sexually transmitted disease (granuloma inguinale, lymphogranuloma venereum)
- Crohn's disease
- Fox-Fordyce disease

Associated Conditions: Dyspareunia, vulvodynia.

Workup and Evaluation

Laboratory: No evaluation indicated.

Imaging: No imaging indicated.

Special Tests: Biopsy of the affected area may be necessary to establish the diagnosis.

Diagnostic Procedures: History, physical, and biopsy of affected area.

Pathologic Findings

Inflammation of the apocrine glands with occlusion of ducts, cystic dilation, and inspissation of keratin material. Multiple draining sinuses and abscesses are common.

MANAGEMENT AND THERAPY

Nonpharmacologic

General Measures: Perineal hygiene, sitz baths, loose-fitting clothing.

Specific Measures: Most effective therapy is based on early, aggressive, wide excision of affected area. Topical therapy with antibiotics, topical steroids, oral contraceptives, antiandrogens, and isotretinoin may be used in early or mild cases.

Diet: No specific dietary changes indicated.

Activity: No restriction. Patients frequently abandon intercourse because of pain, discharge, odor, or embarrassment.

Patient Education: Reassurance, American College of Obstetricians and Gynecologists Patient Education Pamphlet AP088 (*Diseases of the Vulva*).

Drug(s) of Choice

Antibiotics (tetracycline 2 g PO qd, clindamycin topical qd), topical steroids, oral contraceptives, antiandrogens, and isotretinoin (Accutane) 0.5–2.0 mg/kg in two divided doses for 15–20 weeks. A second course may be considered after a 2-month hiatus.

Contraindications: Isotretinoin must not be taken during pregnancy. Therefore, isotretinoin should not be given to women who are or may become pregnant.

Precautions: Isotretinoin should be given with food. Isotretinoin has been associated with the development of pseudotumor cerebri. Periodic assessment of liver function, cholesterol and triglyceride levels, and white blood counts should be carried out on patients receiving isotretinoin therapy.

Interactions: See individual agents.

Alternative Drugs

Dexamethasone or gonadotropin-releasing hormone agonists have been proposed, but costs and side effects limit their use.

FOLLOW-UP

Patient Monitoring: Normal health maintenance, watch for periodic worsening or secondary infection.

Prevention/Avoidance: Meticulous perineal hygiene; keep the affected area dry.

Possible Complications: Secondary infection, abscess formation, scarring, sexual dysfunction.

Expected Outcome: Relapses and chronic infections are common. With surgical excision, results are generally good, but scarring and dyspareunia may persist or result.

MISCELLANEOUS

Pregnancy Considerations: No effect on pregnancy. Isotretinoin should not be given to women who are or may become pregnant.

ICD-9-CM Codes: 705.83.

VULVAR DISEASE

REFERENCES

Basta A, Madej JG Jr. Hidradenoma of the vulva. Incidence and clinical observations. *Eur J Gynecol Oncol* 1990;11:185.

Sherman AL, Reid R. CO_2 laser for suppurative hidradenitis of the vulva. *J Reprod Med* 1991;36:113.

Thomas R, Barnhill D, Bibro M, Hoskins, W. Hidradenitis suppurativa: a case presentation and review of the literature. *Obstet Gynecol* 1985;66:592.

Wilkinson EJ, Stone IK. *Atlas of Vulvar Disease.* Baltimore, Md: Williams & Wilkins; 1995:148.

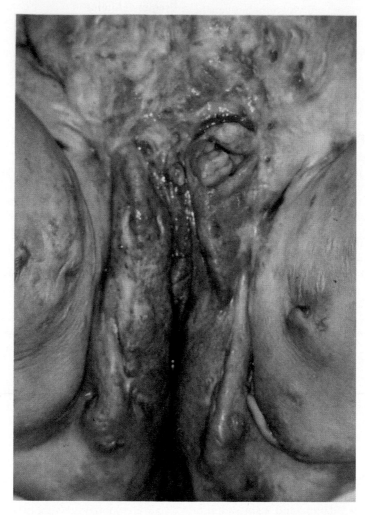

Reproduced from Wilkinson EJ, Stone IK. Atlas of Vulvar Disease. Baltimore, MD, Williams & Wilkins, 1995.

HYMENAL STENOSIS

INTRODUCTION

Description: A thickening or narrowing of the hymenal opening resulting in difficulty in tampon use and intercourse.

Prevalence: Uncommon.

Predominant Age: Congenital, although generally diagnosed in the early reproductive years.

Genetics: No genetic pattern.

ETIOLOGY AND PATHOGENESIS

Causes: Congenital narrowing of the hymen or scarring after trauma or surgery (eg, previous excision).

Risk Factors: Introital surgery (for iatrogenic cases).

CLINICAL CHARACTERISTICS

Signs and Symptoms:
- Insertional dyspareunia
- Difficulty with tampon use
- Narrowing of the vaginal introitus

DIAGNOSTIC APPROACH

Differential Diagnosis:
- Vulvar vestibulitis
- Vaginismus
- Other vulvitis
- Cribriform hymen

Associated Conditions: Dyspareunia, orgasmic or libidinal dysfunction.

Workup and Evaluation

Laboratory: No evaluation indicated.

Imaging: No imaging indicated.

Special Tests: None indicated.

Diagnostic Procedures: History and physical examination.

Pathologic Findings

None.

MANAGEMENT AND THERAPY

Nonpharmacologic

General Measures: Evaluation, reassurance.

Specific Measures: Gentle digital dilation, surgical excision.

Diet: No specific dietary changes indicated.

Activity: No restriction.

Drug(s) of Choice

None.

FOLLOW-UP

Patient Monitoring: Normal health maintenance.

Prevention/Avoidance: None.

Possible Complications: Sexual dysfunction.

Expected Outcome: Generally good, but secondary problems (such as sexual dysfunction) often may persist.

MISCELLANEOUS

Pregnancy Considerations: No effect on pregnancy once achieved. Generally no effect on the route of delivery. Delivery (with or without an episiotomy) often results in improvement or resolution of symptoms.

ICD-9-CM Codes: 623.3.

REFERENCES

Bachmann GA. Superficial dyspareunia and vestibulitis. In: Sciarra JJ, ed. *Gynecology and Obstetrics.* Vol 1. Philadelphia, Pa: JB Lippincott; 1998;77:1.

Smith RP. *Gynecology in Primary Care.* Baltimore, Md: Williams & Wilkins; 1997,517.

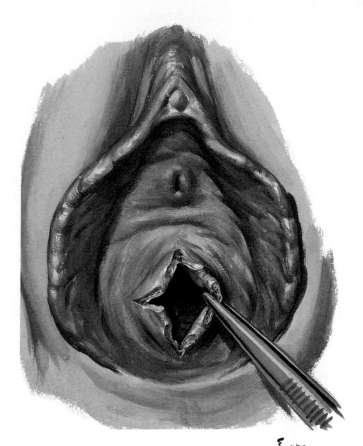

Thick, fibrous hymen
(after cruciate incision)

HYPERPLASTIC VULVAR DYSTROPHY (SQUAMOUS CELL HYPERPLASIA)

INTRODUCTION

Description: Hypertrophic vulvar dystrophy causes a thickening of the vulvar skin over the labia majora, outer aspects of the labia minora, and clitoral areas. Eczematous inflammation or hyperkeratosis may be present.

Prevalence: Common, 40%–45% of non-neoplastic epithelial disorders.

Predominant Age: Middle to late reproductive and beyond.

Genetics: No genetic pattern.

ETIOLOGY AND PATHOGENESIS

Causes: Unknown. Dermal reaction to chronic itch-scratch cycle. Often associated with or worsened by stress.

Risk Factors: Genital atrophy (postmenopausal), recurrent vulvitis.

CLINICAL CHARACTERISTICS

Signs and Symptoms:
- Vulvar itching (almost always present)
- Dusky red to thickened white appearance of the vulva
- Fissuring and excoriations (common)

DIAGNOSTIC APPROACH

Differential Diagnosis:
- Vulvar cancer (premalignant or malignant changes)
- Chronic mycotic vulvitis
- Contact vulvitis
- Psoriasis
- Lichen sclerosus

Associated Conditions: Vulvodynia, vulvar pruritus, and dyspareunia.

Workup and Evaluation

Laboratory: No evaluation indicated.

Imaging: No imaging indicated.

Special Tests: Biopsy may be required to confirm the diagnosis. Cultures for *Candida* or other dermatophytes should be considered.

Diagnostic Procedures: History, physical examination, colposcopy, or biopsy of lesions.

Pathologic Findings

There is thickening of the epithelium with acanthosis, elongation of the epithelial folds, and chronic inflammatory changes (lymphocytes and plasma cells). Hyperkeratosis may be present.

MANAGEMENT AND THERAPY

Nonpharmacologic

General Measures: Perineal hygiene, sitz baths, stress reduction. Reduce or eliminate sources of irritation such as candidiasis or contact allergy. Wearing white cotton gloves (especially at night) reduces the tissue damage caused by scratching.

Specific Measures: Treatment is focused on interrupting the itch-scratch-rash-itch cycle. Topical steroids, perineal soothing agents, and agents to reduce itching are most effective. If significant improvement is not achieved in 3 months, biopsy is indicated.

Diet: No specific dietary changes indicated.

Activity: No restriction.

Patient Education: Reassurance, American College of Obstetricians and Gynecologists Patient Education Pamphlet AP088 (*Diseases of the Vulva*).

Drug(s) of Choice

Fluocinolone acetonide (0.025% or 0.01%), triamcinolone acetonide (0.01%) or betamethasone valerate (Valisone 0.1%), or a similar corticosteroid applied two to three times daily may give relief. Once relief is achieved, treatment should switch to hydrocortisone 2.5% cream or ointment.

For itching: diphenhydramine hydrochloride (Benadryl) or hydroxyzine hydrochloride (Atrax) used at night.

Contraindications: See individual agents.

Precautions: Fluorinated steroids should be used for short periods only and replaced with hydrocortisone or nonsteroidal therapies when possible.

Interactions: See individual agents.

Alternative Drugs

Topical clobetasol propionate (0.05%) may be used if relief of pruritus is not achieved with less potent agents.

Subcutaneous injections of triamcinolone (5 mg suspension mixed with 2 mL of saline) or alcohol (0.1–0.2 mL of absolute alcohol) have been reported but should be reserved for the most intractable disease.

FOLLOW-UP

Patient Monitoring: Constant vigilance is required to watch for possible premalignant or malignant changes that can often mimic these lesions and those of lichen sclerosis.

Prevention/Avoidance: Avoidance of local irritants.

Possible Complications: Vulvar cancer may be overlooked; excoriation is common with secondary infection possible.

Expected Outcome: Generally good if itch-scratch cycle is broken.

MISCELLANEOUS

Pregnancy Considerations: No effect on pregnancy.

ICD-9-CM Codes: 624.3.

REFERENCES

American College of Obstetricians and Gynecologists. *Vulvar Dystrophies*. Washington, DC: ACOG; 1990. ACOG Technical Bulletin 139.

Bousema MT, Romppanen U, Geiger JM, et al. Acitretin in the treatment of severe lichen sclerosus et atrophicus of the vulva: a double-blind, placebo-controlled study. *J Am Acad Dermatol* 1994;30:225.

Cattaneo A, Bracco GL, Maestrini G, et al. Lichen sclerosis and squamous hyperplasia of the vulva. A clinical study of medical treatment. *J Reprod Med* 1991;36:301.

Friedrich EG Jr. Vulvar dystrophy. *Clin Obstet Gynecol* 1985;28:178.

Maloney ME. Exploring the common vulvar dermatoses. *Contemp Obstet/Gynecol* 1988;29:91.

McKay M. Vulvar dermatoses. *Clin Obstet Gynecol* 1991; 34:614.

Nanda VS. Common dermatoses. *Am J Obstet Gynecol* 1995;173:488.

Wilkinson EJ, Stone IK. *Atlas of Vulvar Disease*. Baltimore, Md: Williams & Wilkins; 1995:98.

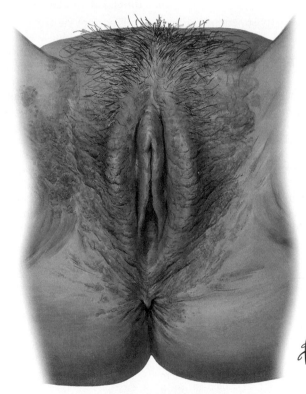

Hyperplastic vulvar dystrophy

IMPERFORATE HYMEN

INTRODUCTION

Description: An imperforate hymen is the most commonly encountered anomaly resulting from abnormalities in the development or canalization of the Müllerian ducts.

Prevalence: Uncommon.

Predominant Age: Generally not diagnosed until puberty.

Genetics: No genetic pattern.

ETIOLOGY AND PATHOGENESIS

Causes: Failure of the endoderm of the urogenital sinus and the epithelium of the vaginal vestibule to fuse and perforate during embryonic development.

Risk Factors: None known.

CLINICAL CHARACTERISTICS

Signs and Symptoms:
- Vaginal obstruction
- Primary amenorrhea
- Cyclic abdominal pain
- Hematocolpos

DIAGNOSTIC APPROACH

Differential Diagnosis:
- Vaginal agenesis
- Hermaphroditism

Associated Conditions: Endometriosis, vaginal adenosis, infertility, chronic pelvic pain, sexual dysfunction, and hematocolpos.

Workup and Evaluation

Laboratory: No evaluation indicated.

Imaging: Ultrasonography to evaluate the upper genital tract.

Special Tests: None indicated.

Diagnostic Procedures: History and physical examination.

Pathologic Findings

None.

MANAGEMENT AND THERAPY

Nonpharmacologic

General Measures: Evaluation, reassurance.

Specific Measures: Incision of hymenal membrane and drainage of vaginal canal.

Diet: No specific dietary changes indicated.

Activity: No restriction.

Drug(s) of Choice

None.

FOLLOW-UP

Patient Monitoring: Normal health maintenance.

Prevention/Avoidance: None.

Possible Complications: Hematocolpos, endometriosis, hymenal scarring and narrowing after surgical excision.

Expected Outcome: Generally good with early resection. Delayed diagnosis is associated with reduced fertility caused by secondary damage (endometriosis).

MISCELLANEOUS

Pregnancy Considerations: No effect on pregnancy, although often associated with conditions such as endometriosis that do affect fertility. Reproductive outlook is best only when diagnosis and treatment occur early.

ICD-9-CM Codes: 752.42.

REFERENCES

Baramki TA. The treatment of congenital anomalies in girls and women. *J Reprod Med* 1984;29:376.

Greiss FC, Mauzy CH. Congenital anomalies in women: an evaluation of diagnosis, incidence, and obstetric performance. *Am J Obstet Gynecol* 1961;82:330.

VULVAR DISEASE

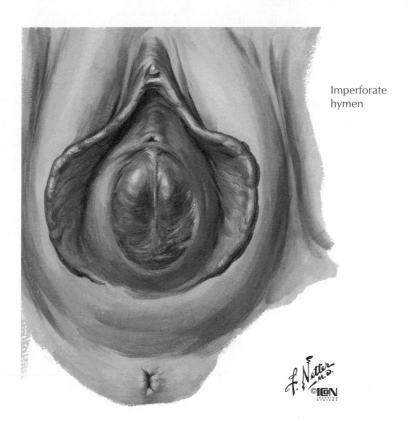

Imperforate
hymen

LABIAL ADHESIONS

INTRODUCTION

Description: Agglutination of the labial folds resulting in fusion in the midline.

Prevalence: 1%–2% of female children.

Predominant Age: Peak 2–6; may be found at any age up to puberty.

Genetics: No genetic pattern.

ETIOLOGY AND PATHOGENESIS

Causes: Local inflammation and the hypoestrogenic environment of preadolescence.

Risk Factors: Labial infections or irritation.

CLINICAL CHARACTERISTICS

Signs and Symptoms:

- Fusion of the labia majora in the midline (extends from just below the clitoris to the posterior fourchette)
- Retention of urine in the vestibule or vagina resulting in irritation, discharge, and odor

DIAGNOSTIC APPROACH

Differential Diagnosis:

- Intersex
- Female circumcision
- Sexual abuse

Associated Conditions: Urinary tract infection.

Workup and Evaluation

Laboratory: No evaluation indicated.

Imaging: No imaging indicated.

Special Tests: None indicated.

Diagnostic Procedures: History and physical examination.

Pathologic Findings

None.

MANAGEMENT AND THERAPY

Nonpharmacologic

General Measures: Evaluation, reassurance, perineal hygiene, and sitz baths.

Specific Measures: Topical estrogen cream, gentle traction to separate the labia (only after estrogen pretreatment; generally not necessary and strongly discouraged). Surgical treatment is almost never required.

Diet: No specific dietary changes indicated.

Activity: No restriction.

Patient Education: Reassurance, American College of Obstetricians and Gynecologists Patient Education Pamphlet AP041 (*Growing Up* [for ages 8–14]).

Drug(s) of Choice

Topical estrogen cream (Premarin vaginal cream, Dienestrol cream)—small portion applied to the vulva bid for 7–10 days. May be continued one to three times a week if desired, although generally not necessary.

Contraindications: Undiagnosed vaginal bleeding.

FOLLOW-UP

Patient Monitoring: Normal health maintenance.

Prevention/Avoidance: Good perineal hygiene.

Possible Complications: Vaginitis, urinary tract infection, urinary retention, or vaginal cyst formation.

Expected Outcome: Excellent.

MISCELLANEOUS

ICD-9-CM Codes: 624.9.

REFERENCES

Slupik R. Pediatric gynecology. In: Sciarra JJ, ed. *Obstetrics and Gynecology.* Vol 1. Philadelphia, Pa: JB Lippincott; 1991;19:14.

Smith RP. *Gynecology in Primary Care.* Baltimore, Md: Williams & Wilkins; 1997:177.

Stovall TG, Murman D. Urinary retention secondary to labial adhesions. *Adolesc Pediatr Gynecol* 1988;1:203.

Wells EC. Simple operation of the vulva. In: Sciarra JJ, ed. *Obstetrics and Gynecology.* Vol 1. Philadelphia, Pa: JB Lippincott; 1998;11:10.

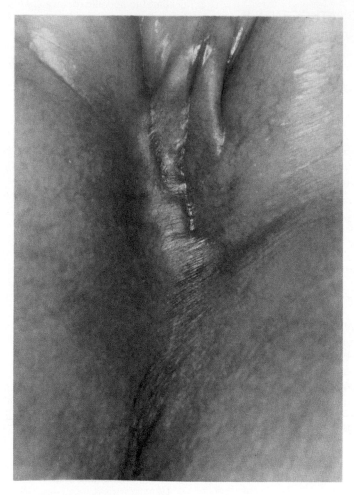

Reproduced from Wilkinson EJ, Stone IK. Atlas of Vulvar Disease. Baltimore, MD, Williams & Wilkins, 1995.

LICHEN PLANUS

INTRODUCTION

Description: A nonneoplastic epithelial disorder that affects glabrous skin, hair-bearing skin and scalp, nails, mucous membranes, or the oral cavity and the vulva.

Prevalence: Unknown, but relatively common.

Predominant Age: 30–60.

Genetics: No genetic pattern.

ETIOLOGY AND PATHOGENESIS

Causes: Unknown. Proposed—autoimmune disorder.

Risk Factors: None known.

CLINICAL CHARACTERISTICS

Signs and Symptoms:

- Red erosion and ulceration of the vulva and inner aspects of the labia minora (may precede oral lesions by years; 33% of patients)
- Loss of the labia minora with scarring, adhesions, and narrowing common (complete obliteration of the vagina possible); dyspareunia and postcoital bleeding common
- Oral lesions—reticulated gray, lacy pattern (Wickham's striae) with gingivitis (vulvar involvement in 50% of patients with oral lesions)

DIAGNOSTIC APPROACH

Differential Diagnosis:

- Amebiasis
- Behçet's syndrome
- Candidiasis
- Dermatophyte infection
- Lichen sclerosus
- Neurodermatitis
- Pemphigus and pemphigoid (cicatricial or bullous type)
- Plasma cell vulvitis
- Psoriasis
- Vulvar intraepithelial neoplasia (VIN III)
- Squamous cell hyperplasia
- Systemic lupus erythematosus

Associated Conditions: Hair loss and a history of papular lesions on the skin (ankle, dorsal surface of the hands, and flexor surfaces of the wrists and forearms).

Workup and Evaluation

Laboratory: No evaluation indicated.

Imaging: No imaging indicated.

Special Tests: Skin biopsy (taken from the nearby intact skin or mucous membranes rather than the ulcer). Direct immunofluorescence testing on fresh tissue.

Diagnostic Procedures: History, physical examination, and biopsy.

Pathologic Findings

Chronic inflammatory cell infiltrate (lymphocytes and plasma cells) involving the superficial dermis and the basal and parabasal epithelium. Liquefaction necrosis with colloid bodies may be present. Prominent acanthosis with a prominent granular layer and hyperkeratosis. Ulceration and bullae may be present. Hyperkeratosis is absent in the vulvar tissues.

MANAGEMENT AND THERAPY

Nonpharmacologic

General Measures: Evaluation, local cleansing, antipruritics.

Specific Measures: Therapy is often difficult, chronic, and prone to failure or relapse. Therapies include steroids, retinoids, griseofulvin, dapsone, cyclosporine, and surgery. Vaginal dilators may be necessary to maintain vaginal caliber.

Diet: No specific dietary changes indicated.

Activity: No restriction.

Patient Education: Reassurance, American College of Obstetricians and Gynecologists Patient Education Pamphlet AP088 (*Diseases of the Vulva*).

Drug(s) of Choice

Topical steroids (betamethasone valerate 0.1% ointment or hydrocortisone 25 mg vaginal suppository daily)

or griseofulvin (250 mg PO bid)

or dapsone (50–100 mg PO qd) (after negative results of screening for glucose-6-phosphate dehydrogenase)

or isotretinoin (Accutane) 0.5–1 mg/kg/d in divided doses (or etretinate [Tegison] 0.75–1 mg/kg/d in two doses)

or cyclosporine (1 mg/kg/d, increased weekly by 0.5 mg/kg/d up to 3–5 mg/kg/d).

Contraindications: Vulvar cancer. Isotretinoin and etretinate are teratogenic and must not be given during pregnancy or if there is a potential for pregnancy.

Precautions: Continued or prolonged use of topical steroids may result in thinning of the skin outside the area of lichen sclerosis with subsequent atrophy and traumatic injury (splitting and cracking). The use of dapsone, isotretinoin, etretinate, or cyclosporin requires careful monitoring of complete blood counts, liver function

VULVAR DISEASE

tests, cholesterol, triglycerides, electrolytes, urea nitrogen, creatinine, and creatinine clearance. Reliable contraception must be maintained if isotretinoin or etretinate is used.

Interactions: See individual agents.

FOLLOW-UP

Patient Monitoring: Because malignant change is possible, long-term follow-up is required.

Prevention/Avoidance: None.

Possible Complications: Vulvar lesions are often chronic and may undergo malignant change.

Expected Outcome: Chronic therapy required with relapses common.

MISCELLANEOUS

Pregnancy Considerations: No effect on pregnancy.

ICD-9-CM Codes: 697.0.

REFERENCES

Eisen D. The vulvovaginal-gingival syndrome of lichen planus. The clinical characteristics of 22 patients. *Arch Dermatol* 1994;130:1379.

Franck JM, Young AW Jr. Squamous cell carcinoma in situ arising within lichen planus of the vulva. *Dermatol Surg* 1995;21:890.

Lewis FM, Shah M, Harrington CI. Vulvar involvement in lichen planus: a study of 37 women. *Br J Dermatol* 1996;135:89.

Mann MS, Kaufman RH. Erosive lichen planus of the vulva. *Clin Obstet Gynecol* 1991;34:605.

Pelisse M. Erosive vulvar lichen planus and desquamative vaginitis. *Semin Dermatol* 1996;15:47.

Wilkinson EJ, Stone IK. *Atlas of Vulvar Disease.* Baltimore, Md: Williams & Wilkins; 1995:27.

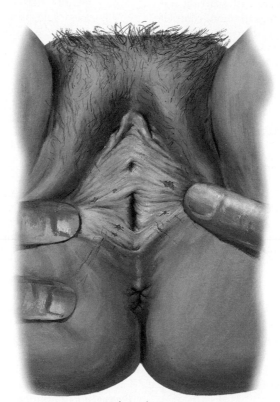

Lichen planus

LICHEN SCLEROSUS

INTRODUCTION

Description: A chronic condition of the vulvar skin characterized by thinning, distinctive skin changes, and inflammation. It is nonneoplastic and involves glabrous skin as well as the vulva. The term "lichen sclerosus et atrophicus" has been dropped because the epithelium is metabolically active, not atrophic.

Prevalence: Common.

Predominant Age: Late reproductive to early menopausal (however, may be seen as early as 6 months).

Genetics: No genetic pattern.

ETIOLOGY AND PATHOGENESIS

Causes: Unknown. Proposed—immunologic (autoimmune), genetic, inactive or deficient androgen receptors, epidermal growth factor deficiency.

Risk Factors: None known.

CLINICAL CHARACTERISTICS

Signs and Symptoms:
- Intense itching common (99%)
- Thinned, atrophic appearing skin, with linear scratch marks or fissures (the skin often has a "cigarette-paper" or parchment-like appearance); these changes frequently extend around the anus in a figure-eight configuration
- Atrophic changes result in thinning, or even loss, of the labia minora and significant narrowing of the introitus
- Fissures, scarring, and synechiae cause marked pain for some patients

DIAGNOSTIC APPROACH

Differential Diagnosis:
- Lichen simplex (hyperplastic vulvar dystrophy)
- Scleroderma
- Vitiligo
- Paget's disease
- Vulvar candidiasis
- Squamous cell hyperplasia or carcinoma (when thickening is present)

Associated Conditions: Dyspareunia, vulvodynia, vulvar pruritus, hypothyroidism.

Workup and Evaluation

Laboratory: Thyroid function studies should be considered because up to one third of patients have coexisting hypothyroidism.

Imaging: No imaging indicated.

Special Tests: Culture or KOH wet preparations of skin scrapings may help to evaluate the possibility of candidiasis.

Diagnostic Procedures: History, physical, and biopsy of affected area.

Pathologic Findings

Loss of normal vulvar architecture with loss of rete pegs, a homogeneous dermis with edema, fibrin, and loss of vascularity, elastic fibers, and dermal collagen. Chronic inflammation is common and spongiosis of the basilar epithelial cells is often present. Ulceration or hypertrophy may be present as a result of rubbing or scratching.

MANAGEMENT AND THERAPY

Nonpharmacologic

General Measures: Evaluation, perineal hygiene, cool sitz baths, moist soaks, or the application of soothing solutions such as Burow's solution. Patients should be advised to wear loose-fitting clothing and keep the area dry and well ventilated. Emollients such as petroleum jelly may help to reduce local drying.

Specific Measures: Topical steroid therapy is preferred over the traditional testosterone cream. Surgical excision is occasionally required if medical therapy fails. This is associated with a high rate of recurrence and the risk of postsurgical scarring.

Diet: No specific dietary changes indicated.

Activity: No restriction.

Patient Education: Reassurance, American College of Obstetricians and Gynecologists Patient Education Pamphlet AP088 (*Diseases of the Vulva*), AP028 (*Vaginitis: Causes and Treatments*), AP020 (*Pain During Intercourse*).

Drug(s) of Choice

Burow's solution (Domeboro, aluminum acetate 5% aqueous solution, three to four times daily for 30–60 minutes).

Crotamiton 10% (Eurax) may be applied topically, twice daily. High-potency prednisolone analogs (clobetasol propionate, Cormax, Temovate) 0.05% bid for 30 days, qhs for 30 days, then qd.

Fluorinated corticosteroids (Valisone 0.1%, Synalar 0.01%) applied two to three times a day for 2 weeks. Lower-potency steroids (hydrocortisone) may be used after initial therapy or in children.

Testosterone propionate in petrolatum (2%) applied two to three times daily for up to 6 months.

Contraindications: Vulvar cancer.

Precautions: Continued or prolonged use of topical steroids may result in thinning of the skin outside the area of lichen sclerosis with subsequent atrophy and traumatic injury (splitting and cracking). Prolonged testosterone propionate therapy may be associated with clitoral enlargement or pain, local burning, or erythema. Rarely hirsutism may result.

Alternative Drugs

In selected patients, intralesional steroids (Kenalog-10) may be used.

Topical progesterone (400 mg in oil with 4 oz of Aquaphor, applied bid) may be substituted for testosterone cream in children.

FOLLOW-UP

Patient Monitoring: Frequent follow-up (3–6 months) is required to watch for recurrence or worsening of symptoms.

Prevention/Avoidance: None.

Possible Complications: Scarring and narrowing of the introitus may be sufficient to preclude intercourse. Excoriation with secondary infections may occur. Areas that become hyperplastic as a result of scratching are thought to be at increased risk for premalignant or malignant changes (squamous cell carcinoma—lifetime risk of 3%–5%).

Expected Outcome: Initial response is generally good, but recurrence is common, often necessitating lifelong therapy.

MISCELLANEOUS

Pregnancy Considerations: No effect on pregnancy (generally not a consideration).

***ICD-9-CM* Codes:** Based on location and severity of disease.

REFERENCES

Bracco GL, Carli P, Sonni L, et al. Clinical and histologic effects of topical treatments of vulvar lichen sclerosus: a critical evaluation. *J Reprod Med* 1993;38:37.

Cattaneo A, Bracco GL, Maestrini G, et al. Lichen sclerosis and squamous hyperplasia of the vulva. A clinical study of medical treatment. *J Reprod Med* 1991;36:301.

Elchalal U, Gilead L, Bardy D, Ben-Schachar L, Anteby SO, Schenker JG. Treatment of vulvar lichen sclerosus in the elderly: an update. *Obstet Gynecol Surv* 1995;50:155.

Hewitt J. Lichen sclerosus. *J Reprod Med* 1986;31:781.

Maloney ME. Exploring the common vulvar dermatoses. *Contemp Ob/Gyn* 1988;29:91.

Mann MS, Kaufman RH. Erosive lichen planus of the vulva. *Clin Obstet Gynecol* 1991;34:605.

Soper DE, Patterson JW, Hurt WG, Fantl JA, Blaylock WK. Lichen planus of the vulva. *Obstet Gynecol* 1988;72:74.

Wilkinson EJ, Stone IK. *Atlas of Vulvar Disease.* Baltimore, Md: Williams & Wilkins; 1995:33.

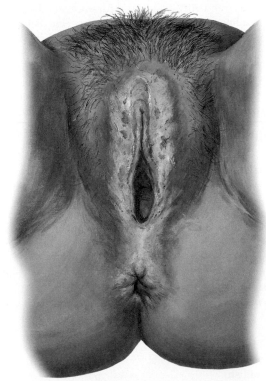

Lichen sclerosus

VULVAR CANCER

INTRODUCTION

Description: Squamous cell cancer of the vulva generally presents as an exophytic ulcer or hyperkeratotic plaque. It may arise as a solitary lesion or develop hidden within hypertrophic or other vulvar skin changes, making diagnosis difficult and often delayed.

Prevalence: Less than 5000 cases per year, 4% of gynecologic malignancies.

Predominant Age: 65–70.

Genetics: No genetic pattern.

ETIOLOGY AND PATHOGENESIS

Causes: Unknown. Thought to be associated with human papillomavirus.

Risk Factors: Infection with human papillomavirus.

CLINICAL CHARACTERISTICS

Signs and Symptoms:
- Itching, irritation, cracking, or bleeding of the vulva, most common on the posterior two thirds of the labia majus
- Ulcerated exophytic lesion or hyperkeratotic plaque (late in disease)

DIAGNOSTIC APPROACH

Differential Diagnosis:
- Hypertorphic vulvar dystrophy
- Lichen sclerosis

Associated Conditions: Hyperplastic vulvar dystrophy.

Workup and Evaluation

Laboratory: No evaluation indicated.

Imaging: No imaging indicated.

Special Tests: Biopsy of any suspicious lesion.

Diagnostic Procedures: History, physical examination, and vulvar biopsy.

Pathologic Findings

Histologic types include squamous cell (90%), basaloid, warty, verrucous, giant cell, spindle cell, acantholytic squamous cell (adenoid squamous), lymphoepithelioma-like, basal cell, Merkel cell.

MANAGEMENT AND THERAPY

Nonpharmacologic

General Measures: Evaluation (generally by biopsy).

Specific Measures: Initial treatment consists of wide local excision (1 cm margins). Subsequent therapy, including node dissections and adjunctive therapy (radiation), is determined by the stage of disease, cell type, and surgical margins.

Diet: No specific dietary changes indicated.

Activity: No restriction. except as dictated by surgical therapy.

Patient Education: American College of Obstetricians and Gynecologists Patient Education Pamphlet AP088 (*Diseases of the Vulva*).

Drug(s) of Choice

None.

FOLLOW-UP

Patient Monitoring: Careful follow-up for recurrence or additional new lesions.

Prevention/Avoidance: None.

Possible Complications: Distant spread and disease progression, secondary infection.

Expected Outcome: If tumor invasion is less than 1 mm, the risk of lymph node involvement is essentially 0 and high success rates may be expected. Five-year survival rates decline with advancing stage: 20% with deep node involvement. Overall 5-year survival is 70%.

MISCELLANEOUS

Pregnancy Considerations: No effect on pregnancy, although the presence of a pregnancy may affect surgical therapeutic options.

ICD-9-CM Codes: Specific to cell type and location.

REFERENCES

American College of Obstetricians and Gynecologists. *Vulvar Dystrophies.* Washington, DC: ACOG; 1990. ACOG Technical Bulletin 139.

American College of Obstetricians and Gynecologists. *Classification and Staging of Gynecologic Malignancies.* Washington, DC: ACOG; 1991. ACOG Technical Bulletin 155.

American College of Obstetricians and Gynecologists. *Vulvar Cancer.* Washington, DC: ACOG; 1993. ACOG Technical Bulletin 186.

DiSaia PJ. Management of superficially invasive vulvar carcinoma. *Clin Obstet Gynecol* 1985;28:196.

Hacker NF, Van der Velden J. Conservative management of early vulvar cancer. *Cancer* 1993;71(suppl):1673.

Kurman RJ, Norris HJ, Wilkinson EJ. In: Rosai J, ed. *Atlas of Tumor Pathology: Tumors of the Cervix, Vagina and Vulva.* Vol 4. Washington, DC: AFIP; 1992.

Wilkinson EJ, Stone IK. *Atlas of Vulvar Disease.* Baltimore, Md: Williams & Wilkins; 1995:162.

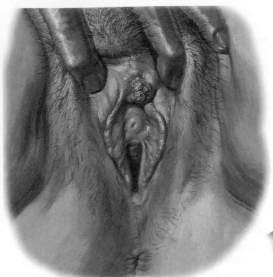

Carcinoma of the clitoris

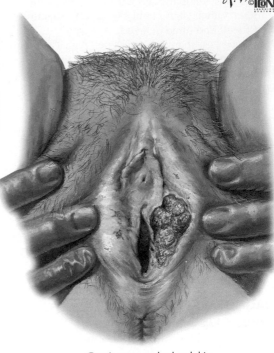

Carcinoma on leukoplakia

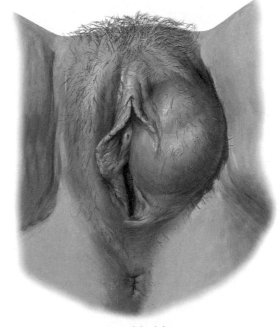

Sarcoma of the labium

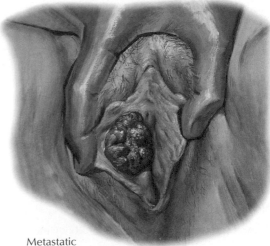

Metastatic
hypernephroma

VULVAR HEMATOMA

INTRODUCTION

Description: Swelling of one or both labia because of interstitial bleeding, most often after blunt trauma.

Predominant Age: Most common in childhood and teen years, may occur at any age.

Genetics: No genetic pattern.

ETIOLOGY AND PATHOGENESIS

Causes: Blunt trauma (straddle injury, sexual abuse, rape, water skiing), vaginal surgery or delivery, varicose veins of vulva.

Risk Factors: Sports activities, uncommonly consensual intercourse.

CLINICAL CHARACTERISTICS

Signs and Symptoms:
- Painful swelling of one or both labia
- Dark blue or black discoloration
- Bleeding from vulva if laceration is present

DIAGNOSTIC APPROACH

Differential Diagnosis:
- Bartholin's gland cyst or abscess
- Varicose veins of vulva
- Lymphogranuloma venereum
- Hydradenitis suppurativa

Associated Conditions: The presence of vaginal lacerations must always be considered.

Workup and Evaluation

Laboratory: No evaluation indicated.

Imaging: No imaging indicated.

Special Tests: None indicated.

Diagnostic Procedures: History and gentle visualization, speculum examination if vaginal trauma also suspected or possible.

Pathologic Findings

None.

MANAGEMENT AND THERAPY

Nonpharmacologic

General Measures: Analgesics (avoid aspirin), pressure, ice packs.

Specific Measures: Surgical drainage for rapidly expanding hematomas or those >10 cm in diameter. Children with vulvar trauma should have a tetanus toxoid booster if none has been given in the preceding 5 years.

Diet: No specific dietary changes indicated.

Activity: Bed rest until condition is stable; return to activity as tolerated.

Drug(s) of Choice

Nonaspirin analgesics.

FOLLOW-UP

Patient Monitoring: Observation for expanding hematoma, hemodynamic monitoring if blood loss severe.

Prevention/Avoidance: Good footwear during sports.

Possible Complications: Chronic expanding hematoma with fibrosis and pain.

Expected Outcome: Most hematomas gradually resolve with conservative management only.

MISCELLANEOUS

Pregnancy Considerations: No effect on pregnancy; rarely may complicate delivery if present before or during labor. More often, delivery precedes hematoma formation.

ICD-9-CM Codes: 624.5, 664.5 (Vulvar hematoma following delivery).

REFERENCES

Naumann RO, Droegemueller W. Unusual etiology of vulvar hematomas. *Am J Obstet Gynecol* 1982;142:357.

Huddock JJ, Dupayne N, McGeary JA. Traumatic vulvar hematomas. *Am J Obstet Gynecol* 1955;70:1064.

Mishell DR, Stenchever MA, Droegemueller W, Herbst AL. *Comprehensive Gynecology.* 3rd ed. St Louis: Mosby; 1997:270, 474.

Niv J, Lessing JB, Hartuv J, Peyser MR. Vaginal injury resulting from sliding down a water chute. *Am J Obstet Gynecol* 1992;166:930.

Ridgeway LE. Puerperal emergency: vaginal and vulvar hematomas. *Obstet Gynecol Clin North Am* 1995; 22:275.

Smith RP. *Gynecology in Primary Care.* Baltimore, Md: Williams & Wilkins; 1997:603.

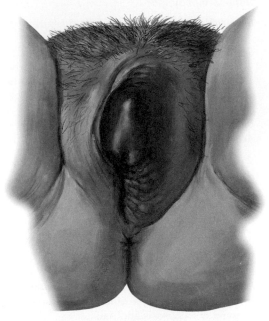

Typical appearance of vulvar hematoma, a hematoma involving one or both labia

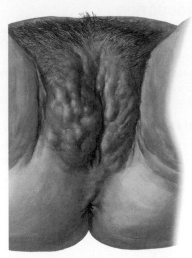

Vulvar varicosities, trauma and childbirth may all contribute to vulvar hematoma formation

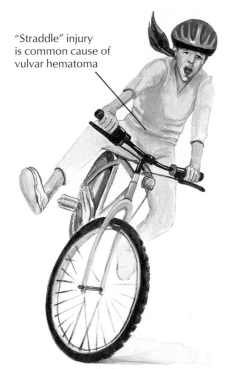

"Straddle" injury is common cause of vulvar hematoma

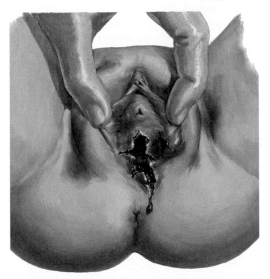

Presence of vulvar hematoma in children most often due to "straddle" injury, but should raise concern of sexual abuse, especially if lacerations are present

VULVAR LESIONS

THE CHALLENGE

The skin of the vulva is subject to all the changes that affect skin elsewhere in the body. In addition, the tissues of the vulva represent a rich ecosystem, with interactions between tissues, fluids, hormones, and microbes.

Scope of the Problem: In gynecologic practices, two to five or more patients a day with these concerns is the norm.

Objectives of Management: To establish a timely diagnosis and management plan for those patients with vulvar lesions.

TACTICS

Relevant Pathophysiology: The skin of the vulva is like that of other areas of the body with stratified squamous epithelium, hair follicles, and sebaceous, sweat, and apocrine glands. Just as in other areas of the body, the vulva is susceptible to inflammatory and dermatologic diseases. Intertrigo, hidradenitis suppurativa, psoriasis, seborrheic dermatitis, Fox-Fordyce disease, Fifth disease, changes caused by Behçet's or Crohn's diseases, viral infections, and parasites may all affect the skin of the vulva. The skin of the vulva is also vulnerable to irritation from vaginal secretions, recurrent urinary loss, or contact with external irritants (such as soap residue, perfumes, fabric softeners, or infestation by pinworms). Changes may occur because of the effects of diabetes or hormonal alterations as well as dermatoses such as hypertrophic dystrophy, lichen sclerosis, psoriasis, and others.

Strategies: The character of the lesion or vulvar findings may be used to establish a working diagnosis for the patient with a vulvar lesion. Processes that result in lesions that occupy a superficial location are very different from those that cause processes deep within the tissues of the vulva. It is important to keep in mind the fact that many conditions that cause vulvar lesions may present in several forms.

Consequently, in any decision tree based on lesion morphology, some diagnoses may be represented at the end of more than one branch (eg, seborrheic keratosis or nevus).

Patient Education: American College of Obstetricians and Gynecologists Patient Education Pamphlet AP088 (*Diseases of the Vulva*).

IMPLEMENTATION

Special Considerations: In addition to the diagnoses discussed in the preceding, several other significant possibilities must always be considered when diffuse symptoms and findings are present: atopic dermatitis, contact dermatitis, fixed drug reaction, and factitial vulvitis. When cystic structures are encountered, the possibility of congenital remnants such as mesothelial cysts (cysts of the canal of Nuck), Wolffian duct remnants, and periurethral cysts must be considered. Lipomas, neurofibromas, rhabdomyomas, schwannomas, and leiomyomas may present as fleshy tumors of the vulva. Of special importance are lesions that involve significant necrosis: necrotizing fasciitis and pyoderma gangrenosum. Both of these processes represent a significant threat to the life and health of the patient and require prompt and aggressive treatment.

REFERENCES

American College of Obstetricians and Gynecologists. *Vulvar Dystrophies.* Washington, DC: ACOG; 1990. ACOG Technical Bulletin 139.

American College of Obstetricians and Gynecologists. *Genital Human Papillomavirus Infections.* Washington, DC: ACOG; 1994. ACOG Technical Bulletin 193.

McKay M. Vulvar dermatoses. *Clin Obstet Gynecol* 1991;34:614.

Nanda VS. Common dermatoses. *Am J Obstet Gynecol* 1995;173:488.

Peckham EM, Maki DG, Patterson JJ, Hafez GR. Focal vulvitis: a characteristic syndrome and cause of dyspareunia. Features, natural history, and management. *Am J Obstet Gynecol* 1986;154:855.

Wilkinson EJ, Stone IK. *Atlas of Vulvar Disease.* Baltimore, Md: Williams & Wilkins; 1995.

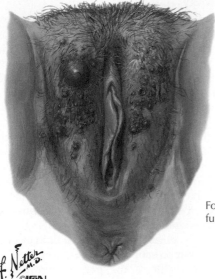

Folliculitis and
furunculosis

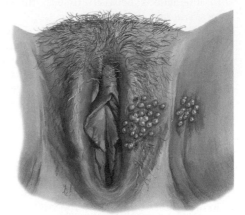

Herpes genitalis

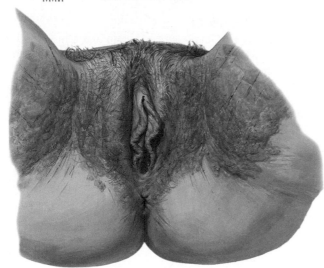

Tinea cruris

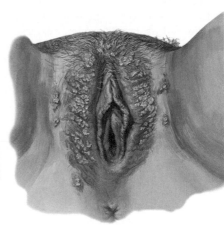

Psoriasis

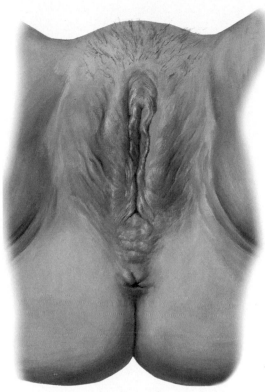

Senile atrophy

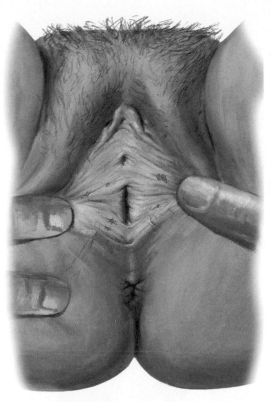

Kraurosis vulvae

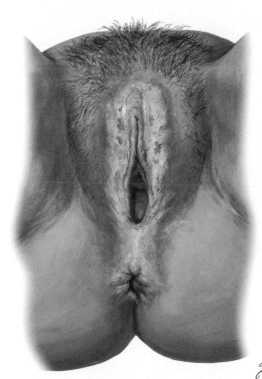

Leukoplakia

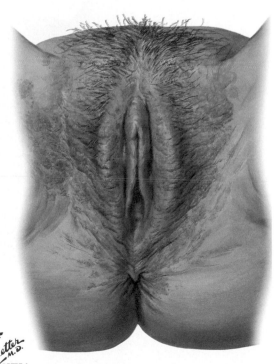

Lichenification

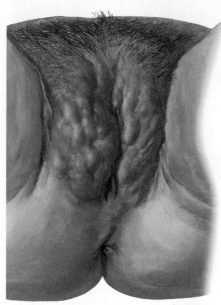

Varicose veins

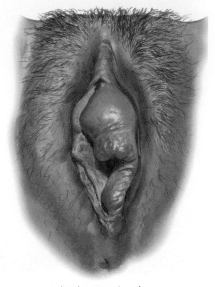

Angioneurotic edema

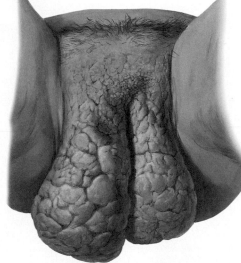

Elephantiasis

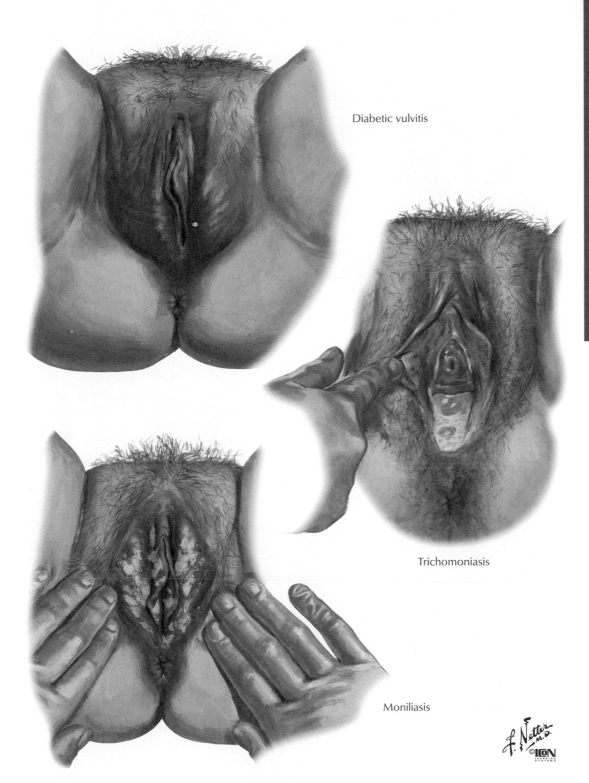

Diabetic vulvitis

Trichomoniasis

Moniliasis

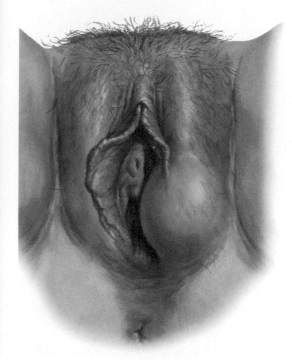

Bartholin's cyst

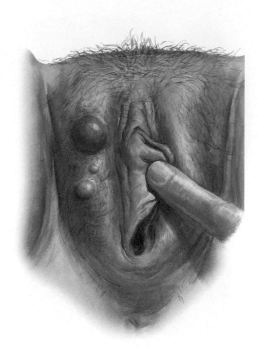

Sebaceous cyst

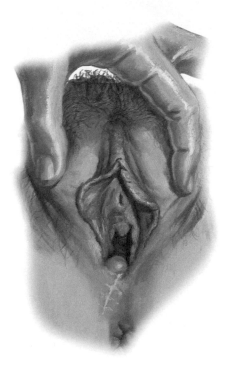

Inclusion cyst

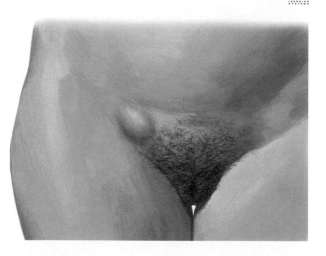

Cyst of Canal of Nuck

VULVAR VESTIBULITIS

INTRODUCTION

Description: An uncommon syndrome of intense sensitivity of the skin of the posterior vaginal introitus and vulvar vestibule, with progressive worsening, which leads to loss of function.

Prevalence: Rare.

Predominant Age: 19–81, median 36.

Genetics: No genetic pattern.

ETIOLOGY AND PATHOGENESIS

Causes: Unknown. High degree of association with human papillomavirus, but no causal link established.

Risk Factors: None known. It has been postulated that the use of oral contraceptives may increase the risk or severity of vulvar vestibulitis and that users should switch to other methods of contraception. Strong evidence for either causation or significant improvement is lacking.

CLINICAL CHARACTERISTICS

Signs and Symptoms:
- Intense pain and tenderness at the posterior introitus and vestibule present for 2–5 years
- Unable to use tampons (33%) or have intercourse (entry dyspareunia, 100%)
- Focal inflammation, punctation, and ulceration of the perineal and vaginal epithelium
- Punctate areas (1–10) of inflammation 3–10 mm in size may be seen between the Bartholin's glands (75%), hymenal ring, and middle perineum

DIAGNOSTIC APPROACH

Differential Diagnosis:
- Vaginismus
- Chronic vulvitis
- Atrophic vaginitis
- Hypertrophic vulvar dystrophy
- Recurrent vaginal infections
- Herpes vulvitis
- Vulvar dermatoses
- Contact (allergic) vulvitis

Associated Conditions: Sexual dysfunction, dyspareunia, and vulvodynia.

Workup and Evaluation

Laboratory: No evaluation indicated.

Imaging: No imaging indicated.

Special Tests: Colposcopy of the vulva (using 3% acetic acid) may reveal the characteristic punctate and acetowhite areas.

Diagnostic Procedures: History, physical examination, mapping of sensitive areas, and colposcopy.

Pathologic Findings

Small inflammatory punctate lesions varying in size from 3 to 10 mm, often with superficial ulceration. The Bartholin's gland openings may be inflamed as well. The area involved may be demarcated by light touching with a cotton-tipped applicator, although the level of discomfort is often out of proportion to the physical findings. Microscopic—inflammation of minor vestibular glands.

MANAGEMENT AND THERAPY

Nonpharmacologic

General Measures: Evaluation, perineal hygiene, cool sitz baths, moist soaks, or the application of soothing solutions such as Burow's solution. Patients should be advised to wear loose-fitting clothing and keep the area dry and well ventilated.

Specific Measures: Topical anesthetics and antidepressants (amitriptyline hydrochloride) may reduce pain and itch. Interferon injections may provide relief in up to 60% of patients. Refractory disease may require surgical resection or laser ablation.

Diet: No specific dietary changes indicated. (Reducing urinary oxylate through dietary means has been suggested, but remains unproved.)

Activity: No restriction (pelvic rest often recommended when symptoms are maximal).

Patient Education: Reassurance, American College of Obstetricians and Gynecologists Patient Education Pamphlet AP088 (*Diseases of the Vulva*), AP020 (*Pain During Intercourse*).

Drug(s) of Choice

Lidocaine (Xylocaine) 2% jelly (or 5% cream) topically as needed.

Antidepressants (amitriptyline hydrochloride [Elavil] 25 mg PO qhs or 10 mg PO tid).

Interferon injections three times weekly for 4 weeks, introducing 1 million units at each of 12 areas (clock face) by the completion of the course.

Contraindications: Interferon injections cannot be given during pregnancy.

Precautions: Patients should be warned that interferon injections are associated with flulike symptoms and a clinical response may not be seen for up to 3 months. Patients should abstain from intercourse during the series of injections.

FOLLOW-UP

Patient Monitoring: Frequent follow-up and monitoring are required. Frustration for both the patient and provider is common.

Prevention/Avoidance: None.

Possible Complications: Secondary infection, sexual dysfunction.

Expected Outcome: Spontaneous remission in one third of patients over the course of 6 months. Chronic, continuing pain state most common. Surgical therapy is associated with 50%–60% success.

MISCELLANEOUS

Pregnancy Considerations: No effect on pregnancy.

ICD-9-CM Codes: 616.10.

REFERENCES

Baggish MS, Miklos JR. Vulvar pain syndrome: a review. *Obstet Gynecol Surv* 1995;50:618.

David GD. The management of vulvar vestibulitis syndrome with the carbon dioxide laser. *J Gynecol Surg* 1989;5:87.

Fischer G, Spurrett B, Fischer A. The chronically symptomatic vulva: aetiology and management. *Br J Obstet Gynaecol* 1995;102:773.

Goetsch MF. Vulvar vestibulitis: prevalence and histologic features in a general gynecologic practice population. *Am J Obstet Gynecol* 1991;164:1609.

Marinoff SC, Turner ML. Vulvar vestibulitis syndrome: an overview. *Am J Obstet Gynecol* 1991;165:1228.

Peckham EM, Maki DG, Patterson JJ, Hafez GR. Focal vulvitis: a characteristic syndrome and cause of dyspareunia. Features, natural history, and management. *Am J Obstet Gynecol* 1986;154:855.

Stewart DE, Reicher AE, Gerulath AH, Boydel KM. Vulvodynia and psychological distress. *Obstet Gynecol* 1994;84:587.

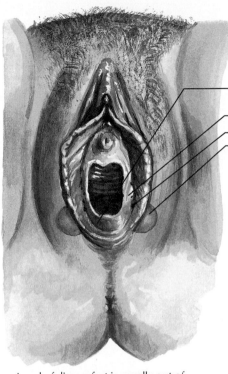

Vulvar vestibulitis is syndrome of intense sensitivity of skin of posterior vaginal introitus and vulvar vestibule resulting in dyspareunia and pain on attempted use of tampons.

Area most commonly involved is posterior to Bartholin's glands.

Opening of minor vestibular glands

Orifice of Bartholin's gland

Bartholin's gland

Level of discomfort is usually out of proportion to degree of physical findings, which include 1 to 10 small (3–10 mm) areas of punctate inflammation, some with ulceration in perineal and vaginal epithelium

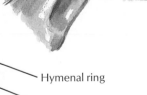

Involved area may be demarcated by light touch with cotton-tipped applicator

JOHN A. CRAIG—AD

D. Mascaro

©ICON

Hymenal ring

Bartholin's gland opening may be inflamed

Punctate erosions on erythematous base found in vestibule and introitus

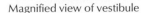

Magnified view of vestibule

Vaginal Disease

CYSTOCELE/URETHROCELE

INTRODUCTION

Description: Loss of support for the anterior vagina, through rupture or attenuation of the pubovesicocervical fascia, manifested by descent or prolapse of the urethra (urethrocele) or bladder (cystocele).

Prevalence: Ten percent to fifteen percent of women, 30%–40% after menopause.

Predominant Age: 40 and older, increasing with age.

Genetics: No genetic pattern.

ETIOLOGY AND PATHOGENESIS

Causes: Loss of normal tissue integrity or tissue disruption as a result of trauma (childbirth, obstetric injury, surgery).

Risk Factors: Multiparity, obesity, chronic cough, heavy lifting, intrinsic tissue weakness or atrophic changes caused by estrogen loss. Some authors include smoking as a risk factor.

CLINICAL CHARACTERISTICS

Signs and Symptoms:
Asymptomatic
Pelvic pressure or "heaviness"
Stress incontinence, frequency, hesitancy, incomplete voiding, or recurrent infections
Bulging of tissue at the vaginal opening
Descent of the anterior vaginal wall during straining
Positive results on Q-tip test

DIAGNOSTIC APPROACH

Differential Diagnosis:
Urethral diverticulum
Skene's gland cyst, tumor, or abscess
Anterior enterocele
Gartner's duct cyst
Urgency incontinence

Associated Conditions: Stress urinary incontinence, pelvic relaxation, uterine prolapse, and other hernias.

Workup and Evaluation

Laboratory: No evaluation indicated; perform urinalysis if urinary tract infection is suspected.

Imaging: No imaging indicated.

Special Tests: "Q-tip test"—a cotton-tipped applicator dipped in 2% lidocaine (Xylocaine) is placed in the middle to upper urethra. Rotation anteriorly with straining (Valsalva's maneuver) is measured. Greater than 30 degree rotation is abnormal.

Diagnostic Procedures: Pelvic examination—best demonstrated by having the patient strain or cough while observing the vaginal opening through the separated labia. When a urethrocele or cystocele is present, a downward movement and forward rotation of the vaginal wall toward the introitus is demonstrated. A Sims speculum or the lower half of a Graves, Peterson, or other vaginal speculum may be used to retract the posterior vaginal wall, facilitating the identification of the support defect.

Pathologic Findings

No characteristic histologic change. Chronic irritation or keratinization secondary to mechanical trauma may be found with complete prolapse.

MANAGEMENT AND THERAPY

Nonpharmacologic

General Measures: Weight reduction, treatment of chronic cough (if present), topical or systemic estrogen replacement or therapy as indicated.

Specific Measures: Pessary therapy, pelvic muscle exercises, surgical repair; limited role for medical therapy.

Diet: No specific dietary changes indicated.

Activity: Avoidance of heavy lifting and straining may slow the rate of progression or risk of recurrence.

Patient Education: Reassurance, American College of Obstetricians and Gynecologists Patient Education Pamphlet AP0012 (*Pelvic Support Problems*), AP081 (*Urinary Incontinence*).

Drug(s) of Choice

None. (Estrogen, either topically or systemically, is often prescribed to improve tissue tone, reduce irritation, and prepare tissues for surgical or pessary therapy.)

Contraindications: Undiagnosed vaginal bleeding, breast cancer.

Precautions: α-Adrenergic blocking agents used to treat hypertension may reduce urethral tone sufficiently to result in stress urinary incontinence in patients with reduced pelvic support. Patients treated with angiotensin-converting enzyme (ACE) inhibitors may develop a cough as a side effect of medication, worsening incontinence symptoms and accelerating the appearance or worsening of a cystourethrocele.

FOLLOW-UP

Patient Monitoring: Normal health maintenance.
Prevention/Avoidance: None.

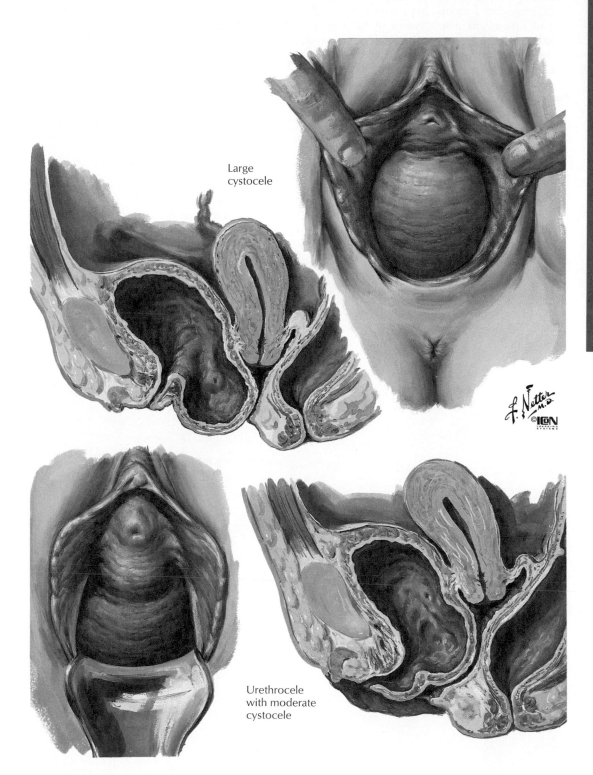

Large
cystocele

Urethrocele
with moderate
cystocele

VAGINAL DISEASE

Possible Complications: Compromise of ureteral drainage may be found in patients with significant downward displacement of the trigone. Recurrent urinary tract infections may occur if the support defect leads to significant residual urine. Vaginal ulceration, bleeding, infection, or pain frequently accompany complete prolapse.

Expected Outcome: Generally favorable reduction in symptoms may be obtained with a carefully chosen and fitted pessary. Surgical therapy is associated with 95% success in long-term correction of the anatomic defect and the associated symptoms.

MISCELLANEOUS

Pregnancy Considerations: No effect on pregnancy, although pregnancy (and vaginal delivery) may cause or contribute to a worsening of pelvic support problems.

ICD-9-CM Codes: 618.0, (618.4 [With uterine prolapse], 618.3 [Complete], 618.2 [Incomplete]).

REFERENCES

American College of Obstetricians and Gynecologists. *Pelvic Organ Prolapse.* Washington, DC: ACOG; 1995. ACOG Technical Bulletin 214.

Federkiw DM, Sand PK, Retzky SS, Johnson DC. The cotton swab test. Receiver-operating characteristic curves. *J Reprod Med* 1995;40:42.

Kinn AC, Lindskog M. Estrogens and phenylpropanolamine in combination for stress urinary incontinence in postmenopausal women. *Urology* 1988;32:273.

Smith RP. *Gynecology in Primary Care.* Baltimore, Md: Williams & Wilkins; 1997:577.

ENTEROCELE

INTRODUCTION

Description: Loss of support for the apex of the vagina, through rupture or attenuation of the pubovesicocervical fascia, manifested by descent or prolapse of the vaginal wall and underlying peritoneum, most commonly after abdominal or vaginal hysterectomy. An enterocele may occur when the uterus is present and tissue damage or weakness allows herniation behind the cervix and between the uterosacral ligaments.

Prevalence: Ten percent to fifteen percent of women, 30%–40% after menopause.

Predominant Age: 40 and older, increasing with age.

Genetics: No genetic pattern.

ETIOLOGY AND PATHOGENESIS

Causes: Loss or rupture of the normal support mechanisms in the pouch of Douglas. There is true herniation of the peritoneal cavity between the uterosacral ligaments and into the rectovaginal septum. Unlike a cystocele, urethrocele, or rectocele, the herniated tissue contains a true sac lined by parietal peritoneum.

Risk Factors: Multiparity, obesity, chronic cough, heavy lifting, intrinsic tissue weakness or atrophic changes resulting from estrogen loss. Some authors include smoking as a risk factor.

CLINICAL CHARACTERISTICS

Signs and Symptoms:
Asymptomatic
Pelvic pressure or "heaviness"
Bulging of tissue at the vaginal opening
Descent of the apical vaginal wall during straining

DIAGNOSTIC APPROACH

Differential Diagnosis:
Urethral diverticulum
Cystocele
Rectocele
Vaginal prolapse (generally includes an enterocele)
Gartner's duct cyst

Associated Conditions: Pelvic relaxation, vaginal prolapse, other hernias, and bowel obstruction (rare).

Workup and Evaluation

Laboratory: No evaluation indicated.

Imaging: No imaging indicated.

Special Tests: When the enterocele prolapses to beyond the introitus, transillumination may reveal loops of small bowel or omentum within the sac.

Diagnostic Procedures: Pelvic examination—best demonstrated by having the patient strain or cough while observing the vaginal opening through the separated labia. Rectovaginal examination differentiates this condition from a rectocele.

Pathologic Findings

No characteristic histologic change. Chronic irritation or keratinization secondary to mechanical trauma may be found when the enterocele descends to the level of the vulva or beyond.

MANAGEMENT AND THERAPY

Nonpharmacologic

General Measures: Weight reduction, treatment of chronic cough (if present), topical or systemic estrogen replacement or therapy as indicated.

Specific Measures: Pessary therapy (generally when the uterus is absent), surgical repair (abdominal or vaginal approach—McCall or Halban repair).

Diet: No specific dietary changes indicated.

Activity: No restriction.

Patient Education: Reassurance, American College of Obstetricians and Gynecologists Patient Education Pamphlet AP0012 (*Pelvic Support Problems*).

Drug(s) of Choice

None. (Estrogen, either topically or systemically, is often prescribed to improve tissue tone, reduce irritation, and prepare tissues for surgical or pessary therapy.)

Contraindications: Undiagnosed vaginal bleeding, breast cancer.

FOLLOW-UP

Patient Monitoring: Normal health maintenance.

Prevention/Avoidance: Maintenance of normal weight, use of surgical techniques at the time of hysterectomy that minimize the risk of enterocele formation (most commonly, this is plication of the uterosacral and cardinal ligaments).

Possible Complications: Bowel obstruction (rare).

Expected Outcome: Generally favorable reduction of symptoms may be obtained with a carefully chosen and fitted pessary. Surgical therapy is associated with 95% success in long-term correction of the anatomic defect and the associated symptoms.

MISCELLANEOUS

Pregnancy Considerations: Generally not a consideration.

ICD-9-CM **Codes:** 618.6.

REFERENCES

American College of Obstetricians and Gynecologists. *Pelvic Organ Prolapse.* Washington, DC: ACOG; 1995. ACOG Technical Bulletin 214.

Smith RP. *Gynecology in Primary Care.* Baltimore, Md: Williams & Wilkins; 1997:577.

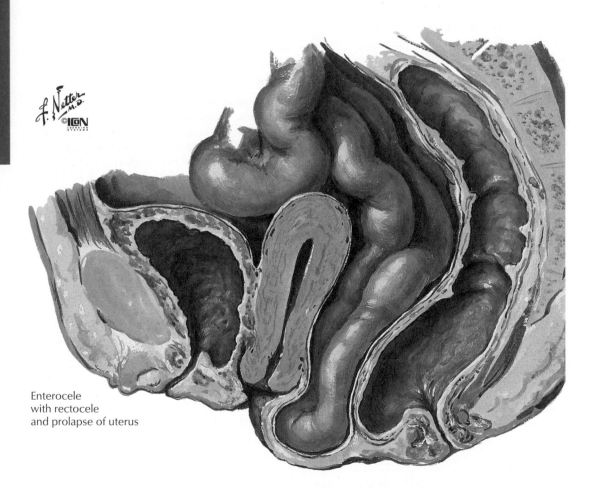

Enterocele
with rectocele
and prolapse of uterus

FISTULAE: GASTROINTESTINAL AND URINARY TRACT

INTRODUCTION

Description: A fistula is an abnormal communication between two cavities or organs. In gynecology, this usually refers to a communication between the gastrointestinal or urinary tracts and genital tract. (Connections directly to the skin are not discussed here.)

Prevalence: Gastrointestinal fistulae are uncommon; urinary tract fistulae are estimated to occur after 1 of 200 abdominal hysterectomies.

Predominant Age: Reproductive and beyond.

Genetics: No genetic pattern.

ETIOLOGY AND PATHOGENESIS

Causes: Urinary tract fistulae may result from surgical or obstetrical trauma, irradiation, or malignancy, although the most common cause by far is unrecognized surgical trauma. Roughly 75% of urinary tract fistulae occur after abdominal hysterectomy. Signs of a urinary fistula (watery discharge) usually occur from 5–30 days after surgery (average 8–12), although they may be present in the immediate postoperative period. Fistulae between the gastrointestinal tract and vagina may be precipitated by the same injuries that cause genitourinary fistulae; most common are obstetric injuries and complications of episiotomies (lower one third of vagina). Fistulae may also follow hysterectomy or enterocele repair (upper one third of vagina). Inflammatory bowel disease or pelvic radiation therapy may hasten fistula formation.

Risk Factors: Gastrointestinal—obstetric tears, puncture wounds, inflammatory bowel disease, intraabdominal surgery, carcinoma, radiation therapy, perirectal abscess. Although Crohn's disease, lymphogranuloma venereum or tuberculosis are recognized risk factors, these are uncommon. Urinary tract—surgery or radiation treatment. Urinary tract fistulae are most common after uncomplicated hysterectomy, although pelvic adhesive disease, endometriosis, or pelvic tumors increase the individual risk.

CLINICAL CHARACTERISTICS

Signs and Symptoms:
Gastrointestinal fistulae—Foul vaginal discharge
Marked vaginal and vulvar irritation
Fecal incontinence and soiling, and the passage of fecal matter or gas from the vagina, pathognomonic
Dyspareunia common
Dark red rectal mucosa or granulation tissue apparent in vaginal canal
Urinary tract fistulae—Continuous incontinence (occasionally made worse by position change or an increase in intraabdominal pressure as with a cough or laugh)
Vaginal and perineal wetness and irritation
Granulation tissue at site of fistula

DIAGNOSTIC APPROACH

Differential Diagnosis:
Gastrointestinal fistulae—Inflammatory bowel disease (Crohn's disease)
Pilonidal sinus
Perianal or other abscess
Rectal carcinoma
Urinary tract fistulae—Overflow incontinence
Urge incontinence

Associated Conditions: Inflammatory bowel disease, bacterial vaginitis, dyspareunia, vaginitis, vulvitis, and urinary tract infection.

Workup and Evaluation

Laboratory: No evaluation indicated. (Evaluation of renal function [serum creatinine] is prudent but not diagnostic.)

Imaging: If inflammatory bowel disease is suspected, lower gastrointestinal series. Intravenous or retrograde pyelography may be useful.

Special Tests: Gastrointestinal fistulae—methylene blue may be instilled in the rectum with a tampon in place; staining indicates a communication. Sigmoidoscopy should be considered. Urinary tract fistulae—a tampon placed in the vagina with dye instilled into the bladder or dye given, usually intravenously, to be excreted by the kidney may be used to help find a fistula. Cystoscopy may help identify vesicovaginal fistulae.

Diagnostic Procedures: History, physical examination, probe of fistulous tract. Anoscopy, proctoscopy, sigmoidoscopy, or intravenous or retrograde pyelography may be helpful. Cystoscopy may be required to evaluate the location of a urinary tract fistula in relation to the ureteral opening and bladder trigone and to exclude the possibility of multiple fistulae.

Pathologic Findings

Inflammation and granulation changes from chronic infection. Tract may be single or multiple. Chronic bacterial vaginitis is generally present. Fistulae may be from the vagina to the bladder (vesicovaginal), to the urethra (urethrovaginal), or

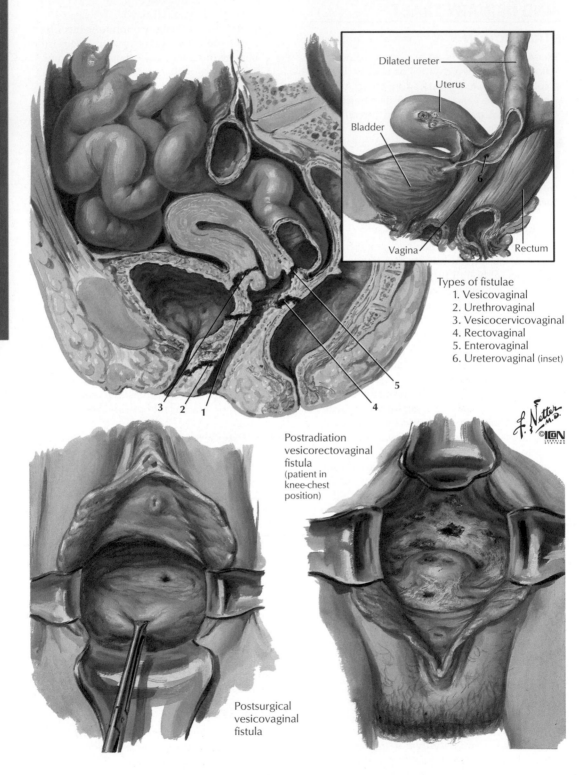

Dilated ureter

Uterus

Bladder

6

Vagina

Rectum

Types of fistulae
1. Vesicovaginal
2. Urethrovaginal
3. Vesicocervicovaginal
4. Rectovaginal
5. Enterovaginal
6. Ureterovaginal (inset)

Postradiation
vesicorectovaginal
fistula
(patient in
knee-chest
position)

Postsurgical
vesicovaginal
fistula

to the ureter (ureterovaginal). Rarely, communication between the bladder and the uterus (vesicouterine) may also occur.

MANAGEMENT AND THERAPY

Nonpharmacologic

General Measures: Gastrointestinal fistulae—evaluation, stool softening, treatment of vaginitis. Urinary tract fistulae—urinary diversion (see the following text), protection of the vulva from continuous moisture (zinc oxide cream or diaper rash preparations).

Specific Measures: Gastrointestinal fistulae—for those that do not heal spontaneously (three fourths of fistulae), the only effective treatment is surgical. When the fistula is small, this is often carried out with the patient under general or spinal anesthesia in an ambulatory surgery unit. Fistulectomy or fistulotomy should not be performed in the presence of tissue edema or inflammation, diarrhea, or active inflammatory bowel disease. Urinary tract fistulae—vesicovaginal fistulae that occur in the immediate postoperative period should be treated by large caliber transurethral catheter drainage. Spontaneous healing is evident within 2–4 weeks (20% of patients). Similarly, in patients with a ureterovaginal fistula, prompt placement of a ureteral stent, left in place for 2 weeks, allows spontaneous healing for roughly 30% of patients. When these conservative therapies fail, full surgical correction is required.

Diet: Low residue diet advisable for patients with a gastrointestinal fistula.

Activity: No restriction. (Pelvic rest after surgical repair, until healing is completed.)

Patient Education: Perianal care, sitz baths, American College of Obstetricians and Gynecologists Patient Education Pamphlet AP081 (*Urinary Incontinence*).

Drug(s) of Choice

Although the only effective treatment is surgical, the use of stool softeners is often beneficial. If diarrhea is present, diphenoxylate hydrochloride (Lomotil) or a similar drug should be used to control symptoms. Treatment of coexisting vaginitis should be instituted.

Urinary antisepsis should be considered when necessary.

FOLLOW-UP

Patient Monitoring: Patients with a gastrointestinal fistula should be closely followed during the postoperative period (hospital discharge is generally delayed until after the first bowel movement). Routine health care. When a ureteral fistula has been repaired, follow-up intravenous pyelography should be planned for 3, 6, and 12 months to check for delayed stricture.

Prevention/Avoidance: Careful surgical and obstetrical techniques including preoperative and perioperative bladder drainage, good visualization, careful dissection, and care in placement of hemostatic sutures.

Possible Complications: Upper genital tract infection, recurrence, ascending urinary tract infection (including pyelonephritis).

Expected Outcome: Healing is generally good after surgical excision, although recurrence, when the original fistulae were caused by underlying disease or radiation therapy, is common.

MISCELLANEOUS

Pregnancy Considerations: No direct effect on pregnancy although some causal processes may result in lower fertility or other effects on reproduction.

ICD-9-CM Codes: 619.1 (Gastrointestinal), 619.0 (Urinary tract).

REFERENCES

Alexander AA, Liu JB, Merton DA, Nagle DA. Fecal incontinence: transvaginal US evaluation of anatomic causes. *Radiology* 1996;199:529.

Alvarez RD. Gastrointestinal complications in gynecologic surgery: a review for the general gynecologist. *Obstet Gynecol* 1988;72:533.

American College of Obstetricians and Gynecologists. *Genitourinary Fistulas.* Washington, DC: ACOG; 1995. ACOG Technical Bulletin 83.

American College of Obstetricians and Gynecologists. *Lower Urinary Tract Operative Injuries.* Washington, DC: ACOG; 1997. ACOG Technical Bulletin 238.

Bassford T. Treatment of common anorectal disorders [review]. *Am Fam Physician* 1992;45:1787.

Gerber GS, Schoenberg HW. Female urinary tract fistulas. *J Urol* 1993;149:229.

Holley RL, Kilgore LC. Urologic complications. In: Orr JW, Jr, Shingleton HM, eds. *Complications in Gynecologic Surgery: Prevention, Recognition, and Management.* Philadelphia, Pa: JB Lippincott; 1994:149.

Meeks GR, Sams JO 4th, Field KW, Fulp KS, Margolis MT. Formation of vesicovaginal fistula: the role of suture placement into the bladder during closure of the vaginal cuff after transabdominal hysterectomy. *Am J Obstet Gynecol* 1997;177:1298.

Smith RP. *Gynecology in Primary Care.* Baltimore, Md: Williams & Wilkins; 1997:577.

Smith RP, Ling FW. *Procedures in Women's Health Care.* Baltimore, Md: Williams & Wilkins; 1997:153, 163, 175, 201.

Symmonds RE. Incontinence: Vesical and urethral fistulas. *Clin Obstet Gynecol* 1984;27:499.

RECTOCELE

INTRODUCTION

Description: Failure of the normal support mechanisms between the rectum and the vagina results in herniation of the posterior vaginal wall and underlying rectum into the vaginal canal and eventually to, and through, the introitus.

Prevalence: Ten percent to fifteen percent of women, 30%–40% after menopause.

Predominant Age: Postmenopausal.

Genetics: No genetic pattern.

ETIOLOGY AND PATHOGENESIS

Causes: Loss of normal tissue integrity or tissue disruption as a result of trauma (childbirth, obstetric injury, surgery).

Risk Factors: Multiparity, obesity, chronic cough, heavy lifting, intrinsic tissue weakness or atrophic changes resulting from estrogen loss. Some authors include smoking as a risk factor.

CLINICAL CHARACTERISTICS

Signs and Symptoms:
Bulging of the posterior vaginal wall
Difficulty passing stool (may require manual splinting of the posterior vaginal wall to have a bowel movement)
Dyspareunia uncommon but may occur

DIAGNOSTIC APPROACH

Differential Diagnosis:
Enterocele
Rectovaginal hematoma
Rectal cancer
Vaginal inclusion cyst (after obstetrical trauma or episiotomy)

Associated Conditions: Stress urinary incontinence, pelvic relaxation, uterine prolapse, other hernias, and vaginal outlet relaxation.

Workup and Evaluation

Laboratory: No evaluation indicated.

Imaging: Transvaginal ultrasonography may be used to assess the presence of an enterocele if not clinically apparent.

Special Tests: None indicated.

Diagnostic Procedures: Pelvic examination—best demonstrated by having the patient strain or cough while observing the vaginal opening through the separated labia. A Sims speculum or the lower half of a Graves, Peterson, or other vaginal speculum (inserted upside down), may be inserted to retract the anterior vaginal wall, facilitating the identification of the support defect.

Pathologic Findings

No characteristic histologic change. Chronic irritation or keratinization secondary to mechanical trauma may be found with complete prolapse.

MANAGEMENT AND THERAPY

Nonpharmacologic

General Measures: Weight reduction, treatment of chronic cough (if present), topical or systemic estrogen replacement or therapy as indicated.

Specific Measures: Pessary therapy, pelvic muscle exercises, surgical repair; limited role for medical therapy.

Diet: No specific dietary changes indicated.

Activity: Avoidance of heavy lifting and straining may slow the rate of progression or risk of recurrence.

Patient Education: Reassurance, American College of Obstetricians and Gynecologists Patient Education Pamphlet AP0012 (*Pelvic Support Problems*).

Drug(s) of Choice

None. (Estrogen, either topically or systemically, is often prescribed to improve tissue tone, reduce irritation, and prepare tissues for surgical or pessary therapy.)

Contraindications: Undiagnosed vaginal bleeding, breast cancer.

FOLLOW-UP

Patient Monitoring: Normal health maintenance.

Prevention/Avoidance: None.

Possible Complications: Laxative abuse/dependence. Vaginal ulceration, bleeding, infection, or pain frequently accompanies complete prolapse.

Expected Outcome: Generally favorable reduction of symptoms may be obtained with a carefully chosen and fitted pessary. Surgical therapy is associated with 95% success in long-term correction of the anatomic defect and the associated symptoms.

MISCELLANEOUS

Pregnancy Considerations: No effect on pregnancy, although pregnancy (and vaginal delivery) may cause or contribute to a worsening of pelvic support problems.

ICD-9-CM Codes: 618.0 (Without uterine prolapse), 618.4 (With uterine prolapse).

REFERENCES

American College of Obstetricians and Gynecologists. *Pelvic Organ Prolapse.* Washington, DC: ACOG; 1995. ACOG Technical Bulletin 214.

Bump RC, Mattiasson A, Bø K, et al. The standardization of terminology of female pelvic organ prolapse and pelvic floor dysfunction. *Am J Obstet Gynecol* 1996;175:10.

Porges RF. Abnormalities of pelvic support. In: Sciarra JJ, ed. *Gynecology and Obstetrics.* Vol 1. Philadelphia, Pa: JB Lippincott; 1994;61:7.

Porges RF. Posterior colpoperineorrhaphy. In: Sciarra JJ, ed. *Gynecology and Obstetrics.* Vol 1. Philadelphia, Pa: JB Lippincott; 1998;63:1.

Smith RP. *Gynecology in Primary Care.* Baltimore, Md: Williams & Wilkins; 1997:577.

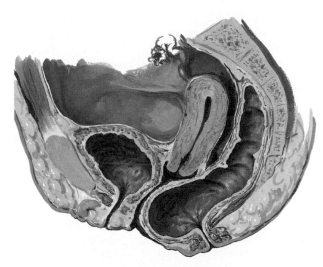

Rectocele

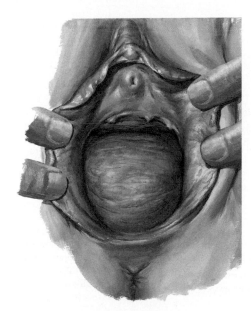

Large rectocele

SARCOMA BOTRYOIDES

INTRODUCTION

Description: A rare form of sarcoma (embryonal rhabdomyosarcoma) generally found in the vagina of young girls. Rarely, these tumors may arise from the cervix. Although the cervical form of sarcoma is histologically similar to the vaginal form, the prognosis for the cervical form is better.

Prevalence: Rare.

Predominant Age: Generally younger than 8 years, two thirds younger than 2, most common neoplasm of the lower genital tract in premenarchal girls.

Genetics: No genetic pattern.

ETIOLOGY AND PATHOGENESIS

Causes: Unknown. Arises in the subepithelial layers of the vagina.

Risk Factors: None known.

CLINICAL CHARACTERISTICS

Signs and Symptoms:
Vaginal bleeding
Vaginal mass (resembles a cluster of grapes, may be hemorrhagic, myxoid, or both)

DIAGNOSTIC APPROACH

Differential Diagnosis:
Urethral prolapse
Vaginal polyp (pseudosarcoma botryoides)
Endodermal sinus tumor (yolk sac tumor)
Precocious puberty
Associated Conditions: None.

Workup and Evaluation

Laboratory: No specific evaluation indicated.

Imaging: No specific imaging indicated, only that necessary to evaluate tumor location and spread.

Special Tests: Biopsy of the mass.

Diagnostic Procedures: Physical examination, histologic tests.

Pathologic Findings

Tumor is often multicentric with loose myxomatous stroma containing malignant pleomorphic cells and eosinophilic rhabdomyoblasts that have characteristic cross-striations (strap cells).

MANAGEMENT AND THERAPY

Nonpharmacologic

General Measures: Evaluation.

Specific Measures: Surgical excision combined with multiagent chemotherapy. Adjunctive radiation therapy has also been advocated, but is generally reserved for those with residual disease.

Diet: No specific dietary changes indicated.

Activity: No restriction.

Drug(s) of Choice

Adjunctive multiagent chemotherapy only.

FOLLOW-UP

Patient Monitoring: Once surgery and chemotherapy have been completed, monitoring for recurrence and general health maintenance.

Prevention/Avoidance: None.

Possible Complications: These are aggressive tumors; dissemination and recurrence are common. Spread is through direct invasion and metastasis to lymph nodes and distant sites (by hematogenous routes). The cause of death is generally by direct local extension.

Expected Outcome: Overall the prognosis is poor. Small series suggest that with the combination of surgical resection and combination chemotherapy, survival in more than 80% may be expected. Among those who survive, normal (eventual) pubertal changes and pregnancy have been reported.

MISCELLANEOUS

Pregnancy Considerations: No effect on pregnancy for those who survive and achieve conception.

ICD-9-CM Codes: M8910/3.

REFERENCES

Blythe JG, Bari WA. Uterine sarcoma: Histology, classification, and prognosis. In: Sciarra JJ, ed. *Gynecology and Obstetrics.* Vol 4. Philadelphia, Pa: JB Lippincott; 1998;22:11.

Copeland LJ, Gershenson DM, Saul PB, Sneige N, Stringer CA, Edwards CL. Sarcoma botryoides of the female genital tract. *Obstet Gynecol* 1985;66:262.

Davos I, Abell MR. Sarcomas of the vagina. *Obstet Gynecol* 1976;47:342.

Hilgers RD. Pelvic exenteration for vaginal embryonal rhabdomyosarcoma: a review. *Obstet Gynecol* 1975; 45:175.

Hilgers RD, Malkasian GD, Soule EH. Embryonal rhabdomyosarcoma (botryoid type) of the vagina. *Am J Obstet Gynecol* 1970;107:484.

Mitchell M, Talerman A, Sholl JS, Okagaki T, Cibils LA. Pseudosarcoma botryoides in pregnancy: report of a case with ultrastructural observations. *Obstet Gynecol* 1987;70:522.

Rutledge F, Sullivan MP. Sarcoma botryoides. *Ann N Y Acad Sci* 1967;124:694.

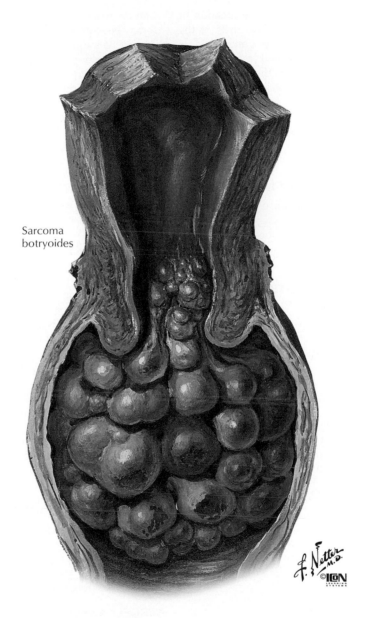

Sarcoma
botryoides

TRANSVERSE VAGINAL SEPTUM

INTRODUCTION

Description: A partial or complete obstruction of the vagina generally found at the junction of the upper third and lower two thirds of the vaginal canal. The septum is generally less than 1 cm in thickness and may or may not have a small opening to the upper genital tract. (The location and thickness are highly variable.)

Prevalence: One of 72,000–75,000 females.

Predominant Age: Present at birth, but generally not diagnosed until puberty.

Genetics: No genetic pattern.

ETIOLOGY AND PATHOGENESIS

Causes: Incomplete canalization of the Müllerian tubercle and sinovaginal bulb.

Risk Factors: Partial septa have been reported in women exposed in utero to diethylstilbestrol (DES).

CLINICAL CHARACTERISTICS

Signs and Symptoms:
Blind, shortened vaginal pouch
Primary amenorrhea
Mucocolpos
Hematocolpos
Hematometra
Foul vaginal discharge (with incomplete septum)
Vaginal/abdominal mass without bulging of the vaginal outlet (hematocolpos and mucocolpos may be associated with urinary tract obstruction if very large)

DIAGNOSTIC APPROACH

Differential Diagnosis:
Vaginal agenesis
Imperforate hymen

Associated Conditions: Endometriosis, infertility, amenorrhea, and hematocolpos.

Workup and Evaluation

Laboratory: No evaluation indicated.

Imaging: Ultrasonography may be used to evaluate the presence and condition of the upper genital tract.

Special Tests: None indicated.

Diagnostic Procedures: Pelvic examination.

Pathologic Findings

None.

MANAGEMENT AND THERAPY

Nonpharmacologic

General Measures: Evaluation, reassurance.

Specific Measures: Transverse vaginal septa must be excised surgically. When the septum is thick, reconstruction with skin grafts or flaps may be required. In extreme cases, a neovagina must be surgically created. (Once drainage of the upper tract is obtained, vaginal reconstruction may be delayed to a later date.)

Diet: No specific dietary changes indicated.

Activity: No restriction.

Patient Education: Reassurance, education about possible effects on fertility and sexual function (for most patients there will be little or no effect).

Drug(s) of Choice

None.

FOLLOW-UP

Patient Monitoring: Once a normal vaginal canal has been restored, normal health maintenance. Patients must be monitored for narrowing of the vagina at the level of the removed septum or vaginal reanastomosis.

Prevention/Avoidance: None.

Possible Complications: In rare patients, a mucocolpos can cause serious and life-threatening compression of surrounding organs leading to hydroureter, hydronephrosis, rectal compression and obstruction, restricted diaphragmatic excursion, compression of the vena cava, and cardiorespiratory failure. Fistulae to the urinary tract may occur. Prolonged obstruction of menstrual outflow is associated with the development of endometriosis and pelvic scarring (often extensive); chronic pelvic pain, dyspareunia and infertility may result. Pregnancy rates for patients with corrected transverse septa range from 25%–50% based on location of the septum and series report.

Expected Outcome: With timely diagnosis and treatment, the prognosis is good.

MISCELLANEOUS

Pregnancy Considerations: No effect on pregnancy once pregnancy is achieved. Pregnancy success is greatest with septa that are lower in the vagina and repaired early. Based on the extent of vaginal reconstruction performed and the degree of subsequent scarring, cesarean delivery may be elected.

ICD-9-CM Codes: 752.49.

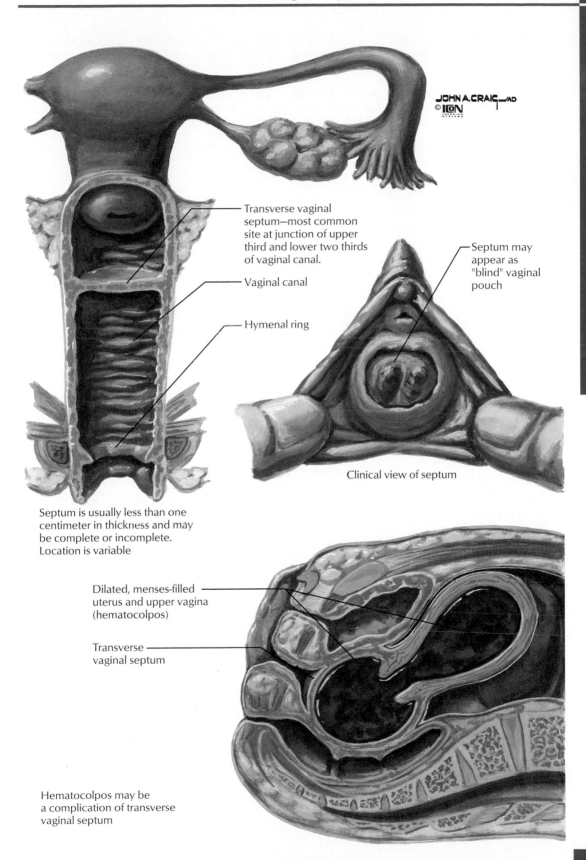

JOHN A. CRAIG—MD
© ICN

Transverse vaginal septum—most common site at junction of upper third and lower two thirds of vaginal canal.

Vaginal canal

Hymenal ring

Septum may appear as "blind" vaginal pouch

Clinical view of septum

Septum is usually less than one centimeter in thickness and may be complete or incomplete. Location is variable

Dilated, menses-filled uterus and upper vagina (hematocolpos)

Transverse vaginal septum

Hematocolpos may be a complication of transverse vaginal septum

REFERENCES

Brenner P, Sedlis A, Cooperman H. Complete imperforate transverse vaginal septum. *Obstet Gynecol* 1965;25:135.

Lilford RJ, Morton K, Dewhurst Sir J. The diagnosis and management of the imperforate vaginal membrane in the pre-pubertal child. *Pediatr Adolesc Gynecol* 1983;1:115.

McKusick VA. Transverse vaginal septum (hydrometrocolpos). *Birth Defects* 1971;7:326.

McKusick VA, Weiboecher RG, Gragg GW. Recessive inheritance of a congenital malformation syndrome. *JAMA* 1968;204:113.

Rock JA, Keenan DL. Surgical correction of uterovaginal anomalies In: Sciarra JJ, ed. *Gynecology and Obstetrics.* Vol 1. Philadelphia, Pa: JB Lippincott; 1998:70:6.

Rock JA, Zacur HA, Dlugi AM, Jones HW Jr, TeLinde RW. Pregnancy success following surgical correction of imperforate hymen and complete transverse vaginal septum. *Obstet Gynecol* 1982;59:448.

VAGINAL CYSTS

INTRODUCTION

Description: Cystic masses in the vaginal wall are uncommon and may arise from either congenital (Gartner's duct cysts) or acquired processes (epithelial inclusion cysts).

Prevalence: One of 200 women.

Predominant Age: Generally from adolescence to middle reproductive years.

Genetics: No genetic pattern.

ETIOLOGY AND PATHOGENESIS

Causes: Congenital (Gartner's duct cyst or remnant, generally found in the anterior lateral vaginal wall), structural (urethral diverticulum, loss of vaginal wall support), acquired (inclusion cyst, >50% of cysts).

Risk Factors: Episiotomy or obstetric laceration, gynecologic surgery.

CLINICAL CHARACTERISTICS

Signs and Symptoms:

Asymptomatic

May be associated with a sense of fullness

Dyspareunia (uncommon)

Difficulty with tampon insertion or retention

Cystic mass lesion (1–5 cm) found generally in the lateral vaginal wall (congenital) or in midline posteriorly (acquired)

DIAGNOSTIC APPROACH

Differential Diagnosis:

Urethral diverticulum

Cystocele

Urethrocele

Rectocele

Bartholin's gland cyst

Vaginal adenosis

Vaginal endometriosis

Perirectal abscess

Vaginal fibromyoma

Associated Conditions: Slightly higher rate of upper genital tract malformations when embryonic remnants persist.

Workup and Evaluation

Laboratory: No evaluation indicated.

Imaging: No imaging indicated.

Special Tests: Vaginal adenosis may be excluded by staining with Lugol's solution (adenosis will not stain).

Diagnostic Procedures: History and physical examination.

Pathologic Findings

Most embryonic cysts are lined by cuboidal epithelium. Stratified epithelium suggests an inclusion (acquired) cyst.

MANAGEMENT AND THERAPY

Nonpharmacologic

General Measures: Evaluation and reassurance.

Specific Measures: Surgical excision if the mass is symptomatic or its cause is uncertain; otherwise no therapy is required.

Diet: No specific dietary changes indicated.

Activity: No restriction.

Patient Education: Reassurance, American College of Obstetricians and Gynecologists Patient Education Pamphlet AP012 (*Pelvic Support Problems*).

Drug(s) of Choice

None.

FOLLOW-UP

Patient Monitoring: Normal health maintenance.

Prevention/Avoidance: None.

Possible Complications: Mechanical irritation or interference with intercourse or childbirth (rare), infection (rare).

Expected Outcome: Some care must be used in the excision of large cysts so that vaginal scarring and stenosis does not occur; otherwise surgical therapy should be successful.

MISCELLANEOUS

Pregnancy Considerations: No effect on pregnancy.

ICD-9-CM Codes: 623.8 (Inclusion), 752.41 (Embryonal).

REFERENCES

Delmore JE, Horbelt DV. Benign neoplasia of the vagina. In: Sciarra JJ, ed. *Gynecology and Obstetrics.* Vol 1. Philadelphia, Pa: JB Lippincott; 1995;10:1.

Deppisch LM. Cysts of the vagina. *Obstet Gynecol* 1975;45:623.

Dmochowski RR, Ganabathi K, Zimmern PE, Leach GE. Benign female periurethral masses. *J Urol* 1994; 152:1943.

Hillard PA. Benign diseases of the female reproductive tract: symptoms and signs. In: Berek JS, Adashi EY, Hillard PA, eds. *Novak's Gynecology.* 12th ed. Baltimore, Md: Williams & Wilkins; 1996:390.

Junaid TA, Thomas SM. Cysts of the vulva and vagina: a comparative study. *Int J Gynaecol Obstet* 1981; 19:239.

Robboy SJ, Ross JS, Prat J, Keh PC, Welch WR. Urogenital sinus origin of mucinous and ciliated cysts of the vulva. *Obstet Gynecol* 1978;51:347.

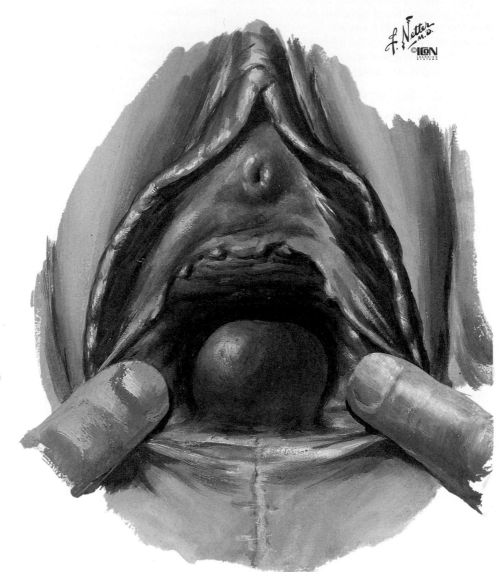

Inclusion
cyst

VAGINAL DRYNESS

INTRODUCTION

Description: Loss of normal vaginal moisture resulting in irritation, itching, or pain with intercourse. This loss may be due to alterations in vaginal physiology caused by infection or the loss of estrogen stimulation (atrophic change). This may also occur situationally because of inadequate or inappropriate sexual stimulation, sexual phobia, or pain.

Prevalence: Common in menopausal women not receiving estrogen replacement therapy.

Predominant Age: Postmenopausal.

Genetics: No genetic pattern.

ETIOLOGY AND PATHOGENESIS

Causes: Loss of estrogen stimulation (menopause), vaginitis, arousal disorders.

Risk Factors: Menopause without estrogen replacement, vaginal infection.

CLINICAL CHARACTERISTICS

Signs and Symptoms:
Sensation of vaginal dryness
Vaginal itching or irritation
Insertional dyspareunia
Dry, inflamed vaginal tissues seen on pelvic examination

DIAGNOSTIC APPROACH

Differential Diagnosis:
Lichen sclerosis
Vaginitis
Vulvar vestibulitis
Libidinal dysfunction/arousal disorders

Associated Conditions: Dyspareunia, vaginitis, and menopause.

Workup and Evaluation

Laboratory: Microscopic examination of vaginal secretions if infection is suspected.

Imaging: No imaging indicated.

Special Tests: A vaginal maturation index may confirm atrophic change but is seldom required.

Diagnostic Procedures: History and physical examination.

Pathologic Findings

Postmenopausal: Thinned vaginal epithelium with loss of rugations. Infection: based on organism present.

MANAGEMENT AND THERAPY

Nonpharmacologic

General Measures: Evaluation, topical moisturizers or lubricants (as needed or long acting).

Specific Measures: Estrogen replacement therapy or treatment of vaginal infection (when appropriate). Counseling regarding sexuality, arousal, foreplay, and coital technique (if needed).

Diet: No specific dietary changes indicated.

Activity: No restriction.

Patient Education: Reassurance, American College of Obstetricians and Gynecologists Patient Education Pamphlet AP047 (*The Menopause Years*), AP066 (*Hormone Replacement Therapy*), AP028 (*Vaginitis: Causes and Treatment*), AP020 (*Pain During Intercourse*)

Drug(s) of Choice

Estrogen replacement therapy when appropriate (see "Menopause")
Water-soluble lubricants for intercourse
Long-acting emollients (Replens)

Contraindications: Known or suspected allergy or intolerance to any agent.

Precautions: Petroleum-based products (e.g., Vaseline) are difficult to remove and may lead to additional irritation.

FOLLOW-UP

Patient Monitoring: Normal health maintenance.

Prevention/Avoidance: Estrogen replacement after menopause.

Possible Complications: Vaginal lacerations and secondary infection, vulvar excoriations, sexual dysfunction.

Expected Outcome: Generally good results with topical and systemic therapy for estrogen loss. Good response to therapy for vaginitis.

MISCELLANEOUS

Pregnancy Considerations: No effect on pregnancy (generally not an issue).

ICD-9-CM Codes: Based on cause.

REFERENCES

Bygdeman M, Swahn ML. Replens versus dienoestrol cream in the symptomatic treatment of vaginal atrophy in postmenopausal women. *Maturitas* 1996;23:259.

Coope J. Hormonal and non-hormonal interventions for menopausal symptoms. *Maturitas* 1996;23:159.

Lamont JA. Dyspareunia and vaginismus. In: Sciarra JJ, ed. *Gynecology and Obstetrics*. Vol 6. Philadelphia, Pa: JB Lippincott; 1998;102:2.

Loprinzi CL, Abu-Ghazaleh S, Sloan JA, et al. Phase III randomized double-blind study to evaluate the efficacy of a polycarbophil-based vaginal moisturizer in women with breast cancer. *J Clin Oncol* 1997;15:969.

Mishell DR. Menopause. In: Mishell DR, Stenchever MA, Droegemueller W, Herbst AL, eds. *Comprehensive Gynecology*. 3rd ed. St Louis, Mo: Mosby; 1997:1163.

Smith RP. *Gynecology in Primary Care*. Baltimore, Md: Williams & Wilkins; 1997:197, 522.

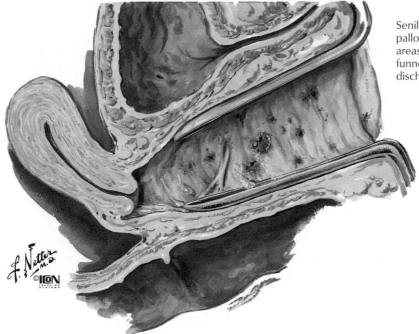

Senile vaginitis early stage: pallor, loss of rugae, denuded areas, petechial hemorrhages, funnel-like narrowing, thin discharge

VAGINAL LACERATIONS

INTRODUCTION

Description: Lacerations of the vaginal wall or introitus are most often the result of sexual trauma (80%, consensual or otherwise).

Prevalence: Uncommon, but specific prevalence is unknown.

Predominant Age: Reproductive.

Genetics: No genetic pattern.

ETIOLOGY AND PATHOGENESIS

Causes: Intercourse (80%), saddle or water skiing injury, sexual assault, penetration by foreign objects.

Risk Factors: Virginity, vaginismus, postpartum and postmenopausal vaginal atrophy, hysterectomy, alcohol or other drug use.

CLINICAL CHARACTERISTICS

Signs and Symptoms:

Vaginal bleeding (may be profuse and prolonged)

Acute pain during intercourse (25%, lacerations of the distal vagina or introitus)

Persistent pain after intercourse (the location of the pain is somewhat dependent on the location of the laceration).

DIAGNOSTIC APPROACH

Differential Diagnosis:

Cervical polyp (as source of bleeding)

Menstrual bleeding

Threatened abortion

Granulation tissue in healing incision (episiotomy, other vaginal surgery)

Sexual abuse/rape

Associated Conditions: Vaginal atrophy, sexual dysfunction, alcohol or drug use/abuse.

Workup and Evaluation

Laboratory: Complete blood count.

Imaging: No imaging indicated.

Special Tests: None indicated.

Diagnostic Procedures: History and physical examination (history is often misleading or false).

Pathologic Findings

The most common site of coital laceration is the posterior fornix, followed by the right and left fornices.

MANAGEMENT AND THERAPY

Nonpharmacologic

General Measures: Rapid assessment and hemodynamic stabilization (when appropriate).

Specific Measures: Surgical closure of the laceration, evaluation of the integrity of the urinary and gastrointestinal tract; may include exploratory laparotomy or laparoscopy in cases of evisceration or peritoneal breach.

Diet: No specific dietary changes indicated.

Activity: Pelvic rest (no tampons, douches, or intercourse) until healing has occurred.

Patient Education: Reassurance, American College of Obstetricians and Gynecologists Patient Education Pamphlet AP083 (*The Abused Woman*), AP020 (*Pain During Intercourse*).

Drug(s) of Choice

Local or general anesthesia for surgical repair. Treatment with an antibiotic is generally not required except if a peritoneal breach is present.

FOLLOW-UP

Patient Monitoring: Normal health maintenance after healing has been completed.

Prevention/Avoidance: Avoidance of alcohol or drug use, careful consensual intercourse, adequate vaginal lubrication.

Possible Complications: Vaginal evisceration, excessive blood loss. In rare cases, death has been reported.

Expected Outcome: Generally good healing, the risk of recurrence is based on cause.

MISCELLANEOUS

Pregnancy Considerations: No effect on pregnancy unless the health or safety of the mother is compromised.

ICD-9-CM Codes: Based on location and cause.

REFERENCES

American College of Obstetricians and Gynecologists. *Operative Vaginal Delivery.* Washington, DC: ACOG; 1994. ACOG Technical Bulletin 196.

Ahnaimugan S, Asuen MI. Coital laceration of the vagina. *Aust N Z J Obstet Gynaecol* 1980;20:180.

Barrett KF, Bledsoe S, Greer BE, Droegemueller W. Tampon-induced vaginal or cervical ulceration. *Am J Obstet Gynecol* 1977;127:332.

Friedel W, Kaiser IH. Vaginal evisceration. *Obstet Gynecol* 1975;45:315.

VAGINAL DISEASE

Haefner HK, Andersen F, Johnson MP. Vaginal laceration following a jet-ski accident. *Obstet Gynecol* 1991;78:986.

Niv J, Lessing JB, Hartuv J, Peyser MR. Vaginal injury resulting from sliding down a water chute. *Am J Obstet Gynecol* 1992;166:930.

Rafla N. Vaginismus and vaginal tears. *Am J Obstet Gynecol* 1988;158:1043.

Smith NC, Van Coeverden de Groot HA, Gunston KD. Coital injuries of the vagina in nonvirginal patients. *S Afr Med J* 1983;64:746.

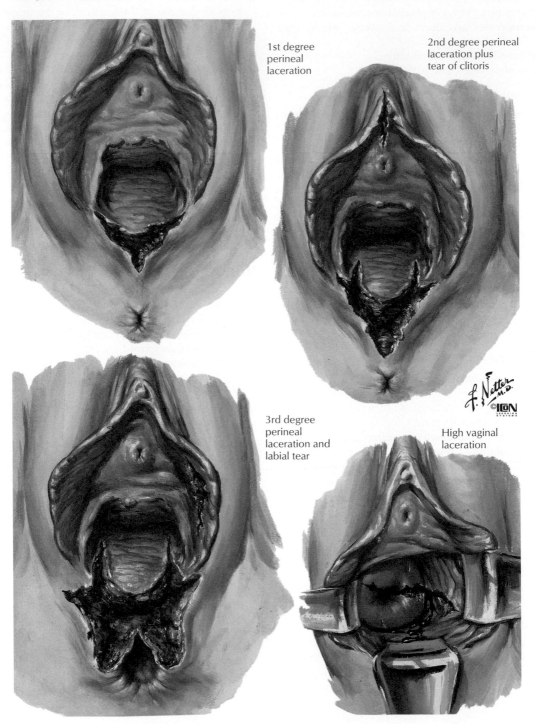

1st degree perineal laceration

2nd degree perineal laceration plus tear of clitoris

3rd degree perineal laceration and labial tear

High vaginal laceration

VAGINAL PROLAPSE

INTRODUCTION

Description: Loss of the normal support mechanism resulting in descent of the vaginal wall down the vaginal canal. In the extreme, this may result in the vagina becoming everted beyond the vulva to a position outside the body. Vaginal prolapse is generally found only after hysterectomy and is a special form of enterocele.

Prevalence: Depends on the severity of the original defect, type of surgery originally performed and other risk factors.

Predominant Age: Late reproductive and beyond.

Genetics: No genetic pattern.

ETIOLOGY AND PATHOGENESIS

Causes: Loss of normal structural support because of trauma (childbirth), surgery, chronic intraabdominal pressure elevation (such as obesity, chronic cough, or heavy lifting), or intrinsic weakness. A recurrence within 1–2 years of surgery is considered a failure of technique.

Risk Factors: Birth trauma, chronic intraabdominal pressure elevation (such as obesity, chronic cough, or heavy lifting), intrinsic tissue weakness, or atrophic changes resulting from estrogen loss.

CLINICAL CHARACTERISTICS

Signs and Symptoms:
Pelvic pressure or heaviness
Mass or protrusion at the vaginal entrance
New onset or paradoxical resolution of urinary incontinence

DIAGNOSTIC APPROACH

Differential Diagnosis:
Cystocele
Urethrocele
Rectocele
Bartholin cyst
Vaginal cyst or tumor

Associated Conditions: Urinary incontinence, pelvic pain, dyspareunia, intermenstrual or postmenopausal bleeding. A cystourethrocele, rectocele, and/or enterocele is almost always present when complete prolapse has occurred.

Workup and Evaluation

Laboratory: No evaluation indicated.

Imaging: No imaging indicated.

Special Tests: Urodynamics testing may be considered if there is altered voiding or continence.

Diagnostic Procedures: History and physical examination.

Pathologic Findings

Tissue change common because of mechanical trauma and desiccation.

MANAGEMENT AND THERAPY

Nonpharmacologic

General Measures: Weight reduction, modification of activity (lifting); address factors such as chronic cough.

Specific Measures: Pessary therapy, surgical repair (culdoplasty, plication of the uterosacral ligaments, sacrospinous ligament fixation, or colpocleisis). When surgical repair is undertaken, attention must also focus on correction of any anterior or posterior vaginal wall support problems.

Diet: No specific dietary changes indicated.

Activity: No restriction, although heavy lifting or strenuous activities may predispose to the development or recurrence of prolapse.

Patient Education: Reassurance, American College of Obstetricians and Gynecologists Patient Education Pamphlet AP012 (*Pelvic Support Problems*), AP081 (*Urinary Incontinence*).

Drug(s) of Choice

Estrogen replacement therapy (for postmenopausal patients) improves tissue tone and healing and is often prescribed before surgical repair or as an adjunct to pessary therapy.

Contraindications: Estrogen therapy should not be used if undiagnosed vaginal bleeding is present.

FOLLOW-UP

Patient Monitoring: Normal health maintenance. If a pessary is used, frequent follow-up (both initially and long-term) is required.

Prevention/Avoidance: Maintenance of normal weight, avoidance of known (modifiable) risk factors.

Possible Complications: Thickening or ulceration of the vaginal tissues, urinary incontinence, kinking of the ureters, and obstipation. Complications of surgical repair include intraoperative hemorrhage, nerve damage (sciatic), damage to the rectum, damage to the ureters, postoperative infection, and complications of anesthesia.

Expected Outcome: Vaginal prolapse tends to worsen with time. If uncorrected, complete

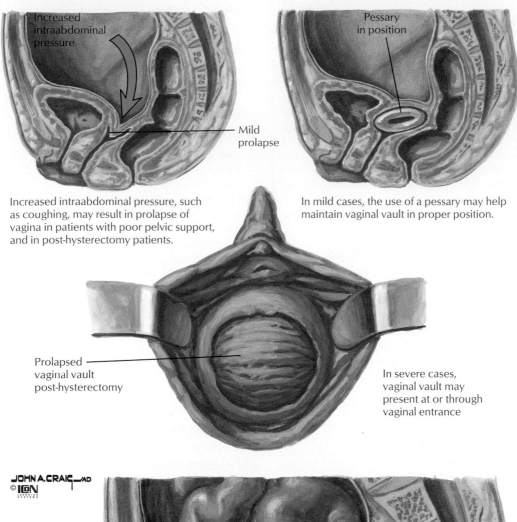

Increased intraabdominal pressure, such as coughing, may result in prolapse of vagina in patients with poor pelvic support, and in post-hysterectomy patients.

In mild cases, the use of a pessary may help maintain vaginal vault in proper position.

Prolapsed vaginal vault post-hysterectomy

In severe cases, vaginal vault may present at or through vaginal entrance

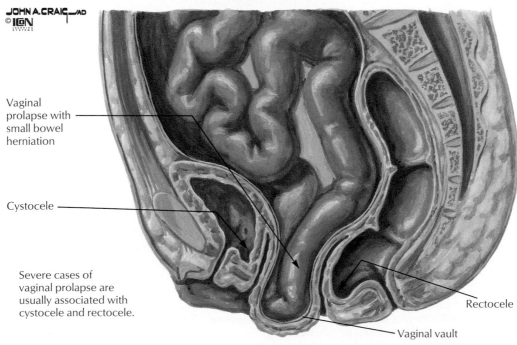

Vaginal prolapse with small bowel herniation

Cystocele

Severe cases of vaginal prolapse are usually associated with cystocele and rectocele.

Rectocele

Vaginal vault

prolapse is associated with vaginal skin changes, ulceration, and bleeding.

MISCELLANEOUS

ICD-9-CM **Codes:** 618.0, 618.5 (Vaginal vault prolapse after hysterectomy).

REFERENCES

American College of Obstetricians and Gynecologists. *Pelvic Organ Prolapse.* Washington, DC: ACOG; 1995. ACOG Technical Bulletin 214.

Birnbaum SJ. Rational therapy for the prolapsed vagina. *Am J Obstet Gynecol* 1973;115:411.

Delancey JOL. Anatomic aspects of vaginal eversion after hysterectomy. *Am J Obstet Gynecol* 1992;166:1717.

Miller DC. Contemporary use of the pessary. In: Sciarra JJ, ed. *Gynecology and Obstetrics.* Vol 1. Philadelphia, Pa: JB Lippincott; 1991;39:1.

Morley GW, Delancey JOL. Sacrospinous ligament fixation for eversion of vagina. *Am J Obstet Gynecol* 1988;158:872.

Nichols DH. Sacrospinous fixation for massive eversion of vagina. *Am J Obstet Gynecol* 1982;142:901.

Percy NM, Perl JI. Total colpectomy. *Surg Gynecol Obstet* 1961;113:174.

Porges RF. Abnormalities of pelvic support. In: Sciarra JJ, ed. *Gynecology and Obstetrics.* Vol 1. Philadelphia, Pa: JB Lippincott; 1993;61:14.

VAGINITIS: ATROPHIC

INTRODUCTION

Description: Atrophy of vaginal tissues caused by the loss of ovarian steroids.

Prevalence: One hundred percent of postmenopausal women who do not receive estrogen replacement.

Predominant Age: 50+ (or after surgical menopause).

Genetics: No genetic pattern.

ETIOLOGY AND PATHOGENESIS

Causes: Loss of estrogen stimulation as a result of surgery, chemotherapy (alkylating agents), radiation, or natural cessation of ovarian function (menopause).

Risk Factors: Loss of ovarian function because of age, chemotherapy, radiation, or surgery.

CLINICAL CHARACTERISTICS

Signs and Symptoms:

Vaginal dryness, burning, and itching

Pain or bleeding with intercourse (may be associated with lacerations)

Thin, shiny, red epithelium with a smooth surface (loss of rugae)

DIAGNOSTIC APPROACH

Differential Diagnosis:

Vaginal infections

Vulvitis (including dermatologic causes)

Chemical vaginitis

Changes after radiation exposure

Lichen sclerosis

Associated Conditions: Menopause, dyspareunia, vulvodynia, atrophic vulvitis, urinary frequency, urinary urgency, urgency incontinence, increased risk of other menopause-related conditions including osteoporosis, increased risk of cardiovascular disease, hot flashes and flushes, or sleep disturbances.

Workup and Evaluation

Laboratory: No evaluation indicated.

Imaging: No imaging indicated.

Special Tests: A vaginal maturation index may be performed, but is generally not required.

Diagnostic Procedures: History and clinical inspection generally sufficient.

Pathologic Findings

Thinned epithelium with loss of rugae and rete pegs (on biopsy).

MANAGEMENT AND THERAPY

Nonpharmacologic

General Measures: Vaginal moisturizers.

Specific Measures: Topical or systemic estrogen (estrogen/progestin) therapy.

Diet: No specific dietary changes indicated.

Activity: No restriction, supplemental lubricants for intercourse (if necessary).

Patient Education: Reassurance, American College of Obstetricians and Gynecologists Patient Education Pamphlet AP047 (*The Menopause Years*), AP066 (*Hormone Replacement Therapy*), AP028 (*Vaginitis: Causes and Treatments*).

Drug(s) of Choice (most common drug dosages shown)

Oral estrogens—conjugated equine estrogens (0.625–1.25 mg/d), diethylstilbestrol, esterified estrogens (0.625–1.25 mg/d), ethinyl estradiol (0.05 mg/d), micronized estradiol (0.5–1 mg/d), piperazine estrone sulfate, estropipate, quinestrol.

Injectable estrogens—conjugated equine estrogens, estradiol benzoate, estradiol cypionate, estradiol valerate (oil), estradiol valerate (oil), estrone (aqueous), ethinyl estradiol, polyestradiol phosphate.

Topical—17β-estradiol (transdermal) (0.05–0.10 μg/d), conjugated equine estrogens (0.625 mg/g), estradiol (0.1 mg/g), estropipate (1.5 mg/g).

Contraindications (Systemic Therapy): Active liver disease, carcinoma of the breast (current), chronic liver damage (impaired function), known sensitivity to topical vehicles, endometrial carcinoma (current), recent thrombosis (with or without emboli), unexplained vaginal bleeding.

Precautions: Up to 25% of estrogen placed in the vagina may be absorbed into the circulation. This amount may be even greater for patients with atrophic changes. Continuous estrogen exposure without periodic or concomitant progestins increases the risk of endometrial carcinoma 6- to 8-fold when the uterus is present.

Interactions: See individual agents.

Alternative Drugs

Topical moisturizers.

FOLLOW-UP

Patient Monitoring: Normal health maintenance. Patients may be at slightly greater risk for vaginal infections or trauma.

Prevention/Avoidance: Estrogen replacement therapy at menopause.

Possible Complications: Reduced resistance to infection, dyspareunia, and traumatic injury during intercourse.

Expected Outcome: Reversal of symptoms, reestablishment of normal physiology.

MISCELLANEOUS

Pregnancy Considerations: Menopause is associated with the loss of fertility.

***ICD-9-CM* Codes:** 627.3 (Postmenopausal atrophic vaginitis).

REFERENCES

American College of Obstetricians and Gynecologists. *Hormone Replacement Therapy.* Washington, DC: ACOG; 1998. ACOG Technical Bulletin 247.

Butler RN, Lewis MI, Hoffman E, Whitehead ED. Love and sex after 60: how to evaluate and treat the sexually active woman. *Geriatrics* 1994;49:33.

Jones KP, ed. Estrogen replacement therapy. *Clin Obstet Gynecol* 1992;35:854.

Smith RP. *Gynecology in Primary Care.* Baltimore, Md: Williams & Wilkins; 1997:281.

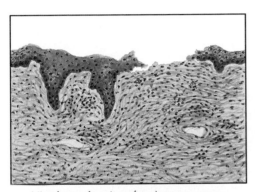

Histology of vagina after the menopause

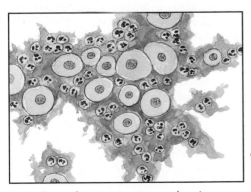

Smear from postmenopausal vagina

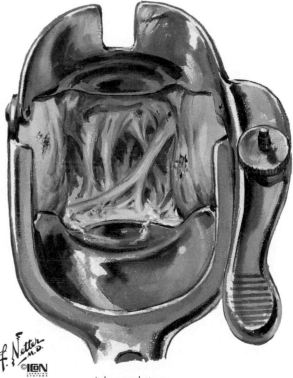

Advanced stage with extensive adhesions

VAGINITIS: BACTERIAL (NONSPECIFIC) AND BACTERIAL VAGINOSIS

INTRODUCTION

Description: Bacterial vaginitis is a vaginal infection caused by an overgrowth of normal or pathogenic bacteria that results in irritation, inflammation, and clinical symptoms. Bacterial vaginosis is a change in vaginal ecology caused by an overgrowth of anaerobic bacteria, often with an absence of clinical symptoms. It should be noted that bacterial vaginosis does not engender an inflammatory response and is therefore technically not a type of vaginitis.

Prevalence: Roughly 6 million cases per year, 50% of "vaginal infections."

Predominant Age: 15–50 (may occur at any age).

Genetics: No genetic pattern.

ETIOLOGY AND PATHOGENESIS

Causes: Bacterial vaginitis—overgrowth of normal or pathologic bacteria with an inflammatory response (which distinguishes this from bacterial vaginosis). Bacterial vaginosis—a polymicrobial process that involves the loss of normal lactobacilli, an increase in anaerobic bacteria (especially *Gardnerella vaginalis, Bacteroides* sp., *Peptococcus* sp., and *Mobiluncus* sp.), and a change in the chemical composition of the vaginal secretions. There is a 1000-fold increase in the number of bacteria present and a 1000:1 anaerobic/aerobic bacteria ratio (normal 5:1), high levels of mucinases; phospholipase A$_2$, lipases, proteases, arachidonic acid, and prostaglandins are all present. Amines (cadaverine and putrescine) are made through bacterial decarboxylation of arginine and lysine. These amines are more volatile at an alkaline pH, such as that created by the addition of 10% KOH or semen (roughly a pH of 7), giving rise to the odor found with the "whiff test" or reported by these patients after intercourse.

Risk Factors: Systemic processes—diabetes, pregnancy, and debilitating disease. Anything that alters the normal vaginal flora—smoking, numbers of sexual partners, vaginal contraceptives used, some forms of sexual expression such as oral sex, antibiotic use, hygiene practices and douching, menstruation, and immunologic status.

CLINICAL CHARACTERISTICS

Signs and Symptoms:
   Bacterial vaginitis—Vulvar burning or irritation
   Increased discharge (often with odor)
   Dysuria
   Dyspareunia
   Edema or erythema of the vulva
   Bacterial vaginosis—Asymptomatic (20%–50% of patients)
   Increased discharge
   Vaginal odor (often more pronounced after intercourse)
   Vulvar burning or irritation
   Uncommon—Dysuria
   Dyspareunia
   Edema or erythema of the vulva

DIAGNOSTIC APPROACH

Differential Diagnosis:
   Chlamydial cervicitis
   Gonococcal cervicitis
   Trichomonas vaginalis infection
   Vaginal candidiasis

Associated Conditions: Other vaginal or sexually transmissible infections, cervicitis, and vulvitis.

Workup and Evaluation

Laboratory: Culture or monoclonal antibody staining may be obtained to evaluate other causes, but are seldom necessary. Evaluation for concomitant sexually transmissible infections should be considered.

Imaging: No imaging indicated.

Special Tests: Vaginal pH 5–5.5, "whiff" test—the addition of 10% KOH to vaginal secretions to liberate volatile amines causing a "fishy" odor (bacterial vaginosis).

Diagnostic Procedures: Physical examination, microscopic examination of vaginal secretions in normal saline. For bacterial vaginosis the diagnosis requires three of the following: homogeneous discharge, pH 5–5.5, clue cells ($\geq$20%), positive "whiff" test.

Pathologic Findings

Increased white blood cells and bacteria when vaginal secretions are viewed under normal saline suggest vaginitis. Clue cells may be present, but are often absent in vaginitis. For bacterial vaginosis clue cells must represent 20% or more of epithelial cells seen.

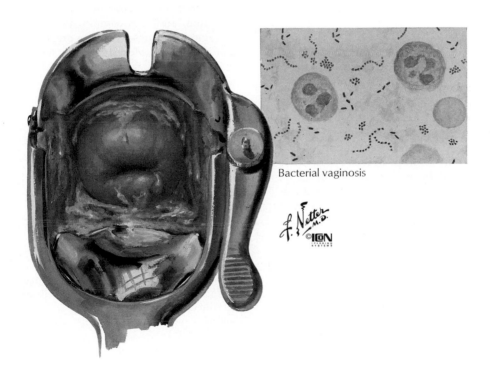

Bacterial vaginosis

VAGINAL DISEASE

MANAGEMENT AND THERAPY

Nonpharmacologic

General Measures: Perineal hygiene, education regarding sexually transmissible infections.

Specific Measures: Medical therapy, vaginal acidification.

Diet: No specific dietary changes indicated.

Activity: No restriction.

Patient Education: Reassurance, American College of Obstetricians and Gynecologists Patient Education Pamphlet AP028 (*Vaginitis: Causes and Treatments*), AP009 (*How to Prevent Sexually Transmitted Diseases*).

Drug(s) of Choice

Oral—metronidazole (Flagyl, Protostat) 500 mg twice daily for 7 days (90%–100% cure), oral ampicillin, 500 mg q6h for 7 days

Topical—clindamycin (5 g of cream, 100 mg of clindamycin) qHS for 7 days, metronidazole (5 g of cream, 37.5 mg of metronidazole) bid for 5 days

Contraindications: Metronidazole is relatively contraindicated in the first trimester of pregnancy.

Precautions: Oral metronidazole is associated with the potential for systemic side effects including a metallic taste in the mouth and stomach upset. Topical metronidazole is currently available in two forms: one for dermatologic use and one for intravaginal use. The pH of these two preparations is very different, making it important to specify the form on the prescription to avoid significant chemical irritation.

Interactions: Because of a disulfiramlike reaction, patients must be warned to avoid alcohol intake during therapy.

Alternative Drugs

Oral—tetracycline, 250–500 mg bid for 7 days, clindamycin, 300–450 mg q6h for 7 days

Topical—topical triple sulfa (cream or suppositories) bid for 7–10 days, vaginal acidification (Aci-jel, Amino-Cerv, boric acid), povidone iodine, as a douche or gel

FOLLOW-UP

Patient Monitoring: Normal health maintenance.

Prevention/Avoidance: It is thought that bacterial vaginosis develops 5–10 days after exposure to the involved bacteria. *Gardnerella* may be found in 90% of male partners of women with bacterial vaginosis. Hence, sexual transmission is postulated, although bacterial vaginosis can occur in virginal women. The role of condoms in prevention is debated.

Possible Complications: Cystitis, cervicitis, infections of the Skene's or Bartholin's glands, increased risk of pelvic inflammatory disease, pelvic pain, and infertility. Increased risk of upper genital tract infections and postoperative infections if surgery is performed while bacterial vaginosis is present. Increased risk of premature delivery, premature rupture of the membranes, and chorioamnionitis when bacterial vaginosis is present during pregnancy.

Expected Outcome: Most treatment failures are actually caused by reinfection or failure to comply with treatment.

MISCELLANEOUS

Pregnancy Considerations: Vaginal infections are associated with an increased risk of prematurity and premature rupture of the membranes.

ICD-9-CM Codes: 616.10.

REFERENCES

American College of Obstetricians and Gynecologists. *Vulvovaginitis.* Washington, DC: ACOG; 1989. Technical Bulletin 135.

Faro S. Bacterial vaginitis. *Clin Obstet Gynecol* 1991;34:582.

Ledger WJ. Historical review of the treatment of bacterial vaginosis. *Am J Obstet Gynecol* 1993;169:474.

Smith RP. *Gynecology in Primary Care.* Baltimore, Md: Williams & Wilkins; 1997:603.

Spiegel CA. Bacterial vaginosis. *Clin Microbiol Rev* 1991;4:485.

Summers P. Vaginitis in 1993. *Clin Obstet Gynecol* 1993;36:105.

Sweet RL. New approaches for the treatment of bacterial vaginosis. *Am J Obstet Gynecol* 1994;169:479.

Thomason JL, Gelbart SM, Scaglione NJ. Bacterial vaginosis: current review with indications for asymptomatic therapy. *Am J Obstet Gynecol* 1991;165:1210.

VAGINITIS: MONILIAL

INTRODUCTION

Description: A vaginal infection caused by ubiquitous fungi found in the air or as common inhabitants of the vagina, rectum, and mouth.

Prevalence: Twenty-five percent to forty percent of "vaginal infections"; 75% of women experience one or more lifetime occurrences.

Predominant Age: 15–50 (rare outside this range except for those receiving estrogen replacement after menopause).

Genetics: No genetic pattern.

ETIOLOGY AND PATHOGENESIS

Causes: *Candida albicans* (80%–95%), *Candida glabrata, Candida tropicalis,* or others (5%–20%).

Risk Factors: Altered vaginal ecosystem (stress, antibiotic use, pregnancy, diabetes, depressed immunity, topical contraceptives, and warm and moist environment).

CLINICAL CHARACTERISTICS

Signs and Symptoms (15% asymptomatic carrier rate):
Vulvar itching or burning (intense)
External dysuria, dyspareunia
Tissue erythema, edema, and excoriations
Thick, adherent, plaque-like, discharge with a white to yellow color (generally odorless)
Vulvar excoriations

DIAGNOSTIC APPROACH

Differential Diagnosis:
Bacterial vaginitis
Bacterial vaginosis
Trichomonas vaginal infection
Contact vulvitis (allergic vulvitis)
Atrophic vulvitis
Vulvar dermatoses
Pinworms

Associated Conditions: Diabetes, immunosuppression or compromise (as risk factors for infection), chronic vulvitis.

Workup and Evaluation

Laboratory: Culture (Nickerson's or Sabouraud media) or monoclonal antibody staining may be obtained but are seldom necessary.

Imaging: No imaging indicated.

Special Tests: Vaginal pH 4–4.5.

Diagnostic Procedures: Physical examination, microscopic examination of vaginal secretions in normal saline and 10% KOH.

Pathologic Findings

Branching and budding of vaginal monilia distinguish monilial vaginitis from lint or other foreign material. The use of 10% KOH lyses white blood cells and renders epithelial cells "ghostlike," making identification easier.

MANAGEMENT AND THERAPY

Nonpharmacologic

General Measures: Perineal hygiene (keep the perineal area clean and dry, avoid tight or synthetic undergarments), education regarding prevention, encourage completion of the prescribed course of therapy.

Specific Measures: Medical therapy.

Diet: No specific dietary changes indicated.

Activity: No restriction.

Patient Education: Reassurance, American College of Obstetricians and Gynecologists Patient Education Pamphlet AP028 (*Vaginitis: Causes and Treatments*).

Drug(s) of Choice

Imidazoles—miconazole (Monistat, 200 mg suppositories, qHS × 3 days, 2% cream, 5g qHS × 7 days), clotrimazole (Femcare, Gyne-Lotrimin, Mycelex, 100 mg inserts, qHS × 7 days, 1% cream, 5 g qHS × 7 days), butoconazole (Femstat, 2% cream, 5 g qHS × 3 days), tioconazole (Vagistat, 6.5% ointment, 4.6 g HS)

Triazoles—terconazole (Terazol, 80 mg suppositories, qHS × 3 days, 0.8% cream, 5 gm qHS × 3 days, 0.4% cream, 5 gm qHS × 7 days), fluconazole (Diflucan, 150 mg PO single dose)

Contraindications: Known or suspected hypersensitivity or allergy. Imidazoles are contraindicated during the first trimester of pregnancy. Fluconazole is a pregnancy category C drug.

Precautions: Topical steroid preparations should be avoided. Use of oral ketoconazole requires baseline and follow-up liver function studies. Gastrointestinal side effects are common with oral therapies.

Interactions: Oral fluconazole should be used with caution in patients taking oral hypoglycemics, coumarin-type anticoagulants, phenytoin, cyclosporine, rifampin, or theophylline.

Alternative Drugs

Povidone iodine (topical), gentian violet (1%), boric acid (600 mg capsules placed high in the vagina twice daily).

FOLLOW-UP

Patient Monitoring: Normal health maintenance, frequent recurrences should suggest host compromise (eg, diabetes, human immunodeficiency virus, anemia).

Prevention/Avoidance: Good perineal hygiene, clothing and activities that allow perineal ventilation (cotton underwear, loose clothing).

Possible Complications: Vulvar excoriation caused by scratching, chronic vulvitis, secondary vaginal or vulvar infections.

Expected Outcome: A small number (<5%) of fungal infections are resistant to imidazole therapy. Organisms causing these infections are generally susceptible to triazoles. Roughly 30% of patients experience a recurrence of symptoms within a month (related to a continuing exposure, a change in host defenses [such as altered cellular immunity], or the ability of the fungus to burrow beneath the epithelium of the vagina).

MISCELLANEOUS

Pregnancy Considerations: Vaginal infections are associated with an increased risk of premature delivery and premature rupture of the membranes.

ICD-9-CM Codes: 112.1.

REFERENCES

American College of Obstetricians and Gynecologists. *Vulvovaginitis.* Washington, DC: ACOG; 1989. Technical Bulletin 135.

American College of Obstetricians and Gynecologists. *Vaginitis.* Washington, DC: ACOG; 1996. ACOG Technical Bulletin 226.

Forssman L, Milsom I. Treatment of recurrent vaginal candidiasis. *Am J Obstet Gynecol* 1985;152:959.

Horowitz BJ. Candidiasis: specification and therapy. *Curr Probl Obstet Gynecol Fertil* 1990;8:233.

Javanovic R, Congema E, Nguyen H. Antifungal agents vs. boric acid for treating chronic mycotic vulvovaginitis. *J Reprod Med* 1991;36:593.

Smith RP. *Gynecology in Primary Care.* Baltimore, Md: Williams & Wilkins; 1997:603.

Summers P. Vaginitis in 1993. *Clin Obstet Gynecol* 1993;36:105.

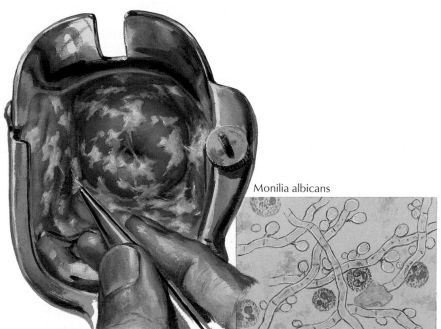

Monilia albicans

VAGINAL DISEASE

VAGINITIS: *TRICHOMONAS*

INTRODUCTION

Description: A vaginal infection by an anaerobic flagellate protozoan, *Trichomonas vaginalis.*

Prevalence: Roughly 3 million cases per year, 25% of "vaginal infections."

Predominant Age: 15–50 (may occur at any age)

Genetics: No genetic pattern.

ETIOLOGY AND PATHOGENESIS

Causes: *Trichomonas vaginalis*, an anaerobic flagellate protozoan.

Risk Factors: Multiple sexual partners, vaginal pH that is less acid (blood, semen, or bacterial pathogens increase the risk).

CLINICAL CHARACTERISTICS

Signs and Symptoms (40% may be asymptomatic):

Vulvar itching or burning

Copious discharge with a rancid odor (generally thin, runny, and yellow-green to gray in color, "frothy" in 25%)

"Strawberry" punctation of the cervix and upper vagina (15%, pathognomonic when present)

Dysuria

Dyspareunia

Edema or erythema of the vulva

DIAGNOSTIC APPROACH

Differential Diagnosis:

Bacterial vaginitis

Bacterial vaginosis

Chlamydial cervicitis

Gonococcal cervicitis

Associated Conditions: Other sexually transmissible infections (specifically gonorrhea and chlamydia).

Workup and Evaluation

Laboratory: Culture or monoclonal antibody testing may be obtained but is seldom necessary. Evaluation for concomitant sexually transmissible infections should be strongly considered.

Imaging: No imaging indicated.

Special Tests: Vaginal pH 6–6.5 or above.

Diagnostic Procedures: Physical examination, microscopic examination of vaginal secretions in normal saline.

Pathologic Findings

Trichomonas is a fusiform protozoon slightly larger than a white blood cell with three to five flagella, which provide active movement, extending from the narrow end.

MANAGEMENT AND THERAPY

Nonpharmacologic

General Measures: Perineal hygiene, education regarding sexually transmissible infections.

Specific Measures: Medical therapy, vaginal acidification.

Diet: No specific dietary changes indicated; avoid alcohol during metronidazole treatment.

Activity: Sexual abstinence until partner(s) are examined and treated.

Patient Education: Reassurance, American College of Obstetricians and Gynecologists Patient Education Pamphlet AP028 (*Vaginitis: Causes and Treatments*), AP009 (*How to Prevent Sexually Transmitted Diseases*).

Drug(s) of Choice

Metronidazole 1 g in AM and PM, 1 day or metronidazole 250 mg q8h for 7 days

Contraindications: Metronidazole is relatively contraindicated in the first trimester of pregnancy.

Precautions: Metronidazole may produce a disulfiramlike reaction, resulting in nausea, vomiting, headaches, or other symptoms if the patient ingests alcohol. Patients should not use metronidazole if they have taken disulfiram in the preceding 2 weeks. Metronidazole must be used with care or the dose must be reduced in patients with hepatic disease.

Interactions: Metronidazole may potentiate the effects of warfarin or coumarin or alcohol (as noted above).

Alternative Drugs

Topical clotrimazole, povidone iodine (topical), hypertonic (20%) saline douches.

FOLLOW-UP

Patient Monitoring: Follow-up serologic testing for syphilis and human immunodeficiency virus infection as indicated.

Prevention/Avoidance: Sexual monogamy, condom use for intercourse.

Possible Complications: Cystitis, infections of the Skene's or Bartholin's glands, increased risk of pelvic inflammatory disease, pelvic pain, infertility, and other sequelae of sexually transmissible infections.

Expected Outcome: Resistance to metronidazole is uncommon. Most treatment failures are actually caused by reinfection or failure to comply with treatment.

VAGINAL DISEASE

MISCELLANEOUS

Pregnancy Considerations: Vaginal infections are associated with an increased risk of prematurity and premature rupture of the membranes.
ICD-9-CM Codes: 131.01.

REFERENCES

American College of Obstetricians and Gynecologists. *Vulvovaginitis.* Washington, DC: ACOG; 1989. Technical Bulletin 135.

American College of Obstetricians and Gynecologists. *Vaginitis.* Washington, DC: ACOG; 1996. ACOG Technical Bulletin 226.

Centers for Disease Control and Prevention. 1998 Guidelines for treatment of sexually transmitted diseases. *MMWR Morb Mortal Wkly Rep* 1998:47(RR-1):74.

Lossick JG. Single-dose metronidazole treatment for vaginal trichomoniasis. *Obstet Gynecol* 1980;56:508.

McLellan R, Spence MR, Brockman M, Raffel L, Smith JL. The clinical diagnosis of trichomoniasis. *Obstet Gynecol* 1982;60:30.

Smith RP. *Gynecology in Primary Care.* Baltimore, Md: Williams & Wilkins; 1997:603.

Summers P. Vaginitis in 1993. *Clin Obstet Gynecol* 1993;36:105.

Thomason JL, Gelbart SM. *Trichomonas vaginalis. Obstet Gynecol* 1989;74:536.

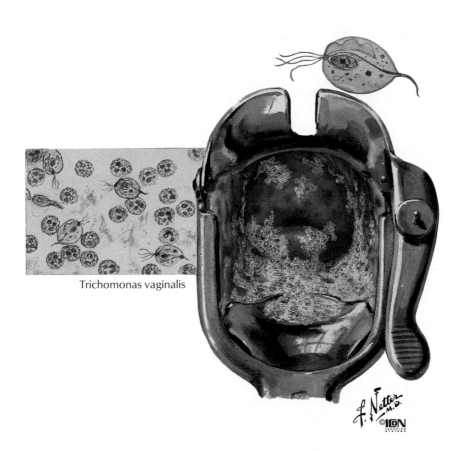

Trichomonas vaginalis

Cervical Disease

ABNORMAL PAP SMEAR: ATYPICAL SQUAMOUS OR GLANDULAR CELLS OF UNDETERMINED SIGNIFICANCE

INTRODUCTION

Description: One of the most perplexing aspects of management under the Bethesda reporting system is how to interpret smears reported as showing atypical squamous or glandular cells of undetermined significance (ASCUS or AGCUS). The category of "atypical glandular cells of undetermined significance" includes a range of findings from benign reactive changes in endocervical or endometrial cells to adenocarcinoma.

Prevalence: ASCUS—approximately 3%–5% of all Pap smears; AGCUS—0.2%–0.4% of all Pap smears.

Predominant Age: Reproductive.

Genetics: No genetic pattern.

ETIOLOGY AND PATHOGENESIS

Causes: The ASCUS diagnosis has been developed to describe squamous cell changes that are more severe than reactive changes, but not as marked as those found in squamous intraepithelial lesions (SIL). This group of changes is not equivalent to those that were previously called "squamous atypias" or "Class II" Pap smears, which accounted for almost 20% of all smears and were associated with cervical changes that ranged from benign inflammation to premalignant lesions. The AGCUS diagnosis reflects benign reactive changes in endocervical or endometrial cells, endometrial hyperplasia, or adenocarcinoma.

Risk Factors: ASCUS—exposure to human papillomavirus (HPV). AGCUS—none known except for those affecting possible pathologic causes (eg, unopposed estrogen therapy as a risk factor for endometrial carcinoma).

CLINICAL CHARACTERISTICS

Signs and Symptoms:
- Asymptomatic

DIAGNOSTIC APPROACH

Differential Diagnosis:
ASCUS—Inflammatory change (cervicitis)
Low-grade squamous intraepithelial lesion (LGSIL) change
AGCUS—Benign reactive changes in endocervical or endometrial cells

Endometrial hyperplasia or adenocarcinoma
Endometritis secondary to an intrauterine contraceptive device
Tuberculous endometritis
Tubal carcinoma

Associated Conditions: ASCUS—HPV infection, vaginitis, cervicitis. AGCUS—dysfunctional uterine bleeding (may be present, but is most often absent).

Workup and Evaluation

Laboratory: No evaluation indicated.

Imaging: No imaging indicated.

Special Tests: Colposcopic examination of the cervix is seldom required for ASCUS smears. It should be considered only if there are high risk factors for progression or multiple recurrences. Ultrasonography (including sonohysterography using saline infusion into the uterine cavity) may be considered for the evaluation of smears classified as AGCUS.

Diagnostic Procedures: Colposcopy, with or without cervical biopsy and endocervical curettage, should be considered for any patient with a Pap smear classified as ASCUS if risk factors are present or the abnormality is persistent or recurrent. Endocervical or endometrial biopsy and/or hysteroscopy may be indicated for AGCUS smears.

Pathologic Findings

Minimal gross findings, mildly elevated numbers of nucleated squamous cells with varying degrees of maturation when ASCUS is present.

MANAGEMENT AND THERAPY

Nonpharmacologic

General Measures: Evaluation of comments made by the cytopathologist. Increased frequency of Pap smears until the abnormality is resolved or further diagnosis is established. (For a followup Pap smear to be "negative," it must have normal or benign findings, but also be "satisfactory for interpretation.")

Specific Measures: Treatment of infection or inflammation (if present). Treatment of atrophic change (if present). If the cytology report accompanying the AGCUS smear indicates a probability of carcinoma, the endocervical canal and endometrial cavity should be evaluated. Cone biopsy and/or hysteroscopy may be required to adequately evaluate these patients.

Diet: No specific dietary changes indicated.

Activity: No restriction.

Cervical Cell Pathology
in Squamous Tissue
●
Grades and Cell Types

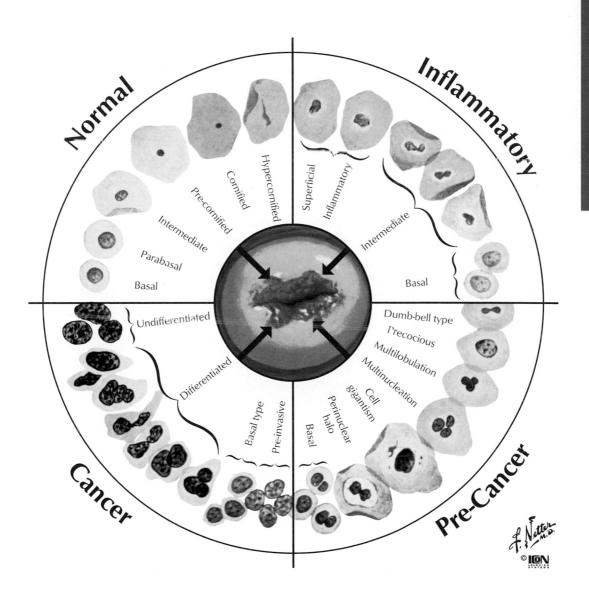

Patient Education: Reassurance, American College of Obstetricians and Gynecologists Patient Education Pamphlet AP033 (*Disorders of the Cervix*), AP085 (*The Pap Test*), AP073 (*Human Papillomavirus Infection*).

Drug(s) of Choice

Based on specific indications.

FOLLOW-UP

Patient Monitoring: Normal health maintenance, increased frequency of Pap smears.

Prevention/Avoidance: Avoidance of HPV infection (ASCUS).

Possible Complications: Progression to more severe squamous abnormalities or occult disease unless a diagnosis is established and treatment is instituted.

Expected Outcome: Sixty percent or more of patients with ASCUS experience a spontaneous return to normal, as seen if their Pap smears are closely followed. When a treatable condition is identified, this response rate is even better.

MISCELLANEOUS

Pregnancy Considerations: No effect on pregnancy. The likelihood of significant pathologic changes with ASCUS abnormalities is small enough that no proscription against pregnancy during the evaluation process is necessary. Although the possibility of significant complica-

tions is small in AGCUS, the underlying causes may be of sufficient concern to mitigate against pregnancy until a diagnosis is established.

ICD-9-CM **Codes:** 795.0 (ASCUS), 622.1 (Cervical atypia), 795.0 (AGCUS).

REFERENCES

American College of Obstetricians and Gynecologists. *Cervical Cytology: Evaluation and Management of Abnormalities.* Washington, DC: ACOG; 1993. ACOG Technical Bulletin 183.

Bose J, Kannan V, Kline TS. Abnormal endocervical cells: really abnormal? Really endocervical? *Am J Clin Pathol* 1994;101:708.

Goff BA, Atanasoff P, Brown E, Muntz HG, Bell DA, Rice LW. Endocervical glandular atypia in Papanicolaou smears. *Obstet Gynecol* 1992;79:101.

Higgins RV, Hall JB, McGee JA, Laurent S, Alvarez RD, Partridge EE. Appraisal of the modalities used to evaluate an initial abnormal Papanicolaou smear. *Obstet Gynecol* 1994;84:174.

Kurman RJ, Henson DE, Herbst AL, Noller KL, Schiffman MH. Interim guidelines for management of abnormal cervical cytology. The 1992 National Cancer Institute Workshop. *JAMA* 1994;271:1866.

Montz FJ, Bradley JM, Fowler JM, Nguyen L. Natural history of the minimally abnormal Papanicolaou smear. *Obstet Gynecol* 1992;80:385.

Smith RP. *Gynecology in Primary Care.* Baltimore, Md: Williams & Wilkins; 1997;305.

Toon PG, Arrand JR, Wilson LP, Sharp DS. Human papillomavirus infection of the uterine cervix of women without cytological signs of neoplasia. *BMJ* 1986;293:1261.

ABNORMAL PAP SMEAR: LOW-GRADE SQUAMOUS INTRAEPITHELIAL LESION AND HIGH-GRADE SQUAMOUS INTRAEPITHELIAL LESION

INTRODUCTION

Description: Low-grade squamous intraepithelial lesions (LGSIL) encompass changes associated with HPV, mild dysplasia, and cervical intraepithelial neoplasia (CIN) I. High-grade squamous intraepithelial lesions (HGSIL) include CIN II and III, as well as carcinoma in situ (CIS).

Prevalence: Less than 5% of Pap smears for low-grade and 2% for high-grade abnormalities.

Predominant Age: Reproductive.

Genetics: No genetic pattern.

ETIOLOGY AND PATHOGENESIS

Causes: HPV has been implicated in the development of cervical dysplasia. Although up to 70% of invasive cervical cancers have HPV serotypes 16 or 18 present, these types may be detected in patients with LGSIL as well. Normal patients have HPV prevalence rates that vary from 10% to 50%, depending on the study technique and population evaluated.

Risk Factors: Exposure to HPV and other sexually transmitted disease; smoking is associated with a higher risk.

CLINICAL CHARACTERISTICS

Signs and Symptoms:
- Asymptomatic

DIAGNOSTIC APPROACH

Differential Diagnosis:
LGSIL—Inflammatory change (cervicitis)
Cervical carcinoma
HGSIL—Cervical CIS
Invasive cervical carcinoma

Associated Conditions: HPV infection, vaginitis, cervicitis, cervical dysplasia, CIS, invasive carcinoma of the cervix, endocervical adenocarcinoma.

Workup and Evaluation

Laboratory: No evaluation indicated.

Imaging: No imaging indicated.

Special Tests: High prevalence, a poor correlation with later risk, and the cost of screening have resulted in the general recommendation that routine HPV screening or serotyping not be carried out.

Diagnostic Procedures: For many patients with LGSIL, colposcopy, colposcopically directed biopsy, and endocervical curettage are appropriate to establish the source of the cytologic abnormality. If colposcopy is inadequate to delineate lesions present or the entire transformation zone cannot be seen, diagnostic conization is required. Colposcopy, colposcopically directed biopsy, and endocervical curettage should be used to evaluate all patients with HGSIL.

Pathologic Findings

Acetowhite areas on colposcopy, early vascular changes leading to mosaicism and punctation. Microscopic—loss of normal maturation, increased nuclear/cytoplasmic ratio, nuclear atypia (mild). Vascular changes leading to mosaicism and punctation (severe) are more typical of HGSIL. Nuclear atypia (moderate to severe) is also a feature of HGSIL.

MANAGEMENT AND THERAPY

Nonpharmacologic

General Measures: Evaluation of comments made by the cytopathologist. Increased frequency of Pap smears until the abnormality is resolved or further diagnosis is established. (For a follow-up Pap smear to be "negative," it must have normal or benign findings, but also be "satisfactory for interpretation.")

Specific Measures: Compliant patients with LGSIL who are at low risk for HPV, sexually transmitted disease, and malignant progression of the lesion (eg, smokers) may be followed by serial Pap smears. If colposcopy is adequate and the histologic abnormality found is mild, obtaining follow-up Pap smears at 4–6 month intervals for 2 years or three normal smears is suitable. When HGSIL is present, the evaluation determines therapy: cryotherapy, electrocautery, electrosurgical loop excision, laser ablation, or conization. Treatment must be based on an accurate diagnosis and the extent of the lesion involved.

Diet: No specific dietary changes indicated.

Activity: No restriction.

Patient Education: Reassurance, American College of Obstetricians and Gynecologists Patient Education Pamphlet AP033 (*Disorders of the Cervix*), AP085 (*The Pap Test*), AP073 (*Human Papillomavirus Infection*).

Cervical Intraepithelial Neoplasia (CIN)

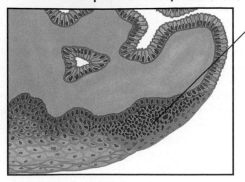

Dysplastic transformation zone

Management of CIN I, II, and III manifested on abnormal Pap smear involves locating source of abnormal cells

Pap smear

Well-Visualized Transformation Zone

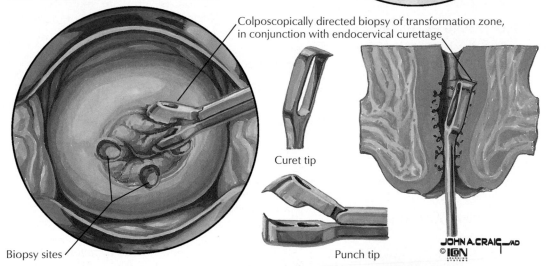

Colposcopically directed biopsy of transformation zone, in conjunction with endocervical curettage

Curet tip

Punch tip

Biopsy sites

JOHN A.CRAIG —AD
©ICON

Nonvisualized Transformation Zone

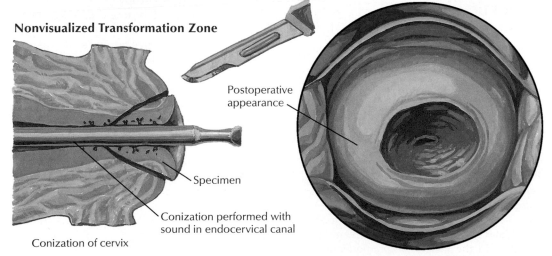

Postoperative appearance

Specimen

Conization performed with sound in endocervical canal

Conization of cervix

Drug(s) of Choice

Based on specific indications, most therapy is surgical or ablative in nature.

FOLLOW-UP

Patient Monitoring: Normal health maintenance, increased frequency of Pap smears.

Prevention/Avoidance: Avoidance of HPV infection.

Possible Complications: Progression to more severe squamous abnormalities.

Expected Outcome: Sixty percent of patients with these findings undergo spontaneous regression of the underlying process, resulting in a return to normal smears. Only 15% of patients with LGSIL progress to HGSIL. HGSIL abnormalities are more likely to progress and warrant aggressive evaluation and treatment.

MISCELLANEOUS

Pregnancy Considerations: No effect on pregnancy. Because of the potential significance of the HGSIL abnormality and the pathologic conditions that cause it, a delay in pregnancy while evaluation is ongoing may be warranted.

ICD-9-CM **Codes:** 622.1 (LGSIL), 233.1 (HGSIL, includes carcinoma in situ).

REFERENCES

American College of Obstetricians and Gynecologists. *Cervical Cytology: Evaluation and Management of Abnormalities.* Washington, DC: ACOG; 1993. ACOG Technical Bulletin 183.

Brinton LA, Hamman RF, Huggins GR, et al. Sexual and reproductive risk factors for invasive squamous cell cervical cancer. *J Natl Cancer Inst* 1987;79:23.

Carmichael JA, Maskens PD. Cervical intraepithelial neoplasia: examination, treatment and follow-up: review. *Obstet Gynecol Surg* 1985;40:545.

Kurman RJ, Henson DE, Herbst AL, Noller KL, Schiffman MH. Interim guidelines for management of abnormal cervical cytology. The 1992 National Cancer Institute Workshop. *JAMA* 1994;271:1866.

Nasiell K, Roger V, Nasiell M. Behavior of mild cervical dysplasia during long-term follow-up. *Obstet Gynecol* 1986;67.665.

Smith RP. *Gynecology in Primary Care.* Baltimore, Md: Williams & Wilkins; 1997:305.

CARCINOMA IN SITU (CERVIX)

INTRODUCTION

Description: Morphologic alteration of the cervical epithelium in which the full thickness of the epithelium is replaced with dysplastic cells (CIN III). This change is generally associated either spatially or temporally with invasive carcinoma.

Prevalence: Less than 2% of Pap smears.

Predominant Age: Early 30s (peak approximately age 32).

Genetics: No genetic pattern.

ETIOLOGY AND PATHOGENESIS

Causes: Unknown.

Risk Factors: Infection by HPV, herpesvirus, or cytomegalovirus, early sexual activity, multiple sexual partners, cigarette smoking (1.5 times risk), oral contraception (2–4 times risk), early childbearing, intrauterine diethylstilbestrol exposure, immunosuppression.

CLINICAL CHARACTERISTICS

Signs and Symptoms:
- Asymptomatic
- Abnormal cervical cytology
- Abnormal colposcopy

DIAGNOSTIC APPROACH

Differential Diagnosis:
- Moderate dysplasia
- Microinvasive and invasive carcinoma

Associated Conditions: HPV infection, condyloma acuminata.

Workup and Evaluation

Laboratory: No evaluation indicated.

Imaging: No imaging indicated.

Special Tests: Colposcopy, colposcopically directed biopsy, and endocervical curettage.

Diagnostic Procedures: Cervical cytologic examination, colposcopy, and biopsy.

Pathologic Findings

The entire thickness of the epithelium is replaced with abnormal (dysplastic) cells, but there is no invasion of the underlying stroma.

MANAGEMENT AND THERAPY

Nonpharmacologic

General Measures: Evaluation of comments made by the cytopathologist.

Specific Measures: Cervical conization and endocervical curettage to confirm the absence of invasion or a more extensive lesion. In those wishing to preserve fertility, this may be curative; in others, standard hysterectomy may be considered. Ablative therapy can only be considered when the entire lesion is visible and invasion has been ruled out.

Diet: No specific dietary changes indicated.

Activity: No restriction.

Patient Education: Reassurance, American College of Obstetricians and Gynecologists Patient Education Pamphlet AP033 (*Disorders of the Cervix*), AP085 (*The Pap Test*), AP073 (*Human Papillomavirus Infection*).

Drug(s) of Choice

None.

Colposcopic Views of Abnormal Cervical Changes

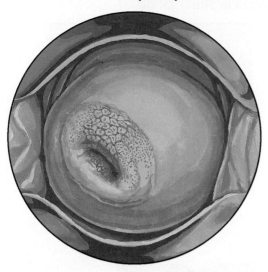

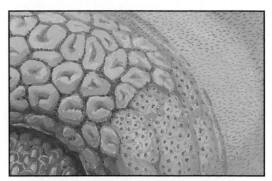

Coarse mosaicism and punctation
in transformation zone

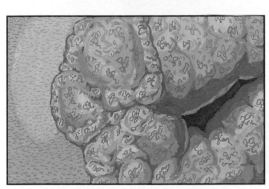

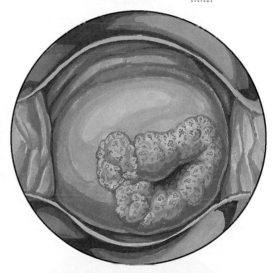

Papilloma of cervix. Some papillomas
may predispose to cervical malignancy

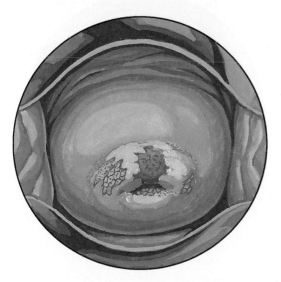

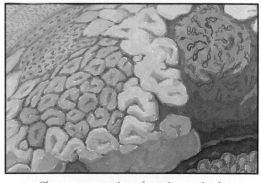

Changes suggestive of carcinoma in situ.
Abnormal vasculature with leukoplakia,
mosaicism, and punctation

JOHN A. CRAIG—AD
© ICN

Management of Carcinoma in Situ (CIN III)

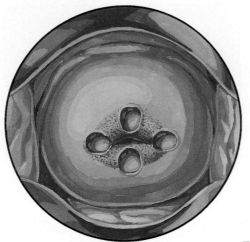

Colposcopy showing biopsy sites
in transformation zone

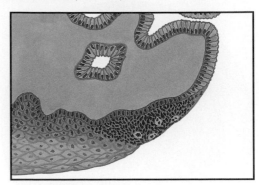

Biopsy specimen showing changes of carcinoma
in situ in transformation zone

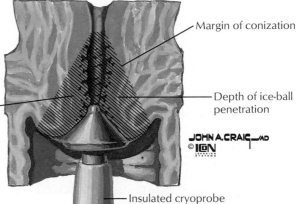

Margin of conization

Depth of ice-ball
penetration

Insulated cryoprobe

Treatment must eradicate transformation
zone and penetrate to a minimum depth
of 5 mm in order to destroy metaplastic
or dysplastic extensions into gland crypts

Treatment modalities include cryosurgery,
CO_2 laser, and radical electrocautery, as
well as conization and hysterectomy

JOHN A. CRAIG—MD
©ICON

Laser burns in
transformation zone

Electrocautery burns

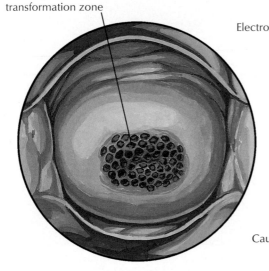

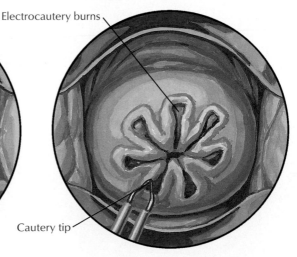

Cautery tip

CO_2 laser therapy

Radical electrocautery

FOLLOW-UP

Patient Monitoring: Follow-up cervical cytologic examination at 3- to 4-month intervals for 1 year, then every 6 months for 1–2 years, then yearly.

Prevention/Avoidance: Reduction or avoidance of known risk factors.

Possible Complications: Advancement of disease or recurrence. Untreated disease is anticipated to progress to invasive carcinoma over the course of 12–86 months in 15%–40% of patients.

Expected Outcome: Low recurrence rates (<10%) for most therapies. When recurrence is found, 75% occur in 21 months.

MISCELLANEOUS

Pregnancy Considerations: No effect on pregnancy. The presence of pregnancy complicates both the diagnosis and treatment: endocervical curettage is generally omitted and definitive therapy is delayed until after delivery; colposcopy is usually repeated every 6–10 weeks until term. In the absence of invasion, vaginal delivery is appropriate.

***ICD-9-CM* Codes:** 233.1.

REFERENCES

American College of Obstetricians and Gynecologists. *Cervical Cytology: Evaluation and Management of Abnormalities.* Washington, DC: ACOG; 1993. ACOG Technical Bulletin 183.

Andersen, Husth M. Cryosurgery for cervical intraepithelial neoplasia: 10-year follow-up. *Gynecol Oncol* 1992;40:240.

Brinton LA, Hamman RF, Huggins GR, et al. Sexual and reproductive risk factors for invasive squamous cell cervical cancer. *J Natl Cancer Inst* 1987;79:23.

Carmichael JA, Maskens PD. Cervical intraepithelial neoplasia: examination, treatment and follow-up: review. *Obstet Gynecol Surg* 1985;40:545.

Kurman RJ, Henson DE, Herbst AL, Noller KL, Schiffman MH. Interim guidelines for management of abnormal cervical cytology. The 1992 National Cancer Institute Workshop. *JAMA* 1994;271:1866.

McIndoe WA, McLean MR, Jones RW, Mullins PR. The invasive potential of carcinoma in situ of the cervix. *Obstet Gynecol* 1991;77:715.

CERVICAL CANCER

INTRODUCTION

Description: Almost all cancers of the cervix are carcinomas—85%–90% squamous carcinoma; 10%–15% adenocarcinoma.

Prevalence: 15,000 cases, 6,000 deaths annually.

Predominant Age: 40s–60s, median 54.

Genetics: No genetic pattern.

ETIOLOGY AND PATHOGENESIS

Causes: Unknown, but associated with early sexual activity, multiple partners, and the presence of sexually transmitted viral infections such as HPV.

Risk Factors: Early sexual activity, multiple sexual partners, HPV, black race, smoking, immunocompromise.

CLINICAL CHARACTERISTICS

Signs and Symptoms:

- None until late in the disease
- Abnormal Pap smear
- Late: vaginal bleeding, dark vaginal discharge, postcoital bleeding, ureteral obstruction, back pain, loss of appetite, weight loss
- Exophytic, friable, bleeding lesion
- Late: supraclavicular or inguinal lymph nodes, leg swelling, ascites, pleural effusion, hepatomegaly

DIAGNOSTIC APPROACH

Differential Diagnosis:

- Cervical eversion
- Cervical erosion
- Cervical polyp
- Condyloma acuminata
- Nabothian cyst

Associated Conditions: HPV, condyloma acuminata, abnormal vaginal bleeding.

Workup and Evaluation

Laboratory: An assessment of renal function is appropriate if ureteral compromise is suspected (advanced disease).

Imaging: Chest radiograph, intravenous pyelogram, and computed tomographic scan are used to assess extent of disease and to assign staging.

Special Tests: Colposcopy and cervical biopsy (conization preferred), biopsy of vaginal or paracervical tissues may be required to assess extent of disease.

Diagnostic Procedures: History, physical examination, and histologic diagnosis (conization, not biopsy).

Pathologic Findings

Squamous cell carcinomas (large cell [keratinizing or nonkeratinizing], small cell, verrucous), adenocarcinoma (endocervical, endometrioid, clear cell, adenoid cystic, adenoma malignum), mixed carcinomas (adenosquamous, glassy cell).

MANAGEMENT AND THERAPY

Nonpharmacologic

General Measures: Timely evaluation and treatment.

Specific Measures: Therapy is based on stage of disease. Radical surgery is used for selected patients with stage I and II disease. Radiation therapy (brachytherapy, teletherapy) is used for stage IB and IIA disease or greater. Postoperative radiation therapy reduces the risk of recurrence by almost 50%.

Diet: No specific dietary changes indicated.

Activity: No restriction.

Patient Education: American College of Obstetricians and Gynecologists Patient Education Pamphlet AP033 (*Disorders of the Cervix*), AP0073 (*Human Papillomavirus Infections*), AP085 (*The Pap Test*), AP110 (*Loop Electrosurgical Excision Procedure*).

Drug(s) of Choice

Chemotherapy does not produce long-term cures but response rates of up to 50% have been obtained with multiagent combinations (cisplatin, doxorubicin, and etoposide; other combinations have also been successful).

FOLLOW-UP

Patient Monitoring: Normal health maintenance, 90% of recurrences occur in the first 5 years.

Prevention/Avoidance: None. Adherence to screening guidelines allow diagnosis and treatment of premalignant changes.

Possible Complications: Risk of nodal involvement is based on stage of disease—pelvic nodes: stage I 15%, stage II 29%, stage III 47%; paraaortic nodes: stage I 6%, stage II 19%, stage III 33%.

Expected Outcome: Survival is based on stage of disease—stage IA 99% 5 year; stage IB 85%–90%; stage IIA 73%–80%; stage IIB 68%; stage IIIA 45%; stage IIIB 36%; stage IVA 15%; stage IVB 2%. One third of patients develop recurrences, half within 3 years after primary therapy (best prognosis for later recurrences).

MISCELLANEOUS

Pregnancy Considerations: Rare in pregnancy. Pregnancy and vaginal delivery do not appear to

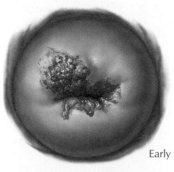

Early carcinoma

Very early squamous cell cancer starting a squamocolumnar junction

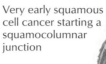

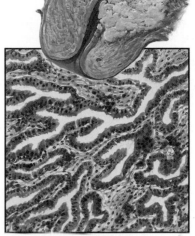

Adenocarcinoma (endocervical)

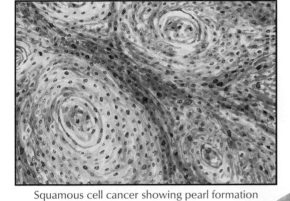

Squamous cell cancer showing pearl formation

Cancer of the cervix with direct extension to vaginal wall, bladder, and rectum

CERVICAL DISEASE

alter the course of disease, although delivery is associated with hemorrhage. Early stages diagnosed late in pregnancy may be watched until after delivery. Advanced disease may require early delivery or interruption of pregnancy to allow aggressive therapy to begin.

***ICD-9-CM* Codes:** 239.5 (unspecified stage; others based on stage).

REFERENCES

American College of Obstetricians and Gynecologists. *Classification and Staging of Gynecologic Malignancies.* Washington, DC: ACOG; 1991. ACOG Technical Bulletin 155.

Clement PB, Scully RE. Carcinoma of the cervix: histologic types. *Semin Oncol* 1982;9:251.

Hacker NF, Berek JS, Lagasse LD. Carcinoma of the cervix associated with pregnancy. *Obstet Gynecol* 1982;59:735.

Leminen A, Paavonen J, Forss M, Wahlstrom T, Vesterinen E. Adenocarcinoma of the uterine cervix. *Cancer* 1990;65:53.

Weiss RS, Lucas WE. Adenocarcinoma of the cervix. *Cancer* 1986;57:1996.

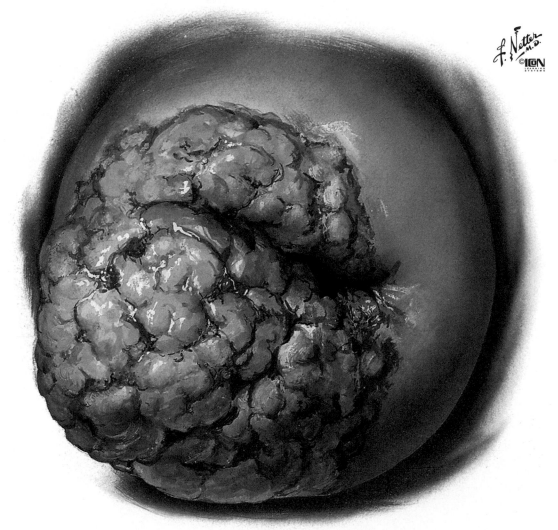

Advanced carcinoma

CERVICAL EROSION

INTRODUCTION

Description: Loss of the epithelial surface on the vaginal portion of the cervix resulting in the exposure of the underlying cervical stroma. Cervical eversion (exposing the dark red columnar epithelium of the endocervix) is often mistaken for or incorrectly labeled as cervical erosion.

Prevalence: Uncommon.

Predominant Age: Reproductive.

Genetics: No genetic pattern.

ETIOLOGY AND PATHOGENESIS

Causes: Generally traumatic. May occur through sexual trauma (fingernail, sexual appliances), iatrogenic process (diaphragm, pessary, biopsy, or other instrumentation), or tampon use.

Risk Factors: None known.

CLINICAL CHARACTERISTICS

Signs and Symptoms:
- Irregularly shaped depressed lesion with a red base and sharp borders
- Bleeding generally absent, although tissues may bleed when touched, resulting in post-coital spotting
- Increased mucoid (clear) discharge may be present

DIAGNOSTIC APPROACH

Differential Diagnosis:
- Cervical eversion (ectopy)
- Herpes simplex cervicitis
- Carcinoma under the surface of the epithelium (barrel lesion)
- Syphilis (primary lesion)
- Chronic cervicitis
- Cervical polyp
- *Chlamydia trachomatis* infection

Associated Conditions: Chronic cervicitis.

Workup and Evaluation

Laboratory: No evaluation indicated.

Imaging: No imaging indicated.

Special Tests: Colposcopy can be used to confirm the diagnosis, but is seldom indicated.

Diagnostic Procedures: Inspection of the cervix.

Pathologic Findings

Loss of surface epithelium. Evidence of inflammation is often present during the healing phase.

MANAGEMENT AND THERAPY

Nonpharmacologic

General Measures: Evaluation and reassurance.

Specific Measures: The use of acidifying agents and topical antibiotics is controversial and generally not necessary.

Diet: No specific dietary changes indicated.

Activity: No restriction.

Patient Education: Reassurance, American College of Obstetricians and Gynecologists Patient Education Pamphlet AP033 (*Disorders of the Cervix*).

Drug(s) of Choice

None.

FOLLOW-UP

Patient Monitoring: Normal health maintenance.

Prevention/Avoidance: None.

Possible Complications: Both overdiagnosis and underdiagnosis; treatment and intervention is generally not warranted and may create additional problems; failure to recognize a more sinister process (cancer) may lead to a delay in treatment.

Expected Outcome: Spontaneous and complete healing is the rule.

MISCELLANEOUS

Pregnancy Considerations: No effect on pregnancy.

ICD-9-CM Codes: 622.0, 616.0 (With chronic cervicitis).

REFERENCES

Barrett KF, Bledsoe S, Greer BE, Droegemueller W. Tampon-induced vaginal or cervical ulceration. *Am J Obstet Gynecol* 1977;127:332.

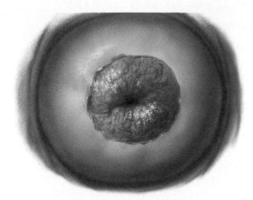

Congenital erosion
in nulliparous cervix

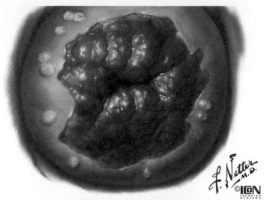

Extensive erosion with proliferation
(papillary erosion); also nabothian cysts

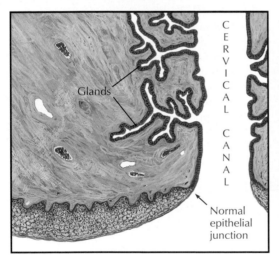

Section through normal portio
vaginalis (schematic)

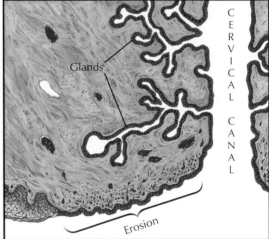

Section through portio vaginalis
showing erosion (schematic)

CERVICAL EVERSION

INTRODUCTION

Description: A turning outward of the endocervical canal so that it is visible and appears as red, inflamed mass at the cervical opening.
Prevalence: Common.
Predominant Age: Reproductive.
Genetics: No genetic pattern.

ETIOLOGY AND PATHOGENESIS

Causes: Chronic cervicitis, estrogen exposure (oral contraceptives).
Risk Factors: Cervicitis, increased estrogen.

CLINICAL CHARACTERISTICS

Signs and Symptoms:
- Generally asymptomatic
- Intermenstrual or postcoital bleeding

DIAGNOSTIC APPROACH

Differential Diagnosis:
- Endocervical polyp
- Endocervical cancer
- Cervicitis
- *Chlamydia trachomatis* infection

Associated Conditions: Cervicitis, intermenstrual and postcoital bleeding.

Workup and Evaluation

Laboratory: No evaluation indicated.
Imaging: No imaging indicated.

Special Tests: Colposcopy confirms the diagnosis but is not required.
Diagnostic Procedures: History and speculum inspection of the cervix.

Pathologic Findings

Normal columnar endocervical epithelium.

MANAGEMENT AND THERAPY

Nonpharmacologic

General Measures: Evaluation and reassurance.
Specific Measures: No therapy required once diagnosis is established.
Diet: No specific dietary changes indicated.
Activity: No restriction.
Patient Education: Reassurance, American College of Obstetricians and Gynecologists Patient Education Pamphlet AP033 (*Disorders of the Cervix*).

Drug(s) of Choice

None.

FOLLOW-UP

Patient Monitoring: Normal health maintenance.
Prevention/Avoidance: None.
Possible Complications: Cervicitis, postcoital bleeding.
Expected Outcome: Normal function without therapy.

MISCELLANEOUS

Pregnancy Considerations: No effect on pregnancy.
ICD-9-CM Codes: 622.0, 616.0 (With chronic cervicitis).

Variations in Location of Transformation Zone

Prepuberal

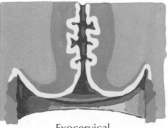

Exocervical

Reproductive

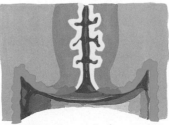

Exocervical

Postmenopausal

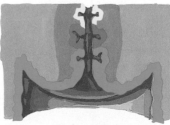

Endocervical

JOHN A.CRAIG—AD
©ICN

CERVICAL POLYPS

INTRODUCTION

Description: Benign fleshy tumors that arise from the cells of the endocervical canal (most common) or the ectocervix.
Prevalence: Four percent of gynecologic patients, most common benign growth of the cervix.
Predominant Age: 40s–50s (multiparous women).
Genetics: No genetic pattern.

ETIOLOGY AND PATHOGENESIS

Causes: Thought to arise as a result of inflammation and the focal hyperplasia and proliferation that it causes.
Risk Factors: More common in multiparous women, history of cervical infection, oral contraceptive use.

CLINICAL CHARACTERISTICS

Signs and Symptoms:
- Asymptomatic (found on routine examination)
- Intermenstrual spotting
- Postcoital spotting
- Smooth, soft, reddish purple to cherry red, friable mass at the cervical os, varying from a few mm to 4 cm in size; may bleed when touched

DIAGNOSTIC APPROACH

Differential Diagnosis:
- Endometrial polyp
- Cervical cancer
- Prolapsed leiomyomata (3%–8% of myomas are cervical)
- Cervical eversion
- Cervical erosion
- Retained products of conception

Associated Conditions: Intramenstrual bleeding, postcoital bleeding, leukorrhea.

Workup and Evaluation

Laboratory: No evaluation indicated.
Imaging: No imaging indicated.
Special Tests: None indicated.
Diagnostic Procedures: Physical examination.

Pathologic Findings

Polypoid growth with a surface epithelium made up of columnar or squamous epithelial cells. The stalk is made up of edematous, loose, often inflamed connective tissue with rich vascularization. The surface may be ulcerated (leading to bleeding). Six histologic types have been described: adenomatous, cystic, fibrous, vascular, inflammatory, and fibromyomatous.

MANAGEMENT AND THERAPY

Nonpharmacologic

General Measures: Evaluation, Pap smear.
Specific Measures: Removal of polyp by gentle traction, twisting, or excision. The base of the polyp may then be treated with chemical cautery, electrocautery, or cryocautery. A polyp may also be cauterized with chemical agents ($AgNO_3$), cryosurgery, or a loop electrosurgical excision procedure. Curettage of the endocervical canal should be considered to rule out a coexisting hyperplasia or cancer.
Diet: No specific dietary changes indicated.
Activity: No restriction.
Patient Education: Reassurance, American College of Obstetricians and Gynecologists Patient Education Pamphlet AP095 (*Abnormal Bleeding*), AP033 (*Disorders of the Cervix*).

Drug(s) of Choice

None.

FOLLOW-UP

Patient Monitoring: Normal health maintenance, no change in Pap smear recommendations.
Prevention/Avoidance: None.
Possible Complications: Malignant change is extremely rare.
Expected Outcome: Excision or cautery is curative.

MISCELLANEOUS

Pregnancy Considerations: No effect on pregnancy.
ICD-9-CM Codes: 622.7.

REFERENCES

Duckman S, Suarez JR, Sese LQ. Giant cervical polyp. *Am J Obstet Gynecol* 1988;159:852.
Pradhan S, Chenoy R, O'Brien PMS. Dilatation and curettage in patients with cervical polyps: a retrospective analysis. *Br J Obstet Gynaecol* 1995;102:415.

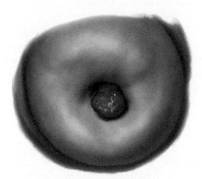

Small cervical polyp

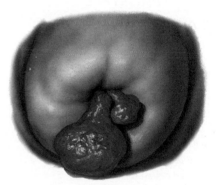

Large and small cervical polyps

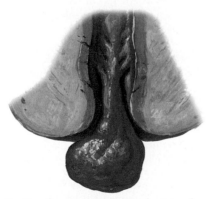

Section showing endocervical origin of a polyp

CERVICAL STENOSIS

INTRODUCTION

Description: A narrowing of the cervical canal, either congenital or acquired, which may result in complete or partial obstruction. Stenosis occurs most often in the region of the internal cervical os.

Prevalence: Uncommon.

Predominant Age: 30–70.

Genetics: No genetic pattern.

ETIOLOGY AND PATHOGENESIS

Causes: Operative damage (cone biopsy, electrocautery, cryocautery), radiation, infection, neoplasia, atrophy, congenital (rare).

Risk Factors: Operative therapy (cone biopsy, cautery), radiation, chronic infection, neoplasia, untreated menopause.

CLINICAL CHARACTERISTICS

Signs and Symptoms:
- Premenopausal—Dysmenorrhea, abnormal bleeding, amenorrhea, infertility
- Boggy uterine enlargement
- Postmenopausal—Asymptomatic
- Hematometra, hydrometra, or pyometra

DIAGNOSTIC APPROACH

Differential Diagnosis:
- Endocervical cancer
- Endometrial cancer
- Uterine leiomyomata

Associated Conditions: Endometriosis, dysmenorrhea, chronic pelvic pain, and infertility.

Workup and Evaluation

Laboratory: Ultrasonography may demonstrate uterine enlargement or hematometra.

Imaging: No imaging indicated.

Special Tests: Inability to pass a 1–2 mm probe beyond the inner cervical os.

Diagnostic Procedures: History, physical examination, sounding of the endocervical canal with a small probe.

Pathologic Findings

None.

MANAGEMENT AND THERAPY

Nonpharmacologic

General Measures: Evaluation, analgesics (nonsteroidal antiinflammatory drugs) for dysmenorrhea.

Specific Measures: Dilation of the cervix with progressive dilators under ultrasound guidance. Placement of a cervical stent for several days after dilation has been advocated, but is not universally accepted.

Diet: No specific dietary changes indicated.

Activity: No restriction.

Patient Education: American College of Obstetricians and Gynecologists Patient Education Pamphlet AP033 (*Disorders of the Cervix*), AP062 (*Dilation and Curettage (D&C)*), AP046 (*Dysmenorrhea*).

Drug(s) of Choice

Symptomatic therapy until definitive surgical dilation.

FOLLOW-UP

Patient Monitoring: Normal health maintenance.

Prevention/Avoidance: Care with surgical technique when cone biopsy or cautery of the cervix is used.

Possible Complications: Retrograde menstruation with the subsequent development of endometriosis, infertility, and chronic pelvic pain. In older patients, the development of hematometra or pyometra.

Expected Outcome: The risk of recurrence is small after dilation (based on causation).

MISCELLANEOUS

Pregnancy Considerations: No effect on pregnancy.

ICD-9-CM Codes: 622.4, 654.6 (Complicating labor), 752.49 (Congenital).

REFERENCES

Baggish MS, Baltoyannis P. Carbon dioxide laser treatment of cervical stenosis. *Fertil Steril* 1987;48:24.

Barbierie RL, Callery M, Perez SE. Directionality of menstrual flow: cervical os diameter as a determinant of retrograde menstruation. *Fertil Steril* 1992;57:727.

Pinsonneault O, Goldstein DP. Obstructing malformations of the uterus and vagina. *Fertil Steril* 1985;44:241.

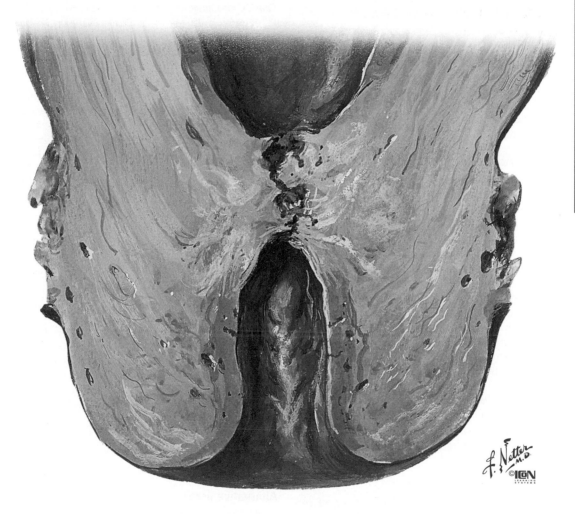

Stricture

CERVICITIS

INTRODUCTION

Description: Inflammation (acute or chronic) of the endocervical glands or the ectocervix.

Prevalence: Ten percent to forty percent of women.

Predominant Age: Reproductive, greatest rate in adolescents to early 20s.

Genetics: No genetic pattern.

ETIOLOGY AND PATHOGENESIS

Causes: Endocervical—*Chlamydia trachomatis* (up to 60% of cases), *Neisseria gonorrhoeae.* Ectocervical—herpes simplex, HPV, *Mycoplasma* species (*Mycoplasma hominis, Ureaplasma urealyticum*), *Trichomonas vaginalis.*

Risk Factors: Exposure to sexually transmissible infections (multiple sexual partners), postpartum period.

CLINICAL CHARACTERISTICS

Signs and Symptoms:

- May be asymptomatic (60%)
- Mucopurulent discharge (yellow discharge with 10 or more white blood cells at ×1000 magnification)
- Cervical erythema or edema, ulceration, and friability

DIAGNOSTIC APPROACH

Differential Diagnosis:

- Vaginitis
- Cervical neoplasia
- Cervical metaplasia
- Cervical erosion
- Cervical eversion

Associated Conditions: Cervical neoplasia, dyspareunia, postcoital bleeding, pelvic inflammatory disease, premature rupture of the membranes in pregnancy, premature labor, and prematurity.

Workup and Evaluation

Laboratory: Cervical culture, Gram's stain of cervical material, enzyme-linked immunosorbent assay (ELISA) or fluorescent monoclonal antibody testing for *Chlamydia.* Consider serum testing for other sexually transmissible infections.

Imaging: No imaging indicated.

Special Tests: None indicated.

Diagnostic Procedures: Inspection, Gram's stain, culture, ELISA assay, or fluorescent monoclonal antibody testing. Colposcopy may be of assistance in selected cases.

Pathologic Findings

Diffuse inflammatory changes, koilocytic changes with HPV infection.

MANAGEMENT AND THERAPY

Nonpharmacologic

General Measures: Diagnosis and management of causal agent.

Specific Measures: In rare patients with consistently negative cultures, cryosurgery of the cervix has been advocated.

Diet: No specific dietary changes indicated.

Activity: No restriction.

Patient Education: Infectious nature of the problem, need for partner evaluation, sexually transmissible infection avoidance, American College of Obstetricians and Gynecologists Patient Education Pamphlet AP033 (*Disorders of the Cervix*), AP009 (*How to Prevent Sexually Transmitted Diseases*), AP071 (*Gonorrhea and Chlamydia*), AP073 (*Human Papillomavirus Infection*), AP028 (*Vaginitis: Causes and Treatments*).

Drug(s) of Choice

Without gonorrhea—doxycycline 100 mg PO bid for 7 days or azithromycin 1 g PO (single dose)

With gonorrhea—ceftriaxone 125 mg IM or (cefixime 400 mg PO or ciprofloxacin 500 mg PO or ofloxacin 400 mg PO) as single dose plus doxycycline 100 mg PO bid for 7 days.

Contraindications: Known or suspected allergy to medication. Doxycycline should not be used during pregnancy or nursing.

Precautions: Doxycycline should not be taken with milk, antacids, or iron-containing preparations.

Interactions: Doxycycline may interact with warfarin or oral contraceptives to reduce their effectiveness.

Alternative Drugs

Without gonorrhea—ofloxacin 300 mg PO bid for 7 days or erythromycin ethylsuccinate 800 mg PO qid for 7 days.

FOLLOW-UP

Patient Monitoring: Repeat cultures for test of cure, annual Pap smears.

Prevention/Avoidance: Use of condoms to reduce the risk of infection.

Possible Complications: Cervical atypia and neoplasia.

Expected Outcome: With treatment, good.

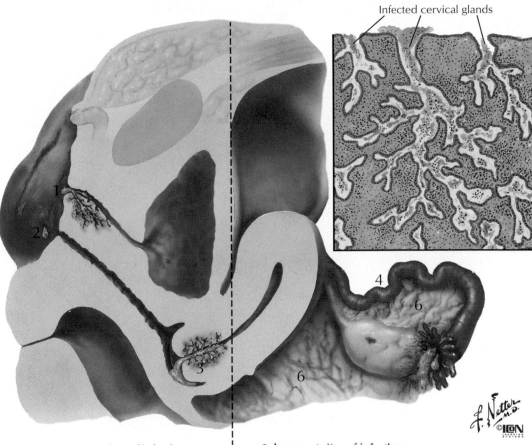

Infected cervical glands

Primary sites of infection
1. Urethra and Skene's gland
2. Bartholin's gland
3. Cervix and cervical glands

Subsequent sites of infection
4. Fallopian tubes (salpingitis)
5. Emergence from tubal ostium (tubo-ovarian abscess and peritonitis)
6. Lymphatic spread to broad ligaments and surrounding tissues (frozen pelvis)

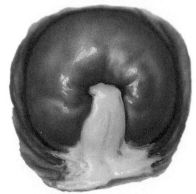

Appearance of cervix
in acute infection

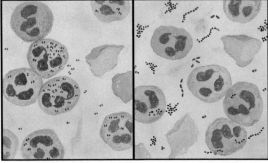

Gonorrheal infection
(Gram's stain)

Non-specific infection
(Gram's stain)

MISCELLANEOUS

Pregnancy Considerations: No effect on pregnancy.

***ICD-9-CM* Codes:** 616.0 (Cervicitis), 098.15 (Acute gonococcal cervicitis), 079.8 (*Chlamydia* infection).

REFERENCES

Centers for Disease Control. Sexually transmitted diseases treatment guidelines. *MMWR Morb Mortal Wkly Rep* 1993;42:56.

Martin DH, Mroczkowski TF, Dalu ZA, et al. A controlled trial of a single dose of azithromycin for the treatment of chlamydial urethritis and cervicitis: the azithromycin for Chlamydial Infections Study Group. *N Engl J Med* 1992;327:921.

NABOTHIAN CYSTS

INTRODUCTION

Description: Retention cysts of the cervix made up of endocervical columnar cells and resulting from closure of a gland opening, tunnel, or cleft by the process of squamous metaplasia.

Prevalence: Normal feature of the adult cervix.

Predominant Age: Reproductive.

Genetics: No genetic pattern.

ETIOLOGY AND PATHOGENESIS

Causes: A cervical gland opening, tunnel, or cleft that becomes covered by the process of squamous metaplasia.

Risk Factors: Chronic inflammation of the cervix.

CLINICAL CHARACTERISTICS

Signs and Symptoms:
- Asymptomatic
- Translucent or opaque, white to blue to yellow, raised bumps on the ectocervix (3 mm–3 cm in diameter)

DIAGNOSTIC APPROACH

Differential Diagnosis:
- Cervical cancer (barrel or undermining type) uncommon

Associated Conditions: None.

Workup and Evaluation

Laboratory: No evaluation indicated.

Imaging: No imaging indicated.

Special Tests: None indicated.

Diagnostic Procedures: Pelvic (speculum) examination.

Pathologic Findings

Mucus-filled cysts lines with columnar epithelium.

MANAGEMENT AND THERAPY

Nonpharmacologic

General Measures: Evaluation and reassurance.

Specific Measures: None necessary.

Diet: No specific dietary changes indicated.

Activity: No restriction.

Patient Education: Reassurance, American College of Obstetricians and Gynecologists Patient Education Pamphlet AP 033 (*Disorders of the Cervix*).

Drug(s) of Choice

None.

FOLLOW-UP

Patient Monitoring: Normal health maintenance.

Prevention/Avoidance: None.

Possible Complications: Distortion or enlargement of the cervix is possible, but unlikely.

MISCELLANEOUS

Pregnancy Considerations: No effect on pregnancy.

ICD-9-CM Codes: 616.0.

REFERENCES

Farrar HK, Nedoss BR. Benign tumors of the uterine cervix. *Am J Obstet Gynecol* 1961;81:124.

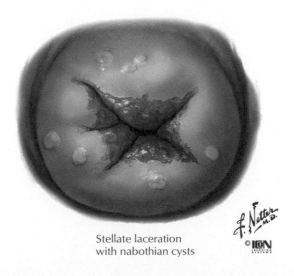

Stellate laceration
with nabothian cysts

Uterine Pathology

ADENOMYOSIS

INTRODUCTION

Description: Endometrial glands and stroma found in the uterine wall (myometrium).

Prevalence: Ten percent to fifteen percent of women; may be 60% in women 40–50 years old.

Predominant Age: 35–50.

Genetics: Familial predisposition (polygenic or multifactorial inheritance pattern).

ETIOLOGY AND PATHOGENESIS

Causes: Adenomyosis is derived from aberrant glands of the basalis layer of the endometrium. These grow by direct extension into the myometrium.

Risk Factors: High levels of estrogen (postulated), high parity, postpartum endometritis (postulated).

CLINICAL CHARACTERISTICS

Signs and Symptoms:
Asymptomatic (40%)
Menorrhagia (40%–50%) often increasing in severity
Dysmenorrhea
Symmetric "woody" enlargement of the uterus (up to 2–3 times normal)
Uterine tenderness that varies with the cycle (worst just before menstruation)

DIAGNOSTIC APPROACH

Differential Diagnosis:
Uterine leiomyomata
Endometrial cancer

Associated Conditions: Coexistent endometriosis (15%), uterine leiomyomata, dyspareunia, salpingitis isthmica nodosa.

Workup and Evaluation

Laboratory: No evaluation indicated, complete blood count if anemia is suspected.

Imaging: No imaging indicated except to rule out other possible pathologic conditions.

Special Tests: Endometrial biopsy is seldom of help in establishing the diagnosis of adenomyosis, although it may be useful to rule out a possible endometrial cancer when that is a consideration.

Diagnostic Procedures: The characteristic history of painful, heavy periods, accompanied by a generous, symmetrical, firm or "woody" uterus suggests, but does not confirm, the diagnosis. Only histologic examination can confirm the diagnosis.

Pathologic Findings

In adenomyosis, endometrial implants (glands and stroma) develop deep within the myometrial wall. Adenomyosis is, therefore, the intramural equivalent of extrauterine endometriosis. Diagnostic criteria require glands to be identified more than 2.5 mm below the basalis layer of the endometrium.

MANAGEMENT AND THERAPY

Nonpharmacologic

General Measures: Analgesics (nonsteroidal antiinflammatory drugs), cyclic hormone therapy, gonadotropin-releasing hormone (GnRH) agonists.

Specific Measures: Hysterectomy is the definitive treatment for adenomyosis.

Diet: No specific dietary changes indicated.

Activity: No restriction.

Patient Education: Reassurance, American College of Obstetricians and Gynecologists Patient Education Pamphlet AP013 (*Important Facts About Endometriosis*), AP046 (*Dysmenorrhea*).

Drug(s) of Choice

There is no satisfactory medical treatment for adenomyosis. All medical therapy is aimed at ameliorating the symptoms or delaying the progression of the condition. Symptoms generally resolve with the loss of ovarian function.

FOLLOW-UP

Patient Monitoring: Normal health maintenance.

Prevention/Avoidance: None.

Possible Complications: Progressive menorrhagia, anemia, chronic pelvic pain.

Expected Outcome: Unless associated with endometriosis, surgical therapy (hysterectomy) is curative.

MISCELLANEOUS

Pregnancy Considerations: No effect on pregnancy.

ICD-9-CM Codes: 617.0.

REFERENCES

Arnold LL, Ascher SM, Simon JA. Familial adenomyosis: a case report. *Fertil Steril* 1994;60:1165.

Azziz R. Adenomyosis: Current perspectives. *Obstet Gynecol Clin North Am* 1989;16:221.

Fedele L, Bianchi S, Dorta M, Arcaini L, Zanotti F, Carinelli S. Transvaginal ultrasonography in the diagnosis of diffuse adenomyosis. *Fertil Steril* 1992;58:94.

Hirata JD, Moghissi KS, Ginsburg KA. Pregnancy after medical therapy of adenomyosis with a gonadotropin-releasing hormone agonist. *Fertil Steril* 1993;59:444.

Popp LW, Schwiedessen JP, Gaetje R. Myometrial biopsy in the diagnosis of adenomyosis uteri. *Am J Obstet Gynecol* 1993;169:546.

Raju GC, Naraynsingh V, Woo J, Jankey N. Adenomyosis uteri: a study of 416 cases. *Aust N Z J Obstet Gynaecol* 1988;28:72.

Siegler AM, Camilien L. Adenomyosis. *J Reprod Med* 1994;39:841.

Possible Locations of Endometrial Implants

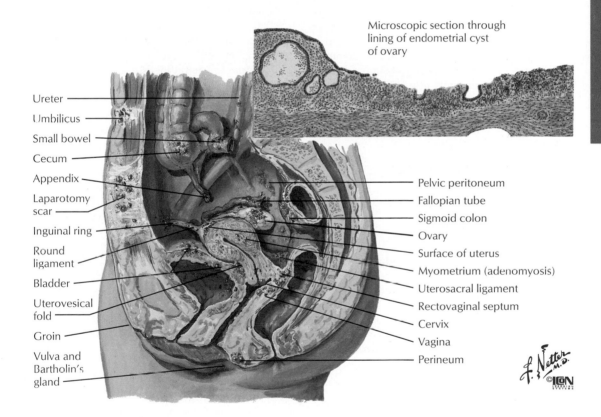

Microscopic section through lining of endometrial cyst of ovary

Ureter
Umbilicus
Small bowel
Cecum
Appendix
Laparotomy scar
Inguinal ring
Round ligament
Bladder
Uterovesical fold
Groin
Vulva and Bartholin's gland

Pelvic peritoneum
Fallopian tube
Sigmoid colon
Ovary
Surface of uterus
Myometrium (adenomyosis)
Uterosacral ligament
Rectovaginal septum
Cervix
Vagina
Perineum

ASHERMAN'S SYNDROME (UTERINE SYNECHIA)

INTRODUCTION

Description: Scarring or occlusion of the uterine cavity after curettage, especially when performed after septic abortion or in the immediate postpartum period.

Prevalence: Rare.

Predominant Age: Reproductive.

Genetics: No genetic pattern.

ETIOLOGY AND PATHOGENESIS

Causes: Endometrial damage (excessive curettage, curettage when infection is present or in the immediate postpartum period—some intrauterine adhesions form in 30% of patients treated by curettage for missed abortion), endometrial infection (tuberculosis or schistosomiasis), scarring after myomectomy or metroplasty.

Risk Factors: Instrumentation of the uterine cavity complicated by infection. Endometrial infection unrelated to instrumentation, such as tuberculosis or schistosomiasis.

CLINICAL CHARACTERISTICS

Signs and Symptoms:
Amenorrhea or hypomenorrhea

DIAGNOSTIC APPROACH

Differential Diagnosis:
Amenorrhea (primary or secondary)
Cervical stenosis

Associated Conditions: Amenorrhea, infertility.

Workup and Evaluation

Laboratory: No evaluation indicated.

Imaging: Sonohysterography or hysterosalpingography.

Special Tests: None indicated.

Diagnostic Procedures: Hysteroscopy.

Pathologic Findings

Intrauterine scarring.

MANAGEMENT AND THERAPY

Nonpharmacologic

General Measures: Evaluation and support.

Specific Measures: Resection of intrauterine scars under hysteroscopic control, followed by intrauterine contraceptive device (IUCD) insertion and estrogen therapy.

Diet: No specific dietary changes indicated.

Activity: No restriction.

Patient Education: Reassurance, American College of Obstetricians and Gynecologists Patient Education Pamphlet AP062 (*Dilatation and Curettage [D&C]*).

Drug(s) of Choice

Estrogen for 1–2 months.
Oral—Conjugated estrogen 1.25 mg qd, diethylstilbestrol 1 mg qd, esterified estrogens 1.25 mg qd, ethinyl estradiol 0.05 mg qd, micronized estradiol 1 mg qd, piperazine estrone sulfate, estropipate 1.25 mg qd.
Topical—17β-estradiol 0.1 mg/d.

Contraindications: Undiagnosed vaginal bleeding.

FOLLOW-UP

Patient Monitoring: Normal health maintenance.

Prevention/Avoidance: Avoidance of excessive curettage, prompt treatment of endometritis after dilatation and curettage.

Possible Complications: Hematocolpos, infertility.

Expected Outcome: Return to normal fertility and menstrual function after treatment.

MISCELLANEOUS

Pregnancy Considerations: Once treated, no effect on future pregnancy.

ICD-9-CM Codes: 621.5.

REFERENCES

Gambone JC, Munro MG. Office sonography and office hysteroscopy. *Curr Opin Obstet Gynecol* 1993; 5:733.

Gimpelson RJ. Office hysteroscopy [review]. *Clin Obstet Gynecol* 1992;35:270.

March CM. Hysteroscopy. *J Reprod Med* 1992;37:293.

March CM, Israel R, March AD. Hysteroscopic management of intrauterine adhesions. *Am J Obstet Gynecol* 1978;130:653.

Siegler AM, Valle RF. Therapeutic hysteroscopic procedures. *Fertil Steril* 1988;50:685.

Smith RS. *Gynecology in Primary Care*. Baltimore, Md: Williams & Wilkins; 1997:405.

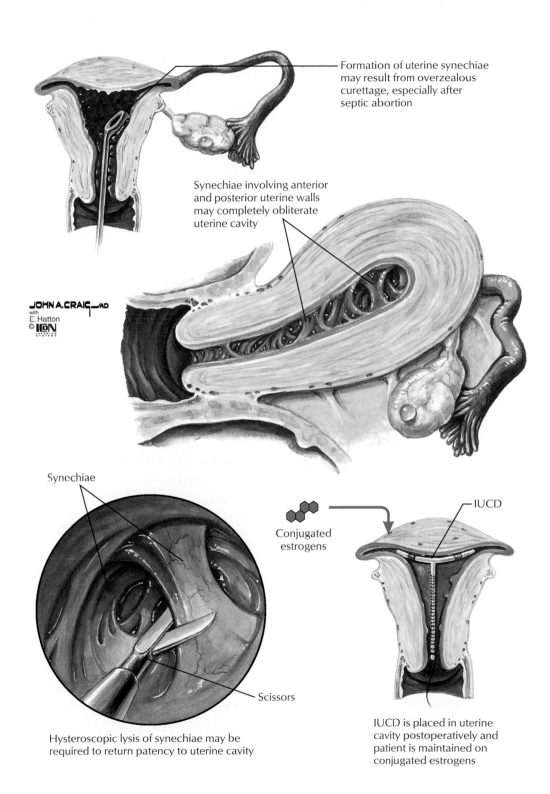

Formation of uterine synechiae may result from overzealous curettage, especially after septic abortion

Synechiae involving anterior and posterior uterine walls may completely obliterate uterine cavity

JOHN A. CRAIG—AD
with
E. Hatton
© ICON

Synechiae

Scissors

Hysteroscopic lysis of synechiae may be required to return patency to uterine cavity

Conjugated estrogens

IUCD

IUCD is placed in uterine cavity postoperatively and patient is maintained on conjugated estrogens

DYSFUNCTIONAL UTERINE BLEEDING

INTRODUCTION

Description: Irregular or intermenstrual bleeding with no clinically identifiable underlying cause.

Prevalence: Ten percent to fifteen percent of all gynecologic visits involve menstrual disturbances.

Predominant Age: Reproductive, greatest in adolescents and climacteric patients.

Genetics: No genetic pattern.

ETIOLOGY AND PATHOGENESIS

Causes: Anovulatory patients—chemotherapy, chronic illness, climacteric changes, endometrial carcinoma, endometrial hyperplasia, hormonal contraception (oral, injectable, intrauterine), iatrogenic (anticoagulation, hormone replacement), idiopathic, medications (anticholinergic agents, monamine oxidase inhibitors, morphine, phenothiazines, reserpine), nutritional disruption (anorexia, bulimia, excess physical activity), obesity, pituitary-hypothalamic-ovarian axis immaturity, pituitary tumor, polycystic ovary syndrome, stress, systemic disease (hepatic, renal, thyroid). Ovulatory patients—anatomic lesions (adenomyosis, cervical neoplasia, cervical polyps, endometrial carcinoma, endometrial polyps, leiomyomata, sarcoma), bleeding at ovulation, coagulopathies (natural or iatrogenic), endometritis, fallopian tube disease (infection, tumor), foreign body (IUCD, pessary, tampon), idiopathic, ingested substances (estrogens, ginseng), leukemia, luteal phase dysfunction, pelvic inflammatory disease (including tuberculosis), pregnancy related (abortion, ectopic, hydatidiform mole, retained products of conception), repeated trauma, systemic disease (hepatic, renal, thyroid).

Risk Factors: Prolonged anovulation.

CLINICAL CHARACTERISTICS

Signs and Symptoms:
Intermenstrual bleeding (painless)
Irregular menstrual cycles (typically prolonged)

DIAGNOSTIC APPROACH

Differential Diagnosis:
Pregnancy
Climacteric changes
Anovulation
Endometrial polyps
Uterine leiomyomata
Endometrial cancer
Endometriosis
Nonuterine sources of bleeding (eg, cervical, vaginal, vulvar, or perineal)
Iatrogenic causes (hormones, oral contraceptives)

Associated Conditions: Anovulation, infertility, endometrial cancer, endometrial polyps or carcinoma, uterine leiomyomata, obesity.

Workup and Evaluation

Laboratory: Testing should be chosen on the basis of the differential diagnoses under consideration.

Imaging: Pelvic ultrasonography or sonohysterography may be of assistance in selected patients.

Special Tests: A menstrual calendar helps document the timing and character of the patient's bleeding. Endometrial biopsy, curettage, or hysteroscopy may be indicated.

Diagnostic Procedures: The diagnosis of dysfunctional uterine bleeding is one of exclusion. History and physical examination often points to possible causes for further evaluation.

Pathologic Findings

Proliferation of the endometrial tissues with irregular shedding evident in some patients; in other patients the endometrium is thin and atrophic.

MANAGEMENT AND THERAPY

Nonpharmacologic

General Measures: Evaluation.

Specific Measures: Focused on underlying causation and desires of patient. If anovulation is the cause and fertility is not desired, periodic progestin therapy may be used to stabilize menstrual cycles and suppress intermenstrual bleeding. Suppression of menstrual cycling (GnRH agonists, long-acting progestin) or hysterectomy may be required for a small number of patients.

Diet: No specific dietary changes indicated.

Activity: No restriction.

Patient Education: Reassurance, American College of Obstetricians and Gynecologists Patient Education Pamphlet AP095 (*Abnormal Uterine Bleeding*), AP049 (*Menstruation*).

Drug(s) of Choice

Medroxyprogesterone acetate 5–10 mg for 1–14 days each month. (In roughly 85% of patients who have ovulated in the past, a single cycle provides adequate response.)

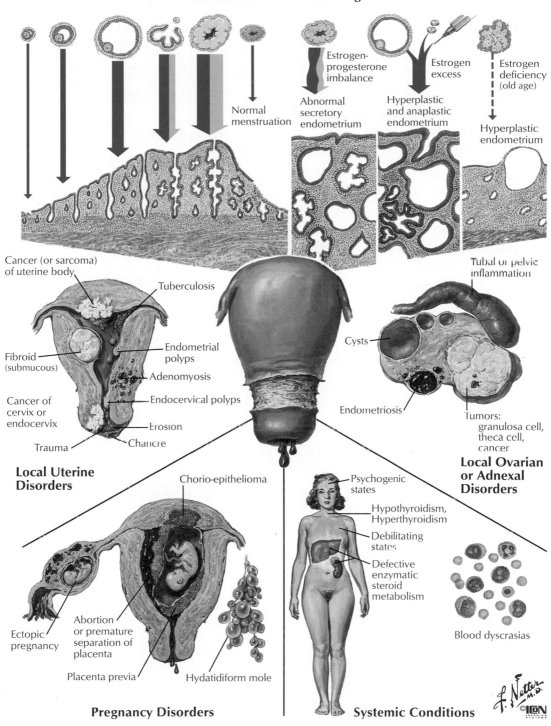

Steroid Withdrawal Bleeding

Normal menstruation

Estrogen-progesterone imbalance

Abnormal secretory endometrium

Estrogen excess

Hyperplastic and anaplastic endometrium

Estrogen deficiency (old age)

Hyperplastic endometrium

Local Uterine Disorders

Cancer (or sarcoma) of uterine body

Tuberculosis

Fibroid (submucous)

Endometrial polyps

Adenomyosis

Endocervical polyps

Cancer of cervix or endocervix

Erosion

Trauma

Chancre

Local Ovarian or Adnexal Disorders

Tubal or pelvic inflammation

Cysts

Endometriosis

Tumors: granulosa cell, theca cell, cancer

Pregnancy Disorders

Chorio-epithelioma

Ectopic pregnancy

Abortion or premature separation of placenta

Placenta previa

Hydatidiform mole

Systemic Conditions

Psychogenic states

Hypothyroidism, Hyperthyroidism

Debilitating states

Defective enzymatic steroid metabolism

Blood dyscrasias

Contraindications: Undiagnosed amenorrhea or bleeding.

Precautions: Progestins should not be used until pregnancy has been ruled out.

Alternative Drugs

Norethindrone acetate 5–10 mg for 10–14 days each month. Combination oral contraceptives may also be used.

FOLLOW-UP

Patient Monitoring: Normal health maintenance.

Prevention/Avoidance: None.

Possible Complications: Anemia, endometrial hyperplasia or carcinoma if left untreated.

Expected Outcome: Return to normal menstrual pattern with correction of underlying pathologic condition or periodic progestin therapy.

MISCELLANEOUS

Pregnancy Considerations: No effect on pregnancy aside from that resulting from causative conditions.

ICD-9-CM **Codes:** 626.8, 626.4 (Irregular menstrual cycle).

REFERENCES

Aksel S, Jones GS. Etiology and treatment of dysfunctional uterine bleeding. *Obstet Gynecol* 1974;44:1.

American College of Obstetricians and Gynecologists. *Dysfunctional Uterine Bleeding.* Washington, DC: ACOG; 1989. ACOG Technical Bulletin 134.

Bayer RL, DeCherney AH. Clinical manifestations and treatment of dysfunctional uterine bleeding. *JAMA* 1993;269:1823.

Cowan BD, Morrison JC. Management of abnormal genital bleeding in girls and women. *N Engl J Med* 1991;324:1710.

Field CS. Dysfunctional uterine bleeding. *Primary Care* 1988;15:561.

Neese RE. Managing abnormal vaginal bleeding. *Postgrad Med* 1991;89:205.

Smith RP. *Gynecology in Primary Care.* Baltimore, Md: Williams & Wilkins; 1997:25, 375.

ENDOMETRIAL CANCER

INTRODUCTION

Description: Malignant change of the endometrial tissues. These are generally of the adenocarcinoma, adenosquamous, clear cell, or papillary serous cell types.

Prevalence: Two percent to three percent lifetime risk, the most frequent malignancy of the female reproductive tract.

Predominant Age: 55–65.

Genetics: No genetic pattern known.

ETIOLOGY AND PATHOGENESIS

Causes: Unopposed (without progestins) estrogen stimulation (polycystic ovary syndrome, obesity, chronic anovulation, and estrogen replacement therapy without concomitant progestin). Selective estrogen receptor modulators with uterine activity (tamoxifen).

Risk Factors: Unopposed estrogen stimulation of the uterus (chronic anovulation, estrogen therapy, and obesity), tamoxifen use, early menarche, late menopause, nulliparity, and breast or colon cancer.

CLINICAL CHARACTERISTICS

Signs and Symptoms:
Postmenopausal bleeding
Abnormal glandular cells on Pap smear (Cervical cytologic tests detect only about 20% of known endometrial carcinomas.)

DIAGNOSTIC APPROACH

Differential Diagnosis:
Endometrial hyperplasia (complex, atypical)
Cervical cancer
Ovarian cancer metastatic to the endometrium
Metachronous Müllerian tumor
Endometriosis
Early pregnancy (younger women)
Granulosa cell tumors

Associated Conditions: Obesity, irregular menstrual bleeding, infertility, breast or colon cancer.

Workup and Evaluation

Laboratory: No evaluation indicated, except for preoperative screening.

Imaging: Chest radiograph (for metastases), transvaginal ultrasonography or sonohysterography may be useful.

Special Tests: Endometrial biopsy (90% accurate).

Diagnostic Procedures: History, physical examination, and endometrial biopsy.

Pathologic Findings

Atypical, hyperplastic glands with little or no stroma. Mitosis common. (See table for staging.)

MANAGEMENT AND THERAPY

Nonpharmacologic

General Measures: Evaluation and staging.

Specific Measures: Surgical exploration with hysterectomy, bilateral salpingo-oophorectomy, cytologic examination of the abdomen and diaphragm, paraaortic node sampling. Radiation to the vaginal cuff reduces local recurrence. Distant metastatic disease is treated with high-dose progestins, cisplatin, and doxorubicin (Adriamycin).

Diet: No specific dietary changes indicated except as dictated by surgical therapy.

Activity: No restriction except as dictated by surgical therapy.

Patient Education: American College of Obstetricians and Gynecologists Patient Education Pamphlet AP097 (*Cancer of the Uterus*), AP008 (*Understanding Hysterectomy*), AP080 (*Preparing*

STAGING FOR ENDOMETRIAL CANCER

Stage I
A—Limited to the endometrium
B—<50% of myometrial depth
C—>50% of myometrial depth
Stage II
A—Endocervical glandular involvement only
B—Cervical stromal involvement
Stage III
A—Serosal and/or adnexal invasion and/or positive peritoneal cytologic test
B—Vaginal metastases
C—Metastases to pelvic and/or paraaortic lymph nodes
Stage IV
A—Invasion of bowel and/or bladder mucosa
B—Distant metastases including abdominal or inguinal lymph nodes
Grade 1—5% or less nonsquamous or nonmorular solid growth pattern
Grade 2—6–50% or less nonsquamous or nonmorular solid growth pattern
Grade 3—>50% or less nonsquamous or nonmorular solid growth pattern

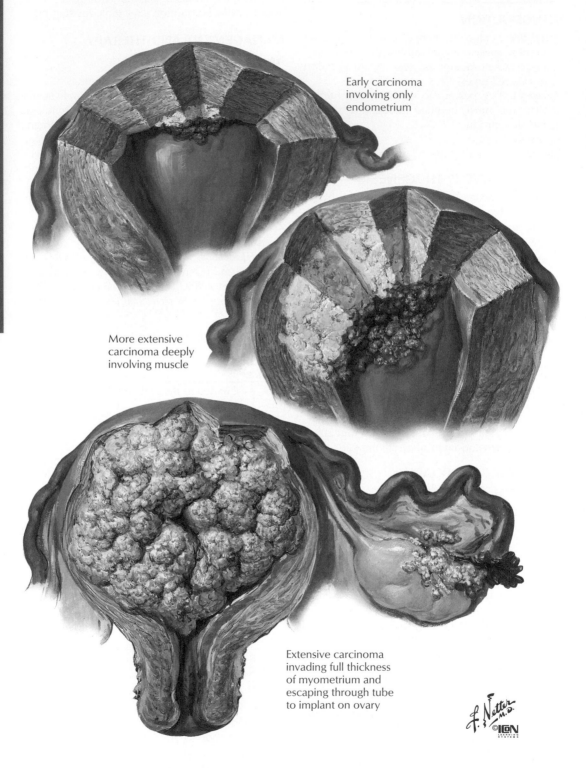

Early carcinoma
involving only
endometrium

More extensive
carcinoma deeply
involving muscle

Extensive carcinoma
invading full thickness
of myometrium and
escaping through tube
to implant on ovary

for Surgery), AP095 (*Abnormal Uterine Bleeding*), AP074 (*Uterine Fibroids*).

Drug(s) of Choice

Hyperplasia and distant metastatic disease: megestrol (Megace) 160 mg PO qd for 3 months. This is generally followed by curettage or other evaluation to assess response.

Doxorubicin (Adriamycin) or cisplatin chemotherapy.

Contraindications: See individual agents.

Precautions: High-dose progestins should be used with caution in patients with congestive heart failure because they may cause fluid retention.

Interactions: See individual agents.

FOLLOW-UP

Patient Monitoring: Follow-up Pap smears from vaginal cuff every 3 months for 2 years then every 6 months for 3 years, then yearly. Chest radiograph annually.

Prevention/Avoidance: Correction of unopposed estrogen states or the addition of progestin.

Possible Complications: Distant spread with progression to death.

Expected Outcome: Five-year survival based on stage and grade—stage I 85%, stage II 60%, stage III 30%, stage IV 10%.

MISCELLANEOUS

Pregnancy Considerations: Generally not a consideration because they are unlikely to coexist.

ICD-9-CM **Codes:** Specific to cell type and location.

REFERENCES

American College of Obstetricians and Gynecologists. *Classification and Staging of Gynecologic Malignancies.* Washington, DC: ACOG; 1991. ACOG Technical Bulletin 155.

American College of Obstetricians and Gynecologists. *Carcinoma of the Endometrium.* Washington, DC: ACOG; 1991. ACOG Technical Bulletin 162.

Cushing KL, Weiss NS, Voigt LF, McKnight B, Beresford SAA. Risk of endometrial cancer in relation to use of low-dose, unopposed estrogens. *Obstet Gynecol* 1998;91:35.

Davies JL, Rosenshein NB, Antunes CMF, Stolley PD. A review of the risk factors for endometrial carcinoma. *Obstet Gynecol Surv* 1981;36:107.

Gallup DG, Stock RJ. Adenocarcinoma of the endometrium in women 40 years or younger. *Obstet Gynecol* 1984;64:417.

Reid PC, Brown VA, Fothergill DJ. Outpatient investigation of postmenopausal bleeding. *Br J Obstet Gynaecol* 1993;100:498.

ENDOMETRIAL HYPERPLASIA: SIMPLE AND COMPLEX

INTRODUCTION

Description: Abnormal proliferation of both the glandular and stromal elements of the endometrium with characteristic alteration in the histologic architecture of the tissues. It is this architectural change that differentiates hyperplasia from normal endometrial proliferation. Simple hyperplasia represents the least significant form of alteration. Complex hyperplasia represents the most significant form of alteration.

Prevalence: Five percent of patients with postmenopausal bleeding have endometrial hyperplasia.

Predominant Age: Late reproductive and early menopausal.

Genetics: No genetic pattern.

ETIOLOGY AND PATHOGENESIS

Causes: Unknown.

Risk Factors: Unopposed estrogen stimulation of the uterus (chronic anovulation, estrogen therapy [4- to 8-fold risk], obesity [3-fold risk]), nulliparity (2- to 3-fold risk), diabetes (2- to 3-fold risk), polycystic ovarian syndrome, tamoxifen use.

CLINICAL CHARACTERISTICS

Signs and Symptoms:
Asymptomatic
Intermenstrual bleeding
Menorrhagia
Postmenopausal bleeding

DIAGNOSTIC APPROACH

Differential Diagnosis:
Complex endometrial hyperplasia
Endometrial adenocarcinoma
Endometrial polyps
Endocervical carcinoma

Associated Conditions: Endometrial polyps, squamous metaplasia, endometrial carcinoma, endometrial polyps.

Workup and Evaluation

Laboratory: No evaluation indicated.

Imaging: Ultrasonography may detect thickening of the endometrial stripe. This test is still being evaluated and must be performed by someone experienced in the technique and its interpretation. It does not take the place of histologic evaluation.

Special Tests: Endometrial biopsy, hysteroscopy, or dilation and curettage.

Diagnostic Procedures: Endometrial biopsy.

Pathologic Findings

Simple hyperplasia—proliferation of both glandular and stromal elements with no atypia. The glands form simple tubules with wide variations in size from small to large cysts. There is little or no outpouching of the epithelium lining the cysts. Complex hyperplasia—proliferation of both glandular and stromal elements. Cellular atypia (characterized by disordered maturation, high nuclear/cytoplasmic ratio, nuclear pleomorphism, mitoses) may be present or absent. Glands are crowded with a "back-to-back" appearance. May be found with coexisting adenocarcinoma. Outpouching in glands is common.

MANAGEMENT AND THERAPY

Nonpharmacologic

General Measures: Prompt evaluation.

Specific Measures: Simple hyperplasia—medical therapy (progestin) is generally adequate. Many use dilation and curettage by itself or in combination with progestin therapy. Complex hyperplasia—for patients with hyperplasia without atypia or selected patients who wish to preserve fertility, high-dose prolonged progestin therapy may be used. All others are treated by hysterectomy (with bilateral salpingo-oophorectomy).

Diet: No specific dietary changes indicated.

Activity: No restriction.

Patient Education: Reassurance, American College of Obstetricians and Gynecologists Patient Education Pamphlet AP095 (*Atypical Uterine Bleeding*), AP097 (*Cancer of the Uterus*), AP062 (*Dilation and Curettage [D&C]*).

Drug(s) of Choice

Simple hyperplasia—medroxyprogesterone acetate (Provera, Cycrin) 10 mg PO qd for 10 days each month, norethindrone acetate (Aygestin) 10 mg PO qd for 10 days each month.

Complex hyperplasia—depo medroxyprogesterone acetate (Depo-Provera) up to 200–1000 mg IM weekly for 5 weeks, followed by 100–400 mg IM monthly, megestrol acetate (Megace) 40–80 mg PO qd for 6–12 weeks. (Some authors have advocated therapy for up to 48 months.) Estrogen replacement therapy may safely be given to those treated by hysterectomy.

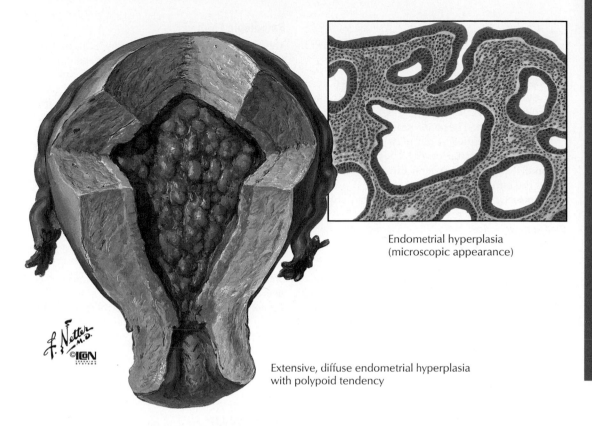

Endometrial hyperplasia
(microscopic appearance)

Extensive, diffuse endometrial hyperplasia
with polypoid tendency

Contraindications: Undiagnosed vaginal bleeding, thrombophlebitis, markedly impaired liver function, known or suspected breast cancer.

Precautions: Progestins should not be used during the first trimester of pregnancy.

Alternative Drugs

Combination oral contraceptives may also be used for simple hyperplasia.

FOLLOW-UP

Patient Monitoring: With simple hyperplasia or for complex hyperplasia managed medically, a follow-up endometrial sampling must be performed after 3 months, then every 6–12 months thereafter.

Prevention/Avoidance: None.

Possible Complications: Progression is uncommon with simple hyperplasia. There is a slight risk associated with endometrial sampling (infection, perforation). Complex hyperplasia, especially with atypia, is associated with coexistent malignancy or the risk of progression to malignant changes (75% of patients). The more atypical the cellular architecture, the greater the risk of malignancy; without atypia 25% of hyperplasia will progress and 50% will persist.

Expected Outcome: Good response to medical therapy can be anticipated for patients with simple hyperplasia. Progression and recurrence are uncommon.

MISCELLANEOUS

Pregnancy Considerations: No effect on pregnancy.

ICD-9-CM Codes: 621.3.

REFERENCES

Copenhaver EH. Atypical endometrial hyperplasia. *Obstet Gynecol* 1959;13:264.

Eichner E, Abellera M. Endometrial hyperplasia treated by progestins. *Obstet Gynecol* 1971;38:739.

Gal D. Endometrial hyperplasia: Diagnosis and management. In: Sciarra JJ, ed. *Gynecology and Obstetrics.* Vol 4. Philadelphia, Pa: JB Lippincott; 1991;12:1.

Gusberg SB, Chen SY, Cohen CJ. Endometrial cancer: factors influencing the choice of treatment. *Gynecol Oncol* 1974;2:308.

Kurman RJ, Kaminski PF, Norris HJ. The behavior of endometrial hyperplasia—a long-term study of "untreated" hyperplasia in 170 patients. *Cancer* 1985;56:403.

Pettersson B, Adami HO, Lindgren A, et al. Endometrial polyps and hyperplasia as risk factors for endometrial carcinoma. *Acta Obstet Gynecol Scand* 1985;64:653.

Wentz WB. Progestin therapy in endometrial hyperplasia. *Gynecol Oncol* 1974;2:362.

UTERINE PATHOLOGY

ENDOMETRIAL POLYPS

INTRODUCTION

Description: Fleshy tumors that arise as local over-growths of endometrial glands and stroma and project beyond the surface of the endometrium. These are most common in the fundus of the uterus, but may occur anywhere in the endometrial cavity. They are generally small (a few millimeters) but may enlarge to fill the entire cavity.

Prevalence: Up to 10% of women (autopsy studies), 20% of uteruses removed for cancer.

Predominant Age: 40–50, infrequent after menopause.

Genetics: No genetic pattern.

ETIOLOGY AND PATHOGENESIS

Causes: Unknown. A role for unopposed estrogen is hypothesized.

Risk Factors: Unopposed estrogen use, tamoxifen therapy.

CLINICAL CHARACTERISTICS

Signs and Symptoms:
Asymptomatic (most)
Abnormal bleeding (most common intermenstrual bleeding and menorrhagia, perimenopausal bleeding). One quarter of women with abnormal bleeding patterns have an endometrial polyp.
Polyps with long pedicles may protrude from the cervix.

DIAGNOSTIC APPROACH

Differential Diagnosis:
Endocervical polyp
Endometrial cancer
Prolapsed leiomyomata
Retained products of conception
Retained (and forgotten) IUCD

Associated Conditions: Endometrial cancer (2-fold increase).

Workup and Evaluation

Laboratory: No evaluation indicated.

Imaging: Sonohysterography generally identifies the polyp. (Special attention should be directed to the fundus, where most polyps arise.)

Special Tests: None indicated.

Diagnostic Procedures: History, physical examination, endometrial sampling, hysteroscopy, or curettage. (Often not diagnosed until the uterus is removed for other reasons.)

Pathologic Findings

Velvety surface with a rich central vascular core. Endometrial glands, stroma, and vascular channels are present with epithelium identified on three sides to establish the pedunculated nature. The endometrial glands are often immature in appearance with a "Swiss cheese" cystic character that is independent of the phase of the cycle. Infection or metaplasia may be present.

MANAGEMENT AND THERAPY

Nonpharmacologic

General Measures: Evaluation.

Specific Measures: Removal by curettage or operative hysteroscopy. (All polyps removed should be examined histologically.)

Diet: No specific dietary changes indicated.

Activity: No restriction.

Patient Education: Reassurance, American College of Obstetricians and Gynecologists Patient Education Pamphlet AP095 (*Abnormal Bleeding*).

Drug(s) of Choice

None.

FOLLOW-UP

Patient Monitoring: Normal health maintenance.

Prevention/Avoidance: Evaluation and treatment of prolonged amenorrhea, treatment of unopposed estrogen states.

Possible Complications: Up to 0.5% of polyps undergo malignant transformation (low grade and stage).

Expected Outcome: Removal is generally curative even when malignant transformation is present.

MISCELLANEOUS

Pregnancy Considerations: No effect on pregnancy.

ICD-9-CM Codes: 621.0.

REFERENCES

Armenia CC. Sequential relationship between endometrial polyps and carcinoma of the endometrium. *Obstet Gynecol* 1967;30:524.

Mishell DR, Stenchever MA, Droegemueller W, Herbst AL. *Comprehensive Gynecology.* 3rd ed. St Louis, Mo: Mosby; 1997:483.

Kurman RJ, Mazur MT. Benign disease of the endometrium. In: Kurman RJ, ed. *Blaustein's Pathology of the Female Genital Tract.* 4th ed. New York, NY: Springer-Verlag, 1994:305.

Peterson WF, Novak ER. Endometrial polyps. *Obstet Gynecol* 1956;8:40.

Salm R. The incidence and significance of early carcinomas in endometrial polyps. *J Pathol* 1972;108:47.

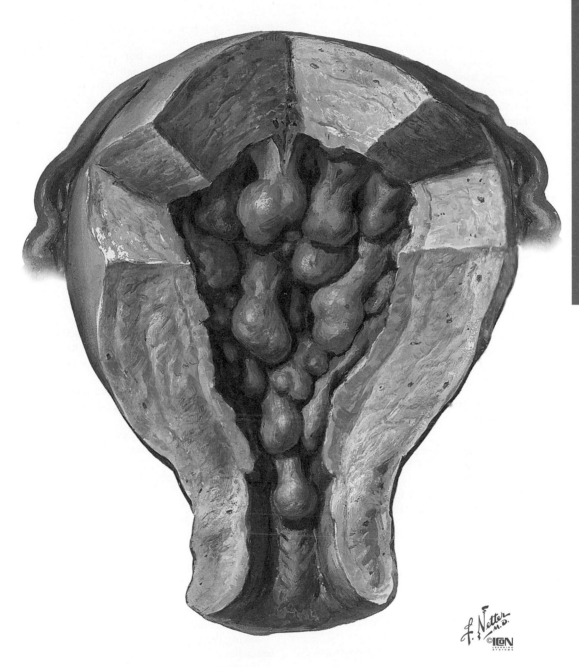

Multiple endometrial polyps

ENDOMETRITIS

INTRODUCTION

Description: A chronic inflammation, usually of infectious origin, of the lining of the uterus. This is a general term that is used for this condition in either nonpregnant or recently pregnant patients; chorioamnionitis is the term commonly used for pregnant patients. Chronic endometritis is often characterized as an intermediate state in ascending infections.

Prevalence: Seventy-five percent of patients with pelvic inflammatory disease, 40% of patients with mucopurulent cervicitis.

Predominant Age: Reproductive.

Genetics: No genetic pattern.

ETIOLOGY AND PATHOGENESIS

Causes: Aseptic inflammation of the endometrium is commonly found in IUCD users. Infection by organisms ascending from the cervix and lower tract are common (most often *Chlamydia trachomatis, Neisseria gonorrhoeae, Ureaplasma urealyticum,* and *Streptococcus agalactiae*). Less common are infections by *Actinomyces israelii* or tuberculosis.

Risk Factors: IUCD use, intrauterine instrumentation (biopsy, hysterosalpingography, biopsy), cervicitis, sexually transmitted disease, retained products of conception.

CLINICAL CHARACTERISTICS

Signs and Symptoms:
Asymptomatic
Dysfunctional uterine bleeding (typically intermenstrual)
Postcoital bleeding
Foul-smelling cervical/vaginal discharge
Pelvic inflammatory disease
Chronic pelvic pain
Tubo-ovarian abscess
Infertility (rare cause)

DIAGNOSTIC APPROACH

Differential Diagnosis:
Accidents of pregnancy
Trophoblastic disease
Endometrial cancer
Estrogen producing tumors or exogenous estrogen
Leiomyomata
Cervical lesion/cervicitis
Forgotten IUCD

Associated Conditions: Chronic pelvic pain, tubo-ovarian abscess, cervicitis, and sexually transmitted disease.

Workup and Evaluation

Laboratory: Complete blood count, cervical cultures for *C trachomatis* and *N gonorrhoeae.* (Tests for other sexually transmitted diseases as indicated.)

Imaging: No imaging indicated. Ultrasonography with saline contrast may demonstrate a thickened endometrium but risks spreading an infection to the fallopian tubes, ovaries, and peritoneal cavity. Consequently, this should be reserved until the possibility of infection has been evaluated.

Special Tests: Endometrial biopsy is generally confirmatory.

Diagnostic Procedures: Endometrial biopsy and culture.

Pathologic Findings

Inflammatory infiltrates (monocytes and plasma cells) in the basal layers and stroma of the endometrium. Sulfur granules may be present in *Actinomyces* infections.

MANAGEMENT AND THERAPY

Nonpharmacologic

General Measures: Evaluation, counseling about sexually transmitted disease (cervicitis).

Specific Measures: Antibiotic therapy (see below), removal of IUCD (if present).

Diet: No specific dietary changes indicated.

Activity: Pelvic rest (no tampons, douches, or intercourse) until therapy has been completed.

Patient Education: American College of Obstetricians and Gynecologists Patient Education Pamphlet AP095 (*Abnormal Uterine Bleeding*), AP099 (*Pelvic Pain*), AP077 (*Pelvic Inflammatory Disease*).

Drug(s) of Choice

Doxycycline (Vibramycin) 200 mg PO initially, 100 mg PO qd for 10 days. If *Actinomyces* is found in a tubo-ovarian abscess, oral penicillin therapy should be continued for 12 weeks.

Contraindications: Known or suspected allergy to tetracycline. Doxycycline is contraindicated in the last half of pregnancy.

Precautions: Photosensitivity may occur in patients taking doxycycline.

Interactions: Doxycycline may enhance the effect of warfarin. Doxycycline absorption is inhibited by most antacids and bismuth subsalicylate (Pepto-Bismol).

Alternative Drugs

Metronidazole or erythromycin may be substituted for doxycycline.

FOLLOW-UP

Patient Monitoring: Normal health maintenance, screening for sexually transmitted disease as needed.

Prevention/Avoidance: Reduce risk of cervicitis or sexually transmitted disease, asepsis during intrauterine procedures.

Possible Complications: Ascending infection resulting in salpingitis, tubo-ovarian abscesses, hydrosalpinx, peritonitis, and chronic pelvic pain.

Expected Outcome: Good with treatment.

MISCELLANEOUS

Pregnancy Considerations: Generally not applicable. *Ureaplasma urealyticum* infection has been implicated as a rare cause of early pregnancy loss.

ICD-9-CM **Codes:** 615.0 (Acute), 615.1 (Chronic), 670 (Following delivery, excludes pregnancy, abortion, ectopic and molar pregnancies).

REFERENCES

Casey BM, Cox SM. Chorioamnionitis and endometritis. *Infect Disease Clin North Am* 1997;11:203.

Michels TC. Chronic endometritis. *Am Fam Physician* 1995;52:217.

Pastorek JG 2nd. Postcesarean endometritis. *Compr Ther* 1995;21:249.

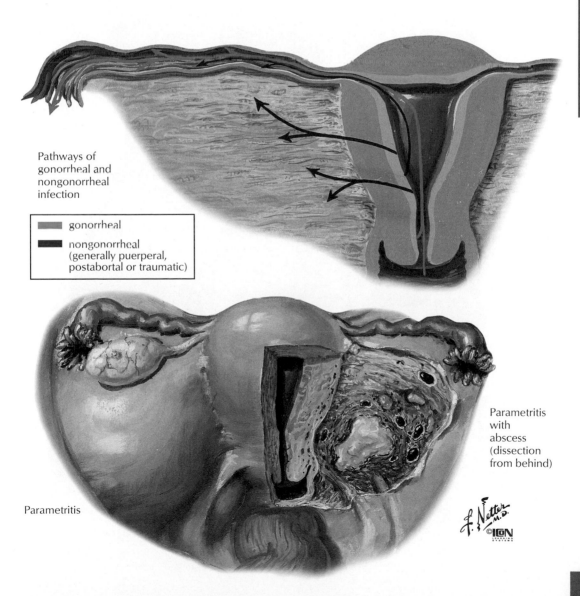

Pathways of gonorrheal and nongonorrheal infection

■ gonorrheal

■ nongonorrheal (generally puerperal, postabortal or traumatic)

Parametritis

Parametritis with abscess (dissection from behind)

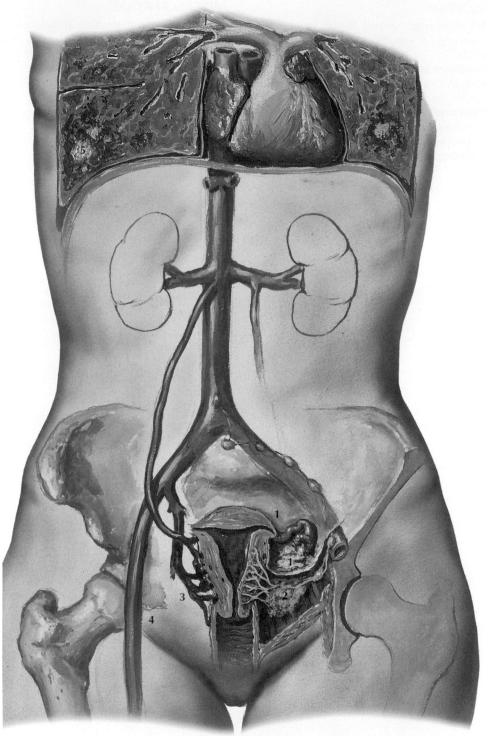

Dissemination of septic endometritis:
(1) Peritonitis
(2) Parametritis (via lymphatics)
(3) Pelvic thrombophlebitis
(4) Femoral thrombophlebitis
(5) Pulmonary infarct or abscess (septic embolus)

HEMATOMETRA

INTRODUCTION

Description: A collection of blood in the body (cavity) of the uterus resulting from obstruction of the normal outflow tract. This obstruction may be due to congenital abnormalities, acquired cervical stenosis, or obstruction by neoplasia.

Prevalence: Uncommon.

Predominant Age: Early reproductive and postmenopausal most common.

Genetics: No genetic pattern.

ETIOLOGY AND PATHOGENESIS

Causes: Obstruction or atresia of the uterine outflow tract (congenital malformation; most common are imperforate hymen and transverse vaginal septum, acquired causes; cervical stenosis from senile atrophy of the endocervix and endometrium, scarring by synechiae, scarring after surgery, radiation, cryocautery, or electrocautery, neoplasia).

Risk Factors: Previous cervical surgery (cone biopsy, cryocoagulation, or electrocautery), menopausal atrophy, cervical neoplasia.

CLINICAL CHARACTERISTICS

Signs and Symptoms:
Asymptomatic (especially in postmenopausal women)
Uterine enlargement (often soft and slightly tender)
Dysmenorrhea, abnormal bleeding, amenorrhea and infertility in premenopausal women
Cyclic abdominal pain

DIAGNOSTIC APPROACH

Differential Diagnosis:
Endometrial hyperplasia/cancer
Endocervical cancer
Pyometra
Leiomyomata
Ovarian neoplasia

Associated Conditions: Cervical cancer, endometrial cancer, tubo-ovarian abscess, and endometriosis.

Workup and Evaluation

Laboratory: No evaluation indicated.

Imaging: Ultrasonography can confirm uterine enlargement and the presence of fluid but cannot define the character of the fluid. The presence of a cervical mass may occasionally be confirmed.

Special Tests: Endometrial biopsy or hysteroscopic evaluation of the uterine cavity should be considered. Gentle probing with a 1–2 mm probe confirms cervical obstruction or stenosis.

Diagnostic Procedures: History, physical examination, ultrasonography, cervical dilation or probing.

Pathologic Findings

Based on cause.

MANAGEMENT AND THERAPY

Nonpharmacologic

General Measures: Evaluation.

Specific Measures: Cervical dilation with or without curettage provides drainage, although it may have to be repeated several times. Antibiotic should be provided to protect against possible colonization by *Bacteroides*, anaerobic *Staphylococcus* and *Streptococcus*, and aerobic coliform bacteria. A mushroom or Foley catheter may be placed to facilitate drainage, but may itself become a source of infection. Definitive therapy is based on cause.

Diet: No specific dietary changes indicated.

Activity: No restriction.

Patient Education: American College of Obstetricians and Gynecologists Patient Education Pamphlet AP095 (*Abnormal Uterine Bleeding*), AP097 (*Cancer of the Uterus*), AP062 (*Dilation and Curettage [D&C]*), AP084 (*Hysteroscopy*).

Drug(s) of Choice

None. Therapy is based on cause and clinical situation. Antibiotic treatment if infection is suspected. (The antibiotic chosen should provide protection against possible colonization by *Bacteroides*, anaerobic *Staphylococcus* and *Streptococcus*, and aerobic coliform bacteria.)

Contraindications: See individual agents.

Precautions: See individual agents.

Interactions: See individual agents.

FOLLOW-UP

Patient Monitoring: Normal health maintenance and periodic reassessment of the cervix and uterus.

Prevention/Avoidance: Avoid unnecessary cervical procedures and limit the scope of therapy when such procedures are necessary. Some authors suggest cervical sounding after such procedures to assess patency although this has not been shown to reduce the incidence of stenosis.

Possible Complications: Infection (leading to pyometra), progression of underlying disease.

Expected Outcome: Based on cause.

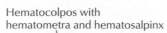

Hematocolpos with
hematometra and hematosalpinx

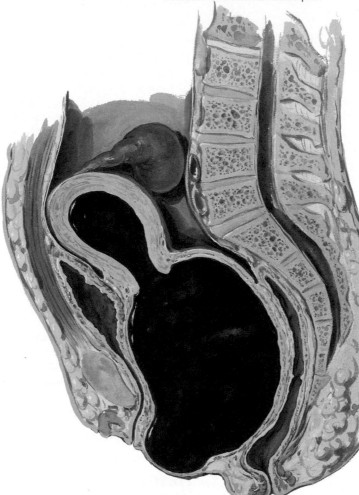

MISCELLANEOUS

Pregnancy Considerations: Incompatible with pregnancy.

***ICD-9-CM* Codes:** 621.4.

REFERENCES

Hatch KD, Fu YS. Cervical and vaginal cancer. In: Berek JS, Adashi EY, Hillard PA, eds. *Novak's Gynecology.* 12th ed. Baltimore, Md: Williams & Wilkins; 1996:1136.

Kinjo K, Kasai T, Ogawa K. Hematometra and ruptured hematosalpinx with ipsilateral renal agenesis presenting as diffuse peritonitis: a case report. *Intens Care Med* 1977;23:354.

Mishell DR, Stenchever MA, Droegemueller W, Herbst AL. *Comprehensive Gynecology.* 3rd ed. St Louis, Mo: Mosby; 1997:482, 484.

Scheerer LJ, Bartolucci L. Transvaginal sonography in the evaluation of hematometra. A report of two cases. *J Reprod Med* 1996;41:205.

Sheih CP, Liao YJ, Liang WW, Lu WT. Sonographic presentation of unilateral hematometra: report of two cases. *J Ultrasound Med* 1995;14:695.

Vernooij CB, Kruitwagen RF, Rodrigus P, Kock HC, Feyen HW. Hematometra after radiotherapy for cervical carcinoma. *Gynecol Oncol* 1997;67:325.

UTERINE PATHOLOGY

INTERMENSTRUAL BLEEDING

INTRODUCTION

Description: Bleeding between otherwise normal menstrual cycles.

Prevalence: Ten percent to fifteen percent of all gynecologic visits involve menstrual disturbances.

Predominant Age: Reproductive, greatest in adolescents and patients who are climacteric.

Genetics: No genetic pattern.

ETIOLOGY AND PATHOGENESIS

Causes: Uterine (pregnancy, endometrial polyps, endometrial hyperplasia, endometrial carcinoma, leiomyomata), cervical (polyps, cervicitis, cervical erosion, cervical dysplasia/neoplasia), vaginal (trauma, infection, atrophy), perineal (vulvar lesions, hemorrhoids).

Risk Factors: None known.

CLINICAL CHARACTERISTICS

Signs and Symptoms:

Intermenstrual bleeding (painless)

Bleeding after intercourse (common)

DIAGNOSTIC APPROACH

Differential Diagnosis:

Pregnancy

Climacteric changes

Anovulation

Endometrial polyps

Uterine leiomyomata

Cervical polyps, lesions, or cervicitis

Endometrial cancer

Endometriosis

Nonuterine sources of bleeding (eg, vaginal, vulvar, or perineal)

Coagulopathy (congenital or acquired)

Iatrogenic (IUCD, medications)

Associated Conditions: Endometrial cancer, endometrial polyps or carcinoma, uterine leiomyomata.

Workup and Evaluation

Laboratory: Testing should be chosen on the basis of diagnoses being considered.

Imaging: No imaging indicated.

Special Tests: A menstrual calendar helps to document the timing and character of the patient's bleeding. Endometrial biopsy, curettage, or hysteroscopy may be indicated.

Diagnostic Procedures: History and physical examination often point to possible causes for further evaluation.

Pathologic Findings

Based on underlying pathologic conditions.

MANAGEMENT AND THERAPY

Nonpharmacologic

General Measures: Evaluation.

Specific Measures: Focused on underlying causation, age of the patient, and contraceptive needs.

Diet: No specific dietary changes indicated.

Activity: No restriction.

Patient Education: Reassurance, American College of Obstetricians and Gynecologists Patient Education Pamphlet AP095 (*Abnormal Uterine Bleeding*), AP049 (*Menstruation*).

Drug(s) of Choice

Based on cause.

FOLLOW-UP

Patient Monitoring: Normal health maintenance.

Prevention/Avoidance: None.

Possible Complications: Anemia.

Expected Outcome: Return to normal menstrual pattern with correction of underlying pathologic condition or periodic progestin therapy.

MISCELLANEOUS

Pregnancy Considerations: No effect on pregnancy aside from that resulting from causative conditions.

ICD-9-CM Codes: 626.6, 626.7 (Postcoital bleeding).

REFERENCES

American College of Obstetricians and Gynecologists. *Dysfunctional Uterine Bleeding.* Washington, DC: ACOG; 1989. ACOG Technical Bulletin 134.

Bayer RL, DeCherney AH. Clinical manifestations and treatment of dysfunctional uterine bleeding. *JAMA* 1993;269:1823.

Cowan BD, Morrison JC. Management of abnormal genital bleeding in girls and women. *N Engl J Med* 1991;324:1710.

Field CS. Dysfunctional uterine bleeding. *Primary Care* 1988;15:561.

Neese RE. Managing abnormal vaginal bleeding. *Postgrad Med* 1991;89:205.

Smith RP. *Gynecology in Primary Care.* Baltimore, Md: Williams & Wilkins; 1997:375.

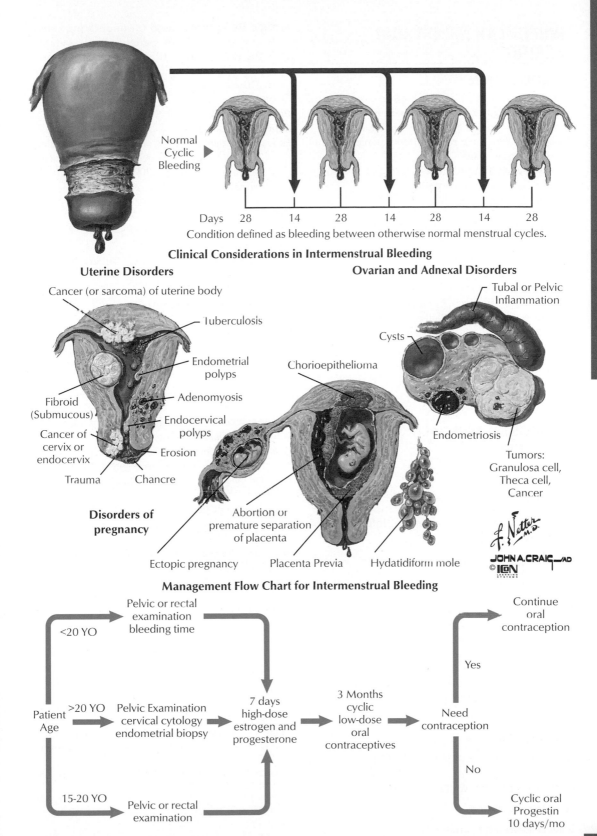

Normal Cyclic Bleeding

Days 28 14 28 14 28 14 28

Condition defined as bleeding between otherwise normal menstrual cycles.

Clinical Considerations in Intermenstrual Bleeding

Uterine Disorders

Cancer (or sarcoma) of uterine body

Tuberculosis

Endometrial polyps

Adenomyosis

Endocervical polyps

Fibroid (Submucous)

Cancer of cervix or endocervix

Erosion

Trauma

Chancre

Disorders of pregnancy

Ectopic pregnancy

Abortion or premature separation of placenta

Placenta Previa

Hydatidiform mole

Chorioepithelioma

Ovarian and Adnexal Disorders

Tubal or Pelvic Inflammation

Cysts

Endometriosis

Tumors: Granulosa cell, Theca cell, Cancer

Management Flow Chart for Intermenstrual Bleeding

Patient Age

<20 YO → Pelvic or rectal examination bleeding time

>20 YO → Pelvic Examination cervical cytology endometrial biopsy

15-20 YO → Pelvic or rectal examination

7 days high-dose estrogen and progesterone

3 Months cyclic low-dose oral contraceptives

Need contraception

Yes → Continue oral contraception

No → Cyclic oral Progestin 10 days/mo

IRREGULAR MENSTRUAL PERIODS

INTRODUCTION

Description: Menstrual cycles that do not follow a rhythmic pattern or whose pattern differs significantly from that expected as "normal."

Prevalence: Ten percent to fifteen percent of all gynecologic visits.

Predominant Age: Reproductive, greatest in adolescents and climacteric patients.

Genetics: No genetic pattern.

ETIOLOGY AND PATHOGENESIS

Causes: Anovulation or oligo-ovulation, climacteric or menopause, hypogonadism, excess estrogen (obese patients, polycystic ovary disease, exogenous estrogen), elevated prolactin, psychosocial conditions (anorexia, bulimia, stress), chronic illness, renal or hepatic failure, thyroid disease.

Risk Factors: Those associated with possible causes.

CLINICAL CHARACTERISTICS

Signs and Symptoms:
Irregular menstrual interval
Variable character of menstrual flow

DIAGNOSTIC APPROACH

Differential Diagnosis:
Climacteric changes
Anovulation
Pregnancy
Ovarian tumors (rare)

Associated Conditions: Anovulation, infertility, and obesity.

Workup and Evaluation

Laboratory: Testing should be chosen on the basis of the different diagnoses under consideration.

Imaging: No imaging indicated.

Special Tests: A menstrual calendar helps to document the timing and character of the patient's bleeding. Endometrial biopsy, curettage, or hysteroscopy may be indicated.

Diagnostic Procedures: History and physical examination often point to possible causes for further evaluation.

Pathologic Findings

Endometrial biopsy may indicate anovulation.

MANAGEMENT AND THERAPY

Nonpharmacologic

General Measures: Evaluation.

Specific Measures: Focused on underlying causation and desires of patient. If anovulation is the cause and fertility is not desired, periodic progestin therapy may be used to stabilize the cycles and suppress intermenstrual bleeding.

Diet: No specific dietary changes indicated.

Activity: No restriction.

Patient Education: Reassurance, American College of Obstetricians and Gynecologists Patient Education Pamphlet AP095 (*Abnormal Uterine Bleeding*), AP049 (*Menstruation*).

Drug(s) of Choice

Medroxyprogesterone acetate 5–10 mg for 1–14 days each month.

Contraindications: Undiagnosed amenorrhea or bleeding.

Precautions: Progestins should not be used until pregnancy has been ruled out.

Alternative Drugs

Norethindrone acetate 5–10 mg for 10–14 days each month. Combination oral contraceptives may also be used.

FOLLOW-UP

Patient Monitoring: Normal health maintenance.

Prevention/Avoidance: None.

Possible Complications: Endometrial hyperplasia or carcinoma if anovulation is left untreated.

Expected Outcome: Return to normal menstrual pattern with correction of underlying pathologic condition or periodic progestin therapy.

MISCELLANEOUS

Pregnancy Considerations: No effect on pregnancy once pregnancy is achieved.

ICD-9-CM Codes: 626.4.

REFERENCES

American College of Obstetricians and Gynecologists. *Dysfunctional Uterine Bleeding.* Washington, DC: ACOG; 1989. ACOG Technical Bulletin 134.

Cowan BD, Morrison JC. Management of abnormal genital bleeding in girls and women. *N Engl J Med* 1991;324:1710.

Field CS. Dysfunctional uterine bleeding. *Primary Care* 1988;15:561.

Fraiser IS. Treatment of ovulatory and anovulatory dysfunctional uterine bleeding with oral progestogens. *Aust N Z J Obstet Gynaecol* 1990;30:353.

Neese RE. Managing abnormal vaginal bleeding. *Postgrad Med* 1991;89:205.

Smith RP. *Gynecology in Primary Care.* Baltimore, Md: Williams & Wilkins; 1997:25, 375.

Neuroendocrine Regulation of Menstrual Cycle

Hypothalamic regulation of pituitary gonadotrophin production and release

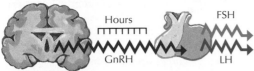

Pulsed release of GnRH by hypothalamus (1 pulse/1–2 hr) permits anterior pituitary production and release of FSH and LH (normal)

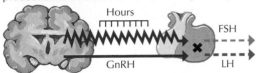

Continuous, excessive, absent, or more frequent GnRH release inhibits FSH and LH production and release (downloading)

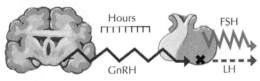

Decreased pulsed release of GnRH decreases LH secretion but increases FSH secretion (slow-pulsing model)

Ovarian feedback modulation of pituitary gonadotropin production and release

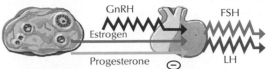

Presence of pulsed GnRH and low estrogen and progesterone levels result in increased levels of pulsed LH and FSH (negative feedback)

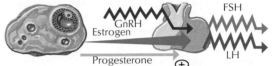

Presence of pulsed GnRH, rapidly increasing levels of estrogen, and small amounts of progesterone results in high pulsed LH and moderately increased pulsed FSH levels (positive feedback)

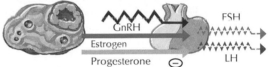

Presence of pulsed GnRH and high levels of estrogen and progesterone results in decreased LH and FSH levels (negative feedback)

Correlation of serum gonadotrophic and ovarian hormone levels and feedback mechanisms

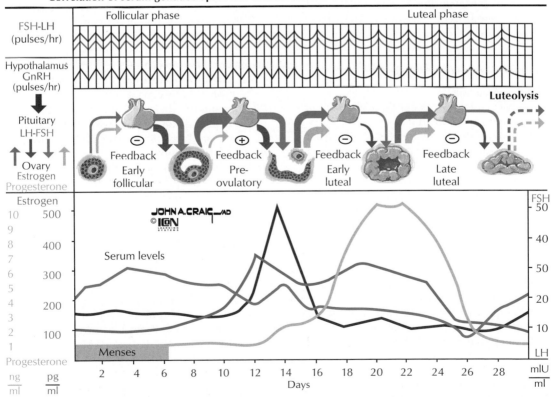

MENORRHAGIA

INTRODUCTION

Description: Heavy menstrual flow. Menorrhagia is generally divided into primary and secondary: Secondary is caused by (secondary to) some clinically identifiable cause; primary is caused by a disturbance of prostaglandin production. Menorrhagia is generally distinguished from acute vaginal bleeding (most often associated with pregnancy and pregnancy complications).

Prevalence: Ten percent to fifteen percent of women experience excessive menstrual flow.

Predominant Age: Reproductive.

Genetics: No genetic pattern.

ETIOLOGY AND PATHOGENESIS

Causes: Secondary—see differential diagnosis following. Primary—overproduction, or an imbalance in the relative ratios of uterine prostaglandins (prostaglandin E_2, prostaglandin I_2, and thromboxane A_2). Some evidence suggests that patients with primary menorrhagia may also have increased fibrinolysis, further enhancing a tendency to bleed.

Risk Factors: Diabetes, obesity, or chronic anovulation (which place the patient at higher risk for endometrial hyperplasia or malignancy), systemic disease, or metabolic disturbances associated with bleeding dyscrasias.

CLINICAL CHARACTERISTICS

Signs and Symptoms:
Menstrual loss of greater than 80 mL, which may result in anemia
Excessive soiling or numbers of menstrual hygiene products used (objective studies have shown a poor correlation with the actual measured blood loss)
Anemia (in the absence of other causes of anemia, anemia is diagnostic for menstrual volumes of greater than 80 mL per cycle)

DIAGNOSTIC APPROACH

Differential Diagnosis:
Uterine leiomyomata (one third of patients will have menorrhagia)
Adenomyosis (40%–50% have menorrhagia)
Endometrial or cervical polyp(s)
Endometrial hypertrophy or hyperplasia
Endometrial cancer
Cervical lesions (including cancer)
Infection (cervicitis, chronic endometritis)
IUCDs

Chronic anovulation
Nongynecologic causes include blood dyscrasia or coagulopathy, hypothyroidism, leukemia, liver disease, systemic lupus erythematosus, thyroid disease
Benign or malignant tumors of ovary (rare)

Associated Conditions: Anemia, toxic shock syndrome (prolonged tampon use).

Workup and Evaluation

Laboratory: Complete blood count, pregnancy test, clotting profile (as indicated).

Imaging: Pelvic ultrasonography (based on diagnosis being considered—limited to the detection of secondary sources).

Special Tests: None indicated.

Diagnostic Procedures: History, physical, and laboratory evaluation.

Pathologic Findings

Based on cause.

MANAGEMENT AND THERAPY

Nonpharmacologic

General Measures: Evaluation, nutritional support.

Specific Measures: Based on cause. Nonsteroidal antiinflammatory agents have been shown to reduce menstrual loss in primary menorrhagia. When taken for this indication, they must be taken continuously for the duration of flow. In patients with intractable menorrhagia or patients being prepared for extirpative surgery or endometrial ablation, therapy with GnRH agonists may be considered.

Diet: No specific dietary changes indicated. Iron supplementation if indicated (either ferrous sulfate or gluconate, 300 mg PO bid to tid).

Activity: No restriction.

Patient Education: American College of Obstetricians and Gynecologists Patient Education Pamphlet AP095 (*Abnormal Bleeding*), AP116 (*Menstrual Hygiene Products*), AP046 (*Dysmenorrhea*).

Drug(s) of Choice

Conjugated estrogen (20–25 mg IV) or intramuscular progestins have been widely advocated.
Oral estrogen (conjugated estrogen 2.5 mg, micronized estradiol 3–6 mg) may be given acutely q2h until the bleeding slows or stops. Estrogen therapy is then maintained for 20–25 additional days, with a progestin added for the last 10 days of treatment.
Combination oral contraceptives containing estradiol and norgestrel (Ovral, 4 tablets a

Primary Menorrhagia

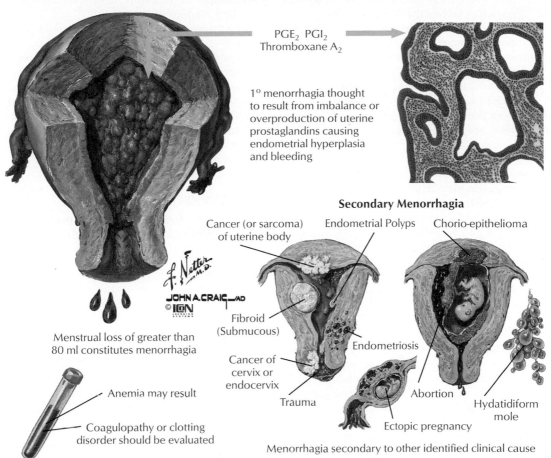

PGE_2 PGI_2
Thromboxane A_2

1° menorrhagia thought to result from imbalance or overproduction of uterine prostaglandins causing endometrial hyperplasia and bleeding

Menstrual loss of greater than 80 ml constitutes menorrhagia

Anemia may result

Coagulopathy or clotting disorder should be evaluated

Secondary Menorrhagia

Cancer (or sarcoma) of uterine body

Endometrial Polyps

Chorio-epithelioma

Fibroid (Submucous)

Endometriosis

Cancer of cervix or endocervix

Trauma

Abortion

Ectopic pregnancy

Hydatidiform mole

Menorrhagia secondary to other identified clinical cause

Management Flowchart for Menorrhagia

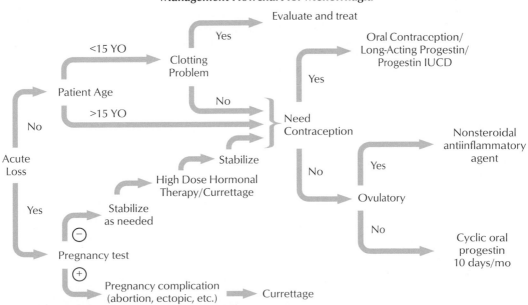

Evaluate and treat

<15 YO — Yes

Clotting Problem

Patient Age

Oral Contraception/ Long-Acting Progestin/ Progestin IUCD

Yes

No

>15 YO

Need Contraception

Acute Loss

No

Nonsteroidal antiinflammatory agent

Yes

Stabilize

High Dose Hormonal Therapy/Currettage

No

Ovulatory

Yes

Stabilize as needed

Yes

No

Pregnancy test

⊖

Cyclic oral progestin 10 days/mo

⊕

Pregnancy complication (abortion, ectopic, etc.) → Currettage

day for 3–5 days or until bleeding stops, followed by 1qd for the duration of the pack or 4 tablets the first day, followed by 3 for 1 day, 2 the next day, and then 1qd for the remainder of the package).

Contraindications: Therapy should not be instituted until the possibility of pregnancy has been evaluated and a working diagnosis has been established.

Precautions: See individual agents.

Interactions: See individual agents.

Alternative Drugs

When the endometrium is reasonably intact, high-dose progestin may be used to stop acute uterine bleeding (medroxyprogesterone acetate 10 mg PO tid or IM depot medroxyprogesterone acetate, 150–300 mg). Nonsteroidal antiinflammatory agents have been shown to reduce menstrual loss 30%–50% when taken for the duration of flow (eg, meclofenamate sodium 100 mg PO tid during flow, mefenamic acid [Ponstel] 250 mg PO tid during flow).

FOLLOW-UP

Patient Monitoring: Normal health maintenance. Watch for anemia. Patients who are at risk for endometrial hyperplasia or neoplasia, or those who do not respond to initial therapy may require endometrial biopsy, hysteroscopy, or diagnostic curettage.

Prevention/Avoidance: Based on cause. If contraception is desired, oral combination contraceptives, or continuously dosed progestins (orally, by injection, or as a medicated intrauterine device), or oral contraceptives (either monophasic or polyphasic) are reasonable options. In patients with intractable menorrhagia or in patients being prepared for extirpative surgery or endometrial ablation, therapy

with GnRH agonists may be considered for a maximum of 6 months. Cost and side effects limit this approach.

Possible Complications: Anemia, hypovolemia (acute loss).

Expected Outcome: Based on cause; most patients respond to conservative therapy. The most successful therapy is directed at the underlying cause. Once acute control has been gained, cyclic estrogen/progestin therapy should be continued for an additional 3 months. During this interval, additional diagnostic studies may be considered and plans laid for long-term management, should it be necessary.

MISCELLANEOUS

Pregnancy Considerations: No effect on pregnancy.

ICD-9-CM Codes: 626.2, 626.3 (Pubertal), 627.0 (Premenopausal).

REFERENCES

Anderson ABM, Haynes PJ, Cuillebaud J, et al. Reduction of menstrual blood loss by prostaglandin synthetase inhibitors. *Lancet* 1976;1:774.

Cohen BJB, Gibor J. Anemia and menstrual blood loss. *Obstet Gynecol Surv* 1980;35:597.

Duncan KM, Hart LL. Nonsteroidal antiinflammatory drugs in menorrhagia. *Ann Pharmacother* 1993;27:1353.

Fraser IS. Hysteroscopy and laparoscopy in women with menorrhagia. *Am J Obstet Gynecol* 1990;165:1264.

Higham JM. The medical management of menorrhagia. *Br J Hosp Med* 1991;45:19.

Liddell H. Menorrhagia. *N Z Med J* 1993;106:255.

Long CA, Gast MJ. Menorrhagia. *Obstet Gynecol Clin North Am* 1990;17:343.

Shaw RW. Treating the patient with menorrhagia. *Br J Obstet Gynaecol* 1994;101(suppl 11):1.

Wood C. Treatment of menorrhagia. *Aust Fam Physician* 1995;24:825.

POSTMENOPAUSAL VAGINAL BLEEDING

INTRODUCTION

Description: Vaginal bleeding that occurs in women who have passed menopause. As a symptom only, postmenopausal bleeding requires evaluation to rule out processes that may threaten the long-term health of the patient.

Prevalence: Common.

Predominant Age: 50 or older.

Genetics: No genetic pattern.

ETIOLOGY AND PATHOGENESIS

Causes: Systemic—estrogen, estrogen/progesterone, thrombocytopenia. Uterine—endometrial cancer, endometrial hyperplasia, endometritis, submucous leiomyomata. Cervical sources—carcinoma, cervical eversion, cervicitis, condyloma, polyps. Vaginal sources—adenosis, atrophic change, carcinoma, foreign bodies (condom, pessary, tampon), infection, lacerations (abortion attempts, coital injury, trauma). Vulvar and extragenital sources—atrophy, condyloma, cystitis/urethritis, gastrointestinal (cancer, diverticulitis, inflammatory bowel disease), hematuria, hemorrhoids, infection, labial varices, neoplasm, trauma, urethral caruncle, urethral diverticula, urethral prolapse/eversion.

Risk Factors: Estrogen replacement therapy, others based on specific pathologic conditions.

CLINICAL CHARACTERISTICS

Signs and Symptoms:
 Painless vaginal bleeding (spontaneous or iatrogenic)
 Pink or dark discharge noted on the underwear or when wiping after urination

DIAGNOSTIC APPROACH

Differential Diagnosis:
 Pregnancy (in the climacteric period or early menopause)
 Iatrogenic bleeding (estrogen, estrogen/progestin)
 Endometrial cancer
 Endometrial disease (hyperplasia, endometritis)
 Vaginal atrophy
 Endometrial polyps
 Cervicitis or cervical lesions (including polyps and cancer)
 Vaginitis
 Retained IUCD

 Nongynecologic sources of bleeding (eg, perineal or rectal)

Associated Conditions: See differential diagnosis.

Workup and Evaluation

Laboratory: No evaluation indicated.

Imaging: Saline infusion ultrasonography (sonohysterography) may allow measurement of endometrial thickness and the possibility of endometrial polyps. The exact role of this technology is yet to be established.

Special Tests: Endometrial biopsy should be strongly considered to evaluate the cause and to check for the possibility of a malignancy.

Diagnostic Procedures: History and physical examination, cervical cytologic examination, endometrial sampling.

Pathologic Findings

Varies with cause.

MANAGEMENT AND THERAPY

Nonpharmacologic

General Measures: Evaluation.

Specific Measures: Based on cause identified.

Diet: No specific dietary changes indicated.

Activity: No restriction.

Patient Education: Reassurance, American College of Obstetricians and Gynecologists Patient Education Pamphlet 047 (*The Menopause Years*), AP066 (*Hormone Replacement Therapy*), AB008 (Menopause packet with 3 titles).

Drug(s) of Choice

(Based on pathophysiologic condition present)

In many cases of postmenopausal bleeding, the endometrium is thin and atrophic. This endometrium is prone to irregular slough, resulting in erratic, although generally light, bleeding. Because the endometrial tissue is so denuded, it does not respond well to progestational agents. Estrogen, alone initially or in combination with progestin therapy, is required to induce initial growth and the development of progestin receptors to effect endometrial stabilization.

FOLLOW-UP

Patient Monitoring: Postmenopausal bleeding should be presumed to indicate the presence of a malignancy, until proved otherwise. The only exception to this is the withdrawal bleeding that occurs as a part of cyclic estrogen-progesterone hormone replacement therapy.

Prevention/Avoidance: None.

Evaluation of Postmenopausal Bleeding

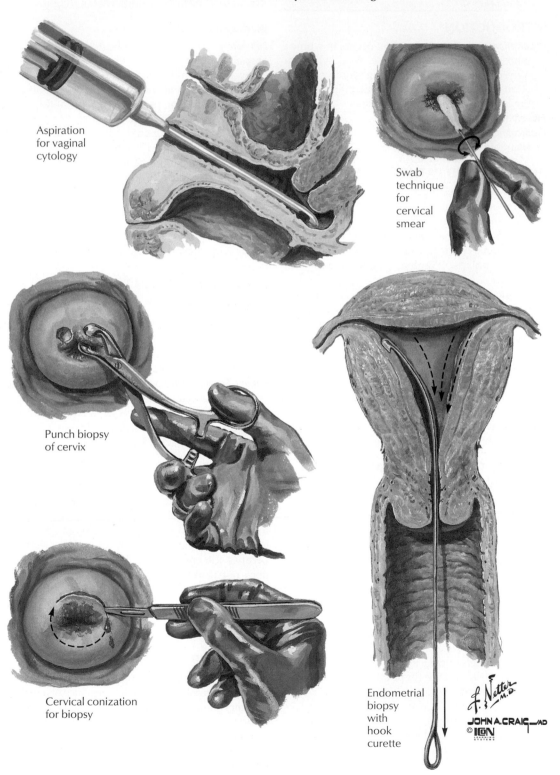

Aspiration for vaginal cytology

Swab technique for cervical smear

Punch biopsy of cervix

Cervical conization for biopsy

Endometrial biopsy with hook curette

UTERINE PATHOLOGY

Possible Complications: Progression of undiagnosed malignancy.

Expected Outcome: If diagnosis is prompt and appropriate therapy is instituted, the outcome should be excellent.

MISCELLANEOUS

Pregnancy Considerations: Not applicable.

ICD-9-CM Codes: 627.1.

REFERENCES

Feldman S, Berkowitz RS, Tosteson ANA. Cost-effectiveness of strategies to evaluate postmenopausal bleeding. *Obstet Gynecol* 1993;81:968.

Ferry J, Farnsworth A, Webster M, Wren B. The efficacy of the Pipelle endometrial biopsy in detecting endometrial carcinoma. *Aust N Z J Obstet Gynaecol* 1993;33:76.

Goldschmit R, Katz Z, Blickstein I, Caspi B, Dgani R. The accuracy of endometrial Pipelle sampling with and without sonographic measurement of endometrial thickness. *Obstet Gynecol* 1993;82:727.

Goldstein SR. Use of ultrasono-hysterography for triage of perimenopausal patients with unexplained uterine bleeding. *Am J Obstet Gynecol* 1994;170:565.

Reid PC, Brown VA, Fothergill DJ. Outpatient investigation of postmenopausal bleeding. *Br J Obstet Gynaecol* 1993;100:498.

SARCOMA (UTERINE)

INTRODUCTION

Description: Sarcomatous change in the tissues of the Müllerian system including the endometrial stroma and myometrium. Mixed Müllerian sarcomas may include elements not native to the genital tract such as cartilage or bone (heterologous type).

Prevalence: One percent to two percent of uterine malignancies, 1 of 800 smooth muscle tumors, 0.67 of 100,000 women older than age 20.

Predominant Age: 40–60, mean age 52.

Genetics: No genetic pattern. Seen more often in black women although there is no racial predisposition.

ETIOLOGY AND PATHOGENESIS

Causes: Etiology unknown.
Risk Factors: Leiomyomata (?).

CLINICAL CHARACTERISTICS

Signs and Symptoms:
Bleeding and passage of tissue
Lower abdominal pain and mass
Rapid enlargement of the uterus
Uterine growth after menopause

DIAGNOSTIC APPROACH

Differential Diagnosis:
Benign leiomyomata
Cervical cancer
Ovarian cancer metastatic to the endometrium
Metachronous Müllerian tumor

Associated Conditions: Breast or colon cancer.

Workup and Evaluation

Laboratory: No evaluation indicated except for preoperative screening.

Imaging: Chest radiograph (for metastases), transvaginal ultrasonography, or sonohysterography may be useful.

Special Tests: None. (Endometrial biopsy results are rarely positive.)

Diagnostic Procedures: Diagnosis rarely made before surgery.

Pathologic Findings

Based on cell type and tissue involved. Most often soft fleshy tumors with a gray-yellow or pink character. Areas of necrosis and hemorrhage are common (75%). Vascular invasion is present in 10%–20% of patients. Higher mitotic rates are associated with greater atypia.

MANAGEMENT AND THERAPY

Nonpharmacologic

General Measures: Evaluation and staging.

Specific Measures: Surgical exploration with hysterectomy, bilateral salpingo-oophorectomy, cytologic examination of the abdomen and diaphragm, and paraaortic node sampling. Radiation to the vaginal cuff reduces local recurrence (although objective evidence of improved survival is lacking).

Diet: No specific dietary changes indicated except as dictated by surgical therapy.

Activity: No restriction except as dictated by surgical therapy.

Patient Education: American College of Obstetricians and Gynecologists Patient Education Pamphlet AP097 (*Cancer of the Uterus*), AP008 (*Understanding Hysterectomy*), AP080 (*Preparing for Surgery*), AP095 (*Abnormal Uterine Bleeding*), AP074 (*Uterine Fibroids*).

Drug(s) of Choice

None. (Adjuvant chemotherapy [vincristine, actinomycin D, and cyclophosphamide or doxorubicin (Adriamycin)] has been advocated but an improvement in prognosis has not been demonstrated.)

FOLLOW-UP

Patient Monitoring: Follow-up Pap smears from vaginal cuff every 3 months for 2 years then every 6 months for 3 years, then yearly. Chest radiograph annually.

Prevention/Avoidance: None.

Possible Complications: Distant spread.

Expected Outcome: Depends on stage of tumor and number of mitotic figures present. Overall survival is approximately 20% at 5 years; patients with stage I and II disease have survival rates of up to 40%.

MISCELLANEOUS

Pregnancy Considerations: Generally not a consideration because they are unlikely to coexist.

ICD-9-CM Codes: Specific to cell type and location.

REFERENCES

Aaro LA, Symmonds RE, Dockerty MB. Sarcoma of the uterus. A clinical and pathologic study of 177 cases. *Am J Obstet Gynecol* 1966;94:101.

American College of Obstetricians and Gynecologists. *Cancer of the Ovary.* Washington, DC: ACOG; 1990. ACOG Technical Bulletin 141.

American College of Obstetricians and Gynecologists. *Classification and Staging of Gynecologic Malignancies.* Washington, DC: ACOG; 1991. ACOG Technical Bulletin 155.

Barter JF, Smith EB, Szpak CA, Hinshaw W, Clarke-Peterson DL. Leiomyosarcoma of the uterus: clinicopathologic study of 21 cases. *Gynecol Oncol* 1985; 21:220.

Gallup DG, Cordray DR. Leiomyosarcoma of the uterus: case report and a review. *Obstet Gynecol Surv* 1979;34:300.

Kempson RL, Bari W. Uterine sarcomas. Classification, diagnosis, and prognosis. *Hum Pathol* 1970;1:331.

Shakfeh AM, Woodruff JD. Primary ovarian sarcomas: report of 46 cases and review of literature. *Obstet Gynecol* 1987;42:331.

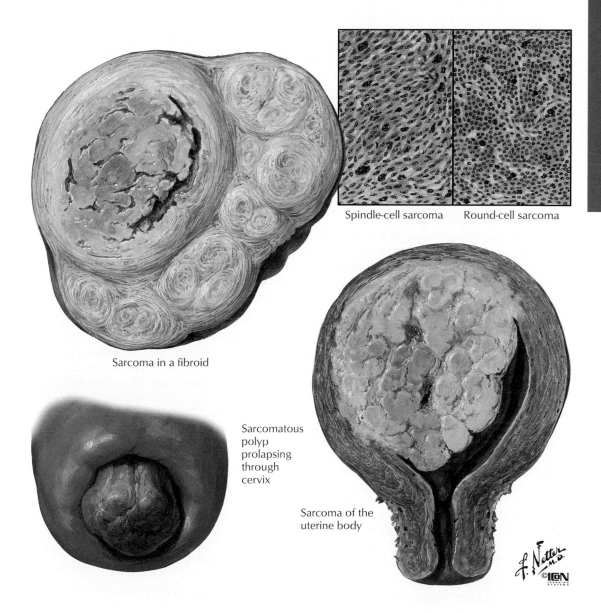

Spindle-cell sarcoma   Round-cell sarcoma

Sarcoma in a fibroid

Sarcomatous polyp prolapsing through cervix

Sarcoma of the uterine body

UTERINE ANOMALIES: BICORNUATE, SEPTATE, AND UNICORNUATE UTERUS

INTRODUCTION

Description: Incomplete formation of the uterus resulting in one or two separate halves or horns or a single uterus with a central septum. (The central septum may divide the uterine cavity either partially or completely. The two resulting halves may be of unequal size or volume.) In its most extensive form, duplication of the cervix and vaginal canal also may occur. These abnormalities are associated with renal agenesis and blind vaginal pouches that may become filled with menstrual fluid after puberty, resulting in a painful mass.

Prevalence: Estimated to be 0.1% of female births. Septate or arcuate uterine anomalies may be present in up to 3% of women.

Predominant Age: Congenital.

Genetics: May be transmitted by polygenic or multifactorial pattern.

ETIOLOGY AND PATHOGENESIS

Causes: Failure of the fusion of the Müllerian ducts, which normally takes place near the beginning of the 10th week of gestation. This may vary from septation of the uterus to complete duplication of the uterus, cervix, and vaginal canal. Most septations are due to a failure of the normal processes of development of the Müllerian system between the 10th and 13th week of gestation when the lower portion of the median septum of the uterus is resorbed, or between the 13th and 20th week when the upper septum (in the uterine body) is resorbed. In utero exposure to diethylstilbestrol has been associated with a T-shaped uterine cavity similar to the arcuate form of a septate uterus. A unicornuate uterus may result from a failure of the normal formation or the destruction of one the Müllerian ducts. This may occur if there is a lack of development of the mesonephric system on the affected side resulting in a failure of the associated Müllerian system. (In these patients, the ipsilateral kidney and ureter are usually absent.)

Risk Factors: None known.

CLINICAL CHARACTERISTICS

Signs and Symptoms:

Asymptomatic

Recurrent abortion (15%–25% of patients with recurrent abortions have uterine abnormalities; there is a 50% risk of pregnancy loss when the uterus is unicornuate)

Premature labor (20% risk for unicornuate uterus)

Uterine pain or rupture in early pregnancy

Abnormal presentation in labor (breech or transverse position)

Inability to stop menstrual flow using tampons (when there is duplication of the vagina as well)

When outflow is obstructed—Hematometra

Dysmenorrhea, abdominal pain, pelvic mass, abrupt blood discharge

DIAGNOSTIC APPROACH

Differential Diagnosis:

Leiomyomata

Adnexal mass

Endometriosis

Chromosomal abnormality resulting in recurrent abortion

Associated Conditions: Endometriosis (75% when outflow obstruction is present), pelvic adhesions, recurrent abortion, infertility, dysmenorrhea, dyspareunia, hematocolpos, and renal anomalies (contralateral pelvic, horseshoe, or absent kidney).

Workup and Evaluation

Laboratory: No evaluation indicated.

Imaging: Hysterosalpingography, ultrasonography, or sonohysterography. Magnetic resonance imaging may be used, but expense and availability limit its utility.

Special Tests: Hysteroscopy or laparoscopy may be required to complete the evaluation.

Diagnostic Procedures: Physical examination, imaging, and direct observation by hysteroscopy and/or laparoscopy. Differentiation between septate and bicornuate uterine anomalies requires visualization of the uterine fundus.

Pathologic Findings

In patients with an unicornuate uterus, a normal ovary and tube are generally present. A normal ovary may be present on the opposite side as well. The septate uterus is characterized by the presence of a fibrous septum of variable length with poor vascularization.

MANAGEMENT AND THERAPY

Nonpharmacologic

General Measures: Evaluation and education.

Specific Measures: Patients with nonobstructive abnormalities require no therapy. Patients with

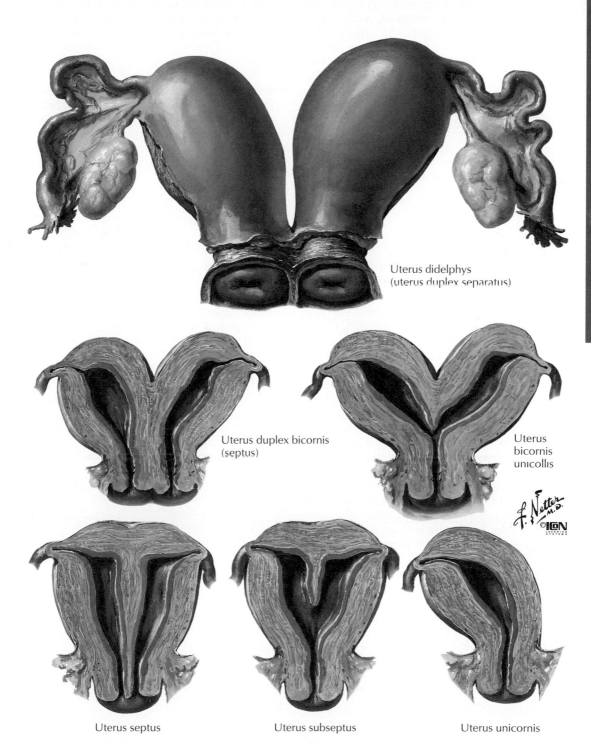

Uterus didelphys
(uterus duplex separatus)

Uterus duplex bicornis
(septus)

Uterus
bicornis
unicollis

Uterus septus

Uterus subseptus

Uterus unicornis

recurrent fetal wastage may be considered for uterine reunification (metroplasty) procedures or the excision of any septum, usually by operative hysteroscopy. Patients with a unicornuate deformity and recurrent fetal wastage should be counseled about adoption or the possibilities of in vitro fertilization with implantation into a host uterus.

Diet: No specific dietary changes indicated.

Activity: No restriction.

Patient Education: Reassurance, American College of Obstetricians and Gynecologists Patient Education Pamphlet AP079 (*If Your Baby Is Breech*), AP100 (*Repeated Miscarriage*), AP090 (*Early Pregnancy Loss: Miscarriage, Ectopic Pregnancy, and Molar Pregnancy*).

Drug(s) of Choice

None. (Estrogen therapy is often given for 1–2 months after resection of a uterine septum, although the need for this is still debated.)

FOLLOW-UP

Patient Monitoring: Normal health maintenance.

Prevention/Avoidance: None.

Possible Complications: Obstruction of the outflow of menstrual blood is associated with a 75% chance of endometriosis with resultant pelvic scarring and infertility. There is an increased risk of ectopic pregnancy and early pregnancy loss (33%–35%).

Expected Outcome: Normal reproduction is frequently possible without intervention (25% of cases) for patients with a bicornuate uterus; metroplasty is associated with an increased likelihood of success when pregnancy failures have occurred (80%–90%). When the only abnormality is a uterine septum, normal reproduction is generally possible without interven-

tion (85% success). For patients with a unicornuate uterus, a live birth rate of 40% may be expected; outcomes are not statistically different from those experienced by women with didelphic uteri.

MISCELLANEOUS

Pregnancy Considerations: Increased risk of pregnancy loss, premature delivery, or fetal malpresentation. The risk of ectopic pregnancy is increased for patients with a unicornuate uterus.

ICD-9-CM **Codes:** 752.2 (Unicornuate or bicornuate uterus), 752.3 (Septate uterus).

REFERENCES

Buttram VC. Müllerian anomalies and their management. *Fertil Steril* 1983;40:159.

Golan A, Langer R, Bukovsky I, Caspi E. Congenital anomalies of the müllerian system. *Fertil Steril* 1981;51:747.

Jones HW. Reproductive impairment and the malformed uterus. *Fertil Steril* 1981;36:137.

Hay D. Uterus unicornis and its relationship to pregnancy. *J Obstet Gynecol Br Emp* 1961;68:371.

Mayo-Smith WW, Lee MJ. MR imaging of the female pelvis. *Clin Radiol* 1995;50:667.

Moutos DM, Damewood MD, Schlaff WD, Rock JA. A comparison of the reproductive outcome between women with a unicornuate uterus and women with a didelphic uterus. *Fertil Steril* 1992;58:88.

Pinsonneault O, Goldstein DP. Obstructing malformations of the uterus and vagina. *Fertil Steril* 1985; 44:241.

Reinhold C, Hricak H, Forstner R, et al. Primary amenorrhea: evaluation with MR imaging. *Radiology* 1997;203:383.

Rock JA, Jones HJ. The double uterus associated with an obstructed hemivagina and ipsilateral renal agenesis. *Am J Obstet Gynecol* 1980;138:339.

Woodward PJ, Wagner BJ, Farley TE. MR imaging in the evaluation of female infertility. *Radiographics* 1993;13:293.

UTERINE LEIOMYOMATA

INTRODUCTION

Description: A benign connective tissue tumor found in or around the uterus, which may be disseminated in rare cases.

Prevalence: Thirty percent of all women, 40%–50% of women older than 50.

Predominant Age: 35–50 or older.

Genetics: No genetic pattern.

ETIOLOGY AND PATHOGENESIS

Causes: Unknown; thought to arise from a single smooth muscle cell. Estrogen, progesterone, and epidermal growth factor all thought to stimulate growth.

Risk Factors: Nulliparity, early menarche, African-Americans (4- to 10-fold increase in risk).

CLINICAL CHARACTERISTICS

Signs and Symptoms:
Uterine enlargement and distortion
Pelvic or abdominal heaviness, low back pain
Pressure on bowel or bladder (ie, frequency, infrequently causing urinary retention or hydroureter to develop)
Dysmenorrhea, menorrhagia, intermenstrual bleeding (30%–40% of patients)
Acute pain (with torsion or degeneration)
Submucous fibroids may prolapse through the cervix

DIAGNOSTIC APPROACH

Differential Diagnosis:
Pregnancy
Adnexal mass
Other pelvic or abdominal tumor
Pelvic kidney
Urachal cyst
Urinary retention

Associated Conditions: Dysmenorrhea, menorrhagia, miscarriage, and infertility (rare).

Workup and Evaluation

Laboratory: No evaluation indicated, hemoglobin or hematocrit if anemia suspected.

Imaging: Ultrasonography only when the diagnosis is uncertain.

Special Tests: None indicated.

Diagnostic Procedures: Pelvic examination is generally sufficient and may be augmented by ultrasonography, but generally is not required.

Pathologic Findings

Localized proliferation of smooth muscle cells surrounded by a pseudocapsule of compressed muscle fibers. Seventy percent to eighty percent of uterine fibroids are found within the wall of the uterus, with 5%–10% lying below the endometrium and less than 5% arising in or near the cervix. Multiple fibroids are found in up to 85% of patients. Myomas may weigh up to 100 pounds.

MANAGEMENT AND THERAPY

Nonpharmacologic

General Measures: Reassurance, observation.

Specific Measures: Surgical therapy (hysterectomy or myomectomy) for uncontrollable symptoms, rapid growth, or uncertain diagnosis. Medical therapy with GnRH agonists may be used temporarily to prepare for surgery, pregnancy, or menopause.

Diet: No specific dietary changes indicated.

Activity: No restriction.

Patient Education: Reassurance, American College of Obstetricians and Gynecologists Patient Education Pamphlet AP074 (*Uterine Fibroids*) or AP008 (*Understanding Hysterectomy*).

Drug(s) of Choice

GnRH agonists (therapy limited to 6 months)—buserelin (Depo-Lupron 3.75 mg IM monthly or Depo-Lupron 3-month 22.5 mg IM every 3 months), goserelin (Zoladex 3.6 mg implant SC monthly or Zoladex 3-month implant SC every 3 months).

Contraindications: Pregnancy or possible pregnancy.

Precautions: Must exclude possibility of pregnancy before medical therapy. GnRH agonists may produce significant symptoms of estrogen withdrawal (menopause).

Interactions: None known.

Alternative Drugs

Synarel nasal solution 2 mg/mL one spray in alternate nostril in AM and PM (not labeled for the treatment of leiomyomata).
Nonsteroidal antiinflammatory drugs may be used to reduce menorrhagia.
Medroxyprogesterone acetate (depot) 100–300 mg IM every 1–3 months may be used to suppress menstruation.

FOLLOW-UP

Patient Monitoring: Watch for development of symptoms. Monitor uterine size.

Prevention/Avoidance: None.

Possible Complications: Possibility of bone loss with prolonged GnRH therapy.

Expected Outcome: Leiomyomata generally stop growing after menopause (even with estrogen replacement). Recurrence after myomectomy is common.

Uterine Leiomyomata

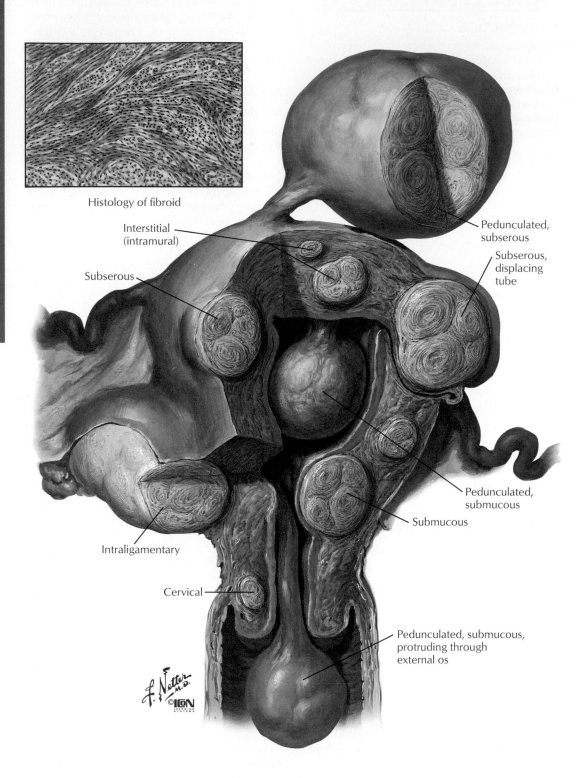

Histology of fibroid

Interstitial (intramural)

Subserous

Pedunculated, subserous

Subserous, displacing tube

Pedunculated, submucous

Submucous

Intraligamentary

Cervical

Pedunculated, submucous, protruding through external os

MISCELLANEOUS

Pregnancy Considerations: May (rarely) interfere with early pregnancy or obstruct delivery. Fibroids may grow rapidly or undergo hemorrhage or necrosis and may occasionally even be a cause for disseminated intravascular coagulopathy. Cesarian section should be considered if the endometrial cavity is entered during myomectomy.

***ICD-9-CM* Codes:** 218.0 (Submucous), 218.1 (Intramural), 218.2 (Subserous), 218.9 (Unspecified).

REFERENCES

American College of Obstetricians and Gynecologists. *Uterine Leiomyomata.* Washington, DC: ACOG; 1994. ACOG Technical Bulletin 192.

American Fertility Society. *Myomas and Reproductive Dysfunction: Guideline for Practice.* Birmingham, Ala: AFS, 1992.

Cramer SF, Horiszny JA, Leppert P. Epidemiology of uterine leiomyomas. *J Reprod Med* 1995;40:595.

Reiter RC, Wagner PL, Gambone JC. Routine hysterectomy for large asymptomatic uterine leiomyomata: a reappraisal. *Obstet Gynecol* 1992;79:481.

Vollenhoven BJ, Lawrence AS, Healy DL. Uterine fibroids: a clinical review. *Br J Obstet Gynaecol* 1990;97:285.

UTERINE PROLAPSE

INTRODUCTION

Description: Loss of the normal support mechanism resulting in descent of the uterus down the vaginal canal. In the extreme, this may result in the uterus descending beyond the vulva to a position outside the body (procidentia).

Prevalence: Some degree of uterine descent is common in parous women.

Predominant Age: Late reproductive and beyond; incidence increases with the loss of estrogen.

Genetics: No genetic pattern.

ETIOLOGY AND PATHOGENESIS

Causes: Loss of normal structural support as a result of trauma (childbirth), surgery, chronic intraabdominal pressure elevation (such as obesity, chronic cough, or heavy lifting), or intrinsic weakness. Most common sites of injury are the cardinal and uterosacral ligaments and the levator ani muscles that form the pelvic floor, which may relax or rupture. Rarely, increased intraabdominal pressure from a pelvic mass or ascites may weaken pelvic support and result in prolapse. Injury to or neuropathy of the S_1 to S_4 nerve roots may also result in decreased muscle tone and pelvic relaxation.

Risk Factors: Birth trauma, chronic intraabdominal pressure elevation (such as obesity, chronic cough, or heavy lifting), intrinsic tissue weakness, or atrophic changes resulting from estrogen loss.

CLINICAL CHARACTERISTICS

Signs and Symptoms:
- Pelvic pressure or heaviness (a sense of "falling out")
- Mass or protrusion at or beyond the vaginal entrance
- New onset or paradoxical resolution of urinary incontinence
- Drying, thickening, chronic inflammation, and ulceration of the exposed tissues, which may result in bleeding, discharge, or odor

DIAGNOSTIC APPROACH

Differential Diagnosis:
- Cystocele
- Urethrocele
- Rectocele
- Enterocele
- Prolapsed uterine leiomyomata
- Bartholin's cyst
- Vaginal cyst or tumor
- Cervical hypertrophy (with normal uterine support)

Associated Conditions: Urinary incontinence, pelvic pain, dyspareunia, intermenstrual or postmenopausal bleeding. Almost always associated with a cystocele, rectocele, and enterocele.

Workup and Evaluation

Laboratory: No evaluation indicated.

Imaging: No imaging indicated.

Special Tests: Urodynamics testing may be considered if voiding or continence is altered.

Diagnostic Procedures: History and physical examination.

Pathologic Findings

Tissue change is common because of mechanical trauma and desiccation.

MANAGEMENT AND THERAPY

Nonpharmacologic

General Measures: Weight reduction, modification of activity (lifting), addressing factors such as chronic cough.

Specific Measures: Minimal prolapse does not require therapy. For those with more severe prolapse or symptoms, pessary therapy (Smith-Hodge, donut, cube, or inflatable ball), surgical repair, or hysterectomy (with colporrhaphy) should be considered. Postmenopausal women should receive estrogen and progesterone replacement therapy for at least 30 days before pessary fitting or surgical repair.

Diet: No specific dietary changes indicated.

Activity: No restriction.

Patient Education: Reassurance, American College of Obstetricians and Gynecologists Patient Education Pamphlet AP012 (*Pelvic Support Problems*), AP081 (*Urinary Incontinence*).

Drug(s) of Choice

Estrogen and progesterone replacement therapy (for postmenopausal patients) improves tissue tone and healing and is often prescribed before surgical repair or as an adjunct to pessary therapy.

Contraindications: Estrogen therapy should not be used if undiagnosed vaginal bleeding is present.

FOLLOW-UP

Patient Monitoring: Normal health maintenance. If a pessary is used, frequent follow-up (both initially and long-term) is required. (Most recommend monthly checks of the vaginal epithelium for lesions and to reassess pessary placement and fit.)

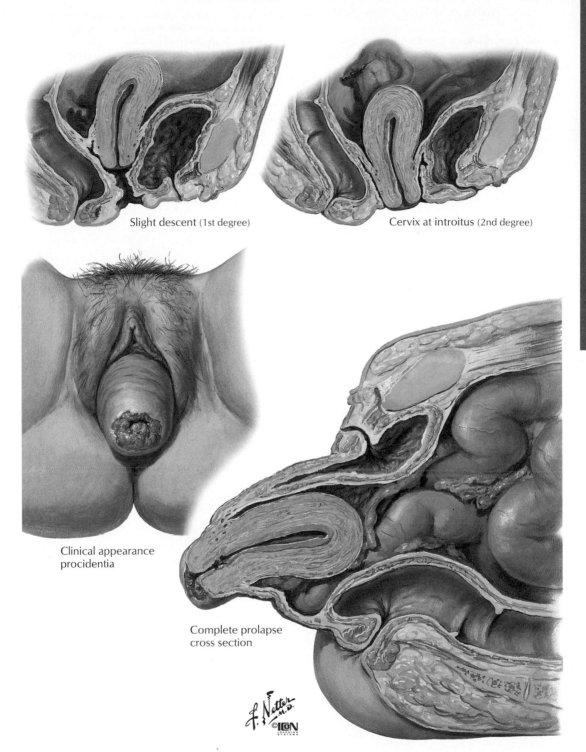

Slight descent (1st degree)

Cervix at introitus (2nd degree)

Clinical appearance
procidentia

Complete prolapse
cross section

Prevention/Avoidance: Maintenance of normal weight, avoidance of known (modifiable) risk factors.

Possible Complications: Thickening or ulceration of the vaginal tissues and cervix, urinary incontinence, kinking of the ureters, obstipation.

Expected Outcome: Uterine descent tends to worsen with time. If uncorrected, complete prolapse is associated with vaginal and cervical skin changes, ulceration, and bleeding.

MISCELLANEOUS

ICD-9-CM Codes: 618.1 (codes 618.2–618.4 are used when cystocele, urethrocele, or rectocele is present).

REFERENCES

American College of Obstetricians and Gynecologists. *Pelvic Organ Prolapse.* Washington, DC: ACOG; 1995. ACOG Technical Bulletin 214.

Beecham CT. Classification of vaginal relaxation. *Am J Obstet Gynecol* 1980;136:957.

Miller DC. Contemporary use of the pessary. In: Sciarra JJ, ed. *Gynecology and Obstetrics.* Vol 1. Philadelphia, Pa: JB Lippincott; 1991;39:1.

Porges RF. Abnormalities of pelvic support. In: Sciarra JJ, ed. *Gynecology and Obstetrics.* Vol 1. Philadelphia, Pa: JB Lippincott; 1993;61:1.

Thomas AG, Brodman ML, Dottino PR, Bodian C, Friedman F Jr, Bogursky E. Manchester procedure vs vaginal hysterectomy for uterine prolapse: a comparison. *J Reprod Med* 1995;40:299.

Obstetrical Conditions

ABNORMALITIES OF PLACENTAL IMPLANTATION

INTRODUCTION

Description: Failure of the normal process of decidua formation results in a placental implantation in which the villi adhere directly to (accreta, 78%), invade into (increta, 17%), or through (percreta, 5%) the myometrium. One portion (partial) or all (total) of the placenta may be involved.

Prevalence: Difficult to assess; estimates vary from 1 in 1667 to 1 in 70,000 pregnancies (average 1 in 7000).

Predominant Age: Reproductive, average 29.

Genetics: No genetic pattern.

ETIOLOGY AND PATHOGENESIS

Causes: Abnormal decidua formation at the time of placental implantation. (Imperfect development of the fibrinoid [Nitabuch's] layer.) Abnormal site of placental implantation (previa, 64% of placenta accreta, cornual or lower uterine segment, or uterine scars such as site of previous cesarean delivery).

Risk Factors: Placenta previa (without previous uterine surgery 5%, with previous surgery 15%–70%), previous cesarean delivery, multigravidity (1 of 500,000 for parity <3, 1 of 2500 for parity >6), older pregnant women, previous uterine curettage, previous uterine sepsis, previous manual removal of the placenta, leiomyomata, uterine malformation, prior abortion.

CLINICAL CHARACTERISTICS

Signs and Symptoms:
Failure of normal placental separation
Abnormally heavy bleeding after delivery of the placenta (may be life-threatening)
History of antepartum hemorrhage

DIAGNOSTIC APPROACH

Differential Diagnosis:
Placenta previa
Uterine rupture with expulsion of the placenta
Uterine rupture at the time of manual removal of the placenta

Associated Conditions: Placenta previa (15%), postpartum hemorrhage.

Workup and Evaluation

Laboratory: Complete blood count after delivery to assess blood loss (which may be excessive).

Imaging: No imaging indicated. (Ultrasonography has been used to make the diagnosis before labor in unusual cases. Low-lying placentas noted in studies performed below 30 weeks may "migrate," leaving the cervix free at term [up to 90% of cases].)

Special Tests: None indicated.

Diagnostic Procedures: Generally diagnosed only at delivery by failure of the normal separation mechanism. Final diagnosis is established histologically.

Pathologic Findings

Absence of the decidua basalis (replaced by loose connective tissue). The decidua parietalis may be normal or absent. The villi may be separated from the myometrial cells by a layer of fibrin.

MANAGEMENT AND THERAPY

Nonpharmacologic

General Measures: Aggressive fluid and blood support as necessary. Oxytocin or other uterotonic agents to promote uterine contractions after placental delivery (if accomplished).

Specific Measures: Most patients require hysterectomy. If the invasion of the myometrium is incomplete and the bladder is spared, conservative management by uterine packing may be possible. Any time the diagnosis is considered, preparations for hysterectomy, including anesthesia, instruments, and adequate blood, should be ready before any attempt is made to free the placenta.

Diet: Nothing by mouth until the patient's condition has been stabilized.

Activity: Bed rest until the patient's condition has been stabilized.

Patient Education: American College of Obstetricians and Gynecologists Patient Education Pamphlet AP038 (*Bleeding During Pregnancy*), AP006 (*Cesarean Birth*), AP025 (*Ultrasound Exams*).

Drug(s) of Choice

Uterotonics should be available and broad-spectrum antibiotics given prophylactically.

FOLLOW-UP

Patient Monitoring: Hemodynamic monitoring during the acute diagnosis and treatment.

Prevention/Avoidance: Patients at high risk may be studied by ultrasonography in an attempt to identify the absence of the subplacental hypoechoic zone or the presence of lacunar blood flow patterns. If present, plans for autologous

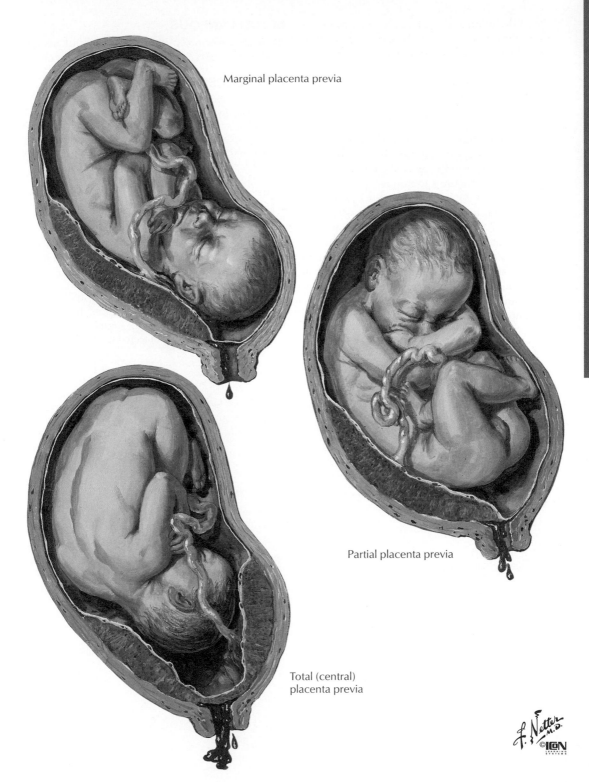

Marginal placenta previa

Partial placenta previa

Total (central)
placenta previa

blood donation and elective cesarean hysterectomy may be made. The absence of these findings does not rule out this possibility.

Possible Complications: Life-threatening hemorrhage may occur; maternal mortality of 2%–6% has been reported for treatment by hysterectomy and up to 30% for conservative management. Coagulopathy secondary to blood loss and replacement is common. Spontaneous rupture of the uterus before labor has been reported. Rupture of the uterus or inversion may occur during attempts to remove the placenta.

Expected Outcome: Most patients go to term with normal fetal development. If the possibility is recognized and appropriate treatment rendered, maternal survival is probable, although loss of the uterus is common. It is hypothesized that small areas of accreta may result in placental cotyledon(s) being torn from the placenta and that these cotyledons may become placental polyps.

MISCELLANEOUS

***ICD-9-CM* Codes:** 667.0 (All types, without hemorrhage), 666.0 (All types, with hemorrhage).

REFERENCES

Breen J, Neubecker R, Gregori C, Franklin J. Placenta accreta, increta and percreta. *Obstet Gynecol* 1977; 49:43.

Clark SL, Koonings PP, Phelan JP. Placenta previa/accreta and prior cesarean section. *Obstet Gynecol* 1985; 66:89.

Cox SM, Carpenter RJ, Cotton DB. Placenta percreta: ultrasound diagnosis and conservative surgical management. *Obstet Gynecol* 1988;72:452.

Fox HG. Placental accreta. *Obstet Gynecol Surv* 1972; 27:475.

Lauria MR, Cotton DB. Modern management of placenta previa and placenta accreta. In: Sciarra JJ, ed. *Gynecology and Obstetrics.* Vol 2. Philadelphia, Pa: JB Lippincott; 1994;49:1.

Morison JE. Placenta accreta: a clinicopathologic review of 67 cases. *Obstet Gynecol Annu* 1978;7:107.

Read JA, Cotton DB, Miller FC. Placenta accreta: changing clinical aspects and outcome. *Obstet Gynecol* 1980; 56:31.

ABORTION

INTRODUCTION

Description: Loss or failure of early pregnancy in several forms: complete, incomplete, inevitable, missed, septic, and threatened. A *complete* abortion is the termination of a pregnancy before the age of viability, typically defined as occurring at less than 20 weeks from the first day of the last normal menstrual period or involving a fetus of weight less than 500 g. Most complete abortions generally occur before 6 weeks or after 14 weeks of gestation. An *incomplete* abortion is the spontaneous passage of some, but not all, of the products of conception, associated with uniform pregnancy loss. A pregnancy in which rupture of the membranes and/or cervical dilatation takes place during the first half of pregnancy is labeled an *inevitable* abortion. Uterine contractions typically follow, ending in spontaneous loss of the pregnancy for most patients. A *missed* abortion is the retention of a failed intrauterine pregnancy for an extended period; however, with ultrasound studies, this can often be detected significantly sooner than it could be on clinical grounds alone. A *septic* abortion is a variant of an incomplete abortion in which infection of the uterus and its contents has occurred. A *threatened* abortion is a pregnancy that is at risk for some reason. Most often, this applies to any pregnancy in which vaginal bleeding or uterine cramping takes place, but no cervical changes have occurred.

Prevalence: Estimates for the frequency of complete abortions are as high as 50%–60% of all conceptions and between 10% and 15% of known pregnancies. Sixty percent of pregnant women hospitalized for bleeding have an incomplete abortion. Less than 2% of fetal losses are missed abortions. Septic abortions occur in 0.40–0.6 of 100,000 spontaneous pregnancy losses. Threatened abortions occur in 30%–40% of pregnant women.

Predominant Age: Reproductive.

Genetics: Some chromosomal abnormalities are associated with reduced or absent fertility and increased risk of fetal loss (eg, translocations).

ETIOLOGY AND PATHOGENESIS

Causes: Endocrine abnormalities (25%–50%)—hyperandrogenism, in utero diethylstilbestrol (DES) exposure, luteal phase defect, thyroid disease. Genetic factors (10%–70%)—Balanced translocation/carrier state, nondisjunction, trisomy (40%–50%, trisomy 16 most common, any possible except trisomy 1), monosomy X (15%–25%), triploidy (15%), tetraploidy (5%). Reproductive tract abnormalities (6%–12%)—Abnormality of placentation, bicornuate or unicornuate uterus, incompetent cervix, intrauterine adhesions (Asherman's syndrome), in utero DES exposure, leiomyomata uteri (submucous), septate uterus. Infection—*Mycoplasma hominis*, syphilis, toxoplasmosis, *Ureaplasma ureolyticus*, possibly *Chlamydia* and herpes. Systemic disease—Chronic cardiovascular disease, chronic renal disease, diabetes mellitus, systemic lupus erythematosus/lupus anticoagulant. Environmental factors—alcohol, anesthetic gases, drug use, radiation, smoking, toxins. Other factors—advanced maternal age, delayed fertilization (old egg), trauma.

Risk Factors: Increasing parity, increasing maternal age, increasing paternal age, a short interval between pregnancies, excessive caffeine consumption (>6 cups of coffee per day). Retention of tissue after pregnancy loss increases the risk of a septic abortion.

CLINICAL CHARACTERISTICS

Signs and Symptoms:
General—vaginal bleeding (may be bright red to dark in color)
Abdominal cramping (generally rhythmic, accompanied by pelvic or low back pressure)
Passage of tissue (complete and incomplete abortion)
Cervical dilation (typical of all types of abortion except missed and threatened)
Cervical dilation with tissue visible at the cervical os (diagnostic of either incomplete or inevitable abortion)
Missed abortion—decreased or minimal uterine growth early in pregnancy
Vaginal bleeding that changes to a dark brown discharge that continues
Loss of early symptoms of pregnancy, such as breast fullness or morning sickness
Disseminated intravascular coagulopathy (DIC) can occur when an intrauterine fetal demise in the second trimester has been retained beyond 6 weeks after the death of the fetus (rare)
Septic abortion—severe hemorrhage (vaginal)
Midline lower abdominal pain
Uterine and perimetrial tenderness
Bacteremia
Septic shock
Renal failure
Threatened abortion—Implantation bleeding
Cervical polyps, cervicitis
Other causes of lower abdominal discomfort (eg, urinary tract infection, constipation)

DIAGNOSTIC APPROACH

Differential Diagnosis:
  Ectopic pregnancy
  Cervical polyps, cervicitis
  Molar pregnancy
  Possibility of trauma, including perforation of the uterus or vagina, when sepsis is present

Associated Conditions: Thirty percent of patients treated by sharp curettage for missed abortion form intrauterine adhesions. Septic abortion is associated with septic shock, ascending infection (myometritis, pelvic inflammatory disease), disseminated intravascular coagulopathy, and renal failure.

Workup and Evaluation

Laboratory: Pregnancy test (if pregnancy has not been confirmed). If serial determinations of quantitative β-human chorionic gonadotropin (β-hCG) do not show at least a 66% increase every 48 hours, the outlook for the pregnancy is poor. Complete blood count (if blood loss has been excessive). Serial determinations of serum β-hCG may be used to confirm pregnancy loss but are not required for diagnosis.

Imaging: Ultrasonography of the uterus may be used to confirm loss of intrauterine contents, the absence of a fetal pole, or failure to grow.

Special Tests: None indicated.

Diagnostic Procedures: If significant cervical dilatation is identified by speculum and bimanual examination or if tissue is seen at the cervix, the diagnosis of inevitable or incomplete abortion is established.

Pathologic Findings

Products of conception (including chorionic villi); in a missed abortion there is the absence of a fetal pole.

MANAGEMENT AND THERAPY

Nonpharmacologic

General Measures: Support and evaluation; analgesia if required. Rh-negative mothers should be treated with Rh immune globulin after completion of the abortion. Because ovulation may occur as early as 2 weeks after an abortion, a discussion of contraception is warranted.

Specific Measures: When there is a complete abortion, immediate considerations include control of bleeding, prevention of infection, pain relief (if needed), and emotional support. Ensuring that all the products of the conception have been expelled from the uterus controls bleeding. Although most patients with an incomplete or inevitable abortion spontaneously pass the remaining tissue (complete abortion), bleeding, cramping, and the risk of infection associated with expectant management generally militate for surgical evacuation. If retained tissue is present or cannot be ruled out, curettage must be performed promptly. When a missed abortion is diagnosed, evacuation of the uterus can be accomplished either through dilatation and evacuation or with the use of prostaglandin suppositories, based on the stage of the pregnancy and other considerations. Septic abortion requires immediate and aggressive management. Broad-spectrum parenteral antibiotics, fluid therapy, and prompt evacuation of the uterus are indicated. Emergency evacuation of the uterine contents is mandatory because of the significant threat it represents. When the diagnosis of threatened abortion is made, intervention should be minimal, even when bleeding is accompanied by low abdominal pain and cramping. If there is no evidence of cervical change, the patient can be reassured and encouraged to continue normal activities. If significant pain or bleeding persist, especially bleeding leading to hemodynamic alterations, evacuation of the uterus should be carried out.

Diet: No specific dietary changes indicated unless immediate surgical therapy is being considered; in that case, nothing by mouth.

Activity: Generally no restriction. When sepsis is present, bed rest is initially required while therapy is instituted. After evacuation is accomplished and fever is reduced, the patient may return to normal activity. Although frequently recommended, a short period of bed rest has no documented benefit for patients with a threatened abortion.

Patient Education: Reassurance, American College of Obstetricians and Gynecologists Patient Education Pamphlet AP038 (*Bleeding During Pregnancy*), AP090 (*Early Pregnancy Loss: Miscarriage, Ectopic Pregnancy, and Molar Pregnancy*), AP062 (*Dilatation and Curettage (D&C)*).

Drug(s) of Choice

May be used to hasten the expulsion of tissue and reduce bleeding—oxytocin 10–20 units/L IV fluids, methylergonovine maleate (Methergine) 0.2 mg IM

Septic abortion—aggressive fluid therapy, antibiotic therapy (ampicillin 1–2 g IV followed by 500 mg IV q4–6h, ampicillin/sulbactam 1.5–3 g IV q6h, or clindamycin 600 mg IV or IM q6h and gentamicin 80 mg IM q8h)

Contraindications: Undiagnosed vaginal bleeding.

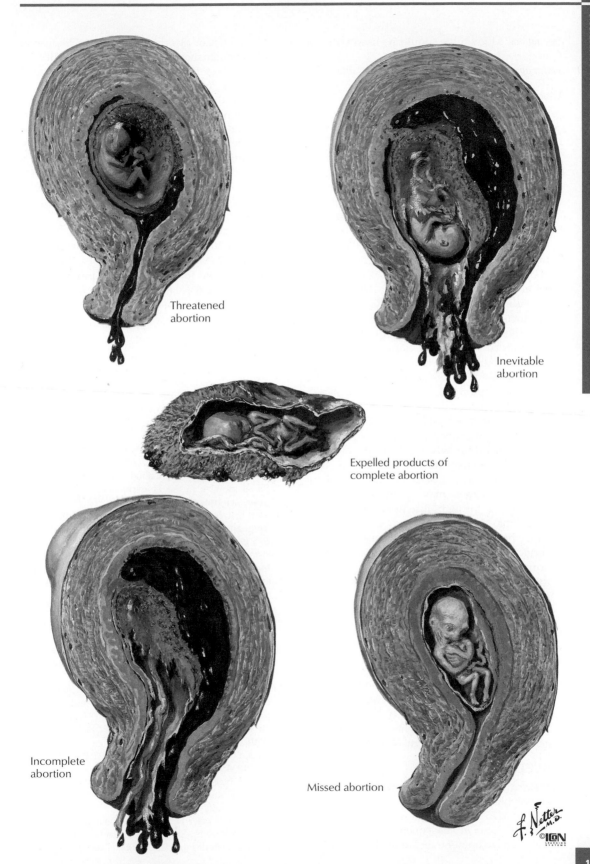

Threatened
abortion

Inevitable
abortion

Expelled products of
complete abortion

Incomplete
abortion

Missed abortion

Precautions: Methergine should be used with care in patients with hypertension.

Interactions: Vasoconstrictors and ergot alkaloids.

Alternative Drugs

Prostaglandin E_2. For septic abortion other broadspectrum antibiotics, singly or in combination.

FOLLOW-UP

Patient Monitoring: Anticipate normal return of menstrual function in 4–6 weeks; contraceptive counseling. Patients with septic abortions must be monitored for the possibility of septic shock.

Prevention/Avoidance: None. Septic abortions may be prevented by the prompt evacuation of the uterus for patients with incomplete or missed abortions.

Possible Complications: Infection (myometritis, pelvic inflammatory disease). Removal of the products of conception, combined with vaginal rest (no tampons, douches, or intercourse), provides adequate protection against infection for most patients.

Expected Outcome: The risk of pregnancy loss subsequent to a spontaneous abortion rises slightly, although much of this increase may be due to selection for those with factors that preclude successful pregnancy. For those with an inevitable abortion who do not spontaneously lose the pregnancy, infection or bleeding often ensue, requiring evacuation of the uterus. Missed abortions may spontaneously abort, progressing through incomplete to complete stages, or may be evacuated. Once the pregnancy has terminated (spontaneous abortion or surgical evacuation of products of conception), normal menses return in 4–6 weeks. With aggressive antibiotic treatment and prompt evacuation of the uterus, the outcome should be good for patients with a septic abortion. Among patients with a threatened abortion, one half go on to lose the pregnancy in a spontaneous abortion. (The risk of failure is greater in those who bleed for 3 or more days.) For those who carry the fetus to viability there is a greater risk for preterm delivery and low fetal birth weight and a higher incidence of perinatal mortality. There does not, however, appear to be a higher incidence of congenital malformations in these newborns.

MISCELLANEOUS

Other Notes: When losses are caused by aneuploidy or polyploidy, they tend to happen earlier in gestation (75% before eight weeks) and are more likely to recur in subsequent pregnancies. Abnormal development, including the zygote, embryo, fetus, or placenta are common. Expulsion of the pregnancy is almost always preceded by the death of the embryo or fetus. For threatened abortion, intercourse is usually proscribed for two to three weeks, or longer, although this probably provides more psychological support than medical effect. Progesterone therapy for threatened abortions is of no benefit and may potentially result in virilization of a fetus, or a missed abortion. It should not be used. Incomplete abortions are more common after the tenth week of gestation when fetal and placental tissues tend to be passed separately.

ICD-9-CM **Codes:** 634.9 (Complete abortion), 637.9 (Incomplete abortion), 634.7 (Inevitable abortion), 632 (Missed abortion), 634.0, 635.0 (Septic abortion following legal termination of pregnancy), 636.0 (Septic abortion following illegal termination of pregnancy), 640.0 (Threatened abortion).

REFERENCES

American College of Obstetricians and Gynecologists. *Early Pregnancy Loss.* Washington, DC: ACOG; 1995. ACOG Technical Bulletin 212.

Batzofin JH, Fielding WI, Friedman EA. Effect of vaginal bleeding in early pregnancy on outcome. *Obstet Gynecol* 1984;63:515.

Boklage CE. Survival probability of human conceptions from fertilization to term. *Int J Fertil* 1990;35:75.

Bromley B, Harlow BL, Laboda LA, Benacerraf BR. Small sac size in the first trimester: a predictor of poor fetal outcome. *Radiology* 1991;178:375.

Funderburk SJ, Guthrie D, Meldrum D. Outcome of pregnancies complicated by early vaginal bleeding. *Br J Obstet Gynecol* 1980;87:100.

Goldstein SR. Embryonic death in early pregnancy: a new look at the first trimester. *Obstet Gynecol* 1994;84:294.

Hakim-Elahie E, Tovell HM, Burnhill MS. Complications of first-trimester abortions: a report of 170,000 cases. *Obstet Gynecol* 1990;76:129.

Hogue CJR. Impact of abortion on subsequent fecundity. *Clin Obstet Gynaecol* 1986;13:95.

Mackenzie WE, Holmes DS, Newton JR. Spontaneous abortion rate in ultrasonographically viable pregnancies. *Obstet Gynecol* 1988;71:81.

Poland BJ, Miller JR, Jones DC, Trimble BK. Reproductive counseling in patients who have had a spontaneous abortion. *Am J Obstet Gynecol* 1977;127:685.

Smith RP. *Gynecology in Primary Care.* Baltimore, Md: Williams & Wilkins; 1997:99.

Stubblefield PG, Grimes DA. Septic abortion. *N Engl J Med* 1994;331:310.

Thom DH, Nelson LM, Vaughan TL. Spontaneous abortion and subsequent adverse birth outcomes. *Am J Obstet Gynecol* 1992;166:111.

Warburton D, Fraser FC. Spontaneous abortion risks in man: data from reproductive histories collected in a medical genetics unit. *Am J Human Genet* 1964;16:1.

ACTIVE MANAGEMENT OF LABOR

THE CHALLENGE

A system of labor management designed to promote effective labor and reduce the need for cesarean delivery.

Scope of the Problem: Cesarean section rate for nulliparous patients approaches 20% in some areas. Active management has been associated with cesarean section rates below 5% for its developers (Ireland).

Objectives of Management: To reduce cesarean delivery rates through a system of management that includes education, strict criteria for labor and abnormal progress, one-on-one care, and the use of high-dose oxytocin (when needed).

TACTICS

Relevant Pathophysiology: As developed in Ireland, active management of labor is based on the following:

Patient education

Strict criteria for the diagnosis of labor, the determination of abnormal progress, and the diagnosis of fetal compromise

One-on-one nursing care during labor

Use of high-dose oxytocin infusion (when needed)

Peer review of all operative deliveries

Strategies: In Ireland, where this technique was developed, active management of labor is restricted to nulliparous patients with singleton pregnancies in vertex presentation with no evidence of fetal compromise. Women are carefully instructed to come to the hospital early in labor. Labor is confirmed by the presence of complete effacement, the passage of the mucous plug, or rupture of the membranes. If these criteria are met, the patient is admitted to the hospital and the membranes ruptured within 1 hour (if not already ruptured). Vaginal examination is performed hourly and administration of high-dose oxytocin is begun if dilation falls below 1 cm/h. Oxytocin is begun at 6 mU/min and the dose is increased every 15 minutes until a maximum of 40 mU/min is reached, active labor is established, or hyperstimulation occurs. As a part of this process, one-on-one nursing care is provided, and fetal status is assessed by auscultation every 5 minutes. Fetal compromise is diagnosed by fetal scalp pH. Cesarean delivery is performed if delivery is not imminent 12 hours after admission or if fetal compromise is diagnosed.

Patient Education: American College of Obstetricians and Gynecologists Patient Education Pamphlet AP004 (*How to Tell When Labor Begins*).

IMPLEMENTATION

Special Considerations: The Irish experience with active management of labor has resulted in a reduced rate of births by cesarean delivery without untoward events. Which elements of the management (education, early amniotomy, intensive nursing, aggressive use of oxytocin, or methods of establishing distress) are directly responsible for this success is unknown. Attempts to apply only some elements of the program have generally not yielded the same reductions in cesarean section rates. It should be noted that conduction (epidural) anesthesia is also less common in Ireland.

REFERENCES

American College of Obstetricians and Gynecologists. *Induction of Labor.* Washington, DC: ACOG; 1995. ACOG Technical Bulletin 217.

American College of Obstetricians and Gynecologists. *Dystocia and the Augmentation of Labor.* Washington, DC: ACOG; 1995. ACOG Technical Bulletin 218.

Boylan P, Robson M, McParland P. Active management of labor. *Am J Obstet Gynecol* 1993;168:295.

Fraser WD, Marcoux S, Moutquin J-M, Christen A, the Canadian Early Amniotomy Study Group. Effect of early amniotomy on the risk of dystocia in nulliparous women. *N Engl J Med* 1993;328:1145.

Frigoletto FD Jr, Lieberman E, Lang JM, et al. A clinical trial of active management of labor. *N Engl J Med* 1995;333:745.

Lopéz-Zeno JA, Peacemen AM, Adashek JA, Socol ML. A controlled trial of a program for the active management of labor. *N Engl J Med* 1992;326:450.

O'Driscoll K, Foley M, MacDonald D. Active management of labor as an alternative to cesarean section for dystocia. *Obstet Gynecol* 1984;63:485.

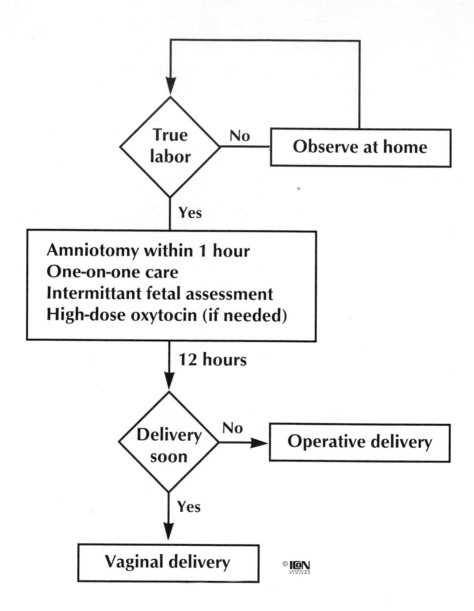

ACUTE FATTY LIVER OF PREGNANCY

INTRODUCTION

Description: A rare complication of pregnancy that results in acute liver failure, often with catastrophic consequences.

Prevalence: One of 10,000–15,000 pregnancies.

Predominant Age: Reproductive.

Genetics: No genetic pattern.

ETIOLOGY AND PATHOGENESIS

Causes: Unknown (mimics other forms of fatty liver failure such as that induced by tetracycline in patients with impaired renal function, Reye's syndrome, hepatotoxicity with sodium valproate, or salicylate intoxication).

Risk Factors: Unknown. More common in nulliparous women, when a male fetus is present, or in multifetal gestation. The risk of recurrence in subsequent pregnancies is low.

CLINICAL CHARACTERISTICS

Signs and Symptoms:

Average gestational age: 37.5 weeks

Gradual onset of malaise, anorexia, nausea and vomiting, epigastric pain, and progressive jaundice

Hypertension, proteinuria, and edema (50% of patients)

Hypofibrinogenemia, prolonged clotting time, hyperbilirubinemia (<10 mg/dL), elevated serum transaminase levels (300–500 U/L), mild thrombocytopenia, hemolysis

DIAGNOSTIC APPROACH

Differential Diagnosis:

Hepatitis

Hemolysis, elevated liver enzymes, low platelet count (HELLP) syndrome

Preeclampsia

Cholestatic jaundice

Cholelithiasis

Associated Conditions: Hypoglycemia and hepatic coma, coagulopathy, renal failure, sepsis, aspiration, circulatory collapse, pancreatitis, and gastrointestinal bleeding are all common.

Workup and Evaluation

Laboratory: Complete blood count, evaluation of liver function, serum bilirubin, clotting studies, serum ammonia.

Imaging: Ultrasonography, computed tomography, or magnetic resonance imaging may demonstrate the fatty metamorphosis, but false-negative results may be as high as 80%.

Special Tests: None indicated.

Diagnostic Procedures: History, physical and laboratory examinations.

Pathologic Findings

Grossly the liver is small, soft, yellow, and greasy. Histologically there are swollen hepatocytes with microvesicular fat and central nuclei and periportal sparing. There may also be lipid accumulation within renal tubular cells.

MANAGEMENT AND THERAPY

Nonpharmacologic

General Measures: Rapid evaluation, supportive measures.

Specific Measures: The only specific measure is delivery, which generally arrests the process. The decision between cesarean or vaginal birth remains uncertain and controversial. Transfusion with fresh-frozen plasma, cryoprecipitate, whole blood, packed red blood cells, and platelets may be necessary if surgery is planned or bleeding ensues. Liver transplantation may have to be considered in selected patients.

Diet: Nothing by mouth.

Activity: Strict bed rest. Often requires admission to intensive care facilities.

Drug(s) of Choice

No specific medications. Other medications based on symptoms and condition.

FOLLOW-UP

Patient Monitoring: Intensive monitoring for circulatory, renal, and hepatic collapse. Often the fetus is severely compromised (often dead at the time of diagnosis) and also requires intensive monitoring.

Prevention/Avoidance: None.

Possible Complications: Often fatal for both mother (75%) and fetus (90%); lower mortality rates have been reported in recent studies. Hypoglycemia and hepatic coma (60% of patients), coagulopathy (55%), renal failure (50%). Sepsis, aspiration, circulatory collapse, pancreatitis, and gastrointestinal bleeding are all common.

Expected Outcome: Often fatal for both mother and fetus. If the diagnosis is established and delivery accomplished in time, recovery is marked by acute pancreatitis and ascites (almost uni-

Hepatic Disease in Pregnancy

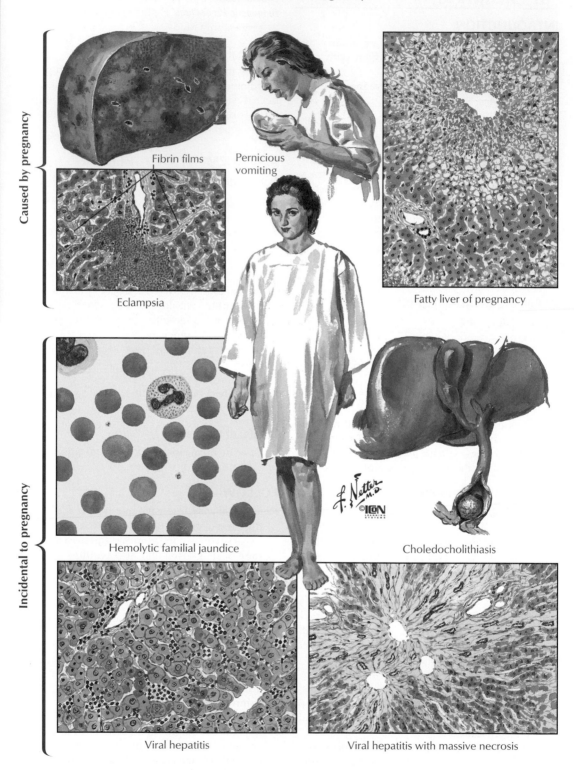

Caused by pregnancy

Fibrin films

Pernicious vomiting

Eclampsia

Fatty liver of pregnancy

Incidental to pregnancy

Hemolytic familial jaundice

Choledocholithiasis

Viral hepatitis

Viral hepatitis with massive necrosis

versal). For these patients eventual recovery is complete and recurrence is rare.

MISCELLANEOUS

ICD-9-CM **Codes:** 646.73.

REFERENCES

Barton JR, Sibai BM, Mabie WC, Shanklin DR. Recurrent acute fatty liver of pregnancy. *Am J Obstet Gynecol* 1990;163:534.

Cunningham FG, MacDonald PC, Gant NF, et al, eds. *Williams Obstetrics.* 20th ed. Stamford, Conn: Appleton & Lange; 1997:1155.

Howard EW, Jones HL. Massive hepatic necrosis in toxemia of pregnancy. *Br J Obstet Gynaecol* 1993;9:74.

MacLean MA, Cameron AD, Cumming GP, Murphy K, Mills P, Hilan KJ. Recurrence of acute fatty liver of pregnancy. *Br J Obstet Gynaecol* 1994;101:453.

Ockner SA, Brunt EM, Cohn SM, Krul ES, Janto DW, Paters MG. Fulminant hepatic failure caused by acute fatty liver of pregnancy treated by orthotopic liver transplantation. *Hepatology* 1990;11:59.

Reyes H, Sandoval L, Wainstein A, et al. Acute fatty liver of pregnancy: a clinical study of 12 episodes in 11 patients. *Gut* 1994;35:101.

Watson WJ, Seeds JW. Acute fatty liver of pregnancy. *Obstet Gynecol* 1990;45:585.

AMNIOTIC FLUID EMBOLISM

INTRODUCTION

Description: A rare but frequently fatal complication of labor in which amniotic fluid containing fetal squamous cells and hair enters the maternal vascular system and becomes lodged in the pulmonary vascular bed. Mechanical obstruction and anaphylaxis combine to produce an often fatal clinical course.

Prevalence: One of 30,000 deliveries (despite its rarity, one of the most common causes of maternal mortality).

Predominant Age: Reproductive (late labor or immediately postpartum).

Genetics: No genetic pattern.

ETIOLOGY AND PATHOGENESIS

Causes: Anaphylaxis induced by fetal squamous cells and hair. Mechanical obstruction of pulmonary vessels by fetal squamous cells and hair. Diffuse intravascular coagulation resulting in coagulopathy.

Risk Factors: Tumultuous labor, reduced uterine tone, premature separation of the placenta, history of allergy or atopy.

CLINICAL CHARACTERISTICS

Signs and Symptoms (Variable):
Respiratory distress followed by
Cyanosis followed by
Cardiovascular collapse followed by
Hemorrhage (DIC with depletion of fibrinogen, platelets, and factors V, VIII, and XIII) followed by coma

DIAGNOSTIC APPROACH

Differential Diagnosis:
Pulmonary embolism (thrombus)
Myocardial infarct
Cardiac arrhythmia

Associated Conditions: Allergy and atopy.

Workup and Evaluation

Laboratory: Coagulation studies, blood gas measurements, renal function studies, all on an ongoing basis.

Imaging: May help in managing pulmonary complications but generally not helpful in establishing the diagnosis.

Special Tests: Continuous monitoring of oxygen saturation and invasive hemodynamic monitoring (pulmonary artery catheter) essential.

Diagnostic Procedures: History and physical examination. Exclusion of other causes.

Pathologic Findings

Fetal squamous cells and lanugo present in the pulmonary vascular space (typical but neither sensitive or specific).

MANAGEMENT AND THERAPY

Nonpharmacologic

General Measures: Aggressive airway control and cardiovascular resuscitation (including myocardial support, inotropic agents and fluids, high-concentration oxygen therapy). The use of vasopressors has been reported to be successful. Correction and support for clotting defects (blood and platelets, fresh-frozen plasma, and cryoprecipitate as indicated).

Specific Measures: None. In women who suffer cardiac arrest before delivery, consideration should be given to perimortem cesarean delivery to improve newborn outcome. In those who have not suffered arrest, maternal considerations generally take precedence.

Diet: Nothing by mouth until condition resolved.

Activity: Bed rest until condition resolved.

Drug(s) of Choice

No specific medications. Other medications as needed for cardiovascular, pulmonary, renal, and coagulation support.

FOLLOW-UP

Patient Monitoring: Intensive hemodynamic monitoring required. Laboratory testing in anticipation of coagulopathy.

Prevention/Avoidance: None.

Possible Complications: Mortality rates with amniotic fluid embolism approximate 50%. Of women who survive, 50% have a life-threatening bleeding diathesis. Renal failure is common, as are pulmonary edema and adult respiratory distress syndrome. Of women who suffer cardiac arrest during the initial phase, only 8% survive neurologically intact. Over half of the neonates that survive have neurologic impairment.

Expected Outcome: Prolonged and complicated course for those who survive.

MISCELLANEOUS

Other Notes: The most devastating effects of amniotic fluid embolism appear to be mediated through the anaphylactic reaction induced. Experimental studies indicate that pretreatment with inhibitors of leukotriene synthesis can prevent the development of symptoms in experimental settings.

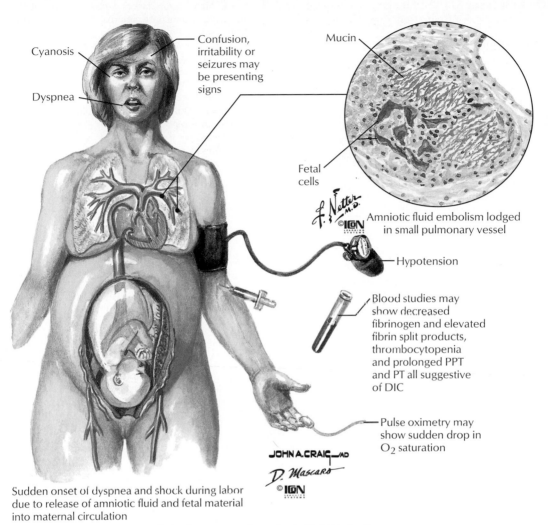

Cyanosis

Dyspnea

Confusion, irritability or seizures may be presenting signs

Mucin

Fetal cells

Amniotic fluid embolism lodged in small pulmonary vessel

Hypotension

Blood studies may show decreased fibrinogen and elevated fibrin split products, thrombocytopenia and prolonged PPT and PT all suggestive of DIC

Pulse oximetry may show sudden drop in O_2 saturation

Sudden onset of dyspnea and shock during labor due to release of amniotic fluid and fetal material into maternal circulation

Clinical Features of Amniotic Fluid Embolism

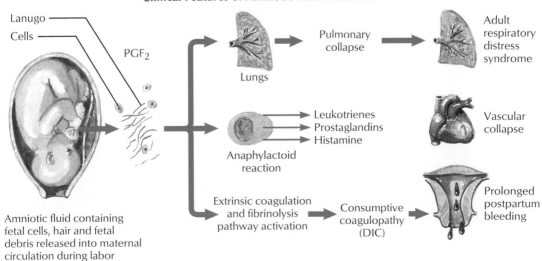

Lanugo

Cells

PGF_2

Lungs

Pulmonary collapse

Adult respiratory distress syndrome

Leukotrienes
Prostaglandins
Histamine

Anaphylactoid reaction

Vascular collapse

Extrinsic coagulation and fibrinolysis pathway activation

Consumptive coagulopathy (DIC)

Prolonged postpartum bleeding

Amniotic fluid containing fetal cells, hair and fetal debris released into maternal circulation during labor

ICD-9-CM Codes: 673.13 (if diagnosed before delivery), 673.11 (if diagnosed after delivery).

REFERENCES

Choi DM, Duffy BL. Amniotic fluid embolism. *Anaesth Intens Care* 1995;23:741.

Clark SL. New concepts of amniotic fluid embolism: a review. *Obstet Gynecol Surv* 1990;45:360.

Clark SL, Hankins GDV, Dudley DA, Dildy GA, Porter TF. Amniotic fluid embolism: analysis of the National Registry. *Am J Obstet Gynecol* 1995;172:1159.

Harvey C, Hankins G, Clark S. Amniotic fluid embolism and oxygen transport patterns. *Am J Obstet Gynecol* 1996;174:304.

Laforga JB. Amniotic fluid embolism. Report of two cases with coagulation disorder. *Acta Obstet Gynecol Scand* 1997;76:805.

Martin RW. Amniotic fluid embolism. *Clin Obstet Gynecol* 1996;39:101.

McDougall RJ, Duke GJ. Amniotic fluid embolism syndrome: case report and review. *Anaesth Intens Care* 1995;23:735.

Syed SA, Dearden CH. Amniotic fluid embolism: emergency management. *J Accid Emerg Med* 1996;13:285.

ANTEPARTUM FETAL TESTING

THE CHALLENGE

To reduce the risk of fetal demise in those at high risk through the use of noninvasive tests that have acceptably low false-positive and false-negative results.

Scope of the Problem: There are roughly 15 fetal or neonatal deaths for every 1000 births in the United States.

Objectives of Management: To identify those fetuses at high risk and those whose status is deteriorating or nonreassuring so that intervention can take place to prevent mortality. Ultimately, the reduction of fetal morbidity and the improvement of neurologic outcome would be ideal as well, but objective studies to support the effectiveness of antepartum fetal testing are lacking.

TACTICS

Relevant Pathophysiology: The nonstress test (NST) and contraction stress test (CST) are based on the premise that when fetal oxygenation is only marginally adequate, the fetus will not possess the normal ability to modulate heart rate in response to fetal movement or to tolerate the stress of placental ischemia induced by uterine contractions. A normal (reactive) NST has two or more accelerations (15 beats/min for 15 seconds) in a 20-minute period. Acoustic stimulation may also be used to startle the fetus and induce a heart rate increase. In the CST, the occurrence of late decelerations occurring with 50% or more contractions (regardless of frequency) is "positive" and suggests fetal risk. The biophysical profile (BPP) is based on the NST, augmented by measures of fetal breathing movements, fetal activity and tone, and quantitation of amniotic fluid volume, rated on a 10-point scale (normal: 8–10/10, equivocal: 6/10, abnormal: ≤5/10).

Strategies: The most commonly used antepartum fetal tests are the NST, CST, BPP, and movement assessment (kick count and others). These may be used individually, in sequence, or in any combination as the individual case demands. Each has advantages and disadvantages; no single test can be said to be definitive. Some possible indications for the use of antenatal fetal testing are shown.

Patient Education: American College of Obstetricians and Gynecologists Patient Education Pamphlet AP098 (*Monitoring Fetal Health During Pregnancy*), AP015 (*Fetal Heart Rate Monitoring*).

IMPLEMENTATION

Special Considerations: The NST is more easily performed than the CST, but has the highest false-positive rate (up to 90% of positive tests) and the highest risk of a false-negative test (1.4 of 1000). The CST requires the induction of contractions by intravenous oxytocin or nipple stimulation. There must be ≥ 3 contractions in a 10-minute test period and no late decelerations. The CST has a lower false-positive rate (50%) and a lower risk of a false-negative result (0.4 of 1000). The BPP has the lowest false-positive and false-negative rates (0–0.6 of 1000), but is the most expensive and requires the most expertise and equipment. All testing must be viewed in the context of the clinical picture. The choice of timing and test must be made on clinical grounds, degree of risk, and the availability and expertise of those who will perform and interpret the test. Normal test results generally warrant further testing in a few days to a week. Positive or nonreassuring test results may suggest the need for a more invasive test (eg, NST to CST, CST to BPP) or more direct intervention in the course of the pregnancy (delivery).

REFERENCES

American College of Obstetricians and Gynecologists. *Antepartum Fetal Surveillance.* Washington, DC: ACOG; 1994. ACOG Technical Bulletin 188.

Anyaegbunam A, Brustman L, Divon M, Langer O. The significance of antepartum variable decelerations. *Am J Obstet Gynecol* 1986;155:707.

Freeman RK, Anderson G, Dorchester W. A prospective multi-institutional study of antepartum fetal heart rate monitoring. II. Contraction stress test versus nonstress test for primary surveillance. *Am J Obstet Gynecol* 1982;57:228.

Manning FA, Harman CR, Morrison I, Mentigoglou SM, Lange IR, Johnson JM. Fetal assessment based on fetal biophysical profile scoring. IV. An analysis of perinatal morbidity and mortality. *Am J Obstet Gynecol* 1990;138:575.

Moore TR, Piacquadio K. A prospective evaluation of fetal movement screening to reduce the incidence of antepartum fetal death. *Am J Obstet Gynecol* 1989;160:1075.

Noninvasive testing used to identify "high-risk" fetus and to elicit signs of deteriorating status to allow intervention and prevent mortality

Testing based on premise that marginal fetal oxygenation limits fetal ability to modulate fetal heart rate in response to fetal movement or to placental ischemia due to uterine contraction. Fetal heart rate should show acceleration to movement or contraction

> Nonstress Test (NST)
> Contraction Stress Test (CST)
> Biophysical Profile (BPP)

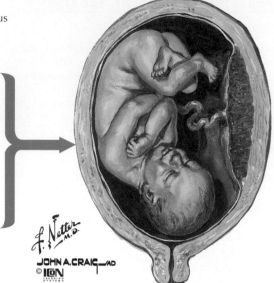

Some Conditions that Suggest Need for Antepartum Testing

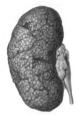
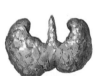
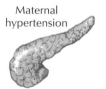
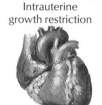
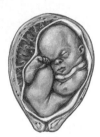

Chronic renal disease	Hyperthyroidism	Type 1 diabetes mellitus	Intrauterine growth restriction / Maternal cyanotic heart disease	Fetal movement

Maternal hypertension

Management Flow Chart for Antepartum Fetal Testing

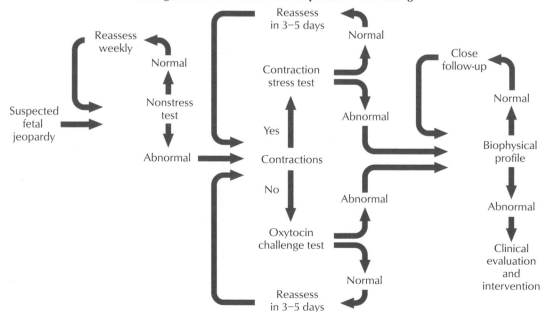

Suspected fetal jeopardy

Reassess weekly — Normal — Nonstress test — Abnormal

Reassess in 3–5 days — Normal — Contraction stress test — Abnormal

Yes — Contractions — No — Oxytocin challenge test

Abnormal / Normal

Reassess in 3–5 days

Close follow-up — Normal — Biophysical profile — Abnormal — Clinical evaluation and intervention

BREECH BIRTH

INTRODUCTION

Description: Presentation of the fetal buttocks, one foot, or both feet at the cervix at the time of labor.

Prevalence: Three percent of term pregnancies, 13% of pregnancies at 30 weeks of gestation.

Predominant Age: Reproductive (maternal).

Genetics: No genetic pattern.

ETIOLOGY AND PATHOGENESIS

Causes: Prematurity, fetal or maternal anomalies (eg, fetal hydrocephalus, maternal uterine anomalies), multiple gestation.

Risk Factors: Prematurity, fetal or uterine anomalies, multiple pregnancies.

CLINICAL CHARACTERISTICS

Signs and Symptoms:
Fetal head located outside the pelvis on abdominal palpation (Leopold's maneuvers)
Fetal heart heard high in the uterus
Buttock, one foot, or both feet palpable on cervical examination

DIAGNOSTIC APPROACH

Differential Diagnosis:
Fetal anomaly (hydrocephalus, anencephaly)
Uterine anomaly (septum, duplication, leiomyomata)
Multiple gestation
Fetal macrosomia

Associated Conditions: Prematurity, placenta previa, placental abruption, premature rupture of the membranes, congenital anomalies (6% versus 2.5% in total population), intracranial hemorrhage, growth retardation, neurologic disorders and mortality, multiple pregnancy, and polyhydramnios.

Workup and Evaluation

Laboratory: No evaluation indicated beyond that usually considered for patients in labor.

Imaging: Ultrasonography may be used to confirm presentation.

Special Tests: Fetal heart rate and uterine activity monitoring.

Diagnostic Procedures: Physical examination (Leopold's maneuvers), ultrasonography.

Pathologic Findings

None.

MANAGEMENT AND THERAPY

Nonpharmacologic

General Measures: Fetal and maternal monitoring and support.

Specific Measures: External version, evaluation for route of delivery. External version is successful in >50% of patients.

Diet: No specific dietary changes indicated; nothing by mouth if the patient is in labor because of the increased risk of operative delivery.

Activity: No restriction.

Patient Education: Reassurance, American College of Obstetricians and Gynecologists Patient Education Pamphlet AP079 (*If Your Baby Is Breech*).

Drug(s) of Choice

None (tocolytics may be used to assist with external version procedures).

FOLLOW-UP

Patient Monitoring: Fetal and maternal monitoring as with normal labor.

Prevention/Avoidance: None.

Possible Complications: Prolapse of umbilical cord, entrapment of the fetal head, birth trauma.

Expected Outcome: Breech deliveries are associated with an increased risk of congenital anomalies, intracranial hemorrhage, growth retardation, neurologic disorders and mortality, but the role of breech presentation and the delivery route are unclear. Much of the morbidity traditionally associated with breech presentation and delivery is due to factors that predispose to breech (congenital anomalies, prematurity).

MISCELLANEOUS

Pregnancy Considerations: The route of delivery must be determined on an individual basis based on fetal and maternal factors, as well as the availability of needed resources and the skill of the obstetrician. Vaginal delivery may be considered if labor is normal, fetal weight is 2000–3800 g, fetal status is normal, the pelvis is adequate, fetal head position is normal, and normal progression of cervical dilation and fetal descent are maintained.

ICD-9-CM Codes: 652.2, 652.1 (With successful version).

REFERENCES

American College of Obstetricians and Gynecologists. *Management of the Breech Presentation.* Washington, DC: ACOG; 1986. ACOG Technical Bulletin 95.

Deformations

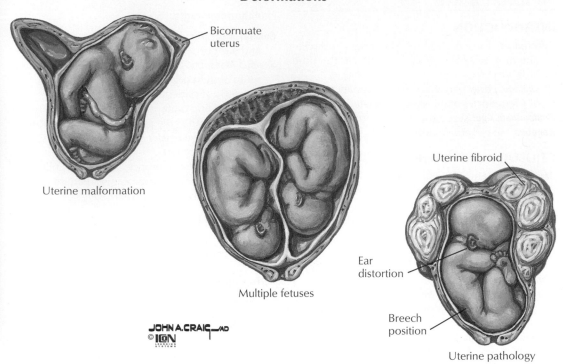

Bicornuate uterus

Uterine malformation

Multiple fetuses

Uterine fibroid

Ear distortion

Breech position

Uterine pathology

JOHN A.CRAIG—AD
©I©N
LEARNING
SYSTEMS

Conditions that cause intrauterine crowding can lead to abnormal fetal positions and thus cause constraint deformities

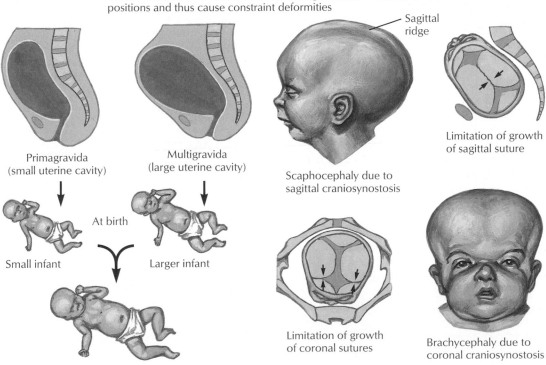

Sagittal ridge

Primagravida (small uterine cavity)

Multigravida (large uterine cavity)

Scaphocephaly due to sagittal craniosynostosis

Limitation of growth of sagittal suture

At birth

Small infant

Larger infant

Limitation of growth of coronal sutures

Brachycephaly due to coronal craniosynostosis

At 6 months

Constraint-related growth deficiency is transient. Small infants rapidly catch up with norm

Early engagement of fetal head may limit sutural growth and result in craniosynostotic skull deformities

Brenner WE. Breech presentation. *Clin Obstet Gynecol* 1978;21:511.

DeCrespigny LJ, Pepperell RJ. Perinatal mortality and morbidity in breech presentations. *Obstet Gynecol* 1979;53:141.

Jenkins DM. Breech delivery. *Clin Obstet Gynecol* 1980;7:561.

Lindqvist A, Nordén-Lindeerg S, Hanson U. Perinatal mortality and route of delivery in term breech presentations. *Br J Obstet Gynaecol* 1997;104:1288.

Luterkort M, Persson PH, Weldner BM. Maternal and fetal factors in breech presentation. *Obstet Gynecol* 1984;64:55.

Premature breech: vaginal delivery or cesarean section? [editorial]. *BMJ* 1979;1:1747.

Wallace RL, VanDorsten JP, Eglinton GS, Meuller E, McCart D, Schifrin BS. External cephalic version with tocolysis. *J Reprod Med* 1984;29:745.

CAPUT SUCCEDANEUM

INTRODUCTION

Description: A characteristic change in the shape of the fetal head that results from the forces of labor acting on the fetal head and the surrounding tissues. This swelling is generally located on the portion of the fetal scalp that was directly under the cervical os.

Prevalence: Typical of most vaginal vertex births; similar swellings on the presenting part are formed with other birth presentations.

Predominant Age: Birth.

Genetics: No genetic pattern.

ETIOLOGY AND PATHOGENESIS

Causes: Pressure by the birth canal and surrounding tissues on the fetal head as it enters and traverses the lower vaginal canal.

Risk Factors: Fetal macrosomia, prolonged labor, contracted maternal pelvis, prolonged maternal expulsive effort (pushing).

CLINICAL CHARACTERISTICS

Signs and Symptoms:

Symmetric swelling of the fetal scalp in a location compatible with that which was directly under the cervical os (upper posterior portion over the right parietal bone in left occiput transverse labors, over the corresponding portion of the left parietal bone in right occiput transverse labors)

Generally with diffuse edges and only a few millimeters in thickness; greater in obstructed or prolonged labors. The periosteal edges provide a sharp demarcation to a cephalohematoma that is not present in caput succedaneum. In addition, cephalohematomas do not cross suture lines.

DIAGNOSTIC APPROACH

Differential Diagnosis:

Cephalohematoma (2%–3% of births)
Molding of the head
Subgaleal hemorrhage

Associated Conditions: Macrosomia, obstructed labor, maternal diabetes.

Workup and Evaluation

Laboratory: No evaluation indicated.

Imaging: No imaging indicated.

Special Tests: None indicated.

Diagnostic Procedures: History and physical examination.

Pathologic Findings

Diffuse tissue edema without bruising.

MANAGEMENT AND THERAPY

Nonpharmacologic

General Measures: Evaluation and reassurance.

Specific Measures: None. Spontaneously regresses in 24–48 hours.

Diet: No specific dietary changes indicated.

Activity: No restriction.

Drug(s) of Choice

None.

FOLLOW-UP

Patient Monitoring: Normal health maintenance.

Prevention/Avoidance: Expeditious labor and delivery.

Possible Complications: Cephalohematoma or intracranial bleeding may be missed.

Expected Outcome: Rapid, spontaneous, and complete resolution.

MISCELLANEOUS

ICD-9-CM **Codes:** 767.1.

REFERENCES

Cunningham FG, MacDonald PC, Gant NF, et al, eds. *Williams Obstetrics.* 20th ed. Stamford, Conn: Appleton & Lange; 1997:325.

Pope BA, Painter MJ. Neurologic sequelae of birth. In: Sciarra JJ, ed. *Gynecology and Obstetrics.* Vol 3. Philadelphia, Pa: JB Lippincott; 1995;99.

**Extracranial Hemorrhage or
Edema in Newborn**

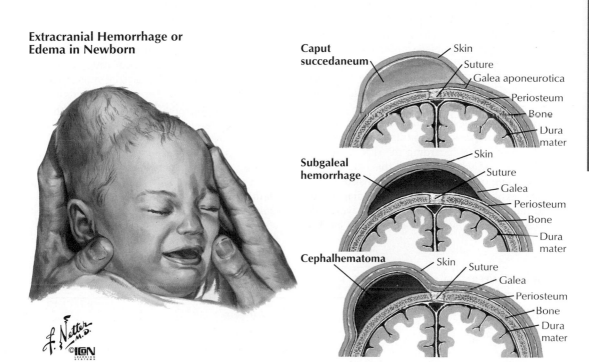

Caput succedaneum
— Skin
— Suture
— Galea aponeurotica
— Periosteum
— Bone
— Dura mater

Subgaleal hemorrhage
— Skin
— Suture
— Galea
— Periosteum
— Bone
— Dura mater

Cephalhematoma
— Skin
— Suture
— Galea
— Periosteum
— Bone
— Dura mater

CARDIOVASCULAR DISEASE IN PREGNANCY

THE CHALLENGE

Cardiac disease is one of the major causes of nonobstetric maternal mortality. Whereas in the past patients with congenital heart disease did not survive to reproductive age, it is now common for these patients to face a pregnancy, be it planned or unplanned.

Scope of the Problem: Cardiac disease complicates approximately 1% of all pregnancies. Mitral valve prolapse may be found in 5%–7% of pregnant women. The type and severity of risk vary with the type of lesion and the functional abilities of the patient (see table). Patients with valvular disease have an increased risk for thromboembolic disease, subacute bacterial endocarditis, cardiac failure, and pulmonary edema during and after pregnancy.

Objectives of Management: Identify patients at risk because of cardiovascular conditions, provide realistic counseling regarding the risk to mother and fetus, and work to reduce this risk. The basis of antepartum management consists of frequent evaluations of maternal cardiac status and fetal well-being, combined with avoidance of conditions or actions that increase cardiac workload. The latter includes the treatment or avoidance of anemia, prompt treatment of any infection or fever, limitation of strenuous activity, and adherence to appropriate weight gain.

TACTICS

Relevant Pathophysiology: By midpregnancy there is a 40% increase in cardiac output; this increase in demand may be potentially fatal. Cardiac output shows an additional increase in the immediate postpartum period, as up to 500 mL of additional blood enters the maternal circulation because of uterine contractions and rapid loss of uterine volume. Cardiac complications, such as peripartum cardiomyopathy, may occur up to 6 months after delivery. Valvular heart disease is the most commonly encountered cardiac complication of pregnancy with rheumatic valvular disease the most frequent type. The severity of the associated valvular lesion determines the degree of risk associated with pregnancy. Roughly 90% of these patients have mitral stenosis, which may result in worsening obstruction as cardiac output increases during the pregnancy. When severe or associated with atrial fibrillation, the risk of cardiac failure during pregnancy is increased.

Strategies: The New York Heart Association classification of heart disease is a useful guide to the

CARDIAC (MATERNAL) MORTALITY ASSOCIATED WITH PREGNANCY

Group I (mortality < 1%)	Atrial septal defect
	Bioprosthetic valve
	Mitral stenosis (functional class I and II)
	Patent ductus arteriosus
	Pulmonic/tricuspid disease
	Tetralogy of Fallot, corrected
	Ventricular septal defect
Group II (mortality 5%–15%)	Aortic stenosis
	Coarctation of aorta, without valvular involvement
IIA	Marfan's syndrome with normal aorta
	Mitral stenosis (functional class III and IV)
	Previous myocardial infarction
	Uncorrected tetralogy of Fallot
IIB	Artificial valve
	Mitral stenosis with atrial fibrillation
Group III (mortality 25%–50%)	Coarctation of aorta, with valvular involvement
	Marfan's syndrome with aortic involvement
	Pulmonary hypertension

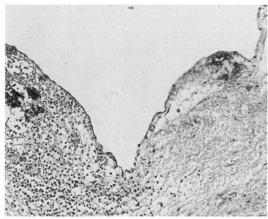

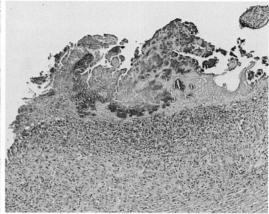

Deposit of platelets and organisms (stained dark), edema and leukocytic infiltration in very early bacterial endocarditis of aortic valve

Development of vegetations containing clumps of bacteria on tricuspid valve

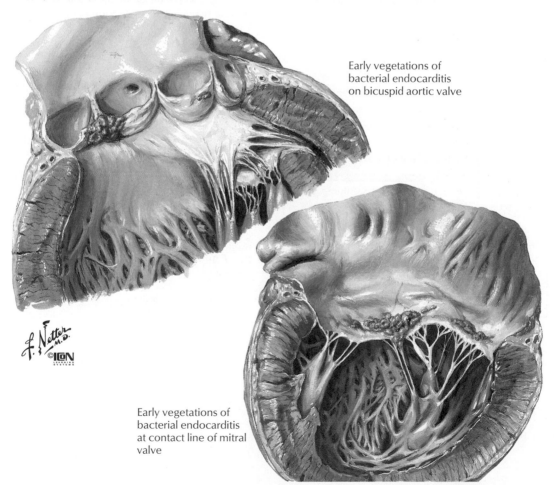

Early vegetations of bacterial endocarditis on bicuspid aortic valve

Early vegetations of bacterial endocarditis at contact line of mitral valve

risk of pregnancy (see table). Patients with class I or II disease, such as those with septal defects, patent ductus arteriosus, or mild mitral or aortic valvular disease, generally do well during pregnancy, although their fetuses are at greater risk for prematurity and low birth weight. Patients with class III or IV disease caused by primary pulmonary hypertension, uncorrected tetralogy of Fallot, Eisenmenger syndrome, or other conditions, rarely do well, with pregnancy inducing a significant risk of death, often in excess of 50%. Patients with this degree of cardiac decompensation should be advised to avoid pregnancy or consider termination based on careful consultation with specialists in both cardiology and high-risk obstetrics.

IMPLEMENTATION

Special Considerations: Most patients with mitral valve prolapse do well. The rare patient with left atrial and ventricular enlargement may de-

NEW YORK HEART ASSOCIATION CLASSIFICATION OF HEART DISEASE

Class I	No cardiac decompensation
Class II	No symptoms of decompensation at rest Minor limitations of physical activity
Class III	No symptoms of decompensation at rest Marked limitations of physical activity
Class IV	Symptoms of decompensation at rest Discomfort with any physical activity

velop dysfunction during the course of pregnancy. The severity of the disease and impact on the atrium and ventricle may be assessed by echocardiography. Peripartum cardiomyopathy is rare, but uniformly severe. Occurring in the last month of pregnancy or during the first 6 months after delivery, it is similar to other cardiomyopathies in symptoms and findings. Most often, a specific cause is not identified, and the cause remains unknown. This process presents an especially grave risk, necessitating early suspicion and aggressive consultative management. Patients at highest risk are those in their 30s, who are multiparous, of black race, who have delivered twins, or who have had preeclampsia. Unusual cardiac conditions, such as idiopathic hypertrophic subaortic stenosis and the structural anomalies associated with Marfan's syndrome, are associated with maternal moralities of 25%–50% or higher. The presence of such conditions demands realistic preconception counseling, and early transfer for specialized care, should a pregnancy occur.

REFERENCES

American College of Obstetricians and Gynecologists. *Cardiac Disease in Pregnancy.* Washington, DC: ACOG; 1992. ACOG Technical Bulletin 168.

Easterling TR, Chadwick HS, Otto CM, Benedetti TJ. Aortic stenosis in pregnancy. *Obstet Gynecol* 1988;72:113.

Landon MB, Samuels P. Cardiac and pulmonary disease. In: Gabbe SG, Niebyl JR, Simpson JL, eds. *Obstetrics: Normal and Problem Pregnancies.* 2nd ed. New York, NY: Churchill Livingstone; 1991:1057.

Schaefer G, Arditi LI, Solomon HA, Ringland JE. Congenital heart disease and pregnancy. *Clin Obstet Gynecol* 1968;11:1048.

Szekely P, Turner R, Snaith L. Pregnancy and the changing pattern of rheumatic heart disease. *Br Heart J* 1973;35:1293.

Veille JC. Peripartum cardiomyopathies: a review. *Am J Obstet Gynecol* 1984;148:805.

CERVICAL INCOMPETENCE

INTRODUCTION

Description: Cervical incompetence is characterized by asymptomatic dilation of the internal os during pregnancy. This generally leads to dilation of the entire cervical canal during the second trimester with subsequent risk of rupture of the membranes and/or expulsion of the fetus.

Prevalence: One of 57 to 1 of 1730 pregnancies; appears to be declining.

Predominant Age: Reproductive.

Genetics: No genetic pattern.

ETIOLOGY AND PATHOGENESIS

Causes: Congenital tissue defect, damage from cervical dilation at the time of dilatation and curettage or other manipulation, damage caused by surgery (conization), uterine anomalies (uterus didelphys).

Risk Factors: In utero exposure to DES, uterine anomalies.

CLINICAL CHARACTERISTICS

Signs and Symptoms:

History of second trimester pregnancy loss accompanied by spontaneous rupture of the membranes without labor, or rapid, painless, preterm labor.

DIAGNOSTIC APPROACH

Differential Diagnosis:

Uterine anomalies

Chorioamnionitis

Chromosomal anomaly (balanced translocation)

Associated Conditions: Premature rupture of the membranes, premature (preterm) delivery, and recurrent second trimester pregnancy loss.

Workup and Evaluation

Laboratory: No evaluation indicated beyond that for routine prenatal care.

Imaging: Ultrasonography before cervical cerclage to ensure normal fetal development. Although cervical length can be measured by ultrasonography, routine use of this has not proven to be an effective screening tool.

Special Tests: None indicated. (Frequent vaginal examinations beginning around the time of previous cervical change or the second trimester, whichever is earlier.)

Diagnostic Procedures: History.

Pathologic Findings

Painless dilation of the cervix.

MANAGEMENT AND THERAPY

Nonpharmacologic

General Measures: Evaluation, frequent prenatal visits with monitoring for cervical change.

Specific Measures: Cervical cerclage (placement of a concentric nonabsorbable suture at the level of the inner cervical os) is performed between 10 and 14 weeks of gestation. When the suture is placed vaginally, it is generally removed at 38 weeks of gestation. If labor occurs before this point, the suture must be removed immediately. Cervical cerclage is occasionally performed transabdominally. These sutures are intended to remain permanently and preclude vaginal delivery. The use of lever pessaries (such as the Smith-Hodge) has been reported to give outcomes similar to that obtained by cerclage, but this modality is infrequently used. Bleeding, uterine contractions, obvious infection, or rupture of the membranes are contraindications to cerclage. Because of scarring after cerclage, about 15% of patients require cesarean delivery.

Diet: No specific dietary changes indicated.

Activity: Restriction of activity is often suggested, but evidence that this alters the outcome of pregnancy is lacking. After 24 weeks of pregnancy, bed rest may be the only therapy available because cerclage may start labor.

Patient Education: American College of Obstetricians and Gynecologists Patient Education Pamphlet AP100 (*Repeated Miscarriage*), AP110 (*Loop Electrosurgical Excision Procedure*).

Drug(s) of Choice

None. (Prophylactic antibiotics have not been shown to be effective.)

FOLLOW-UP

Patient Monitoring: Frequent prenatal visits with monitoring for cervical change in patients thought to be at high risk. If a cerclage is placed, planned removal of cerclage at 38 weeks of gestation is advisable.

Prevention/Avoidance: Care to avoid overdilation of the cervix when surgical manipulation is required.

Possible Complications: Continued fetal loss, chorioamnionitis, cervical avulsion, or uterine rupture if labor occurs and the cerclage is not removed.

Expected Outcome: With correct diagnosis and cervical cerclage, fetal survival increases from 20% to 80%.

MISCELLANEOUS

ICD-9-CM Codes: 622.5.

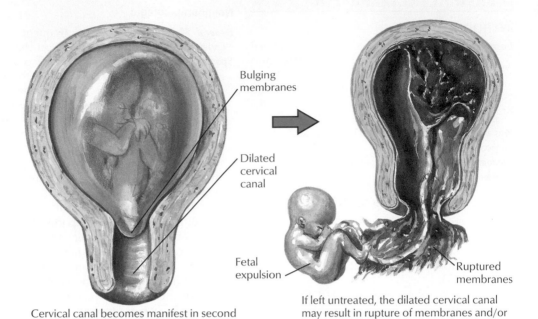

Bulging membranes

Dilated cervical canal

Fetal expulsion

Ruptured membranes

Cervical canal becomes manifest in second trimester as dilation of cervical canal

If left untreated, the dilated cervical canal may result in rupture of membranes and/or fetal expulsion

Surgical Management of Cervical Incompetence (Cerclage)

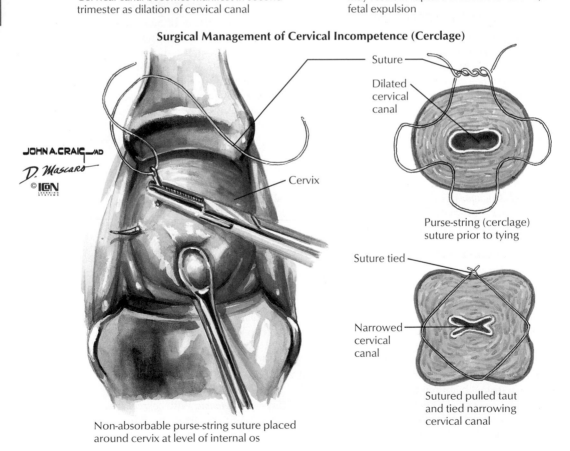

Suture

Dilated cervical canal

Cervix

Purse-string (cerclage) suture prior to tying

Suture tied

Narrowed cervical canal

Sutured pulled taut and tied narrowing cervical canal

Non-absorbable purse-string suture placed around cervix at level of internal os

OBSTETRICAL CONDITIONS

REFERENCES

Aarts JM, Brons JT, Bruinse HW. Emergency cerclage: a review. *Obstet Gynecol Surv* 1995;50:459.

American College of Obstetricians and Gynecologists. *Preterm Labor.* Washington, DC: ACOG; 1995. ACOG Technical Bulletin 206.

American College of Obstetricians and Gynecologists. *Early Pregnancy Loss.* Washington, DC: ACOG; 1995. ACOG Technical Bulletin 212.

Ansari AH, Reynolds RA. Cervical incompetence: a review. *J Reprod Med* 1987;32:161.

Schorr SJ, Morales WJ. Obstetric management of incompetent cervix and bulging fetal membranes. *J Reprod Med* 1996;41:235.

Witter FR. Negative sonographic findings followed by rapid cervical dilation due to cervical incompetence. *Obstet Gynecol* 1984;64:136.

CHOLECYSTITIS IN PREGNANCY

INTRODUCTION

Description: Cholelithiasis and cholecystitis complicate more than 3% of pregnancies.

Prevalence: Cholelithiasis—3%–4% of pregnancies; cholecystitis—0.25% of pregnancies.

Predominant Age: Reproductive.

Genetics: Some races at greater risk (eg, Pima Indians).

ETIOLOGY AND PATHOGENESIS

Causes: The metabolic alteration leading to cholesterol stones is thought to be a disruption in the balance between hydroxymethylglutaryl coenzyme A (HMG-CoA) reductase and cholesterol 7α-hydroxylase. HMG-CoA controls cholesterol synthesis, while cholesterol 7α-hydroxylase controls the rate of bile acid formation. Patients who form cholesterol stones have elevated levels of HMG-CoA and depressed levels of cholesterol 7α-hydroxylase. This change in ratio increases the risk of precipitation of cholesterol. During pregnancy, there is an increased rate of bile synthesis and a reduced rate of gallbladder emptying, increasing the risk of stone formation and obstruction.

Risk Factors: Cholecystitis is associated with increased maternal age, multiparity, multiple gestation, and a history of previous attacks.

CLINICAL CHARACTERISTICS

Signs and Symptoms (Unchanged by Pregnancy):
May be confused with symptoms of pregnancy
Fatty food intolerance
Variable right upper quadrant pain with radiation to the back or scapula
Nausea or vomiting (often mistaken for "indigestion" or "morning sickness")
Fever is usually associated with cholangitis

DIAGNOSTIC APPROACH

Differential Diagnosis:
Labor
Preeclampsia
Placental accident (abruption)
Cholestasis of pregnancy
Gastroenteritis
Esophageal reflux
Malabsorption
Irritable bowel syndrome
Peptic ulcer disease
Coronary artery disease
Pneumonia
Appendicitis

Associated Conditions: Jaundice, cirrhosis, pancreatitis, ileus, and premature labor.

Workup and Evaluation

Laboratory: Supportive, but often not diagnostic—complete blood count, serum bilirubin, amylase, alkaline phosphatase, and aminotransferase concentrations.

Imaging: Ultrasonography of the gallbladder (96% accurate in making the diagnosis of sludge or stone in the gallbladder).

Special Tests: None indicated.

Diagnostic Procedures: History, physical examination, ultrasonography, and laboratory investigation.

Pathologic Findings

None.

MANAGEMENT AND THERAPY

Nonpharmacologic

General Measures: Watchful waiting, dietary modifications aimed at reducing cholesterol and fatty food exposure.

Specific Measures: Cholelithiasis may be treated with oral therapy; surgical extirpation may be required. Cholecystectomy during pregnancy is associated with a 5% fetal loss rate, which rises to approximately 60% if pancreatitis is present at the time of surgery.

Diet: Nothing by mouth during acute attacks or until the diagnosis is established; reduced fatty food and cholesterol at other times.

Activity: No restriction.

Drug(s) of Choice

Ursodeoxycholic acid (Actigall) 8–10 mg/d as two to three doses. When cholecystitis is present, intravenous fluids, nasogastric suction, analgesics and antibiotics (cephalosporin) are appropriate.

Contraindications: Known allergy, acute cholecystitis, abnormal liver function, calcified stones (not cholesterol based).

Interactions: See warning for individual agents.

FOLLOW-UP

Patient Monitoring: Normal prenatal care once acute episode is resolved.

Prevention/Avoidance: None.

Possible Complications: Acute cholecystitis, pancreatitis, ascending cholangitis, peritonitis, internal fistulization (to the gastrointestinal tract), premature labor or delivery.

Expected Outcome: Cholecystitis—generally good with either oral or surgical therapy.

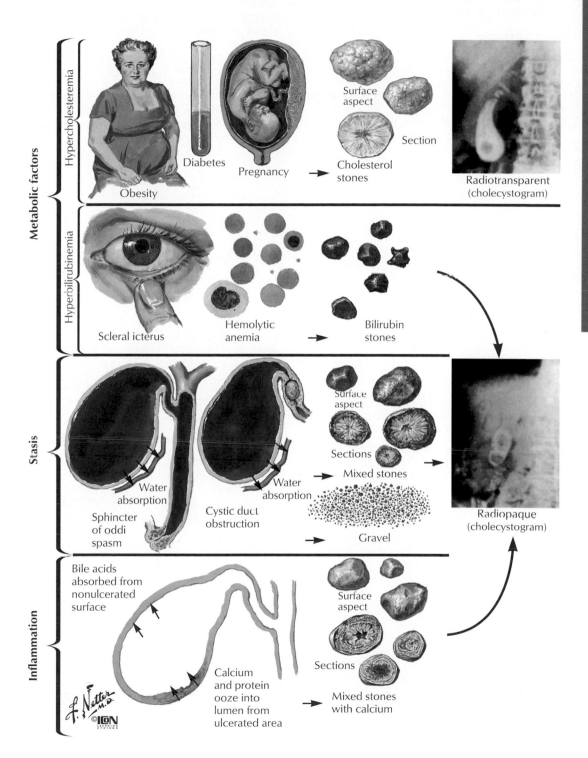

Metabolic factors

Hypercholesteremia

Obesity

Diabetes

Pregnancy → Cholesterol stones

Surface aspect

Section

Radiotransparent (cholecystogram)

Hyperbilirubinemia

Scleral icterus

Hemolytic anemia → Bilirubin stones

Stasis

Sphincter of oddi spasm

Water absorption

Cystic duct obstruction

Water absorption

Surface aspect

Sections

Mixed stones →

Gravel

Radiopaque (cholecystogram)

Inflammation

Bile acids absorbed from nonulcerated surface

Calcium and protein ooze into lumen from ulcerated area → Mixed stones with calcium

Surface aspect

Sections

OBSTETRICAL CONDITIONS

MISCELLANEOUS

ICD-9-CM **Codes:** 574.2 (others based on obstruction or inflammation).

REFERENCES

Block P, Kelley TR. Management of gallstone pancreatitis during pregnancy and the postpartum period. *Surg Gynecol Obstet* 1989;168:426.

Davis A, Katz VL, Cox R. Gallbladder disease in pregnancy. *J Reprod Med* 1995;40:759.

Dixon NF, Faddis DM, Silberman H. Aggressive management of cholecystitis during pregnancy. *Am J Surg* 1987;154:294.

Landers D, Carmona R, Crombleholme W, Lim R. Acute cholecystitis in pregnancy. *Obstet Gynecol* 1987; 69:131.

Smith RP, Nolan TE: Gallbladder disease and women: etiology, diagnosis and therapy. *Female Patient* 1992; 17:99.

Stauffer RA, Adams A, Wygal J, Lavery JP. Gallbladder disease in pregnancy. *Am J Obstet Gynecol* 1982; 144:661.

Valdivieso V, Covarrubias C, Siegel F, Cruz F. Pregnancy and cholelithiasis: pathogenesis and natural course of gallstones diagnosed in early puerperium. *Hepatology* 1993;17:1.

CONTRACTION STRESS TESTING

THE CHALLENGE

Fetal health may be assessed using the contraction stress test or oxytocin challenge test. This test is somewhat analogous to an exercise stress test for the evaluation of adult cardiac function in that problems or weaknesses that are normally compensated for at rest may become apparent with stress. In the contraction stress test, the fetal-placental-maternal unit is stressed through uterine contractions. The resulting periodic deprivation of uterine blood flow can be used to evaluate the robustness of the fetal condition.

Scope of the Problem: Three percent to twelve percent of pregnancies are at risk because of gestations that extend beyond term. More pregnancies may be compromised by maternal disease states that affect fetal health or placental function (eg, hypertension, diabetes).

Objectives of the Test: To assess fetal health and reserve.

TACTICS

Relevant Pathophysiology: During uterine contractions, uterine intramural pressure exceeds perfusion pressure, resulting in transient ischemia and loss of blood delivery to the intervillous spaces. When the fetus and placenta are healthy, this loss of blood flow causes no change in fetal tissue oxygenation, and there is no compensatory or reactive change in fetal heart rate. When the fetal-placental or placental-maternal relationships have been degraded, this brief loss of perfusion may be sufficient to cause a reduction in heart rate in the same way as that seen in labor when late decelerations are found.

Strategies: If uterine contractions are occurring spontaneously, the contraction stress test may proceed directly. To perform the oxytocin challenge test there must be no contraindications to the use of oxytocin. Fetal heart rate and uterine activity monitoring is established and contractions are induced using oxytocin or through intermittent nipple stimulation. Con-tractions must occur at a rate of 3 per 10 minutes for at least three 10-minute periods. A normal stress test should show normal fetal heart rate variability and the absence of periodic decelerations. Accelerations with fetal activity are reassuring.

Patient Education: Reassurance, American College of Obstetricians and Gynecologists Patient Education Pamphlet 098 (*Monitoring Fetal Health During Pregnancy*), AP015 (*Fetal Heart Rate Monitoring*).

IMPLEMENTATION

Special Considerations: If contractions are occurring spontaneously at a rate of at least 3 per 10 minutes, the term "contraction stress test" is generally used, whereas the term "oxytocin challenge test" is used when contractions must be induced through oxytocin administration. Like most tests of fetal status, the contraction stress test has a moderate false-positive rate. Consequently, the interpretation of a positive test must be made in the perspective of other information about the mother and fetus, including the results of other tests such as the nonstress test or biophysical profile. (See also "Antepartum Testing.")

REFERENCES

American College of Obstetricians and Gynecologists. *Antepartum Fetal Surveillance.* Washington, DC: ACOG; 1994. ACOG Technical Bulletin 188.

American College of Obstetricians and Gynecologists. *Fetal Heart Rate Patterns: Monitoring, Interpretation, and Management.* Washington, DC: ACOG; 1995. ACOG Technical Bulletin 207.

Freeman RK, Anderson G, Dorchester W. A prospective multi-institutional study of antepartum fetal heart rate monitoring. II. Contraction stress test versus nonstress test for primary surveillance. *Am J Obstet Gynecol* 1982;57:228.

Manning FA, Harman CR, Morrison I, Mentigoglou SM, Lange IR, Johnson JM. Fetal assessment based on fetal biophysical profile scoring. IV. An analysis of perinatal morbidity and mortality. *Am J Obstet Gynecol* 1990;138:575.

Moore TR, Piacquadio K. A prospective evaluation of fetal movement screening to reduce the incidence of antepartum fetal death. *Am J Obstet Gynecol* 1989; 160:1075.

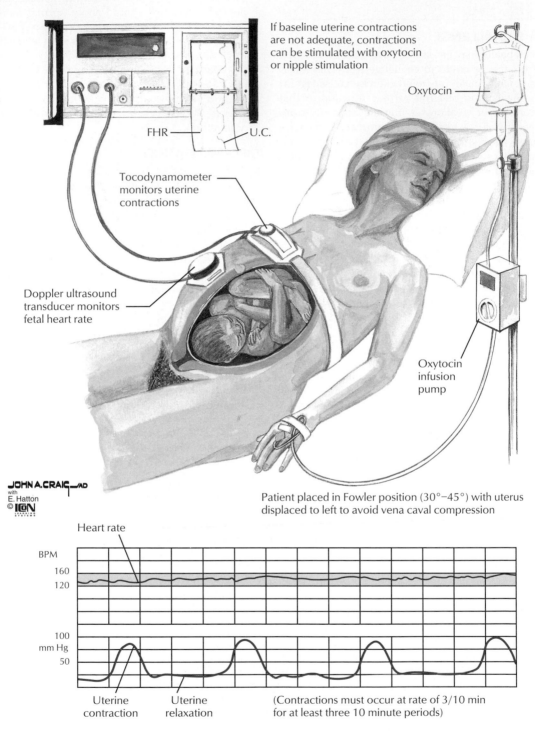

If baseline uterine contractions are not adequate, contractions can be stimulated with oxytocin or nipple stimulation

Oxytocin

FHR

U.C.

Tocodynamometer monitors uterine contractions

Doppler ultrasound transducer monitors fetal heart rate

Oxytocin infusion pump

JOHN A. CRAIG __AD
with
E. Hatton
© ICON

Patient placed in Fowler position (30°–45°) with uterus displaced to left to avoid vena caval compression

Heart rate

BPM

160
120

100
mm Hg
50

Uterine contraction

Uterine relaxation

(Contractions must occur at rate of 3/10 min for at least three 10 minute periods)

Portion of a "normal" (negative) contraction stress test exhibiting absence of heart rate decelerations following uterine contractions

DEPRESSION: POSTPARTUM

INTRODUCTION

Description: A cluster of symptoms characterized by disturbance of mood, a loss of sense of control, intense mental, emotional, and physical anguish, and a loss of self-esteem associated with childbirth.

Prevalence: Eight percent to ten percent of delivering women, true psychosis—1–2 of 1000 deliveries.

Predominant Age: Reproductive.

Genetics: No genetic pattern, although there is a proposed family tendency.

ETIOLOGY AND PATHOGENESIS

Causes: Unknown.

Risk Factors: History of major depression, premenstrual syndrome, prior postpartum depression, perinatal loss, early childhood loss (parent, sibling), physical or sexual abuse, socioeconomic deprivation, family predisposition, lifestyle stress, unplanned pregnancy. There is a 50% recurrence rate for subsequent pregnancies.

CLINICAL CHARACTERISTICS

Signs and Symptoms:

Five of the following must be present—
depressive mood the majority of time; diminished interest in normal or pleasurable activities; significant involuntary change in weight; insomnia or hypersomnia; psychomotor agitation or retardation; fatigue or loss of energy; feelings of worthlessness or guilt; diminished ability to think or concentrate; recurrent thoughts of death

Begins 2–12 months after delivery; lasts 3–14 months

DIAGNOSTIC APPROACH

Differential Diagnosis:

Normal grief reaction

Transient mood change ("postpartum blues")

Substance abuse

Eating disorders or other non-mood psychiatric disorders

Associated Conditions: None.

Workup and Evaluation

Laboratory: No evaluation indicated.

Imaging: No imaging indicated.

Special Tests: Beck Depression Inventory may be used to screen for depression.

Diagnostic Procedures: History, suspicion.

Pathologic Findings

None.

MANAGEMENT AND THERAPY

Nonpharmacologic

General Measures: Support, reassurance, and assistance with transition to motherhood.

Specific Measures: Psychotherapy, antidepressants, electroshock therapy.

Diet: No specific dietary changes indicated.

Activity: No restriction.

Patient Education: Reassurance, family support, American College of Obstetricians and Gynecologists Patient Education Pamphlet AP091 (*Postpartum Depression*).

Drug(s) of Choice

Selective serotonin reuptake inhibitors (fluoxetine [Prozac] 10–40 mg daily, paroxetine [Paxil] 20–50 mg daily, sertraline [Zoloft] 50–150 mg daily)

For symptoms of appetite loss, loss of energy or interest in pleasure, psychomotor retardation, thoughts of hopelessness, guilt, or suicide: cyclic antidepressants (eg, amitriptyline, clomipramine, doxepin, imipramine, nortriptyline, bupropion, and others)

For symptoms of increased appetite, sleepiness, high levels of anxiety, phobias, obsessive-compulsive disorders: monoamine oxidase (MAO) inhibitors (eg, isocarboxazid, phenelzine, tranylcypromine)

Contraindications: See individual agents.

Precautions: Use in pregnancy must be carefully weighed versus the potential effects (teratogenic) on the fetus. Some agents are associated with delayed cardiac conduction and disturbances in rhythm. Tricyclic agents, paroxetine, sertraline, and venlafaxine must be tapered over 2–4 weeks to discontinue.

Interactions: Virtually all agents may produce fatal interactions with MAO inhibitors or antiarrhythmic medications. MAO inhibitors can also adversely interact with vasoconstrictors, decongestants, meperidine, and other narcotics.

ALTERNATIVE THERAPY

Electroshock therapy may still play a role in the treatment of major depression and mania in those who do not respond to other therapies or are at high risk for suicide.

FOLLOW-UP

Patient Monitoring: Follow up at 6 weeks, 3 and 6 months, and as needed.

Prevention/Avoidance: None.

Patient may have prior history of depression, premenstrual tension, or prior postpartum depression

Condition begins 2–12 months postdelivery and may last 3–14 months

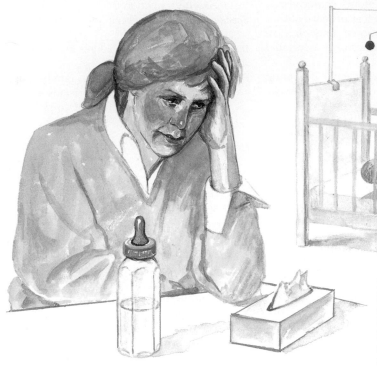

Postpartum depression is characterized by a disturbance of mood; a loss of sense of control; intense mental, emotional, and physical anguish; and a loss of self-esteem associated with childbirth

Diagnostic Criteria
(must meet five of the following factors)

1.) Depressed mood for majority of time

2.) Decreased interest in pleasurable activities

3.) Significant involuntary weight loss

4.) Psychomotor agitation or retardation

5.) Feelings of guilt or worthlessness

6.) Decreased concentration

7.) Recurrent thoughts of death

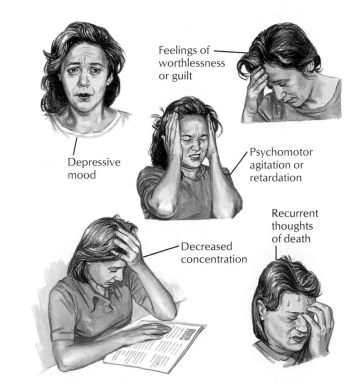

Feelings of worthlessness or guilt

Depressive mood

Psychomotor agitation or retardation

Decreased concentration

Recurrent thoughts of death

JOHN A. CRAIG—MD

C. Machado—M.D.

with
E. Hatton
© ICN

Possible Complications: Progressive loss of function, suicide.

Expected Outcome: Generally good response for mild to moderate depression with psychotherapy and medication; severe depression in 45%–65% of patients responds to medication. Recurrence rates are approximately 50% after a single episode, 70% after two episodes, and 90% with three or more episodes.

MISCELLANEOUS

Pregnancy Considerations: Tends to recur with subsequent pregnancies. Prophylactic treatment after delivery should be considered for these patients.

ICD-9-CM Codes: 648.4.

REFERENCES

American College of Obstetricians and Gynecologists. *Depression in Women.* Washington, DC: ACOG; 1993. ACOG Technical Bulletin 182.

American College of Obstetricians and Gynecologists. *Grief Related to Perinatal Death.* Washington, DC: ACOG; 1985. ACOG Technical Bulletin 86.

Beck A. *Depression Inventory.* Philadelphia, Pa: Center for Cognitive Therapy, 1991.

McGrath E, Ketia GP, Strickland BR, Russo NF. *Women and depression: risk factors and treatment issues.* Washington, DC: American Psychological Association, 1990.

Notman MT. Depression in women. Psychoanalytic concepts. *Psychiatr Clin North Am* 1989;12:221.

Nurnberg HG. An overview of somatic treatments of psychotic depression during pregnancy and postpartum. *Gen Hosp Psychiatry* 1989;11:328.

O'Hara MW. Postpartum mental disorders. In: Sciarra JJ, ed. *Gynecology and Obstetrics.* Vol 3. Philadelphia, Pa: JB Lippincott; 1998;3:1.

DIABETES MELLITUS IN PREGNANCY

THE CHALLENGE

To diagnose and manage disturbances of glucose metabolism to minimize the risk to mother and fetus associated with diabetes. Diabetes and pregnancy have profound effects on each other, making a familiarity with the interactions between mother, fetus, and the diabetic process a requirement to provide optimal care.

Scope of the Problem: Diabetes mellitus is the most common medical complication of pregnancy, affecting 2%–3% of patients. Patients with type I diabetes are at greater risk for maternal complications (diabetic ketoacidosis, glucosuria, hyperglycemia, polyhydramnios, preeclampsia, pregnancy-induced hypertension, preterm labor, retinopathy, urinary tract infections, uterine atony). The offspring of diabetic women have a 3-fold greater risk of congenital anomalies (3%–6%) than those of nondiabetic mothers (1%–2%). Most common among these anomalies are cardiac and limb deformities. Other fetal complications include fetal demise, hydramnios, hyperbilirubinemia, hypocalcemia, hypoglycemia, macrosomia, polycythemia, prematurity, respiratory distress syndrome, and spontaneous abortion.

Objectives of Management: To return serum glucose levels to as close to normal as possible through a combination of diet, exercise, and insulin (for selected patients). Optimal management of diabetes begins before pregnancy. Optimal management also requires patient and family education and involvement. For the established diabetic patient, this teaching is directed to the need for tighter control and more frequent monitoring. The woman with newly diagnosed diabetes requires general instruction about her disease as well as the unique aspects of diabetes during pregnancy.

TACTICS

Relevant Pathophysiology: Human placental lactogen, made in abundance by the growing placenta, promotes lipolysis and decreases glucose uptake and gluconeogenesis. This antiinsulin effect is sufficient to tip borderline patients into a diabetic state or prompt readjustments in the insulin dosage used by insulin-dependent diabetics. Estrogen, progesterone, and placental insulinase further complicate the management of diabetes, making diabetic ketoacidosis more common. High renal plasma flow and diffusion rates that exceed tubular reabsorption result in a physiologic glucosuria of approximately 300 mg/d. This physiologic glucosuria, combined with the poor correlation between urinary glucose and blood glucose levels, make the urinary glucose screening useless to detect or monitor diabetes during pregnancy.

Strategies: The severity of diabetes may be classified by either the American Diabetes Association (ADA) classification or by the White classification schemes, although the latter has been rendered less useful by improvements in fetal assessment, neonatal care, and the metabolic management of the pregnant patient. The use of these classifications makes comparisons of published data meaningful and may help to predict the relative risk to the pregnant mother and fetus. Patients with ADA type 2 disease are often overweight and their diabetes may be controlled with strict diet or with minimal insulin therapy. Gestational diabetes is reversible, although these patients have a greater incidence of glucose intolerance in subsequent pregnancies or with aging. Because of the increased risk of fetal anomalies, a determination of maternal serum α-fetoprotein and early ultrasonographic studies are of greater importance for these patients.

Patient Education: American College of Obstetricians and Gynecologists Patient Education Pamphlet AP051 (*Diabetes and Pregnancy*).

IMPLEMENTATION

Special Considerations: Screening for gestational diabetes is carried out by measurement of plasma glucose level 1 hour after ingestion of a 50-g glucose load, performed between 24 and 32 weeks of gestation. The upper limit of normal for such a test is 140 mg/dL (7.8 mmol/L). If a patient's value exceeds this threshold, a formal 3-hour glucose tolerance test is performed. About 15% of patients have an abnormal screening test, and about the same proportion have an abnormal 3-hour test. For a 3-hour glucose tolerance test, the patient must ingest a minimum of 150 g/d of glucose for the 3 days preceding the test. A fasting glucose level is determined, and a 100-g glucose load is consumed. Plasma glucose levels are then measured at 1, 2, and 3 hours. If two or more values are abnormal, the diagnosis of gestational diabetes may be made. If only one value is abnormal, the test is considered equivocal and should be repeated in 4–6 weeks.

Diabetes in Pregnancy

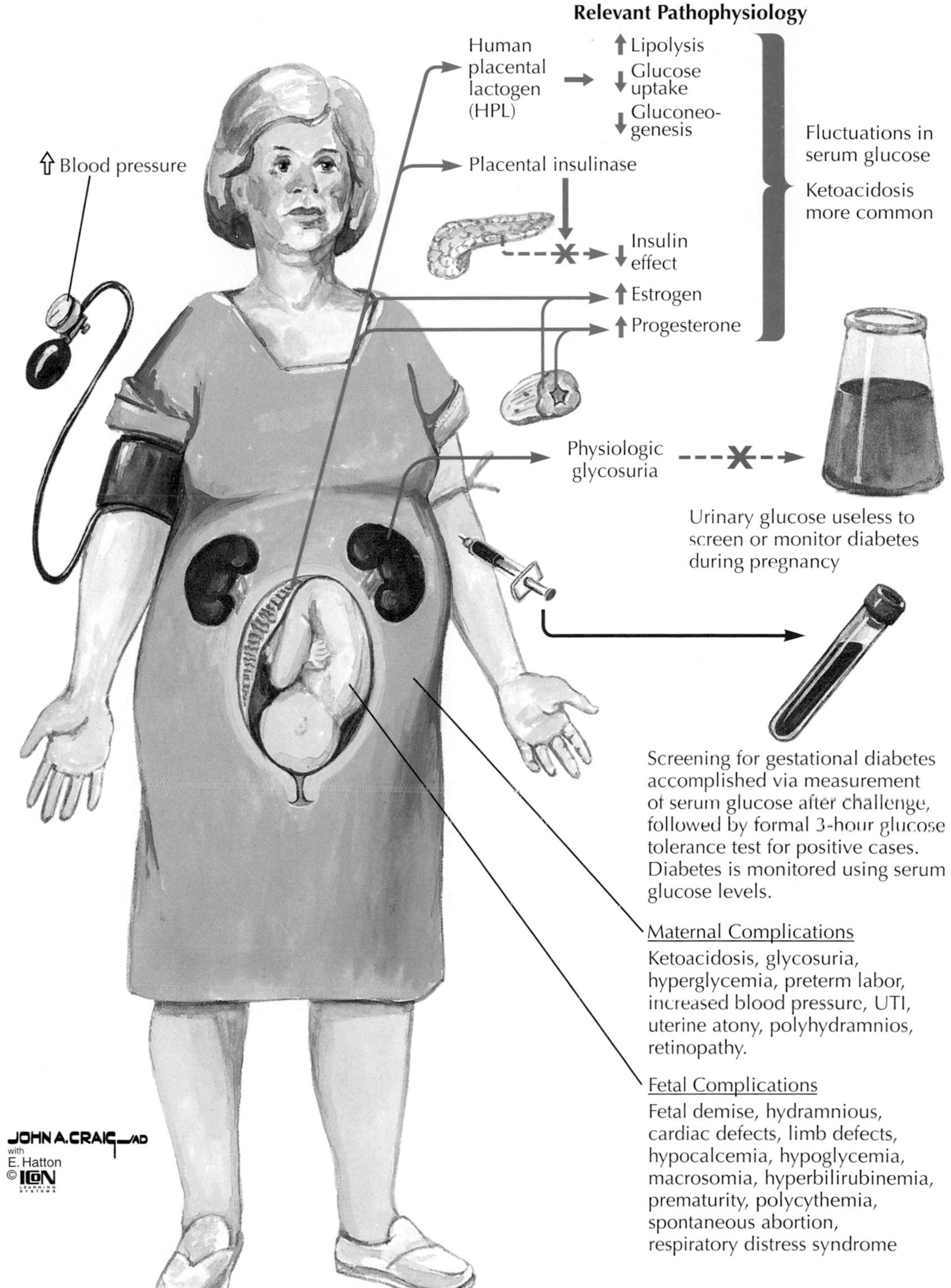

Relevant Pathophysiology

Human placental lactogen (HPL) → ↑ Lipolysis
↓ Glucose uptake
↓ Gluconeo-genesis

Placental insulinase

↓ Insulin effect

↑ Estrogen

↑ Progesterone

} Fluctuations in serum glucose

Ketoacidosis more common

↑ Blood pressure

Physiologic glycosuria - - - ✗ - - ▶

Urinary glucose useless to screen or monitor diabetes during pregnancy

Screening for gestational diabetes accomplished via measurement of serum glucose after challenge, followed by formal 3-hour glucose tolerance test for positive cases. Diabetes is monitored using serum glucose levels.

Maternal Complications
Ketoacidosis, glycosuria, hyperglycemia, preterm labor, increased blood pressure, UTI, uterine atony, polyhydramnios, retinopathy.

Fetal Complications
Fetal demise, hydramnious, cardiac defects, limb defects, hypocalcemia, hypoglycemia, macrosomia, hyperbilirubinemia, prematurity, polycythemia, spontaneous abortion, respiratory distress syndrome

JOHN A.CRAIG—AD
with
E. Hatton
© ICON
LEARNING SYSTEMS

Management objectives involve efforts to return serum glucose levels to as close to normal as possible through a combination of diet, exercise, and insulin (as indicated), and tight control in established diabetic patients.

REFERENCES

American College of Obstetricians and Gynecologists. *Diabetes in Pregnancy*. Washington, DC: ACOG; 1994. ACOG Technical Bulletin 200.

American Diabetes Association. Position statement: screening for diabetes. *Diabetes Care* 1989;12:588.

Carpenter MW, Coustan DR. Criteria for screening test for gestational diabetes. *Am J Obstet Gynecol* 1982;144:768.

Cousins L. Pregnancy complications among diabetic women: review 1965–1985. *Obstet Gynecol Surv* 1987; 42:140.

Freinkel N, Dooley SL, Metzger BE. Care of the pregnant women with insulin-dependent diabetes mellitus. *N Engl J Med* 1985;313:96.

Landon MB, Gabbe SG. Antepartum fetal surveillance and delivery timing in diabetic pregnancies. *Clin Diabetes* 1990;8:33.

Metzger BE. Summary and recommendations of the Third International Workshop-Conference on Gestational Diabetes Mellitus. *Diabetes* 1991;40(suppl 2):197.

FETAL ALCOHOL SYNDROME

INTRODUCTION
Description: A syndrome of malformations found in infants born to mothers who have consumed alcohol during pregnancy. Abnormalities include structural malformations (predominately facial), growth restriction, and neurologic abnormalities including mental retardation.

Prevalence: Estimates vary from 6 of 10,000 births (1993) to 1–2 of 1,000 births (2000).

Predominant Age: Reproductive for mothers, infants diagnosed at birth.

Genetics: No genetic pattern.

ETIOLOGY AND PATHOGENESIS
Causes: Alcohol consumption during pregnancy (generally >3 oz/day). There does not appear to be a lower limit of safety nor are the effects confined to one part of pregnancy. The severity of the effects does appear to be proportional to the amount and duration of exposure. Clinically identifiable effects are generally not seen with sporadic exposures of less than 1 oz of alcohol per day, although absolute safety cannot be assured even at this dose.

Risk Factors: Alcohol use during pregnancy.

CLINICAL CHARACTERISTICS
Signs and Symptoms:
Facial deformities—Microcephaly, short palpebral fissures, flat midface, underdeveloped philtrum and thinned upper lip; low nasal bridge, epicanthal folds, minor ear anomalies, small teeth with faulty enamel, foreshortened nose and micrognathia may also be seen; two or more abnormal facial features must be present to make the diagnosis
Cardiac malformations
Deformities of joints, limbs, and fingers
Vision difficulties including nearsightedness (myopia)
Intrauterine and extrauterine growth restriction
Mental retardation and developmental abnormalities, brain and spinal defects
Abnormal behavior such as short attention span, hyperactivity, poor impulse control, extreme nervousness, and anxiety

DIAGNOSTIC APPROACH
Differential Diagnosis:
Other chromosomal or congenital syndromes

Associated Conditions: Maternal—other substance abuse (tobacco, drugs), sexually transmitted disease. Fetal—dental caries, cardiac defects, and ophthalmic problems (vision correction often necessary).

Workup and Evaluation
Laboratory: No evaluation indicated.

Imaging: Ultrasonography may be used to assess fetal growth and development. Some cardiac anomalies may be detected while in utero; absence does not exclude effects.

Special Tests: None indicated.

Diagnostic Procedures: History (maternal) and physical examination of newborn.

Pathologic Findings
None.

MANAGEMENT AND THERAPY
Nonpharmacologic
General Measures: For the mother—counseling, alcohol and substance abuse programs. For the fetus—evaluation, special education and support, surveillance for dental caries (more common in these children) and cardiac and ophthalmic problems.

Specific Measures: None.

Diet: Reduction or elimination of alcohol for the duration of pregnancy.

Activity: No restriction.

Patient Education: Diet and alcohol counseling, American College of Obstetricians and Gynecologists Patient Education Pamphlet AP104 (*Drugs and Pregnancy: Alcohol, Tobacco, and Other Drugs*).

Drug(s) of Choice
None.

FOLLOW-UP
Patient Monitoring: Normal health maintenance, surveillance for dental caries (more common in these children) and cardiac and ophthalmic problems.

Prevention/Avoidance: Reduction or elimination of alcohol use during pregnancy. No safe level of exposure has been demonstrated although sporadic use of less than 1 oz of alcohol per day has not been associated with the syndrome.

Possible Complications: Higher rate of spontaneous miscarriage in heavy users of alcohol.

Expected Outcome: Infants affected by fetal alcohol syndrome vary from mildly to profoundly

Fetal Alcohol Syndrome

Clinical Features

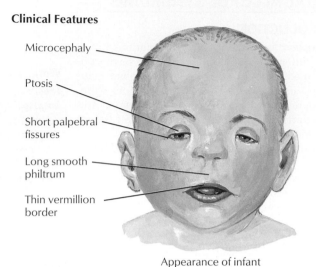

Microcephaly

Ptosis

Short palpebral fissures

Long smooth philtrum

Thin vermillion border

Appearance of infant

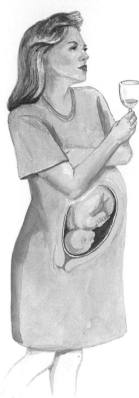

Alcohol consumption in excess of 3 oz/day during pregnancy is considered "high risk." Although identifiable effects are seldom seen with consumption less than 1 oz/day, there is no assurance of safety at that level

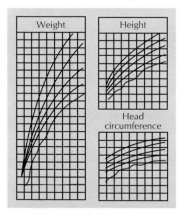

Weight	Height
	Head circumference

Developmental deficiency is common. Prognosis is most influenced by degree of maternal alcohol consumption, extent and severity of malformation pattern, including growth retardation

Atrial septal defect

Ventricular septal defect

Abnormal palmer crease

Cardiac and skeletal anomalies are common

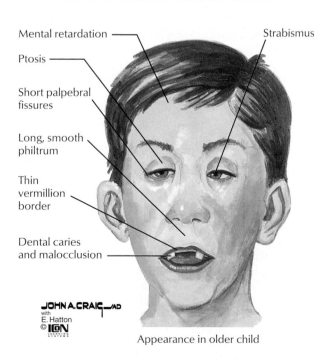

Mental retardation

Strabismus

Ptosis

Short palpebral fissures

Long, smooth philtrum

Thin vermillion border

Dental caries and malocclusion

JOHN A.CRAIG—AD
with
E. Hatton
©ICON

Appearance in older child

mentally retarded. Similarly, structural anomalies are variable, but lifelong.

MISCELLANEOUS

ICD-9-CM **Codes:** 760.71.

REFERENCES

American College of Obstetricians and Gynecologists. *Substance Abuse in Pregnancy.* Washington, DC: ACOG; 1994. ACOG Technical Bulletin 195.

American Medical Association, Council on Scientific Affairs. Fetal Effects of Maternal Alcohol Use. *JAMA* 1983;249:2517.

Autti-Rämö I, Korkman M, Hilakivi-Clark L, Lehtonen M, Halmesmäki E, Granström ML. Mental development of 2-year-old children exposed to alcohol in utero. *J Pediatr* 1992;120:740.

Centers for Disease Control and Prevention. Update: trends in fetal alcohol syndrome–United States, 1979–1993. *MMWR Morb Mortal Wkly Rep* 1995;44:249.

Holzman C, Paneth N, Little R, Pinto-Martin J, Neonatal Brain Hemorrhage Study Team. Perinatal brain injury in premature infants born to mothers using alcohol in pregnancy. *Pediatrics* 1995;94:66.

Jones KL, Smith DW, Ulleland CN, Streissguth AP. Patterns of malformation in offspring of chronic alcoholic mothers. *Lancet* 1973;1:1267.

GESTATIONAL TROPHOBLASTIC DISEASE

INTRODUCTION

Description: Gestational trophoblastic diseases include choriocarcinoma and molar pregnancy. They are abnormalities of pregnancy that arise entirely from abnormal placental proliferation. They are classified as being either complete, in which no fetus is present, or incomplete, in which both fetus and molar tissues are present.

Prevalence: Molar pregnancy—1 of 1000–1500 pregnancies; choriocarcinoma—1 of 20,000 pregnancies.

Predominant Age: Greatest during the early and late reproductive years.

Genetics: Complete—mostly 46,XX (paternal in origin). Incomplete—triploid (69,XXY or 69,XXX) (all of paternal origin).

ETIOLOGY AND PATHOGENESIS

Causes: Unknown.

Risk Factors: Maternal age (older than 40: 5.2 times risk), Asians living in Southeast Asia, folate deficiency, prior molar pregnancy (2% recurrence rate).

CLINICAL CHARACTERISTICS

Signs and Symptoms:
- Present as a pregnancy, but associated with more profound hormonal changes, leading to exaggerated symptoms of pregnancy in many patients
- Uterine size that is inappropriate for dates (larger or smaller)
- Painless vaginal bleeding (95%)
- Hypertension, preeclampsia, proteinuria, nausea and vomiting, visual changes, tachycardia, and shortness of breath all possible (pregnancy-induced hypertension in the first trimester of pregnancy is virtually diagnostic)

DIAGNOSTIC APPROACH

Differential Diagnosis:
- Choriocarcinoma
- Missed abortion
- Threatened abortion

Associated Conditions: Hyperemesis, hypertension, preeclampsia, proteinuria, nausea and vomiting, visual changes, tachycardia, and shortness of breath. Bilateral adnexal masses (theca lutein cysts) occur in 15%–20% of patients.

Workup and Evaluation

Laboratory: Complete blood count, quantitative measurement of β-human chorionic gonadotropin (β-hCG) (to establish risk and serial to follow success of therapy), the patient's blood type and Rh status should be established, to allow for Rh immune globulin therapy (if needed) or blood replacement. Clotting function studies are advisable before evacuation of the uterus.

Imaging: Ultrasonography can establish the diagnosis. A baseline chest radiograph to check for metastatic disease should be obtained.

Special Tests: Absence of fetal heart sounds (in complete mole).

Diagnostic Procedures: History and physical examination. Edematous trophoblastic fragments may be passed vaginally through a partially dilated cervical os, alerting the clinician to the diagnosis.

Pathologic Findings

Edematous trophoblastic fronds. Karyotype: incomplete; triploid (80%); complete; 46,XX (95%).

MANAGEMENT AND THERAPY

Nonpharmacologic

General Measures: Evaluation and diagnosis, general supportive measures.

Specific Measures: The treatment of molar pregnancies is surgical: evacuation of the uterine contents. This is most often accomplished via suction curettage. Because of the large size of some molar pregnancies and a tendency toward uterine atony, concomitant oxytocin administration is advisable and blood for transfusion must be immediately available, should it be needed.

Diet: No specific dietary changes indicated.

Activity: No restriction.

Drug(s) of Choice

None. (Oxytocin or methylergonovine maleate [Methergine] is used to help contract the uterus during surgical evacuation.) Primary or recurrent malignant trophoblastic disease is generally treated with chemotherapy (methotrexate, actinomycin D, chlorambucil, or cyclophosphamide [Cytoxan], singly or in combination).

FOLLOW-UP

Patient Monitoring: Once the uterus has been emptied, the patient must be closely followed for at least 1 year for the possibility of recurrent benign or malignant disease. Any change in the patient's examination, an increase in β-hCG titers, or a failure of the β-hCG level to fall below 10 mIU/mL by 12 weeks after evacuation must be evaluated for the possibility of recurrent benign or malignant disease.

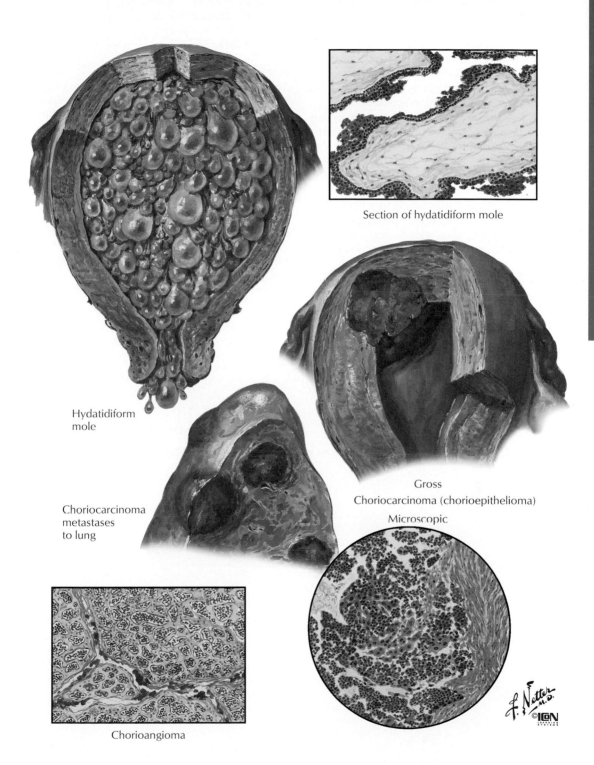

Section of hydatidiform mole

Hydatidiform mole

Choriocarcinoma metastases to lung

Gross
Choriocarcinoma (chorioepithelioma)

Microscopic

Chorioangioma

Prevention/Avoidance: None.

Possible Complications: Gestational trophoblastic neoplasia is notable for the possibility of malignant transformation, although less than 10% of patients develop malignant changes. In general, the larger or more advanced the molar pregnancy, the greater the risk of pulmonary complications, bleeding, trophoblastic emboli, or fluid overload during evacuation.

Expected Outcome: Roughly 80% of molar pregnancies follow a benign course after initial therapy. Between 15% and 25% of patients develop invasive disease, and 3%–5% eventually have metastatic lesions. The prognosis for patients with primary or recurrent malignant trophoblastic disease is generally good (90% cure rate). The theca lutein cysts often found in molar pregnancies may take several months to regress after evacuation of the uterine contents.

MISCELLANEOUS

Pregnancy Considerations: Pregnancy should be delayed for at least 1 year after a molar pregnancy to avoid confusion between normal pregnancy and recurrent disease. These patients have no higher rate of abortions, stillbirths, congenital anomalies, prematurity, or other complications of pregnancy with future gestations.

ICD-9-CM Codes: 630, 236.1 (Invasive or malignant).

REFERENCES

American College of Obstetricians and Gynecologists. *Management of Gestational Trophoblastic Disease.* Washington, DC: ACOG; 1993. ACOG Technical Bulletin 178.

Craighill MC, Cramer DW. Epidemiology of complete molar pregnancy. *J Reprod Med* 1984;29:784.

Goldstein DP, Berkowitz RS, Bernstein MR. Reproductive performance after molar pregnancy and gestational trophoblastic tumors. *Clin Obstet Gynecol* 1984;27:221.

Messerli ML, Lilienfeld AM, Parmeley T, Woodruff JD, Rosenshein NB. Risk factors for gestational trophoblastic neoplasia. *Am J Obstet Gynecol* 1985;153:294.

Romero R, Horgan JG, Kohorn EI, Kadar N, Taylor KJW, Hobbins JC. New criteria for the diagnosis of gestational trophoblastic disease. *Obstet Gynecol* 1985;66:553.

Wong LC, Choo YC, Ma HK. Methotrexate with citrovorum factor rescue in gestational trophoblastic disease. *Am J Obstet Gynecol* 1985;152:59.

GINGIVITIS IN PREGNANCY

INTRODUCTION

Description: Elevated hormone levels during pregnancy may induce gingival hyperplasia, pedunculated gingival growths, and pyogenic granuloma. Despite concerns directed elsewhere during pregnancy, the practitioner must watch for this common problem and address it when present.

Prevalence: Common (some estimate up to 90% of population affected).

Genetics: No genetic pattern.

ETIOLOGY AND PATHOGENESIS

Causes: Hormonally induced hypertrophy (may occur with combination oral contraceptives as well). Inadequate plaque removal. Fusiform bacillus or spirochete infection. Allergic reactions

Risk Factors: Increased hormones (pregnancy, oral contraceptives), poor dental hygiene, mouth breathing, diabetes mellitus, HIV infection, and malocclusion.

CLINICAL CHARACTERISTICS

Signs and Symptoms:
Mouth odor
Gum swelling and redness (especially at the base of the tooth)
Change in gum contours
Bleeding when brushing or flossing
Edema of interdental papillae

DIAGNOSTIC APPROACH

Differential Diagnosis:
Diabetes mellitus
Desquamative gingivitis
Leukemia
Drug reaction (phenytoin)
HIV infection

Associated Conditions: Periodontis, glossitis.

Workup and Evaluation

Laboratory: No evaluation indicated.

Imaging: No imaging indicated.

Special Tests: Smear to identify causative agent. Culture may also be performed.

Diagnostic Procedures: History and physical examination.

Pathologic Findings

Acute or chronic inflammation, broken crepuscular epithelium, hyperemia, polymorphonuclear infiltrates.

MANAGEMENT AND THERAPY

Nonpharmacologic

General Measures: Evaluation, encourage good oral hygiene, smoking cessation, warm saline rinses (bid), periodic dental care.

Specific Measures: Removal of irritating factors (plaque).

Diet: Assure adequate nutrition.

Activity: No restriction.

Patient Education: Reinforce the need for periodic dental care.

Drug(s) of Choice

Penicillin V 250–500 mg PO q6h, topical corticosteroids (triamcinolone in Orabase)

Contraindications: Known or suspected allergy.

Precautions: Watch for possible overgrowth of vaginal fungal flora if penicillin is used.

Interactions: See individual agents.

Alternative Drugs

Other antibiotics based on smear or culture results.

FOLLOW-UP

Patient Monitoring: Normal health maintenance.

Prevention/Avoidance: Good dental hygiene (daily brushing and flossing), periodic evaluation and cleaning.

Possible Complications: Severe periodontal disease, tooth loss.

Expected Outcome: Generally improves after delivery if hormonal change is the cause; can recur if dental hygiene is not maintained.

MISCELLANEOUS

ICD-9-CM Codes: 523.1.

REFERENCES

Pihlstrom BL, Ammons WF. Treatment of gingivitis and periodontitis. Research, Science and Therapy Committee of the American Academy of Periodontology. *J Periodontol* 1997;68:1246.

Robinson PJ. Gingivitis: a prelude to periodontitis? *J Clin Dent* 1995;6:41.

Scully C, Porter SR. The clinical spectrum of desquamative gingivitis. *Semin Cutan Med Surg* 1997;16:308.

Wang PH, Chao HT, Lee WL, Yuan CC, Ng HT. Severe bleeding from a pregnancy tumor. A case report. *J Reprod Med* 1997;42:359.

Warren PR, Chater BV. An overview of established interdental cleaning methods. *J Clin Dent* 1996;7:65.

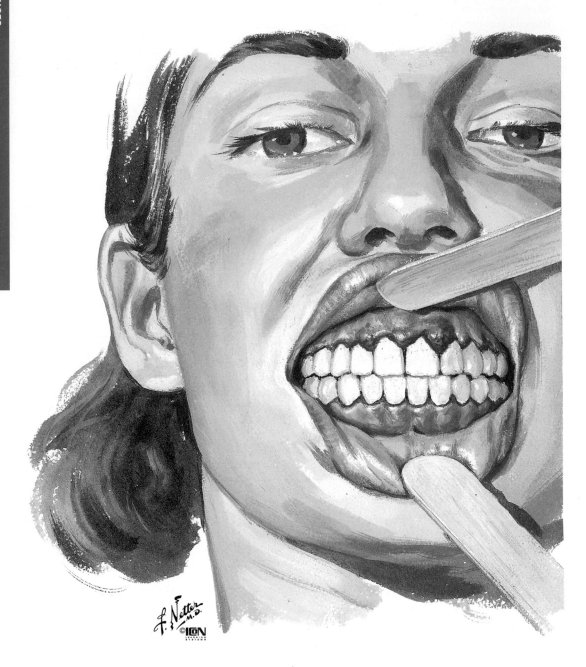

HELLP SYNDROME

INTRODUCTION

Description: Hemolysis, elevated liver enzymes, low platelet count (HELLP) syndrome is a variant of pregnancy-induced hypertension and preeclampsia, which is dominated by hepatic and hematologic changes.

Prevalence: Six percent to eight percent of pregnancies.

Predominant Age: Reproductive.

Genetics: No genetic pattern.

ETIOLOGY AND PATHOGENESIS

Causes: Unknown. Genetic, endocrine/metabolic (including altered prostaglandin production), uteroplacental ischemia, immunologic.

Risk Factors: Nulliparity, age older than 40, black race, family history of pregnancy-induced hypertension (PIH), renal disease, antiphospholipid syndrome, diabetes mellitus, multiple gestation. Chronic hypertension increases the risk of PIH.

CLINICAL CHARACTERISTICS

Signs and Symptoms:
Preeclampsia or eclampsia with hemolysis, thrombocytopenia, elevated hepatic transaminase levels (any or all; blood pressure may be normal in up to 20% of patients)
Right upper quadrant or epigastric pain

DIAGNOSTIC APPROACH

Differential Diagnosis:
Preeclampsia or eclampsia
Secondary hypertension
Improper blood pressure measurement (wrong cuff size, position, technique) resulting in false elevation of readings
Multiple pregnancy
Molar pregnancy
Primary hepatic disease

Associated Conditions: Intrauterine growth restriction, prematurity.

Workup and Evaluation

Laboratory: Liver and renal function studies (eg, enzymes, renal clearance, 24-hour urinary protein), platelet counts, clotting studies. (Platelet counts of >50,000/mm3 generally are not associated with spontaneous bleeding.)

Imaging: Ultrasonography to monitor fetal growth (frequently restricted).

Special Tests: Assessment of fetal lung maturation may be performed, but if maternal disease is severe, management is based on maternal factors and not fetal maturation.

Diagnostic Procedures: Measurement of blood pressure, laboratory confirmation.

Pathologic Findings

HELLP syndrome is a multiorgan process, including the renal, hepatic, hematologic, and nervous systems.

MANAGEMENT AND THERAPY

Nonpharmacologic

General Measures: Evaluation, support, and preparation for delivery.

Specific Measures: Patients with HELLP syndrome often represent the sickest patients with preeclampsia or eclampsia. The only true treatment is delivery. The presence of HELLP syndrome generally militates against conservative treatment for any but the briefest stabilization period.

Diet: No specific dietary changes indicated.

Activity: No restriction.

Patient Education: American College of Obstetricians and Gynecologists Patient Education Pamphlet AP034 (*High Blood Pressure During Pregnancy*).

Drug(s) of Choice

For mild to moderate chronic hypertension, α-methyldopa is considered first-line therapy.

During labor or labor induction, magnesium sulfate is often used to reduce the chance of seizures (4 g IV over 20 minutes, then 2–3 g/h IV continuous infusion; therapeutic range 4–8 mg/dL).

If blood pressure >180 torr systolic or 110 torr diastolic: hydralazine HCl 5–10 mg IV bolus q20min as needed or labetalol 20 mg IV bolus q10min as needed to a maximum of 300 mg in 24 hours. (Sodium nitroprusside may be used for extreme disease.)

Contraindications: Angiotensin-converting enzyme inhibitors are teratogenic and are contraindicated in pregnancy. Diuretics should be avoided in pregnancy because of the possibility of adverse fetal effects caused by reduced plasma volume. (Despite the common occurrence of edema, these patients have constricted circulatory volume.)

Precautions: Central hemodynamic monitoring should be considered if blood pressure is high or potent agents are used.

OBSTETRICAL CONDITIONS

Alternative Drugs

Verapamil or nifedipine may also be used to acutely reduce blood pressure.

FOLLOW-UP

Patient Monitoring: Increased maternal and fetal surveillance, antenatal testing.

Prevention/Avoidance: The value of low-dose aspirin therapy or calcium supplementation remains unproved.

Possible Complications: Maternal—cardiac decompensation, stroke, pulmonary edema and respiratory failure, renal failure, seizures and seizure-related injuries, intracranial hemorrhage, coma, and death (0.5%–5% mortality). Fetal risk (growth restriction and death) is directly proportional to both the degree of proteinuria and the level of maternal diastolic blood pressure.

Expected Outcome: HELLP syndrome generally resolves after delivery, but the risk of recurrence with future pregnancies or elevated blood pressure in later life is increased.

MISCELLANEOUS

ICD-9-CM **Codes:** 642.5

REFERENCES

American College of Obstetricians and Gynecologists. *Hypertension in Pregnancy.* Washington, DC: ACOG; 1996. ACOG Technical Bulletin 219.

Martin JN Jr, Blake PG, Pery KG Jr, McCaul JF, Hess LW, Martin RW. The natural history of HELLP syndrome: patterns of disease progression and regression. *Am J Obstet Gynecol* 1991;164:1500.

Pritchard JA, Weisman R Jr, Ratnoff OD, Vosburgh GJ. Intravascular hemolysis, thrombocytopenia and other hematologic abnormalities associated with severe toxemia of pregnancy. *N Engl J Med* 1954;250:87.

Sibai BM, Ramadan MK, Usta I, Salama M, Mercer BM, Friedman SA. Maternal morbidity and mortality in 442 pregnancies with hemolysis, elevated liver enzymes, and low platelets (HELLP syndrome). *Am J Obstet Gynecol* 1993;169:1000.

Weinstein L. Syndrome of hemolysis, elevated liver enzymes and low platelet count: a severe consequence of hypertension in pregnancy. *Am J Obstet Gynecol* 1982;142:159.

Clinical triad

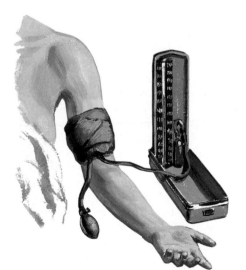

Elevated blood pressure

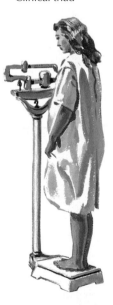

Excessive weight gain

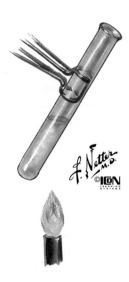

Albuminuria

HEPATITIS IN PREGNANCY

INTRODUCTION

Description: Hepatitis is one of the most serious infections that occurs during pregnancy.

Prevalence: Hepatitis—0.1%–1.5% of pregnancies (one third of Americans have antibodies to hepatitis A).

Predominant Age: Reproductive.

Genetics: No genetic pattern.

ETIOLOGY AND PATHOGENESIS

Causes: There are five different forms of hepatitis that may be involved. Hepatitis A is caused by an RNA virus that is transmitted by fecal-oral contamination and accounts for 30%–50% of acute disease. Hepatitis B is caused by a small DNA virus that accounts for 40%–45% of occurrences. It is estimated that acute hepatitis B occurs in 1–2 of 1000 pregnancies and chronic infections are present in 5–15 of 1000 pregnancies. Hepatitis B is transmitted by parenteral and sexual contact. Hepatitis B is easily transmitted sexually: 25% of people who have sexual contact with an infected person become infected. Hepatitis C (non-A, non-B) accounts for 10%–20% of cases and is caused by a single-stranded RNA virus spread by parenteral exposure. Hepatitis D is caused by an RNA virus that requires coinfection with the hepatitis B virus. Significant mortality and long-term consequences may occur from this less common infection. Hepatitis E and other forms of non-A, non-B hepatitis are uncommon, but may occur during pregnancy as well.

Risk Factors: Groups at greatest risk for hepatitis B are intravenous drug users, hemophiliacs, homosexuals, and health care workers. Poor hand-washing habits, multiple sexual partners, a history of sexually transmitted disease, tattoos, and multiple blood transfusions (hepatitis C) increase the risk of infection as well.

CLINICAL CHARACTERISTICS

Signs and Symptoms (Unchanged by Pregnancy):
Fever (60%), malaise (70%), fatigue, anorexia (50%), nausea (80%)
Variable right upper quadrant pain (50%)
Upper abdominal tenderness with hepatomegaly
Dark urine (85%) and acholic stools
Jaundice a possibility in up to 60%
Coagulopathy or encephalopathy (fulminant infections only)

DIAGNOSTIC APPROACH

Differential Diagnosis:
Acute fatty liver of pregnancy
Toxic hepatic injury
Cholestasis of pregnancy
Severe preeclampsia
Mononucleosis
Cytomegalovirus hepatitis
Lupoid hepatitis
Viral enteritis

Associated Conditions: Jaundice, cirrhosis, pancreatitis, nephritis, ileus, and premature labor.

Workup and Evaluation

Laboratory: Hepatitis during pregnancy is diagnosed in the same manner as for nonpregnant patients; serum chemistry abnormalities indicate active hepatic disease (marked elevation of alanine aminotransferase, aspartate aminotransferase, and bilirubin), and immunochemical analysis indicates the presence of infection and the phase of the clinical course (see table). In severe cases, coagulation studies should be performed. Routine screening of all pregnant patients is recommended.

SEROLOGIC TESTS FOR VIRAL HEPATITIS

Virus	Acute Infection	Carrier State
Hepatitis A	Hepatitis A IgM antibody	None
Hepatitis B	HBsAg	
	HBeAg	
	HBcAg IgM antibody	HBsAg
Hepatitis C	Hepatitis C antibody	Persistent evidence of liver dysfunction
Hepatitis D	D antigen	D antigen
	Hepatitis D IgM antibody	Hepatitis D IgM antibody

HBsAg, hepatitis B surface antigen; HBeAg, hepatitis B e antigen (indicates high rates of viral replication); HBcAg, hepatitis B core antigen.

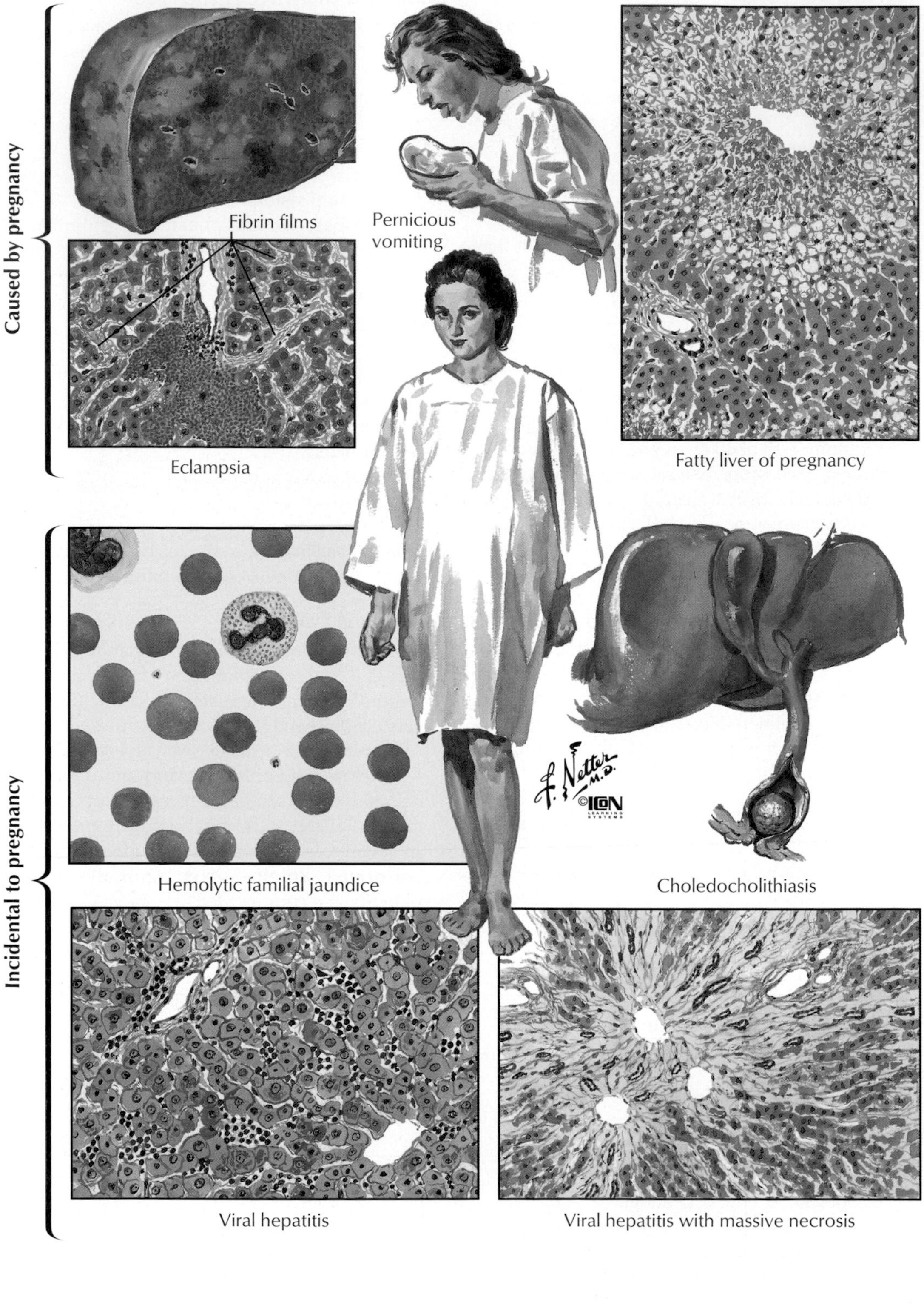
Caused by pregnancy
Fibrin films
Pernicious
vomiting
Eclampsia
Fatty liver of pregnancy
Incidental to pregnancy
Hemolytic familial jaundice
Choledocholithiasis
Viral hepatitis
Viral hepatitis with massive necrosis
F. Netter M.D.
©ICON LEARNING SYSTEMS

Imaging: None indicated.

Special Tests: Percutaneous liver biopsy may be helpful but is generally not required.

Diagnostic Procedures: History, physical examination, ultrasonography (limited value), and laboratory investigation.

Pathologic Findings

Viral hepatitis is distinguished from other hepatic injuries by the characteristic pattern of injury and infiltrate.

MANAGEMENT AND THERAPY

Nonpharmacologic

General Measures: Patients with encephalopathy or coagulopathy or who are severely debilitated should be hospitalized. Nutritional support is generally required. Fluid intake and electrolyte levels must be maintained. The upper abdomen should be protected from trauma. Sexual contact should be avoided until the partner(s) receive prophylaxis.

Specific Measures: No specific measures have been shown to alter the natural course of these infections. Prophylaxis should be considered for anyone at risk (eg, travel to endemic area, sexual partners). Acute exposure should be treated with immune globulin (see *Follow-Up*).

Diet: Maintain good nutrition.

Activity: The upper abdomen should be protected from trauma.

Patient Education: Patients should be instructed regarding risk factors and modes of spread to limit risk for family contacts and future recurrences, American College of Obstetricians and Gynecologists Patient Education Pamphlet AP125 (*Protecting Yourself Against Hepatitis B*).

Drug(s) of Choice

Those necessary for support only; others of limited or unproved value.

FOLLOW-UP

Patient Monitoring: Normal prenatal care once the acute episode is resolved. Continued monitoring for chronic liver dysfunction or carrier state (where applicable).

Prevention/Avoidance: Active immunization of those at risk before a pregnancy is planned. Patients exposed to hepatitis A may be given γ-globulin in the same manner as that for nonpregnant patients. Patients exposed to hepatitis B or those found to be carriers may receive either active immunization with hepatitis vaccine or passive immunization with hepatitis B immune globulin (HBIG). To be effective, HBIG should be given within 48 hours of exposure. The infants of these mothers should receive both forms of immunization. Infants born to hepatitis B-infected mothers should be given immune globulin (HBIg) 0.5 mL and hepatitis B vaccine (separate site) within 12 hours of birth, with follow up vaccinations at 1 and 6 month of age.

Possible Complications: Mortality from acute hepatitis varies with the type of hepatitis and severity of infection but is generally in the range of 2–10 of 1000 cases. Serious complications of hepatitis A are uncommon. Vertical transmission of hepatitis B to the developing fetus can pose a significant risk. The majority of untreated infants become chronic carriers, capable of infecting others. These infants are also at increased risk of cirrhosis and hepatic cancer. Neonatal infection rates vary with gestation and are highest in the third trimester (exposure to blood and fluids at delivery). Patients with the envelope antigen have an 80% chance of vertical transmission of the infection. Hepatitis D leads to chronic hepatitis in 80% of patients with rapid appearance of cirrhosis in 15%; mortality approaches 25%. Chronic liver disease and liver failure may follow infection with hepatitis B, C, or D.

Expected Outcome: Eighty-five percent to ninety percent of patients experience complete resolution of symptoms; 10%–15% of hepatitis B patients become chronic carriers (10%–15% of these develop serious long-term liver problems including cirrhosis and hepatocellular carcinoma). Patients with hepatitis C or D have a >80% risk of chronic hepatitis with cirrhosis and liver failure in 20%–25%.

MISCELLANEOUS

ICD-9-CM **Codes:** 647.6.

REFERENCES

American College of Obstetricians and Gynecologists. *Hepatitis in Pregnancy.* Washington, DC: ACOG; 1992. ACOG Technical Bulletin 174.

Centers for Disease Control: Protection against viral hepatitis. Recommendations of the Immunization Practices Advisory Committee. *MMWR Morb Mortal Wkly Rep* 1990;39:1.

Centers for Disease Control: Prevention of perinatal transmission of hepatitis B virus. Recommendations of the Immunization Practices Advisory Committee. *MMWR Morb Mortal Wkly Rep* 1988;37:341.

Floreani A, Paternoster D, Zappalà F, et al. Hepatitis C virus infection in pregnancy. *Br J Obstet Gynaecol* 1996;103:325.

Sweet RL. Hepatitis B infection in pregnancy. *Obstet Gynecol Rep* 1990;2:128.

Thaler MM, Park C-K, Landers DV, et al. Vertical transmission of hepatitis C virus. *Lancet* 1991;338:17.

INTRAUTERINE GROWTH RESTRICTION

INTRODUCTION

Description: Symmetric or asymmetric reduction in the size and weight of the growing fetus in utero, compared with that expected for a fetus of comparable gestational age. This may occur for many reasons, but most occurances represent signs of significant risk of fetal death or jeopardy to the fetus. Some authors advocate identifying fetuses with growth between the 10th and 20th percentiles as suffering "diminished" growth and at intermediate risk for complications.

Prevalence: Problems of consistent definition make estimates difficult; by most definitions 5%–10% of pregnancies.

Predominant Age: Reproductive.

Genetics: No genetic pattern.

ETIOLOGY AND PATHOGENESIS

Causes: Idiopathic (50%). Maternal disease—hypertension, drug or alcohol use, smoking, dilantin, coumarin, propranolol, steroids, poor nutrition, inflammatory bowel disease, low maternal weight (<50 kg), high altitude, hemoglobinopathy, cyanotic heart disease, multiple pregnancy, irradiation. Placental disease or abnormalities—placenta previa, fibrosis, chronic infection, partial abruption or infarction. Fetal factors—congenital anomalies, chromosomal factors, chronic fetal infections.

Risk Factors: Chronic maternal disease (hypertension, renal disease, cardiovascular disease), impaired placental function, congenital anomalies, history of recurrent abortion, fetal death, or preterm labor.

CLINICAL CHARACTERISTICS

Signs and Symptoms:
Uterine size less than dates
Oligohydramnios
Fetal growth that falls below the 10th percentile for gestational age or demonstrates reduced growth velocity on serial examinations

DIAGNOSTIC APPROACH

Differential Diagnosis:
Inaccurate gestational age
Congenital anomalies
Multiple gestation
Constitutionally small infants (small for gestational age [SGA])

Extrauterine gestation

Associated Conditions: Prematurity, intrauterine fetal death, congenital anomalies, and oligohydramnios.

Workup and Evaluation

Laboratory: No evaluation indicated unless suggested by maternal disease.

Imaging: Ultrasonography with fetal biometry compared with curves specific to the location and population served. The diagnosis must also be based on serial examinations that provide information about the growth of the individual fetus.

Special Tests: When found in advanced gestations: fetal nonstress and contraction stress testing or biophysical profiling. The role of Doppler flow studies continues to be evaluated.

Diagnostic Procedures: Physical examination, ultrasonography. (Physical examination may miss up to two thirds of cases; ultrasonography can exclude or verify growth restriction in 90% and 80% of cases, respectively.) Intrauterine growth restriction must be distinguished from constitutionally SGA infants, who are not at increased risk. Asymmetric restrictions in growth argues against a constitutional cause. Early intrauterine insults are more likely to result in symmetric growth restriction; later insults result in asymmetry. Similarly, intrinsic factors generally cause symmetric restriction; extrinsic factors generally cause asymmetric restriction.

Pathologic Findings

Reduced fetal fat stores and reduced overall size compared with that expected for gestational age.

MANAGEMENT AND THERAPY

Nonpharmacologic

General Measures: Evaluation, ultrasonography with biometry. Cessation of tobacco and alcohol use (if present).

Specific Measures: Based on cause and stage of gestation. Early delivery is often necessary. (The majority of fetal deaths occur after 36 weeks of gestation.) Constitutionally small infants require no intervention.

Diet: No specific dietary changes indicated unless deficiencies identified.

Activity: No restriction except as dictated by maternal disease or fetal condition.

Patient Education: American College of Obstetricians and Gynecologists Patient Education Pamphlet AP098 (*Monitoring Fetal Health During Pregnancy*), AP025 (*Ultrasound Exams*).

Intrauterine Growth Restriction (IUGR)

Causes

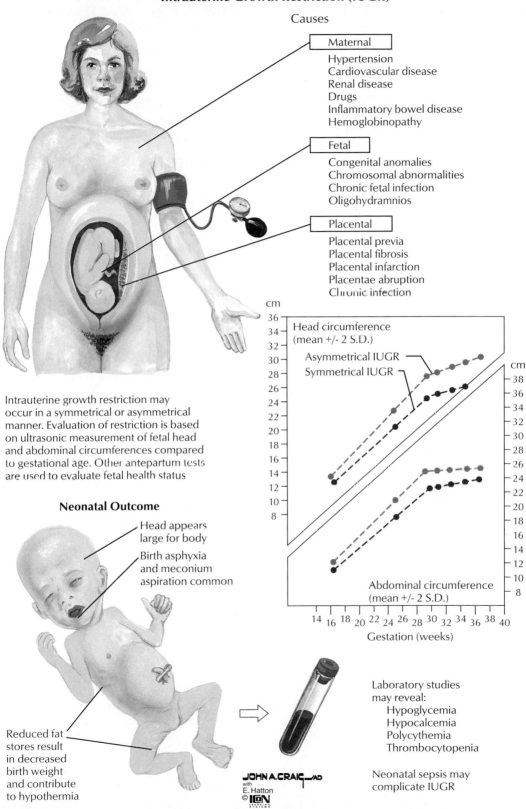

Maternal

Hypertension
Cardiovascular disease
Renal disease
Drugs
Inflammatory bowel disease
Hemoglobinopathy

Fetal

Congenital anomalies
Chromosomal abnormalities
Chronic fetal infection
Oligohydramnios

Placental

Placental previa
Placental fibrosis
Placental infarction
Placentae abruption
Chronic infection

Intrauterine growth restriction may occur in a symmetrical or asymmetrical manner. Evaluation of restriction is based on ultrasonic measurement of fetal head and abdominal circumferences compared to gestational age. Other antepartum tests are used to evaluate fetal health status

cm
36
34   Head circumference
32   (mean +/- 2 S.D.)
30   Asymmetrical IUGR   cm
28   Symmetrical IUGR   38
26   36
24   34
22   32
20   30
18   28
16   26
14   24
12   22
10   20
8   18
                                 16
                                 14
                                 12
          Abdominal circumference 10
          (mean +/- 2 S.D.)   8

14 16 18 20 22 24 26 28 30 32 34 36 38 40
Gestation (weeks)

Neonatal Outcome

Head appears
large for body

Birth asphyxia
and meconium
aspiration common

Reduced fat
stores result
in decreased
birth weight
and contribute
to hypothermia

JOHN A.CRAIG—AD
with
E. Hatton
© ICON

Laboratory studies
may reveal:
Hypoglycemia
Hypocalcemia
Polycythemia
Thrombocytopenia

Neonatal sepsis may
complicate IUGR

Drug(s) of Choice
None.

FOLLOW-UP

Patient Monitoring: Enhanced fetal assessment, antenatal fetal testing (including nonstress testing, biophysical profiles, and contraction stress tests). Patients at risk because of maternal disease should have early assessment of fetal growth (biparietal diameter, head circumference, abdominal circumference, and femur length) with frequent remeasurement as the pregnancy progresses. This may need to be done as often as every 2–3 weeks in severe cases. Careful fetal monitoring during labor.

Prevention/Avoidance: Management of maternal disease.

Possible Complications: Progressive deterioration of fetal status and intrauterine fetal demise. (There is an 8- to10-fold increase in the risk of perinatal mortality: Growth restriction is the second most important cause of perinatal morbidity after preterm delivery.) Long-term physical and neurologic sequelae are common. The risk of adverse outcome is generally proportional to the severity of growth restriction present. The presence of risk factors for intrauterine growth restriction increases the risk of fetal death by 2-fold in growth-restricted fetuses. The most immediate fetal morbidities are birth asphyxia, meconium aspiration, sepsis, hypoglycemia, hypocalcemia, hypothermia, polycythemia, thrombocytopenia, and pulmonary hemorrhage.

Expected Outcome: With early detection, progressive fetal growth can often be achieved, although many pregnancies may require early delivery or other interventions to ensure fetal well-being.

MISCELLANEOUS

ICD-9-CM Codes: 656.5.

REFERENCES

Alexander GR, Kimes JH, Kaufman RB, Mor J, Kogan M. A United States national reference for fetal growth. *Obstet Gynecol* 1996;87:163.

Cunningham FG, MacDonald PC, Gant NF, et al, eds. *Williams Obstetrics.* 20th ed. Stamford, Conn: Appleton & Lange; 1997:839.

Depp R. Care of the high-risk mother. In: Sciarra JJ, ed. *Gynecology and Obstetrics.* Vol 3. Philadelphia, Pa: JB Lippincott; 1990;1:16.

Gabbe SG. Intrauterine growth retardation. In: Gabbe SG, Neibyl JR, Simpson JL, eds. *Obstetrics: Normal and Problem Pregnancies.* 2nd ed. New York, NY: Churchill Livingstone; 1991:923.

Galbraith RS, Karchmar EJ, Piercy WN, Low JA. The clinical prediction of intrauterine growth retardation. *Am J Obstet Gynecol* 1979;133:281.

Tamura RK, Sabbagha RE. Altered fetal growth. In: Sciarra JJ, ed. *Gynecology and Obstetrics.* Vol 3. Philadelphia, Pa: JB Lippincott; 1990;74:1.

OLIGOHYDRAMNIOS

INTRODUCTION

Description: An abnormal reduction in the amount of amniotic fluid surrounding the fetus. At term, there should be about 800 mL of amniotic fluid present.

Prevalence: Rare in early pregnancy, common in post-term pregnancies (12%–25% at 41 weeks).

Predominant Age: Reproductive.

Genetics: No genetic pattern.

ETIOLOGY AND PATHOGENESIS

Causes: Unknown. Generally associated with a reduction in fetal urine production (renal agenesis, urinary tract obstruction, and fetal death), chronic amniotic leak, maternal disease (hypertension, diabetes, uteroplacental insufficiency, preeclampsia).

Risk Factors: Fetal chromosomal or congenital abnormalities (see box), fetal growth restriction or demise, postterm pregnancy, multiple gestation (twin-twin transfusion), maternal hypertension, diabetes, preeclampsia, and prostaglandin synthetase inhibitors.

Anomalies Associated with Oligohydramnios

- Amniotic band syndrome
- Cardiac anomalies: tetralogy of Fallot, septal defects
- Central nervous system: holoprosencephaly, meningocele, encephalocele, microcephaly
- Chromosomal: triploidy, trisomy 18, Turner's syndrome
- Cloacal dysgenesis
- Cystic hygroma
- Diaphragmatic hernia
- Genitourinary tract: renal agenesis, renal dysplasia, urethral obstruction (posterior urethral valve), bladder exstrophy, Meckel-Gruber syndrome, ureteropelvic junction obstruction, prune-belly syndrome
- Hypothyroidism
- Multiple gestation: twin-twin transfusion syndrome, twin reverse arterial perfusion sequence (TRAP)
- Musculoskeletal: sirenomelia, sacral agenesis, absent radius, facial clefting
- VACTERL (vertebral, anal, cardiac, tracheoesophageal, renal, limb) association

CLINICAL CHARACTERISTICS

Signs and Symptoms:
  Uterine size smaller than normal for stage of pregnancy
  Reduced amniotic fluid measured by ultrasonography

DIAGNOSTIC APPROACH

Differential Diagnosis:
  Inaccurate gestational age
  Intrauterine growth restriction
  Fetal anomalies
  Premature rupture of the membranes

Associated Conditions: Fetal—renal and urinary tract anomalies, intrauterine fetal growth restriction, pulmonary hypoplasia, musculoskeletal defects (clubfoot, amniotic bands, amputations), meconium-stained amniotic fluid. Fetal anomalies are present in 15–25% of cases. Maternal—chronic disease (diabetes, hypertension).

Workup and Evaluation

Laboratory: No evaluation indicated.

Imaging: Amniotic fluid index calculated by adding the vertical depths of the largest pockets of amniotic fluid in each quadrant of the uterus (average at term = 12.5 cm, 95th percentile = 21.4). Borderline values should always be rechecked before any intervention is undertaken. Fetal anomalies may also be documented.

Special Tests: Nonstress or contraction stress testing to evaluate fetal health.

Diagnostic Procedures: Physical examination, ultrasonography.

Pathologic Findings

Reduced amniotic fluid (other findings based on cause).

MANAGEMENT AND THERAPY

Nonpharmacologic

General Measures: Evaluation. Mild degrees may be managed expectantly.

Specific Measures: Amnioinfusion (the introduction of normal saline via an intrauterine catheter placed through the partially dilated cervix during labor) has been used to reduce the incidence of umbilical cord compression during labor. This does not reduce the risk of meconium aspiration.

Events in Oligohydramnios

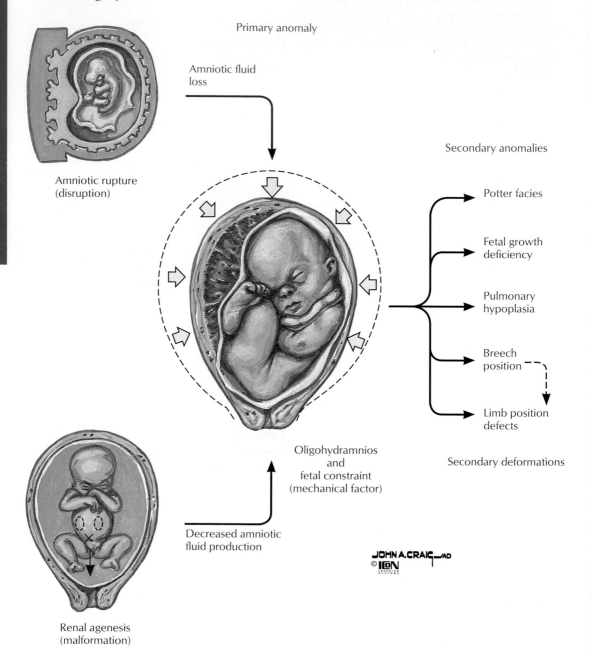

Primary anomaly

Amniotic fluid loss

Amniotic rupture (disruption)

Secondary anomalies

Potter facies

Fetal growth deficiency

Pulmonary hypoplasia

Breech position

Limb position defects

Oligohydramnios and fetal constraint (mechanical factor)

Secondary deformations

Decreased amniotic fluid production

Renal agenesis (malformation)

JOHN A.CRAIG—AD
© ICON
LEARNING SYSTEMS

Diet: No specific dietary changes indicated.

Activity: No restriction.

Patient Education: Reassurance. American College of Obstetricians and Gynecologists Patient Education Pamphlet AP069 (*Postdate Pregnancy*), AP025 (), AP098 (*Monitoring Fetal Health During Pregnancy*).

Drug(s) of Choice

None.

FOLLOW-UP

Patient Monitoring: Intensive fetal surveillance is required.

Prevention/Avoidance: None.

Possible Complications: Amniotic band syndrome (including partial limb amputation), pulmonary hypoplasia, premature labor, clubfoot, and meconium-stained amniotic fluid. The prognosis is inversely related to gestational age: the earlier the oligohydramnios occurs, the worse the outcome.

Expected Outcome: When oligohydramnios occurs in term or post-term pregnancies, it is associated with fetuses that do not tolerate labor well (5–7 times increase in rate of cesarean delivery).

MISCELLANEOUS

ICD-9-CM **Codes:** 658.0, affecting the fetus, 761.2, due to premature rupture of the membranes, 658.1

REFERENCES

Baron C, Morgan MA, Garite TJ. The impact of amniotic fluid volume assessed intrapartum on perinatal outcome. *Am J Obstet Gynecol* 1995;173:167.

Hallak M, Kirshon B, Smith EO, Cotton DB. Amniotic fluid index. Gestational age-specific values for normal human pregnancy. *J Reprod Med* 1993;38:853.

Lameier LN, Katz VL. Amnioinfusion: a review. *Obstet Gynecol Surv* 1993;48:829.

McCurdy CM, Seeds JW. Oligohydramnios: problems and treatments. *Semin Perinatol* 1993;17:183.

Peipert JF, Donnenfeld AE. Oligohydramnios: a review. *Obstet Gynecol Surv* 1991;46:325.

Queenan JT. Polyhydramnios and oligohydramnios. *Contemp Ob/Gyn* 1991;36:60.

PLACENTA PREVIA

INTRODUCTION

Description: Implantation of the placenta in a location that leaves part or all of the cervical os covered. This is associated with potentially catastrophic maternal bleeding and obstruction of the uterine outlet. Several degrees are recognized: total, partial, marginal, and low-lying placenta. These degrees may vary with cervical dilation or gestational age.

Prevalence: Seen in 0.3%–0.5% of deliveries.

Predominant Age: Reproductive, average 29.

Genetics: No genetic pattern.

ETIOLOGY AND PATHOGENESIS

Causes: Implantation by the zygote low in the uterine cavity (in close proximity to the cervical os). Defective decidual vascularization, resulting from inflammation or atrophy, has been implicated.

Risk Factors: Multiparity, advance maternal age (>35: 1% of deliveries, >40: 2%), prior cesarean delivery (2–5 times increase), induced abortion, smoking (2 times increase), cocaine use, multiple gestation, high altitude, and prior abortion.

CLINICAL CHARACTERISTICS

Signs and Symptoms:

Painless vaginal bleeding (70%, generally not present until late second or early third trimester); may be catastrophic in amount although initial episodes are rarely fatal; blood is maternal in origin

Uterine hyperactivity possibly present with bleeding (20%)

Heavy or prolonged bleeding after delivery

DIAGNOSTIC APPROACH

Differential Diagnosis:

Bloody show of early labor

Placental abruption

Vasa previa

Low lying placenta

Associated Conditions: Placenta accreta (15%–25% of patients), increta, or percreta and prematurity.

Workup and Evaluation

Laboratory: Complete blood count, type and cross match blood products for possible replacement.

Imaging: Ultrasonography (transabdominal) to determine placental location and condition, fetal status. (False-positive sonography results may occur with a full bladder; suspicious studies should be repeated with the bladder empty. Low-lying placentas noted in studies performed below 30 weeks may "migrate," leaving the cervix free at term [up to 90% of cases].)

Special Tests: Kleihauer-Betke test for fetal-maternal transfusion, clot tube to assess possibility of coagulopathy, Apt test to identify fetal blood loss (such as from a vasa previa).

Diagnostic Procedures: History, ultrasonography. (Pelvic examination is contraindicated until the location of the placenta can be ascertained.)

Pathologic Findings

Placental implantation in the lower uterine segment.

MANAGEMENT AND THERAPY

Nonpharmacologic

General Measures: Evaluation, hemodynamic stabilization, fetal assessment. *NO* vaginal examinations, until the location and degree of placental obstruction can be determined, if placenta previa is suspected.

Specific Measures: If bleeding is heavy or the placenta obstructs delivery, cesarean delivery is indicated. Marginal (low-lying) placental implantation may be managed conservatively if it occurs long before term. Bleeding from the placental site may be heavy, requiring extensive measures (including hysterectomy) to control bleeding.

Diet: No specific dietary changes indicated unless active bleeding is present or the patient's condition is unstable.

Activity: Bed rest is generally indicated.

Patient Education: American College of Obstetricians and Gynecologists Patient Education Pamphlet AP038 (*Bleeding During Pregnancy*), AP006 (*Cesarean Birth*), AP025 (*Ultrasound Exams*).

Drug(s) of Choice

Fluid and blood product replacement as needed. Steroid therapy to accelerate fetal lung maturation has been advocated for patients remote from term, but a meta-analysis of studies available does not document a positive effect on fetal respiratory distress syndrome or mortality. Oxytocin, methylergonovine maleate (Methergine), and prostaglandin (E_2) therapy to assist with uterine contraction after delivery. Rh (D) immune globulin should be given as indicated in Rh-negative mothers. If tocolysis is required, $MgSO_4$ is preferred.

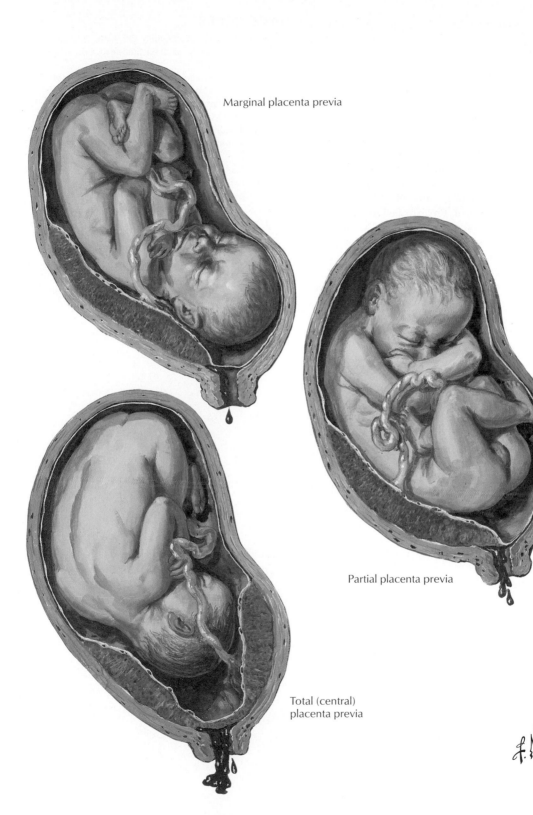

Marginal placenta previa

Partial placenta previa

Total (central)
placenta previa

OBSTETRICAL CONDITIONS

Contraindications: β-Mimetic agents should not be used if there is significant maternal blood loss or hypotension.

FOLLOW-UP

Patient Monitoring: Normal health maintenance.
Prevention/Avoidance: None.
Possible Complications: Catastrophic maternal hemorrhage, fetal anoxia. Coagulation defects may occur as a result of heavy or prolonged blood loss. Significant bleeding from the placental site may result in maternal compromise and extensive measures (including hysterectomy) to achieve control. Preterm delivery represents the greatest source of morbidity for the fetus. Roughly 35% of infants whose mothers require transfusion require transfusion themselves.
Expected Outcome: Generally good—25%–30% of patients complete 36 weeks of gestation despite labor or repetitive bleeding.

MISCELLANEOUS

ICD-9-CM **Codes:** 641.1.

REFERENCES

Cunningham FG, MacDonald PC, Gant NF, et al, eds. *Williams Obstetrics.* 20th ed. Stamford, Conn: Appleton Lange; 1997:755.

Benedetti TJ. Obstetric hemorrhage. In: Gabbe SG, Neibyl JR, Simpson JL, eds. *Obstetrics: Normal and Problem Pregnancies.* 2nd ed. New York, NY: Churchill Livingstone; 1991:584.

Comeau J, Shaw L, Marcell CC, Lavery JP. Early placenta previa and delivery outcome. *Obstet Gynecol* 1983; 61:577.

Drost S, Keil K. Expectant management of placenta previa: cost-benefit analysis of outpatient treatment. *Am J Obstet Gynecol* 1994;170:1254.

Iyasu S, Saftlas AK, Rowley DL, Koonin LM, Lawson HW, Atrask AK. The epidemiology of placenta previa in the United States, 1979 through 1987. *Am J Obstet Gynecol* 1993;168:1424.

McClure N, Dornal JC. Early identification of placenta previa. *Br J Obstet Gynaecol* 1990;97:959.

Miller DA, Diaz FG, Paul RH. Incidence of placenta previa with previous cesarean. *Am J Obstet Gynecol* 1996;174:345.

PLACENTAL ABRUPTION

INTRODUCTION

Description: Premature separation of an otherwise normally implanted placenta before delivery of the fetus.

Prevalence: One percent of deliveries.

Predominant Age: Reproductive.

Genetics: No genetic pattern.

ETIOLOGY AND PATHOGENESIS

Causes: Pregnancy-induced hypertension (most common), trauma to the abdomen, decompression of an overdistended uterus (loss of amniotic fluid, delivery of a twin), cocaine use.

Risk Factors: Pregnancy-induced hypertension (most common). Prior abruption: 15% chance if one prior episode, 20%–25% for two or more prior events Others: smoking >1 pack/day, multiparity, alcohol abuse, cocaine use, hydramnios, maternal hypertension, premature rupture of the membranes, external trauma, uterine leiomyomata, and multiple gestation.

CLINICAL CHARACTERISTICS

Signs and Symptoms:
Vaginal bleeding (not universal)
Abdominal, back, or uterine pain
Uterine irritability, tachysystole, tetany, elevated baseline intrauterine pressure
Fetal bradycardia or late decelerations
Maternal hypotension or signs of volume loss (postural hypotension, shock)

DIAGNOSTIC APPROACH

Differential Diagnosis:
Uterine rupture
Placenta or vasa previa
Bloody show
Other sources of abdominal pain

Associated Conditions: Hypertension, preeclampsia, eclampsia, intrauterine fetal demise, postpartum hemorrhage, tumultuous labor, premature delivery, and fetal bradycardia.

Workup and Evaluation

Laboratory: Complete blood count, assessment of clotting function (bleeding time, prothrombin time, partial thromboplastin time, fibrinogen, D-dimer assay).

Imaging: Ultrasound may show signs of a retroplacental clot or collection of blood, but absence does not rule out abruption.

Special Tests: Kleihauer-Betke test for fetal-maternal transfusion, clot tube to assess possibility of coagulopathy, Apt test to identify fetal blood loss (vasa previa).

Diagnostic Procedures: History, physical examination, and laboratory evaluation. Fetal heart rate and uterine activity monitoring.

Pathologic Findings

Bleeding into the decidua basalia with hematoma formation, leading to progressive separation of the placenta and pressure necrosis. Acute anemia, evidence of clotting activation and consumption, histologically normal placenta.

MANAGEMENT AND THERAPY

Nonpharmacologic

General Measures: Prompt evaluation, fluid support, cross-match blood or blood products, Rh typing (if not known).

Specific Measures: Fetal and uterine activity monitoring, monitoring of maternal condition (pulse, blood pressure, pulse oxygenation).

Diet: Nothing by mouth until the diagnosis is established and the patient's condition is stabilized.

Activity: Bed rest until the diagnosis is established and the patient's condition is stabilized.

Patient Education: Reassurance, American College of Obstetricians and Gynecologists Patient Education Pamphlet AP038 (*Bleeding During Pregnancy*).

Drug(s) of Choice

None. (Oxygen and intravenous fluids are commonly prescribed, Rh immune globulin if indicated.)

Contraindications: Tocolytics should not be used until a diagnosis is established.

FOLLOW-UP

Patient Monitoring: Close attention to vaginal bleeding, fetal well-being, and maternal circulatory status.

Prevention/Avoidance: Eliminate modifiable risk factors.

Possible Complications: Consumptive coagulopathy, maternal mortality 0.5%–1% and fetal mortality 20%–70% based on the size of the separation, the cause and gestational age; 10%–15% neurologic sequelae in fetal survivors.

Expected Outcome: Small abruption may be managed conservatively; larger separations may jeopardize mother and fetus and frequently require immediate delivery.

MISCELLANEOUS

ICD-9-CM Codes: 641.2.

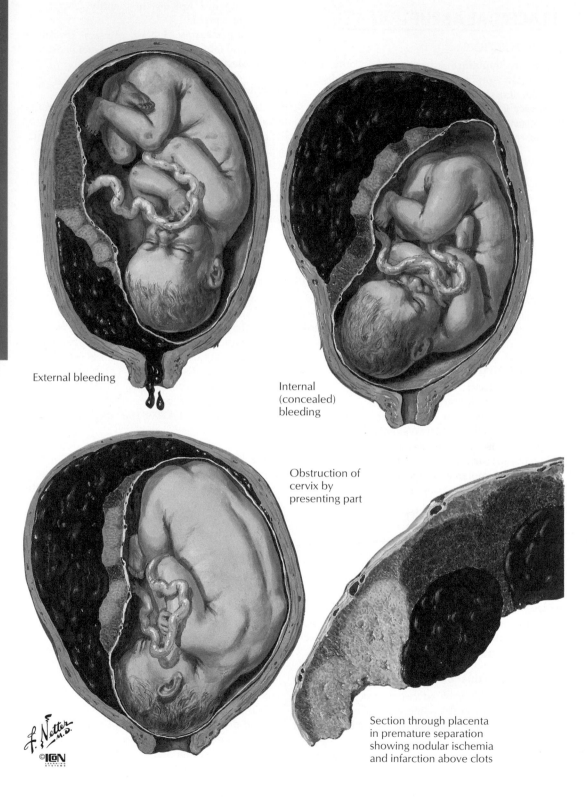

External bleeding

Internal
(concealed)
bleeding

Obstruction of
cervix by
presenting part

Section through placenta
in premature separation
showing nodular ischemia
and infarction above clots

REFERENCES

Abdella TN, Sibai BM, Hays MJ Jr, Anderson GD. Perinatal outcome in abruptio placentae. *Obstet Gynecol* 1984;63:365.

Ananth CV, Savitz DA, Williams MA. Placental abruption and its association with hypertension and prolonged rupture of the membranes: a methodologic review and meta-analysis. *Obstet Gynecol* 1996;88:309.

Kettel LM, Branch DW, Scott JR. Occult placental abruption after maternal trauma. *Obstet Gynecol* 1988;71:449.

Knab DR. Abruptio placentae. An assessment of the time and method of delivery. *Obstet Gynecol* 1978: 52:625.

Naeye RL. Abruptio placentae and placenta previa: frequency, perinatal mortality, and cigarette smoking. *Obstet Gynecol* 1980;55:701.

Pritchard JA, Cunningham FG, Pritchard SA, Mason RA. On reducing the frequency of severe abruptio placentae. *Am J Obstet Gynecol* 1991;165:1345.

OBSTETRICAL CONDITIONS

POLYHYDRAMNIOS

INTRODUCTION

Description: An abnormal increase in the amount of amniotic fluid surrounding the fetus. This diagnosis is generally reserved for volumes >2 l. (At term, there should be about 800 mL of amniotic fluid present.) This fluid may accumulate gradually over time (chronic hydramnios) or acutely over the course of several days (more common in early pregnancy).

Prevalence: In 0.9%–1.6% of women, some increase in amniotic fluid is seen during pregnancy (80% mild, 5% severe).

Predominant Age: Reproductive.

Genetics: No genetic pattern.

ETIOLOGY AND PATHOGENESIS

Causes: Idiopathic (two thirds), maternal diabetes, multiple gestation, fetal anomalies (50% of patients with severe hydramnios: central nervous system, gastrointestinal tract, chromosomal).

Risk Factors: Fetal anomalies that impair swallowing or alter urine production, multiple gestation (twin-twin transfusion), maternal diabetes, erythroblastosis.

CLINICAL CHARACTERISTICS

Signs and Symptoms:
Uterine size larger than normal for stage of pregnancy
Increased amniotic fluid measured by ultrasonography (amniotic fluid index [AFI] >24 cm)
Dyspnea (especially when supine)
Lower extremity and vulvar edema
Premature labor
Difficulty palpating fetal parts or hearing fetal heart tones

DIAGNOSTIC APPROACH

Differential Diagnosis:
Inaccurate gestational age
Normal multiple gestation
Fetal anomalies
Ascites
Ovarian cyst

Associated Conditions: Anencephaly, esophageal atresia, prematurity, umbilical cord prolapse, and placental abruption.

Workup and Evaluation

Laboratory: No evaluation indicated.

Imaging: AFI calculated by adding the vertical depths of the largest pockets of amniotic fluid in each quadrant of the uterus (average at term = 12.5 cm, 95th percentile = 21.4). Fetal anomalies may also be documented.

Special Tests: None indicated.

Diagnostic Procedures: Physical examination, ultrasonography.

Pathologic Findings

None.

MANAGEMENT AND THERAPY

Nonpharmacologic

General Measures: Evaluation. Mild conditions may be managed expectantly. If dyspnea or abdominal pain is present, hospitalization may be required.

Specific Measures: Indomethacin therapy has been shown to be of help in some patients. Therapeutic amniocentesis may be used to transiently relieve maternal symptoms and in some cases allow prolongation of the gestation. (If performed, the rate of withdrawal should be about 500 mL/h and limited to 1500–2000 mL total volume.) Bed rest, diuretics, and salt and water restrictions are ineffective.

Diet: No specific dietary changes indicated.

Activity: No restriction except for those imposed by the enlarged uterus.

Patient Education: Reassurance, American College of Obstetricians and Gynecologists Patient Education Pamphlet AP025 (*Ultrasound Exams*), AP098 (*Monitoring Fetal Health During Pregnancy*).

Drug(s) of Choice

Indomethacin 1.5–3.0 mg/kg/d.

Contraindications: Aspirin-sensitive asthma, inflammatory bowel disease, or ulcers.

Precautions: Use of nonsteroidal antiinflammatory agents has been associated with premature closure of the ductus arteriosus. This is generally transient and may be monitored by ultrasonography.

Alternative Drugs

None.

FOLLOW-UP

Patient Monitoring: Normal health maintenance.

Prevention/Avoidance: None.

Possible Complications: Premature labor and delivery (40%), abruptio placenta, maternal pulmonary compromise, umbilical cord prolapse.

Expected Outcome: Mild to moderate increases in fluid are not associated with significant risk.

Severe polyhydramnios is often associated with significant fetal anomalies. Perinatal mortality is as high as 25%–30% in some studies. In general, the more severe the hydramnios, the greater the fetal risk.

MISCELLANEOUS

***ICD-9-CM* Codes:** 657, affecting the fetus, 761.3

REFERENCES

Carlson DE, Platt LD, Medearis AL, Hornestein J. Quantifiable polyhydramnios: diagnosis and management. *Obstet Gynecol* 1990;75:989.

Damato N, Filly RA, Goldstein RB, Callen PW, Goldberg J, Golbus M. Frequency of fetal anomalies in sonographically detected polyhydramnios. *J Ultrasound Med* 1993;12:11.

Hallak M, Kirshon B, Smith EO, Cotton DB. Amniotic fluid index. Gestational age-specific values for normal human pregnancy. *J Reprod Med* 1993;38:853.

Kramer WB, Van den Veyver IB, Kirshorn B. Treatment of polyhydramnios with indomethacin. *Clin Perinatol* 1994;21:615.

Many A, Hill LM, Lazebnik N, Martin JG. The association between polyhydramnios and preterm delivery. *Obstet Gynecol* 1995;86:389.

Queenan JT. Polyhydramnios and oligohydramnios. *Contemp Ob/Gyn* 1991;36:60.

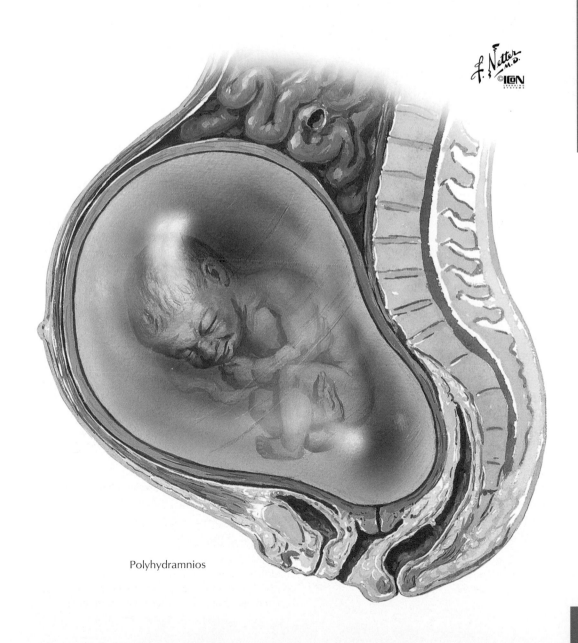

Polyhydramnios

PREECLAMPSIA AND ECLAMPSIA (TOXEMIA OF PREGNANCY)

INTRODUCTION

Description: Pregnancy can induce hypertension or aggravate existing hypertension. Edema and proteinuria (one or both) are characteristic pregnancy-induced changes. If preeclampsia is untreated, convulsions (eclampsia) may occur. Chronic hypertension may be worsened by or superimposed on pregnancy-induced changes.

Prevalence: Five percent of all births, 250,000 cases/yr, results in 150 maternal deaths (18%) and 3000 fetal deaths/yr.

Predominant Age: Rare before 20 weeks of gestation.

Genetics: Multifactorial, runs in families.

ETIOLOGY AND PATHOGENESIS

Causes: Unknown, genetic, endocrine/metabolic (including altered prostaglandin production), uteroplacental ischemia, immunologic.

Risk Factors: Prior history, body mass index >32.3, black race, nulliparity, age older than 35 (2- to 3-fold increase) or younger than 18, multifetal pregnancy, fetal hydrops, hydatidiform mole.

CLINICAL CHARACTERISTICS

Signs and Symptoms:

Hypertension without proteinuria or edema (pregnancy-induced hypertension)

Hypertension with proteinuria or edema (preeclampsia) (severe preeclampsia: headache, abdominal pain, weight gain, visual disturbances, thrombocytopenia, oliguria, hemoconcentration, pulmonary edema)

Hypertension, proteinuria, or edema and seizures (grand mal type) (eclampsia)

DIAGNOSTIC APPROACH

Differential Diagnosis:

Chronic (essential) hypertension
Transient hypertension
Chronic renal disease
Acute or chronic glomerulonephritis
Coarctation of the aorta
Cushing's disease
Systemic lupus erythematosus
Periarteritis nodosa
Obesity
Epilepsy
Encephalitis
Cerebral aneurysm or tumor
Lupus cerebritis
Hysteria

Associated Conditions: Hypertension, heart disease, stroke, placental infarcts, and placental abruption.

Workup and Evaluation

Laboratory: Liver and renal function studies (eg, enzymes, renal clearance, 24-hour urinary protein measurement).

Imaging: Ultrasonography to monitor fetal growth (frequently restricted).

Special Tests: Assessment of fetal lung maturation may be performed, but if maternal disease is severe, management is based on maternal factors and not fetal maturation.

Diagnostic Procedures: History, physical examination (with blood pressure), urinalysis (or "dipstick"), laboratory assessment.

Pathologic Findings

Results of 24-hour urinary protein measurement >300 mg, blood pressure >140/90 or significantly elevated over baseline, characteristic renal glomerular lesions (capillary endotheliosis), premature aging of the placenta, increased vascular reactivity, elevated liver enzymes, thrombocytopenia.

MANAGEMENT AND THERAPY

Nonpharmacologic

General Measures: Aggressive evaluation, frequent prenatal visits, increased fetal surveillance (fetal growth). Hospitalization is required for all but the most benign conditions (mild PIH, stable chronic hypertension with normal fetal growth).

Specific Measures: The only true treatment for preeclampsia or eclampsia is delivery. Management of symptoms may be used to get both mother and baby into optimal condition for delivery.

Diet: No specific dietary changes indicated except as dictated by labor or other management. (A low-salt diet has been advocated but is unproved.)

Activity: Bed rest with severe conditions or for women in the process of delivery.

Patient Education: American College of Obstetricians and Gynecologists Patient Education Pamphlet AP034 (*High Blood Pressure During Pregnancy*).

Drug(s) of Choice

Drug treatment of mild preeclampsia has generally been disappointing. Glucocorticoids are often given to encourage fetal lung maturation. Drugs such as labetalol or nifedipine have been given as

Clinical triad

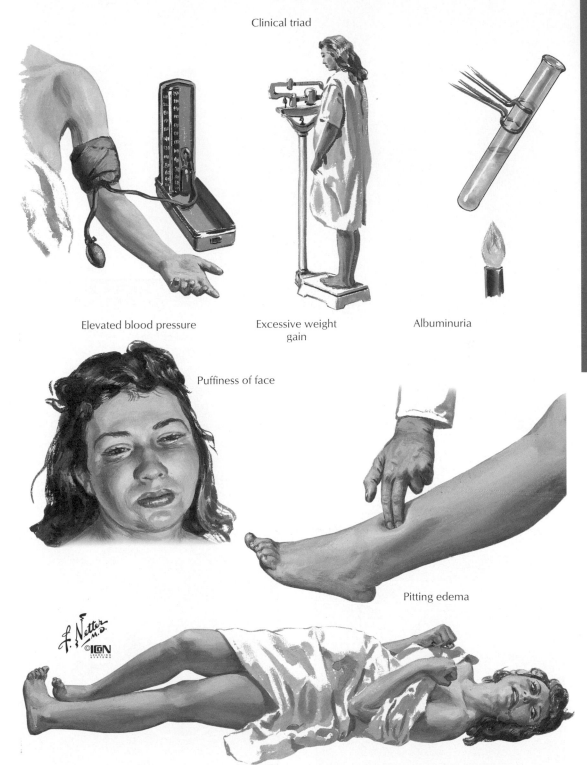

Elevated blood pressure

Excessive weight gain

Albuminuria

Puffiness of face

Pitting edema

Convulsion in true eclampsia

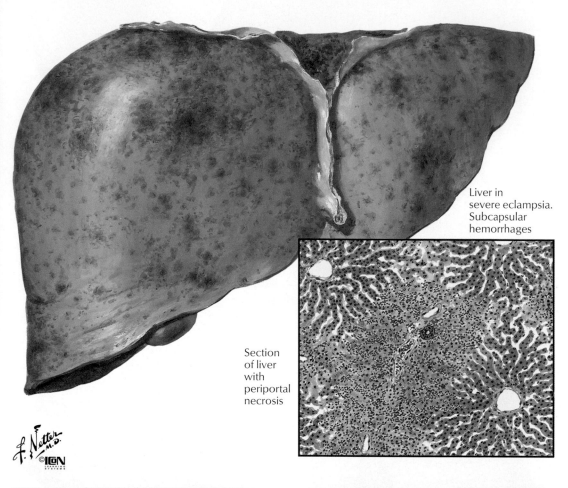

Liver in
severe eclampsia.
Subcapsular
hemorrhages

Section
of liver
with
periportal
necrosis

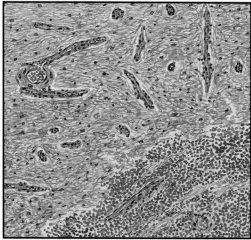

Hemorrhage and
necrosis in brain

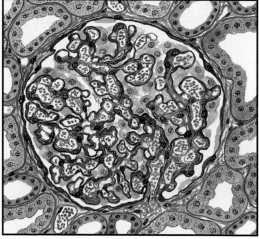

Fibrin deposition and swelling
of epithelial cells in glomerulus

part of conservative management protocols. These have generally resulted in prolongation of the gestation and improved fetal outcome, but no reduction in catastrophic events such as placental abruption. Magnesium sulfate is often given intravenously during labor to stabilize blood pressure and reduce the risk of seizures. Intravenous hydralazine may be used to lower blood pressure acutely during labor.

Contraindications: Angiotensin-converting-enzyme inhibitors are contraindicated in pregnancy.

Precautions: Excessive levels (>10 mEg/L) of magnesium sulfate may result in respiratory paralysis and cardiac arrest.

Interactions: See individual agents.

Alternative Drugs

Verapamil, nimodipine, diazoxide, and nitroglycerin have all been studied or advocated at some time. (Prophylactic treatment with aspirin has not been proved to be effective in preventing preeclampsia.)

FOLLOW-UP

Patient Monitoring: Increased maternal and fetal surveillance (more frequent prenatal visits, laboratory tests, and ultrasonography evaluations).

Prevention/Avoidance: Early detection and treatment. The risk of eclampsia may be reduced by aggressive management of preeclampsia. (The use of prophylactic aspirin remains controversial and unproven.)

Possible Complications: Maternal—cardiac decompensation, stroke, pulmonary edema and respiratory failure, renal failure, seizures and seizure-related injuries, intracranial hemorrhage, coma,

death (0.5%–5% mortality). Fetal risk (growth restriction and death) is directly proportional to both the degree of proteinuria and the level of diastolic blood pressure. The risk to both mother and fetus increases dramatically in eclampsia.

Expected Outcome: Generally PIH, preeclampsia, and eclampsia improve after delivery. Eclamptic seizures may occur up to 10 days after delivery but are uncommon beyond 48 hours.

MISCELLANEOUS

ICD-9-CM **Codes:** 642.4 (Mild preeclampsia), 642.5 (Severe preeclampsia), 642.6 (Eclampsia), 642.7 (With superimposed preexisting hypertension).

REFERENCES

American College of Obstetricians and Gynecologists. *Hypertension in Pregnancy.* Washington, DC: ACOG; 1996. ACOG Technical Bulletin 219.

Bhalla AK, Dhall GI, Dhall K. A safer and more effective treatment regimen for eclampsia. *Aust N Z J Obstet Gynaecol* 1994;34:144.

Cunningham FG, Lindheimer MD. Hypertension in pregnancy. Current concepts. *N Engl J Med* 1992;326:927.

Davery DA, MacGillivray I. The classification and definition of the hypertensive disorders of pregnancy. *Am J Obstet Gynecol* 1988;158:892.

Dekker GA, Sibai BM. Early detection of preeclampsia. *Am J Obstet Gynecol* 1991;165:160.

O'Brien WF. Predicting preeclampsia. *Obstet Gynecol* 1990;75:445.

Redman CWG, Roberts JM. Management of preeclampsia. *Lancet* 1993;341:1451.

Sibai BM, Ewell M, Levine RJ, et al. Risk factors associated with preeclampsia in healthy nulliparous women. *Am J Obstet Gynecol* 1997;177:1003.

PUERPERAL INFECTION

INTRODUCTION

Description: Although the term *puerperal infection* can be used to describe any infection during or after labor, it generally applies to infection of the uterus and surrounding tissues after delivery. This can vary from mild to life-threatening in severity. Some of the most severe infections may appear within hours of delivery and are often opportunistic and not associated with reliable risk factors. Vigilance and aggressive diagnosis and treatment are required.

Prevalence: Ten percent to twenty percent if antibiotic prophylaxis is given during delivery; 50%–90% without antibiotic prophylaxis.

Predominant Age: Reproductive.

Genetics: No genetic pattern.

ETIOLOGY AND PATHOGENESIS

Causes: Colonization and infection of the tissues of the uterus, peritoneum, or surrounding organs. The most common organisms are group B streptococci, other facultative streptococci, *Gardnerella vaginalis,* and *Escherichia coli, Bacteroides,* and *Peptostreptococcus* species. Infection by clostridia or group A streptococci may result in rapidly progressive soft tissue (subcutaneous tissue, muscle, or myometrial) infection. Abscesses usually contain both aerobic and anaerobic bacteria such as *Bacteroides* species (*Bacteroides bivius, Bacteroides disiens,* or *Bacteroides fragilis*). Approximately 50% of ascending uterine infections involve *Chlamydia trachomatis.*

Risk Factors: Cesarean delivery (10- to 20-fold increase), invasive procedures during labor, prolonged rupture of the membranes, prolonged labor, multiple examinations, retained placental fragments, urinary catheter, intravenous line(s), low socioeconomic status, and chronic disease (diabetes).

CLINICAL CHARACTERISTICS

Signs and Symptoms:

Fever (90% >38.5°C by 24 hours) and tachycardia (often developing rapidly after delivery)

Uterine tenderness (may be absent)

Signs of septic or cardiovascular shock (hypotension, anxiety, disorientation, prostration)

Impaired renal function (<20 mL/h urine production)

Altered white blood count (<1,000 or ≥ 25,000)

Hemolysis or hemoconcentration

DIAGNOSTIC APPROACH

Differential Diagnosis:

Urinary tract infections including pyelonephritis (5% of patients, classical signs are routinely absent, urinalysis shows large numbers of white blood cells and cultures are positive)

Wound infection

Atelectasis or pneumonitis

Infection in intravenous line or site, contaminated fluids

Disturbed abscess (old tubo-ovarian or appendiceal abscess)

Septic thrombophlebitis

Necrotizing fasciitis

Transfusion reaction (when applicable)

Amniotic fluid or pulmonary embolism

Cardiogenic shock (drugs, cardiac disease, aortic dissection)

Toxic shock syndrome

Mastitis (2% of patients)

Associated Conditions: Septic shock, adult respiratory distress syndrome, acute renal failure, and disseminated intravascular coagulation.

Workup and Evaluation

Laboratory: Complete blood count, endometrial culture obtained by protected swab (if amniotic fluid or endometrial culture obtained at the time of delivery [within 24 hours] is not available). Blood cultures (are positive in 15%–25% of febrile patients, but do not reflect the severity of the infection). Tissue culture (direct or by needle aspiration, when wound infections is suspected) and Gram's stain.

Imaging: Ultrasonography may be useful in evaluating the possibility of pelvic abscess or gas formation. Computed tomography and magnetic resonance imaging are useful for a more wide-ranging assessment.

Special Tests: Frozen section histopathologic evaluation may be useful if necrotizing fasciitis is suspected.

Diagnostic Procedures: History, physical examination, cultures.

Pathologic Findings

Evidence of inflammation and/or necrosis (based on tissue involved and severity of infections).

MANAGEMENT AND THERAPY

Nonpharmacologic

General Measures: Evaluation, fluid replacement or resuscitation, antipyretics and analgesics (once a diagnosis has been established). Close moni-

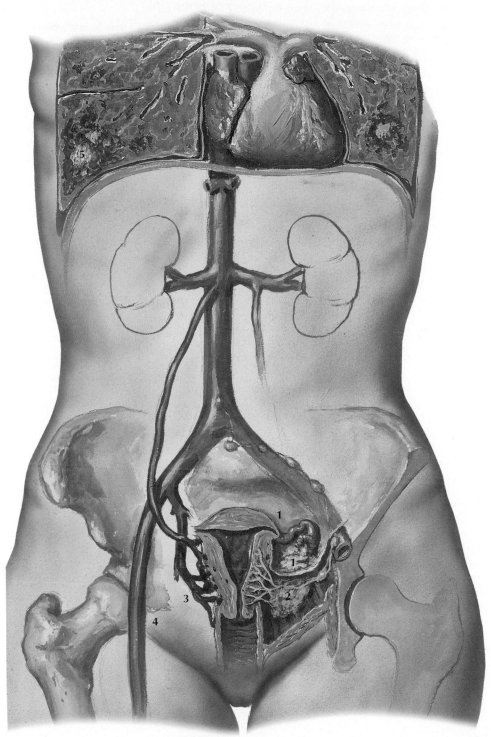

Dissemination of septic endometritis:
(1) Peritonitis
(2) Parametritis (via lymphatics)
(3) Pelvic thrombophlebitis
(4) Femoral thrombophlebitis
(5) Pulmonary infarct or abscess (septic embolus)

toring, including intensive care, may be required when infection is severe. Consultation with an infectious disease specialist may be desirable. Low grade (<38°C) or intermittent fevers may not require treatment when present in the first 24 hours.

Specific Measures: Aggressive antibiotic therapy. Based on response, removal of infected products (if present), surgical exploration, abscess drainage (percutaneous or open), debridement, or hysterectomy may be required. (Virtually all postpartum septic shock is caused by surgically treatable processes.) Because of the expanded blood and tissue volume at and after delivery, antibiotic dosages must be increased by 40% over those used outside of pregnancy.

Diet: For acutely ill patients, nothing by mouth until condition is stabilized. For other patients, no specific dietary changes indicated.

Activity: Bed rest until patient's condition is stable, then a progressive return to normal activity.

Patient Education: Reassurance, American College of Obstetricians and Gynecologists Patient Education Pamphlet AP006 (*Cesarean Birth*).

Drug(s) of Choice

Antibiotics should be chosen to provide protection against Gram-negative facultative and anaerobic bacteria. Moderate infections require double antibiotic treatment; severe infections should be treated with triple therapy: an aminoglycoside or first-generation cephalosporin (for facultative bacteria); clindamycin, imipenem-cilastatin, or metronidazole (anaerobic bacteria); and penicillin or ampicillin (clostridia and synergistic action with aminoglycosides on enterococci). β-Lactam antibiotics (penicillin or cephalosporin) should be given in dosages of 8–12 g/d.

Contraindications: See individual agents.

Precautions: Antibiotic dosages must be increased by up to 40% because of the altered physiologic state of pregnancy.

Interactions: See individual agents.

FOLLOW-UP

Patient Monitoring: When severe infections are present, intensive monitoring (including placement in an intensive care unit) is required. This may include central venous access and monitoring, pulse oximetry, careful (frequent if not continuous) blood pressure monitoring.

Prevention/Avoidance: Careful attention to antisepsis, reduced numbers of vaginal examinations when the amniotic membranes have been ruptured, careful tissue handling during operative procedures, use of prophylactic antibiotics when risk factors are identified. Changing intravenous sites every 48 hours reduces the risk of infection.

Possible Complications: Progression of infection, abscess formation, septic thrombophlebitis, septic shock, adult respiratory distress syndrome, renal failure, cardiovascular collapse, death. If septic shock occurs, mortality rates of 20%–30% are common. Coagulopathy may develop. Necrotizing fasciitis is possible.

Expected Outcome: With timely diagnosis and appropriate therapy a complete recovery with no long-term sequelae should be expected. Roughly, 90% of patients respond rapidly to antibiotic therapy (and/or percutaneous drainage of abscesses).

MISCELLANEOUS

ICD-9-CM Codes: 670.0.

REFERENCES

Casey BM, Cox SM. Chorioamnionitis and endometritis. *Infect Dis Clin North Am* 1997;11:203.

Eschenbach DA. Serious postpartum infections. In: Sciarra JJ, ed. *Gynecology and Obstetrics*. Vol 3. Philadelphia, Pa: JB Lippincott; 1986;39:1.

Eschenbach DA, Wager GP. Puerperal infection. *Clin Obstet Gynecol* 1980;23:1003.

Pastorek JG 2nd. Postcesarean endometritis. *Compr Ther* 1995;21:249.

RH INCOMPATIBILITY

INTRODUCTION

Description: Isoimmunization to any fetal blood group not possessed by the mother is possible. The most common example is the Rh (D) factor. What was once a common cause for intrauterine fetal death has largely been eradicated by prophylactic administration of immune globulin to those at risk.

Prevalence: Uncommon since the routine use of D immune globulin therapy.

Predominant Age: Reproductive.

Genetics: Rh (D)-negative mothers.

ETIOLOGY AND PATHOGENESIS

Causes: Antibody formation against the D antigen.

Risk Factors: Any process that exposes the woman to blood carrying the D antigen including blood transfusion, miscarriage, ectopic or normal pregnancy, trauma, amniocentesis during pregnancy, and others.

CLINICAL CHARACTERISTICS

Signs and Symptoms:
  Elevated serum titers of anti-D immunoglobulin (IgM)
  Fetal hydrops, erythroblastosis fetalis, hemolytic disease of the newborn
  Intrauterine fetal demise

DIAGNOSTIC APPROACH

Differential Diagnosis:
  Other isoimmunizations (most frequently Lewis, Kell, or Duffy antigens)
  Iron deficiency anemia (maternal)
  Hemoglobinopathy

Associated Conditions: Polyhydramnios.

Workup and Evaluation

Laboratory: Serum antibody titers (at first visit, 20 weeks, and approximately every 4 weeks thereafter), testing of partner's (baby's father) antibody status.

Imaging: Ultrasonography is useful to establish gestational age and monitor amniotic fluid volume and fetal growth.

Special Tests: Amniocentesis or umbilical cord blood sampling if titers are elevated or there has been a prior affected pregnancy.

Diagnostic Procedures: Serum titers, amniocentesis or umbilical cord blood sampling.

MANAGEMENT AND THERAPY

Nonpharmacologic

General Measures: Evaluation, increased surveillance.

Specific Measures: When antibody titers are ≤ 1:8, no intervention is required. When titers are ≥ 1:16 in albumin or 1:32 by an indirect Coombs' test, amniocentesis or umbilical cord blood sampling should be considered. In severely affected fetuses, intrauterine transfusion may be required.

Diet: No specific dietary changes indicated.

Activity: No restriction.

Patient Education: American College of Obstetricians and Gynecologists Patient Education Pamphlet AP027 (*The Rh Factor: How It Can Affect Your Pregnancy*), AP107 (*Amniocentesis and Chorionic Villus Sampling*).

Drug(s) of Choice

None if isoimmunization has taken place. Prophylaxis (with Rh-positive father): D immune globulin—50 μg for miscarriage before 13 weeks of gestation or after chorionic villus sampling; 300 μg after amniocentesis or ectopic pregnancy; at 28–30 weeks of gestation in unsensitized patients or after normal delivery. (20 μg/1 mL of D-positive cells [2 mL of whole blood] infused or lost into the patient's circulation.)

Contraindications: Patients who are already sensitized to the D antigen should not receive D immune globulin.

FOLLOW-UP

Patient Monitoring: Normal prenatal care with increased surveillance of fetal growth and health.

Prevention/Avoidance: All patients should have their Rh type established and be tested for isoimmunization (indirect Coombs' test) at the first prenatal visit. Those who are Rh-negative should receive D immune globulin after delivery, amniocentesis, fetal demise, miscarriage, ectopic pregnancy, or any other time exposure to Rh-positive cells may have occurred. Prophylactic administration between 28 and 30 weeks of gestation is also wise.

Possible Complications: Isoimmunization with subsequent immune damage to fetal red cells leading to lysis, anemia, hydrops, and fetal death.

Expected Outcome: With prophylaxis, the risk of isoimmunization is estimated to be 0.3%.

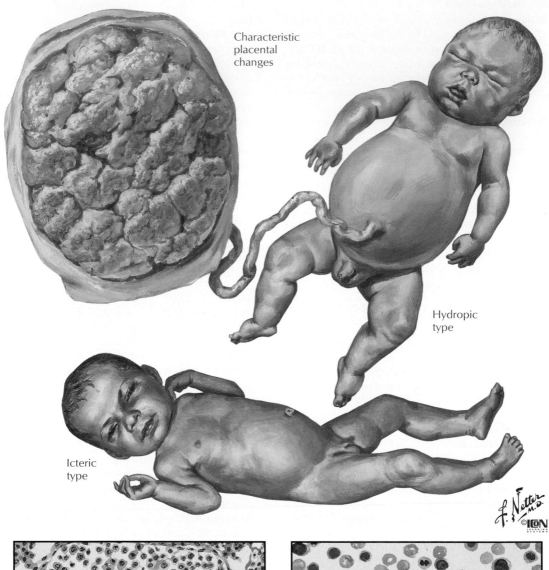

Characteristic
placental
changes

Hydropic
type

Icteric
type

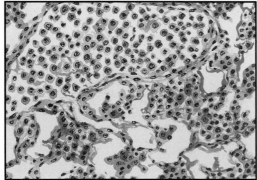

Erythropoiesis in lung

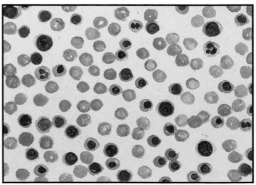

Blood smear showing erythroblastosis

MISCELLANEOUS

ICD-9-CM **Codes:** 656.1.

REFERENCES

American College of Obstetricians and Gynecologists. *Prevention of D Isoimmunization.* Washington, DC: ACOG; 1990. ACOG Technical Bulletin 147.

American College of Obstetricians and Gynecologists. *Management of Isoimmunization in Pregnancy.* Washington, DC: ACOG; 1996. ACOG Technical Bulletin 227.

Chitkara U, Wilkins I, Lynch L, Mehalek K, Berkowitz RL. The role of sonography in assessing severity of fetal anemia in Rh- and Kell-isoimmunized pregnancies. *Obstet Gynecol* 1988;71:393.

Parer JT. Severe Rh isoimmunization—current methods of in utero diagnosis and treatment. *Am J Obstet Gynecol* 1988;158:1323.

Queenan JT, Tomai TP, Ural SH, King JC. Deviation in amniotic fluid optical density at a wavelength of 450 nm in Rh-immunized pregnancies from 14 to 40 weeks' gestation: a proposal for clinical management. *Am J Obstet Gynecol* 1993;168:1370.

TRAUMA IN PREGNANCY

INTRODUCTION

Description: Trauma and violence are the leading causes of death for women of reproductive age and of maternal death from nonobstetric causes. The most common cause of fetal death in automobile accidents is death of the mother. The altered physiologic state of pregnancy and the need to treat two patients simultaneously alters the management of even simple trauma.

Prevalence: One of 12 pregnancies.

Predominant Age: Reproductive.

Genetics: No genetic pattern.

ETIOLOGY AND PATHOGENESIS

Causes: Motor vehicle accidents (most common), falls, direct assault (battering most common).

Risk Factors: Failure to use a safety restraint while driving, abusive relationship, low socioeconomic status, drug or alcohol use and abuse.

CLINICAL CHARACTERISTICS

Signs and Symptoms:

Varies with type of trauma—blunt trauma, trauma associated with covert internal injuries such as retroperitoneal hemorrhage or splenic rupture with bowel injuries less common, penetrating, fetal injury (two thirds)

Abruptio placenta (1%–5% of minor trauma, 40%–50% of major trauma)—vaginal bleeding, uterine tenderness, tetany, or contractions suggest abruption

Uterine rupture (0.6%) as the result of substantial force to the abdomen

Direct fetal injury rare in blunt trauma

Because of increased blood volume during pregnancy, signs of blood loss may be delayed.

DIAGNOSTIC APPROACH

Differential Diagnosis:

Based on type of trauma and organs potentially involved

Associated Conditions: Rh isoimmunization.

Workup and Evaluation

Laboratory: Based on normal management of trauma.

Imaging: As needed for the management of trauma (unchanged by the pregnancy, trauma takes precedence). Ultrasonography for gestational age assessment, placental location, intrauterine death, and others. (Not reliable for assessment of fetal injury.)

Special Tests: Peritoneal lavage under direct vision may be used to evaluate intraperitoneal hemorrhage. Kleihauer-Betke test for fetal-maternal hemorrhage.

Diagnostic Procedures: History, physical examination, imaging studies, and exploratory surgery when indicated.

Pathologic Findings

Based on the nature of the trauma.

MANAGEMENT AND THERAPY

Nonpharmacologic

General Measures: Rapid assessment and stabilization (eg, administration of fluids and oxygen, cardiac and fetal heart rate monitoring based on gestational age), assessment of status (blood pressure, oxygen saturation, urinary output). Tetanus prophylaxis should be provided as needed.

Specific Measures: The uterus should be displaced leftward, off the vena cava. All penetrating abdominal injuries must be explored surgically. The decision to deliver the fetus surgically must be based on gestational age, fetal and maternal injuries, and the risk of death of the fetus if left in utero. Prophylaxis for Rh isoimmunization should be given if fetal-maternal hemorrhage is likely.

Diet: Nothing by mouth until the patient has been fully evaluated.

Activity: Bed rest until the patient has been fully evaluated.

Patient Education: American College of Obstetricians and Gynecologists Patient Education Pamphlet AP018 (*Car Safety for You and Your Baby*), AP055 (*Travel During Pregnancy*), AP083 (*The Abused Woman*).

Drug(s) of Choice

Based on injuries sustained. D immunoglobulin 300 μg IM for each 30 mL of fetal blood thought to have been transfused to the mother (for Rh incompatibility prophylaxis).

Precautions: Tocolytics should only be administered after abruption has been ruled out because medication side effects such as tachycardia may confuse the clinical picture. Vasopressors should be withheld until appropriate fluid resuscitation has been given.

FOLLOW-UP

Patient Monitoring: Aggressive monitoring as appropriate for the trauma sustained, fetal heart rate monitoring.

Blunt Trauma in Pregnancy
Causes and Prevention

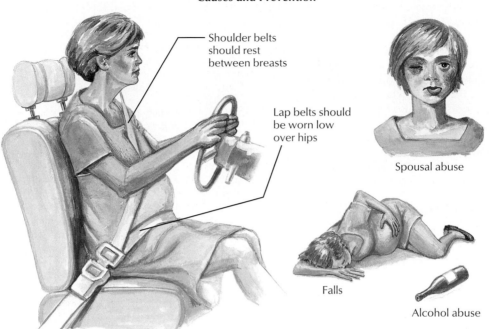

Shoulder belts should rest between breasts

Lap belts should be worn low over hips

Spousal abuse

Falls

Alcohol abuse

Automobile accidents are most common cause of injury. Proper seat belt use can decrease injury

JOHN A.CRAIG—AD
with
E. Hatton
© I¢¢N

Clinical Considerations in Trauma

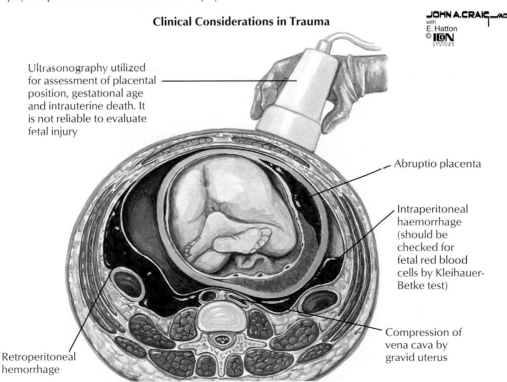

Ultrasonography utilized for assessment of placental position, gestational age and intrauterine death. It is not reliable to evaluate fetal injury

Abruptio placenta

Intraperitoneal haemorrhage (should be checked for fetal red blood cells by Kleihauer-Betke test)

Compression of vena cava by gravid uterus

Retroperitoneal hemorrhage

Prevention/Avoidance: The greatest injuries are seen when a pregnant women is not using safety restraints during an automobile accident; injury is not usually caused by the restraints. (Approximately 15% of pregnant women use safety restraints while driving.) Lap belts should be worn low over the hips and shoulder restraints should rest comfortably between the breasts. The use of approved infant seats to transport the newborn home and for all subsequent travel must also be encouraged in the strongest terms.

Possible Complications: Based on injuries sustained.

Expected Outcome: Based on trauma sustained; maternal generally good, fetal mortality 50%–75% for penetrating injuries involving the uterus.

MISCELLANEOUS

***ICD-9-CM* Codes:** 760.5.

REFERENCES

American College of Obstetricians and Gynecologists. *Trauma During Pregnancy.* Washington, DC: ACOG; 1991. ACOG Technical Bulletin 161.

American College of Obstetricians and Gynecologists. *Automobile Passenger Restraints for Children and Pregnant Women.* Washington, DC: ACOG; 1991. ACOG Technical Bulletin 151.

Helton AS, McFarlane J, Anderson ET. Battered and pregnant: a prevalence study. *Am J Public Health* 1987;77:1337.

Kanthor HA. Car safety for infants: effectiveness of prenatal counseling. *Pediatrics* 1976;58:320.

Kettel LM, Branch DW, Scott JR. Occult placental abruption after maternal trauma. *Obstet Gynecol* 1988; 71:449.

Pearlman MD, Tintinalli JE, Lorenz RP. Blunt trauma during pregnancy. *N Engl J Med* 1990;323:1609.

Pearlman MD, Tintinalli JE, Lorenz RP. A prospective controlled study of outcome after trauma during pregnancy. *Am J Obstet Gynecol* 1990;162:1502.

UTERINE ATONY (POSTPARTUM)

INTRODUCTION

Description: Loss of uterine tone after delivery that often presents as postpartum hemorrhage.

Prevalence: Hemorrage is seen in 5% of deliveries, mostly because of atony; milder degrees are more common.

Predominant Age: Reproductive.

Genetics: No genetic pattern.

ETIOLOGY AND PATHOGENESIS

Causes: Loss of the normal uterine contractile forces.

Risk Factors: Multiparity (grand multiparity), uterine overdistention (multiple birth, polyhydramnios), prolonged labor, prolonged oxytocin stimulation, muscle relaxant agents ($MgSO_4$, tocolytics), rapid labor, chorioamnionitis, retained placental tissue.

CLINICAL CHARACTERISTICS

Signs and Symptoms:

Bright red vaginal bleeding

Loss of uterine tone palpable on abdominal examination

Tachycardia, hypotension, and vascular collapse possible

DIAGNOSTIC APPROACH

Differential Diagnosis:

Retained placental fragments

Genital tract lacerations (cervical, vaginal)

Uterine rupture

Uterine inversion

Coagulopathy

Associated Conditions: Uterine inversion and postpartum hemorrhage.

Workup and Evaluation

Laboratory: Hemoglobin or hematocrit to monitor status and volume of blood loss.

Imaging: Ultrasonography may be used to identify retained placental products but is generally not necessary.

Special Tests: None indicated.

Diagnostic Procedures: Physical examination (abdomen and vagina).

Pathologic Findings

Hemoglobin and hematocrit concentrations will not reflect the volume of blood lost until after equilibration has taken place at 6–24 hours.

MANAGEMENT AND THERAPY

Nonpharmacologic

General Measures: Uterine atony should be suspected in any patient with excessive bleeding after delivery of placenta. If initial treatments do not appear to alter patient's bleeding, other diagnoses should be considered while measures to treat atony continue. Rapid evaluation, fluid support or resuscitation (through large-bore access), massage of the uterine fundus. Type and cross-match blood for possible transfusion. The bladder should be drained to allow the uterus to contract and to assess urinary output.

Specific Measures: Uterotonic agents (see below), uterine exploration (manual), uterine artery ligation (O'Leary stitch), hypogastric artery ligation, uterine packing, hysterectomy.

Diet: Nothing by mouth until a diagnosis is established and effective treatment is rendered.

Activity: Bed rest until a diagnosis is established and effective treatment is rendered.

Drug(s) of Choice

Oxytocin 10–20 U/L of intravenous fluids—100–300 mL given as rapid infusion until uterine tone is reestablished, then 100–150 mL/h for the next several hours (Concentrations as high as 20–40 U/L may be used)

Methylergonovine maleate (Methergine) 0.2 mg IM, may repeat in 5 minutes (produces tetanic contractions)

15-Methylprostaglandin $F_2\alpha$ (carboprost tromethamine, Hemabate) 0.25 mg IM or 0.25–1 mg in 10 mL of normal saline injected into the myometrium (may repeat once)

Iron replacement therapy

Broad-spectrum antibiotic treatment should be considered, especially if uterine packing is used

Contraindications: Prostaglandin therapy is contraindicated in patients with asthma. Methergine should not be used in the presence of hypertension and may not be given intravenously.

Precautions: The volume of fluids administered should be monitored closely to avoid inadvertent fluid overload. The placement of a bladder catheter to assess urinary output and to keep the bladder decompressed is desirable. When prostaglandins are used, side effects such as di-

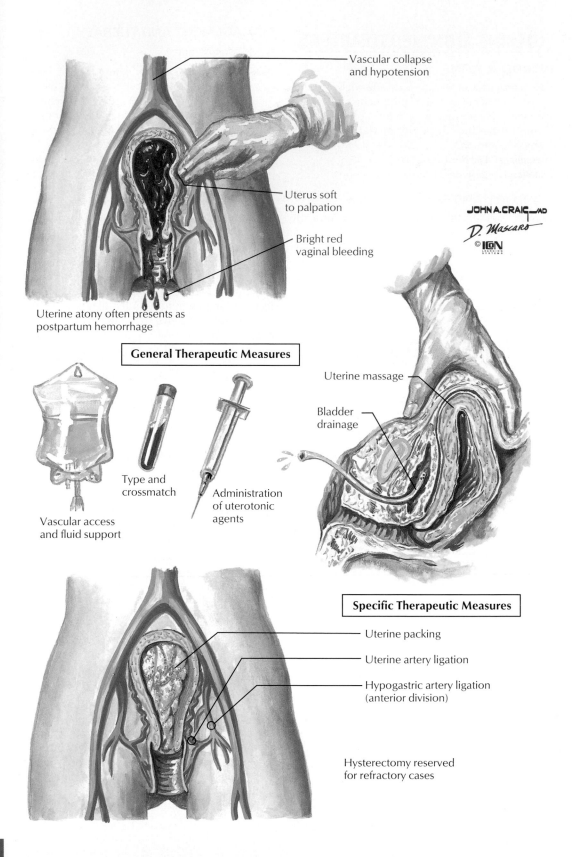

Vascular collapse
and hypotension

Uterus soft
to palpation

Bright red
vaginal bleeding

Uterine atony often presents as
postpartum hemorrhage

JOHN A. CRAIG—MD
D. Mascaro
©ICN

General Therapeutic Measures

Type and
crossmatch

Administration
of uterotonic
agents

Vascular access
and fluid support

Uterine massage

Bladder
drainage

Specific Therapeutic Measures

Uterine packing

Uterine artery ligation

Hypogastric artery ligation
(anterior division)

Hysterectomy reserved
for refractory cases

arrhea, hypertension, vomiting, fever, flushing, and tachycardia are common.

Interactions: Magnesium sulfate and some halogenated anesthetic agents promote atony and work against uterotonic agents.

Alternative Drugs

Prostaglandin E$_2$ vaginal suppositories have been used, but newer agents and the techniques shown above are more effective and are more readily available.

FOLLOW-UP

Patient Monitoring: Normal postpartum care, follow-up complete blood count as needed.

Prevention/Avoidance: Anticipation of possible uterine atony, fundal massage, and oxytocin stimulation after delivery.

Possible Complications: Hysterectomy, hemorrhagic shock, and cardiovascular collapse.

Expected Outcome: Most conditions respond to simple measures (uterine massage, oxytocin, methylergonovine maleate [Methergine]) if ad-

ministered for the appropriate problem and in a timely way.

MISCELLANEOUS

***ICD-9-CM* Codes:** 666.1.

REFERENCES

American College of Obstetricians and Gynecologists. *Diagnosis and Management of Postpartum Hemorrhage.* Washington, DC: ACOG; 1990. ACOG Technical Bulletin 143.

Andersen HF, Hopkins M. Postpartum Hemorrhage. In: Sciarra JJ, ed. *Gynecology and Obstetrics.* Vol 2. Philadelphia, Pa: JB Lippincott; 1996;80:1.

Hayashi RH, Castillo MS, Noah ML. Management of severe postpartum hemorrhage with a prostaglandin F-2-alpha analogue. *Obstet Gynecol* 1984;63:806.

Hertz RH, Sokol RJ, Dierker LJ. Treatment of postpartum uterine atony with prostaglandin E2 vaginal suppositories. *Obstet Gynecol* 1980;56:129.

Oleen MA, Mariano JP. Controlling refractory atonic postpartum hemorrhage with Hemabate sterile solution. *Am J Obstet Gynecol* 1990;162:205.

Thorsteinsson VT, Kempers RD. Delayed postpartum bleeding. *Am J Obstet Gynecol* 1970;107:565.

UTERINE RUPTURE

INTRODUCTION

Description: Breech of the uterine wall (new or after previous uterine surgery such as cesarean delivery) that may result in significant maternal or fetal morbidity or mortality. This should be distinguished from uterine scar dehiscence in which there is separation of an old scar that does not penetrate the uterine serosa or result in complications. Rupture of an intact uterus (without scars) does occur on rare occasions (1 in 15,000 deliveries) and is generally associated with significant uterine distension (polyhydramnios, multiple gestation).

Prevalence: Found in 0.5%–1.5% of patients with a previous cesarean delivery and 5% of patients for whom vaginal birth after cesarean delivery fails. Roughly 7% of emergency cesarean hysterectomies are for rupture.

Predominant Age: Reproductive.

Genetics: No genetic pattern.

ETIOLOGY AND PATHOGENESIS

Causes: Abnormal healing of a previous uterine scar, mechanical disruption of the uterine wall weakened by previous surgery, congenital anomalies, or abnormalities of placentation. (The uterine wall may also be breached by injudicious manual removal of the placenta or manual exploration of the uterus after delivery of the placenta.) Traumatic rupture of the uterus may occur with blunt trauma to the abdomen such as occurs to an unrestrained passenger during an automobile accident. (The proper use of automobile lap and shoulder belts significantly reduces the risk of injury to both mother and fetus.)

Risk Factors: Previous uterine surgery (cesarean delivery; greatest for vertical incisions, myomectomy, septoplasty), multiple gestation, grand multiparity (20-fold increase), fetal malpresentation, polyhydramnios, oxytocin stimulation (unproved), congenital anomalies, and disuse or misuse of vehicle passenger restraints.

CLINICAL CHARACTERISTICS

Signs and Symptoms:
Abrupt fetal distress (80% of cases)
Abrupt loss of station (presenting part may cease to be present in the vagina)
Vaginal bleeding (may not be present)
Abdominal pain (may not be present; pain may be referred to the chest or diaphragm)
Maternal circulatory collapse
Uterine activity may persist despite expulsion of the fetus

DIAGNOSTIC APPROACH

Differential Diagnosis:
Uterine dehiscence
Placental abruption
Umbilical cord prolapse (causing abrupt fetal distress)
Adnexal torsion
Pulmonary or amniotic fluid embolism
Abdominal pregnancy

Associated Conditions: Fetal demise.

Workup and Evaluation

Laboratory: Interoperative and postoperative blood counts. Evaluation of clotting when significant bleeding has occurred.

Imaging: Ultrasonography may demonstrate uterine dehiscence, but the need for clinical intervention often precludes the examination.

Special Tests: Intensive fetal and maternal monitoring may be indicated.

Diagnostic Procedures: History and physical examination (vaginal and abdominal).

Pathologic Findings

Separation of previous uterine scar or a new failure of the uterine wall muscle.

MANAGEMENT AND THERAPY

Nonpharmacologic

General Measures: Rapid evaluation, supportive measures as needed (fluids, blood products).

Specific Measures: Immediate operative delivery (most often by laparotomy), surgical exploration with the possibility of repair or hysterectomy. Ligation of one or both hypogastric arteries may be necessary.

Diet: Nothing by mouth once the diagnosis is made (pending surgical intervention).

Activity: Strict bed rest (pending surgical intervention).

Patient Education: American College of Obstetricians and Gynecologists Patient Education Pamphlet AP070 (*Vaginal Birth After Cesarean Delivery*).

Drug(s) of Choice

None. (Supportive measures including fluids, blood products, and anesthetics [for immediate

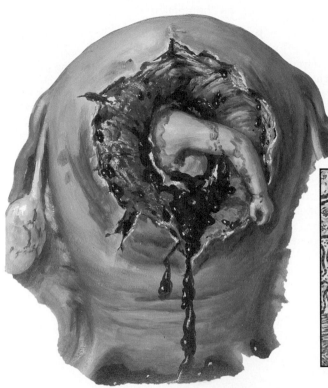

Rupture through scar
of classic cesarean section

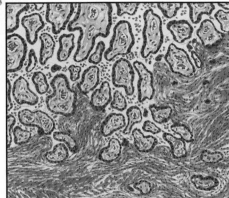

Placenta accreta

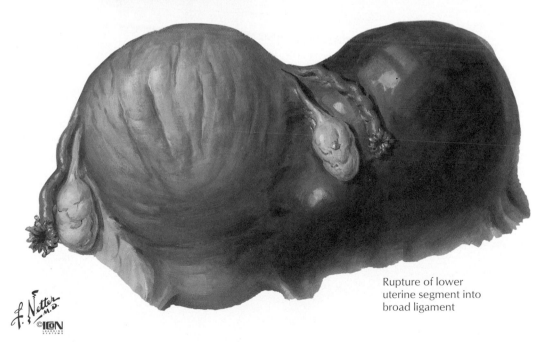

Rupture of lower
uterine segment into
broad ligament

OBSTETRICAL CONDITIONS

delivery] as needed. Prophylactic antibiotics are often recommended.)

FOLLOW-UP

Patient Monitoring: Fetal and maternal monitoring must be maintained for those at risk and intensified when the diagnosis is considered.

Prevention/Avoidance: Care in all uterine manipulations (eg, manual removal of the placenta, version, external pressure during delivery).

Possible Complications: Maternal morbidity or mortality possible (significantly reduced by fetal and maternal monitoring). Damage to the cervix, vagina, or bladder may occur as a part of the rupture. Fetal demise may occur in up to 50%–75% of fundal incision ruptures and 10%–15% of lower uterine segment ruptures. Long-term neurologic sequelae are common in infants who survive. Vertical uterine scars are associated with the greatest morbidity and mortality when a rupture occurs.

Expected Outcome: When diagnosed early and acted upon promptly, a good outcome can be expected. (If the uterus is repaired and preserved, the risk of recurrence in a subsequent pregnancy is roughly 20%.)

MISCELLANEOUS

***ICD-9-CM* Codes:** 665.1 (During labor), 665.0 (Before labor), 763.8 (Affecting the fetus or newborn), 867.4 (Traumatic).

REFERENCES

Benito CW, Smullian JC, Gray SE, Scorza WE. A case control study of uterine rupture during pregnancy. *Am J Obstet Gynecol* 1996;174:485.

Eden RD, Parker RT, Gall SA. Rupture of the pregnant uterus: a 53 year review. *Obstet Gynecol* 1986;68:671.

Farmer RM, Kirschbaum T, Potter D, Strong TH, Medearis AL. Uterine rupture during trial of labor after previous cesarean delivery. *Am J Obstet Gynecol* 1991;165:996.

Golan A, Sandbank O, Rubin A. Rupture of the pregnant uterus. *Obstet Gynecol* 1980;56:349.

Levrant SG, Wingate M. Midtrimester uterine rupture. *J Reprod Med* 1996;41:186.

Miller DA, Paul RH. Rupture of the unscarred uterus. *Am J Obstet Gynecol* 1996;174:345.

Plauche WC, Von Almen W, Mueller R. Catastrophic uterine rupture. *Obstet Gynecol* 1984;64:792.

Rosen MG, Dickinson JC, Westhoff CL. Vaginal birth after cesarean: a meta-analysis of morbidity and mortality. *Obstet Gynecol* 1991;77:465.

Adnexal Disease

ADENOFIBROMA

INTRODUCTION

Description: An epithelial tumor that consists of glandular elements and large amounts of stromal (fibrous) elements. Adenofibromas are most commonly found as ovarian masses. Adenofibromas may also occur in the cervix or uterine body.

Prevalence: Uncommon.

Predominant Age: Peri- and postmenopausal.

Genetics: No genetic pattern.

ETIOLOGY AND PATHOGENESIS

Causes: Unknown.

Risk Factors: None known.

CLINICAL CHARACTERISTICS

Signs and Symptoms:

Asymptomatic (often an incidental finding after oophorectomy)

Adnexal mass (adenofibromas are bilateral in 25% of cases)

Fibrous cervical or endometrial polyp

DIAGNOSTIC APPROACH

Differential Diagnosis:

Thecoma (fibroma)

Stromal and germ cell tumors

Brenner tumor

Endometrioma

Benign cystic teratoma

Serous or mucinous cystadenoma

Metastatic tumors

Pedunculated leiomyomata

Endocervical polyp

Associated Conditions: None.

Workup and Evaluation

Laboratory: No specific evaluation indicated; evaluate as with other adnexal or cervical masses.

Imaging: Ultrasonography may suggest a solid tumor.

Special Tests: None indicated.

Diagnostic Procedures: Histopathology.

Pathologic Findings

Fibrous and epithelial elements make up this tumor. The epithelial components may be serous, mucinous, clear cell, or endometrioid. Epithelial or fibrous elements may predominate, changing the gross character of the tumor.

MANAGEMENT AND THERAPY

Nonpharmacologic

General Measures: Evaluation and diagnosis.

Specific Measures: Simple surgical excision. Adenofibromas that are borderline or of low malignant potential do exist. These tumors must be treated based on their size, location, and histologic evaluation, but may require more extensive surgical therapy.

Diet: No specific dietary changes indicated.

Activity: No restriction.

Patient Education: Reassurance, American College of Obstetricians and Gynecologists Patient Education Pamphlet AP075 (*Ovarian Cysts*), AP096 (*Cancer of the Ovary*).

Drug(s) of Choice

None.

FOLLOW-UP

Patient Monitoring: Normal health maintenance.

Prevention/Avoidance: None.

Possible Complications: Torsion of solid ovarian tumors. Adenofibromas that are borderline or of low malignant potential may spread or recur.

Expected Outcome: Surgical excision is generally curative.

MISCELLANEOUS

Pregnancy Considerations: No effect on pregnancy.

ICD-9-CM Codes: Based on location and predominant cell type.

REFERENCES

Czernobilsky B. Common epithelial tumors of the ovary. In: Kurman RJ, ed. *Blaustein's Pathology of the Female Genital Tract.* 3rd ed. New York, NY: Springer-Verlag; 1987.

Fenoglio CM, Richart RM. Common epithelial ovarian tumors. In: Sciarra JJ, ed. *Gynecology and Obstetrics.* Vol 4. Philadelphia, Pa: JB Lippincott; 1989;30:10.

Fleischer AC. Transabdominal and transvaginal sonography of ovarian masses. *Clin Obstet Gynecol* 1991;34:433.

Herman JR, Locher GW, Goldhirsch A. Sonographic patterns of ovarian tumors: prediction of malignancy. *Obstet Gynecol* 1987;69:777.

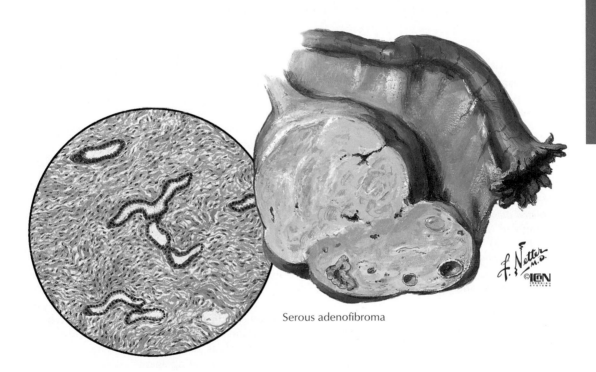

Serous adenofibroma

CLEAR CELL CARCINOMA

INTRODUCTION

Description: An ovarian tumor made up of cells containing large amounts of glycogen that gives them a clear or "hobnailed" appearance. These tumors may also arise in the endocervix, endometrium, and vagina.

Prevalence: Five percent to eleven percent of ovarian cancers.

Predominant Age: 40–78.

Genetics: No genetic pattern.

ETIOLOGY AND PATHOGENESIS

Causes: Unknown. May arise from mesonephric or müllerian elements.

Risk Factors: None known.

CLINICAL CHARACTERISTICS

Signs and Symptoms

Asymptomatic

Pelvic mass (up to 30 cm)—partially cystic with yellow, gray, and hemorrhagic areas

Papillary projections generally present, giving the mass a velvety appearance; 40% of tumors are bilateral

DIAGNOSTIC APPROACH

Differential Diagnosis:

Benign adnexal masses (corpus luteum, follicular cyst)

Nongynecologic pelvic masses

Hepatic, renal, or cardiac disease resulting in weight loss and ascites

Endometriosis

Hydrosalpinx

Ectopic pregnancy (reproductive-age women)

Pedunculated leiomyomata

Pelvic or horseshoe kidney

Gastrointestinal malignancy

Associated Conditions: None.

Workup and Evaluation

Laboratory: As indicated before surgery. (Serum testing for tumor markers, such as CA-125, lipid-associated sialic acid, carcinoembryonic antigen, α-fetoprotein, and others, should be reserved for following the progress of patients with known malignancies and not for prognostic evaluation.)

Imaging: No imaging indicated.

Special Tests: A frozen section histologic evaluation should be considered for any ovarian mass that appears suspicious for malignancy.

Diagnostic Procedures: History, physical examination, and imaging. Final diagnosis is established by histologic evaluation.

Pathologic Findings

Usually found as a malignant tumor. Despite the presence of hobnail cells that are similar to those seen in the endometrium, cervix, and vagina of women exposed to diethylstilbestrol (DES) in utero, there is no evidence that DES has a role in clear cell ovarian tumors.

MANAGEMENT AND THERAPY

Nonpharmacologic

General Measures: Evaluation, supportive therapy based on symptoms.

Specific Measures: Requires surgical exploration and extirpation, including the uterus and contralateral ovary. Adjunctive chemotherapy (platinum-based and paclitaxel [Taxol]) or radiation therapy is often included based on the location and stage of the disease.

Diet: No specific dietary changes indicated, except those imposed by advanced disease.

Activity: No restriction except that imposed by advanced disease.

Patient Education: American College of Obstetricians and Gynecologists Patient Education Pamphlet AP096 (*Cancer of the Ovary*), AP075 (*Ovarian Cysts*).

Drug(s) of Choice

None, except as adjunctive or symptomatic therapy. Preoperative bowel cleansing (mechanical or with antibiotics) is often recommended as a precaution should bowel resection become necessary at the time of surgical staging and resection.

Contraindications: See individual agents.

Precautions: Alkylating agents are associated with an increased risk of future leukemia (10% by 8 years after therapy).

INTERACTIONS: See individual agents.

FOLLOW-UP

Patient Monitoring: Careful follow-up for recurrent pelvic disease or enlargement of the remaining ovary (if any). This is generally performed by pelvic examination, augmented with ultrasonography in selected patients. In those suspected of having recurrent disease and other selected patients, second-look surgery may be desirable to assess progress and discover occult disease.

Prevention/Avoidance: None.

Clear Cell Carcinoma of Ovary

Pelvic mass (up to 30 cm)
Partially cystic
40% bilateral
predominately

Papillary
projections

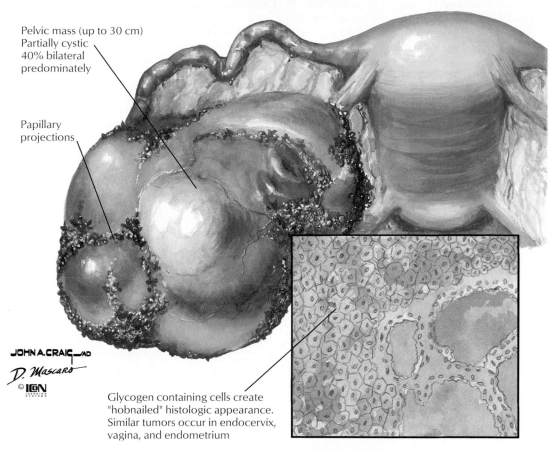

JOHN A. CRAIG—AD

D. Mascaro

© ICON
LEARNING SYSTEMS

Glycogen containing cells create
"hobnailed" histologic appearance.
Similar tumors occur in endocervix,
vagina, and endometrium

Surgical Management

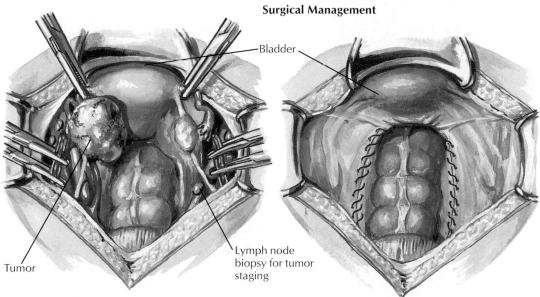

Bladder

Tumor

Lymph node
biopsy for tumor
staging

Total abdominal hysterectomy
with bilateral salpingo-oophorectomy

Closure of pelvic peritoneum
postoperative appearance

Possible Complications: Rapid spread and progressive deterioration of the patient's condition.

Expected Outcome: Typically aggressive course with rapid disease progression and spread. Clear cell ovarian carcinoma has the worst prognosis of all ovarian malignancies, with a 5-year survival rate of <40%. (The 5-year survival rate is modified by stage of disease at diagnosis: limited to one ovary, 80%; higher stage disease, 11%).

MISCELLANEOUS

Pregnancy Considerations: No direct effect on pregnancy. (Generally not an issue.)

***ICD-9-CM* Codes:** M8310/3.

REFERENCES

American College of Obstetricians and Gynecologists. *Cancer of the Ovary.* Washington, DC: ACOG; 1990. ACOG Technical Bulletin 141.

American College of Obstetricians and Gynecologists. *Classification and Staging of Gynecologic Malignancies.* Washington, DC: ACOG; 1991. ACOG Technical Bulletin 155.

Fenoglio CM, Richart RM. Common epithelial ovarian tumors. In: Sciarra JJ, ed. *Gynecology and Obstetrics.* Vol. 4. Philadelphia, Pa: JB Lippincott; 1989;30:24.

Fleischer AC. Transabdominal and transvaginal sonography of ovarian masses. *Clin Obstet Gynecol* 1991;34:433.

Hameed K, Burslem MRG, Tupper WRC. Clear cell carcinoma of the ovary. *Cancer* 1969;24:452.

DERMOID CYST

INTRODUCTION

Description: The most common ovarian tumor in young, reproductive-age women is the cystic teratoma, or dermoid, which originates from a germ cell. These tumors may be benign or malignant (1%–2% malignant, usually in women older than 40).

Prevalence: Fifteen percent to twenty-five percent of ovarian tumors.

Predominant Age: 20s to 30s (75%), most younger than 40.

Genetics: No genetic pattern.

ETIOLOGY AND PATHOGENESIS

Causes: Unknown. Thought to arise from a single germ cell during the first meiotic division at roughly 13 weeks of fetal life. They routinely have a chromosomal makeup of 46,XX.

Risk Factors: None known.

CLINICAL CHARACTERISTICS

Signs and Symptoms:

Asymptomatic (50%–60%)

Adnexal mass (80% <10 cm in diameter, bilateral in 10%–15% of patients)—the contents of cystic teratomas are of low density; they are often found "floating" anterior to the uterus or broad ligament, displacing the uterus posteriorly

May present with pain secondary to torsion or bleeding into the cyst, a sense of pelvic heaviness, or dysmenorrhea

Thyroid storm (when thyroid tissue predominates: struma ovarii) or carcinoid syndrome (rare)

DIAGNOSTIC APPROACH

Differential Diagnosis:

Functional cysts (follicle, corpus luteum)
Epithelial tumors (cystic or solid)
Ectopic pregnancy
Tubo-ovarian abscess
Endometrioma
Hydrosalpinx
Paratubal cyst
Appendiceal abscess

Associated Conditions: None.

WORK UP AND EVALUATION

Laboratory: No evaluation indicated.

Imaging: Ultrasonography (abdominal or transvaginal may be of assistance, but usually is not required). Thirty percent to fifty percent of teratomas have calcifications and may be detected by radiographic examination.

Special Tests: None indicated.

Diagnostic Procedures: History, physical examination, imaging. May be found incidentally at laparotomy or laparoscopy.

Pathologic Findings

These tumors are derived from primary germ cells and include tissues from all three embryonic germ layers (ectoderm, mesoderm, and endoderm). Consequently, these often contain hair, sebaceous material, cartilage, bone, teeth, or neural tissue. On rare occasions, functional thyroid tissue may be present. Cystic teratomas contain malignant elements in only about 1%–2% of cases.

MANAGEMENT AND THERAPY

Nonpharmacologic

General Measures: Evaluation, support for acute symptoms.

Specific Measures: Surgical exploration and resection.

Diet: No specific dietary changes indicated.

Activity: No restriction.

Patient Education: Reassurance, American College of Obstetricians and Gynecologists Patient Education Pamphlet AP075 (*Ovarian Cysts*).

Drug(s) of Choice

None.

FOLLOW-UP

Patient Monitoring: Normal health maintenance.

Prevention/Avoidance: None.

Possible Complications: Most common—torsion (3%–12%). Possible—infection, rupture, and malignant transformation (squamous carcinoma, 1%–2%). (The risk of malignant transformation is greatest when these tumors are found in postmenopausal women.) Recurrence of teratomas is as high as 3.4% in some studies. Rupture of a dermoid can result in an intense chemical peritonitis, and is a surgical emergency. Slow leakage may mimic disseminated carcinoma.

Expected Outcome: Based on the size and location of the tumor, it is often possible to conserve some or most of the ovary while the tumor itself is resected.

MISCELLANEOUS

Pregnancy Considerations: No effect on pregnancy. Ten percent of dermoids are diagnosed during pregnancy and account for 20%–40% of ovar-

Dermoid Cyst

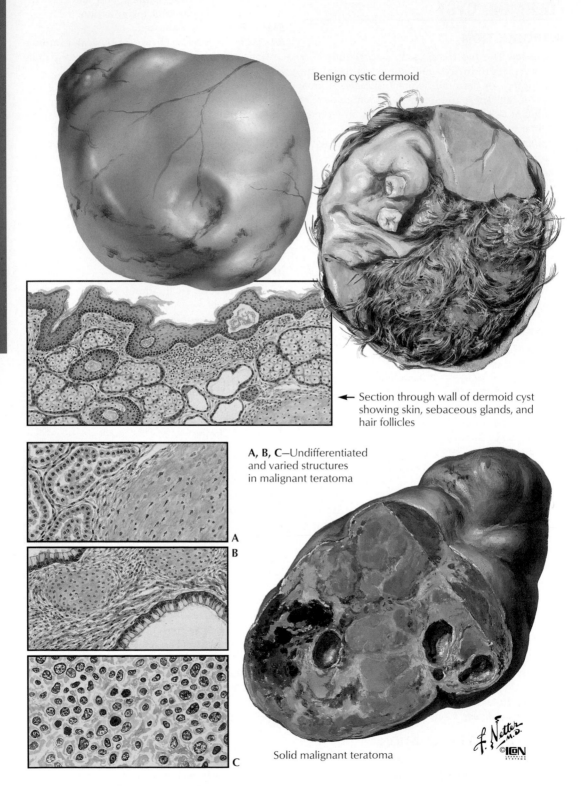

Benign cystic dermoid

← Section through wall of dermoid cyst showing skin, sebaceous glands, and hair follicles

A, B, C—Undifferentiated and varied structures in malignant teratoma

A

B

C

Solid malignant teratoma

ian tumors found during pregnancy. Rupture of the cyst, while rare, is more common during pregnancy.

ICD-9-CM Codes: M9084/0.

REFERENCES

Fleischer AC. Transabdominal and transvaginal sonography of ovarian masses. *Clin Obstet Gynecol* 1991;34:433.

Howard FM. Surgical management of benign cystic teratoma: laparoscopy vs. laparotomy. *J Reprod Med* 1995;40:495.

Linder D, McCau BK, Hecht F. Parthenogenic origin of benign ovarian teratomas. *N Engl J Med* 1975;292:63.

Mais V, Guerriero S, Ajossa S, Angiolucci M, Paoletti AM, Melis GB. Transvaginal ultrasonography in the diagnosis of cystic teratoma. *Obstet Gynecol* 1995; 85:48.

Pantoja E, Noy MA, Axtmayer RW, Colon FE, Pelegrina I. Ovarian dermoids and their complications: comprehensive historical review. *Obstet Gynecol Surv* 1975;30:1.

Parazzini F, La Vecchia C, Negri E, Moroni S, Villa A. Risk factors for benign ovarian teratomas. *Br J Cancer* 1995;71:664.

Petersen WF, Prevost EC, Edmunds FT, Hundley JM, Morriss FK. Benign cystic teratomas of the ovary. *Am J Obstet Gynecol* 1955;70:368.

DYSGERMINOMA

INTRODUCTION

Description: An ovarian tumor made up of germ cells and stroma that appear analogous in structure to the seminomas found in the male testes. Although rare, these tumors are the most common malignant germ cell tumors.

Prevalence: Rare, 1%–2% of ovarian malignancies.

Predominant Age: Older than 30 (10% in prepubertal girls).

Genetics: No genetic pattern.

ETIOLOGY AND PATHOGENESIS

Causes: Unknown. (May differentiate from primitive germ cells.)

Risk Factors: None known.

CLINICAL CHARACTERISTICS

Signs and Symptoms:

Asymptomatic

Adnexal mass (bilateral in 5%–10%), lobulated, solid and soft or firm, with a gray-white or cream-colored cut surface.

DIAGNOSTIC APPROACH

Differential Diagnosis:

Benign adnexal masses (corpus luteum, follicular cyst)

Endometriosis

Hydrosalpinx

Paratubal cyst

Appendiceal abscess

Ectopic pregnancy

Pedunculated leiomyomata

Pelvic or horseshoe kidney

Nongynecologic pelvic masses

Associated Conditions: None.

WORK UP AND EVALUATION

Laboratory: As indicated before surgery. β-Human chorionic gonadotropin is often elevated (several thousand units), as is lactic dehydrogenase. (Serum testing for tumor markers such as CA-125, lipid-associated sialic acid, carcinoembryonic antigen, α-fetoprotein, and others should be reserved for following the progress of patients with known malignancies and not for prognostic evaluation.)

Imaging: Preoperative evaluation (computed tomography [CT] or ultrasonography) for possible lymph node enlargement or intraabdominal spread is indicated for patients for whom malignancy is a significant possibility.

Special Tests: None indicated.

Diagnostic Procedures: History, physical examination, and imaging. Final diagnosis is established by histologic evaluation.

Pathologic Findings

Primitive germ cells with stroma infiltrated by lymphocytes (analogous to seminomas in the testes). Areas of malignant cells are found in 10%–15% of tumors.

MANAGEMENT AND THERAPY

Nonpharmacologic

General Measures: Evaluation, supportive therapy based on symptoms.

Specific Measures: Surgical exploration and resection. When the tumor is confined to one ovary, preservation of the uterus and other ovary is possible to preserve fertility. These tumors are very sensitive to radiation therapy, which may be used as an adjunct or to treat recurrent disease. Multiagent chemotherapy has fewer side effects and is often the preferred adjunct.

Diet: No specific dietary changes indicated, except those imposed by advanced disease.

Activity: No restriction except that imposed by advanced disease.

Patient Education: American College of Obstetricians and Gynecologists Patient Education Pamphlet AP096 (*Cancer of the Ovary*), AP075 (*Ovarian Cysts*).

Drug(s) of Choice

Adjunctive or symptomatic therapy. Combination chemotherapy in selected patients (vincristine, actinomycin D, and cyclophosphamide or bleomycin, etoposide, and cisplatin).

FOLLOW-UP

Patient Monitoring: Careful follow-up for recurrent pelvic disease or enlargement of the remaining ovary (if any). This is generally performed by pelvic examination, augmented with ultrasonography in selected patients. In patients suspected of having recurrent disease and other selected patients, second-look surgery may be desirable to assess progress and discover occult disease.

Prevention/Avoidance: None.

Possible Complications: Tumor progression or growth. These tumors tend to spread by lymphatic channels. Recurrence of tumor is found in 20% of patients, but recurrent disease generally responds well to additional surgery, chemotherapy, or radiation.

Expected Outcome: The prognosis is good for patients with pure dysgerminomas less than 15 cm in size. With limited disease and no indication of spread at the time of surgery (stage I) there is a >90% 5-year survival.

MISCELLANEOUS

Pregnancy Considerations: No effect on pregnancy. May be discovered during pregnancy.

ICD-9-CM Codes: Specific to cell type and location.

REFERENCES

American College of Obstetricians and Gynecologists. *Cancer of the Ovary.* Washington, DC: ACOG; 1990. ACOG Technical Bulletin 141.

American College of Obstetricians and Gynecologists. *Classification and Staging of Gynecologic Malignancies.* Washington, DC: ACOG; 1991. ACOG Technical Bulletin 155.

Assadourian LA, Taylor HB. Dysgerminoma: an analysis of 105 cases. *Obstet Gynecol* 1969;33:370.

Fleischer AC. Transabdominal and transvaginal sonography of ovarian masses. *Clin Obstet Gynecol* 1991;34:433.

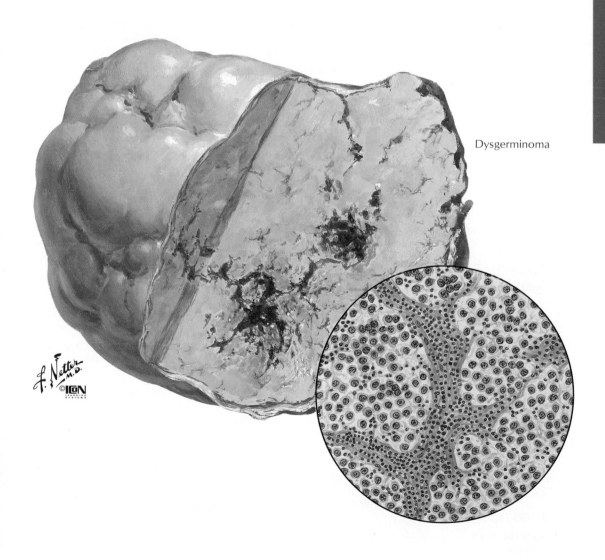

Dysgerminoma

ECTOPIC PREGNANCY

INTRODUCTION

Description: Pregnancy that implants outside of the endometrial cavity (fallopian tube, ovary, abdominal cavity, or cervix).

Prevalence: Ten to fifteen of 1000 pregnancies; varies with age, race, and location (highest in Jamaica and Vietnam).

Predominant Age: 25–34 (>40%).

Genetics: No genetic pattern.

ETIOLOGY AND PATHOGENESIS

Causes: Tubal damage or altered motility that results in the fertilized egg being improperly transported, resulting in implantation outside the uterine cavity. The most common cause is acute salpingitis (50%). In the majority of the remaining patients (40%), no risk factor is apparent. Abnormal embryonic development may play a role.

Risk Factors: Tubal damage (pelvic infections 6-fold increased risk), prior ectopic pregnancy (10-fold increased risk), prior female sterilization, age (age 35–44, 3-fold greater rate of extrauterine gestations than for women aged 15–24), nonwhite race (1.5-fold increased risk), assisted reproduction, cigarette smoking (30+/day: 3- to 5-fold increased risk), intrauterine contraceptive device (IUCD) use, and endometriosis.

CLINICAL CHARACTERISTICS

Signs and Symptoms:

Normal signs and symptoms of pregnancy (amenorrhea, uterine softening)

Acute abdominal pain (dull, crampy, or colicky)

Evidence of intraabdominal bleeding including hypotension and collapse

Adnexal mass (with or without tenderness)

Vaginal bleeding

Signs of peritoneal irritation

Absence of a gestational sac on ultrasonography with β-human chorionic gonadotropin (β-hCG) level >2500 mIU/mL

Abdominal pregnancy may be asymptomatic until term

DIAGNOSTIC APPROACH

Differential Diagnosis:

Appendicitis

Degenerating fibroid

Dysfunctional uterine bleeding

Endometriosis

Gastroenteritis

Mesenteric thrombosis

Ovulation

Ruptured corpus luteum cyst

Salpingitis

Septic abortion (fever >38°C or a white blood count >20,000 WBC/dl are rare in patients with ectopic pregnancies; the presence of either should suggest the possibility of a pelvic infection, including septic abortion)

Threatened or incomplete abortion

Torsion of an adnexal mass

Associated Conditions: Pelvic inflammatory disease, infertility, and recurrent abortion.

Workup and Evaluation

Laboratory: Serial quantitative β-hCG levels (if patient's condition permits). Serum progesterone (low) may be of diagnostic help if <6 weeks gestation.

Imaging: Ultrasonography (transvaginal preferred), may be augmented by color-flow Doppler studies.

Special Tests: Culdocentesis has largely been replaced by ultrasonography.

Diagnostic Procedures: History and physical examination, serum β-HCG level and ultrasonography.

Pathologic Findings

Placental villi invading tissue other than the endometrium. Most ectopic pregnancies are tubal, with the ampulla (78%) and isthmus (12%) the most common locations.

MANAGEMENT AND THERAPY

Nonpharmacologic

General Measures: Rapid assessment and general support when intraabdominal bleeding is present.

Specific Measures: Expeditious diagnosis. Surgical intervention generally required for symptomatic patients (salpingostomy, salpingectomy). Medical therapy may be considered for asymptomatic or mildly symptomatic patients.

Diet: In acute rupture, nothing by mouth in anticipation of possible surgical intervention. If medical therapy is used, avoid folate supplements and folate-containing preparations (eg, multivitamins, prenatal vitamins).

Activity: No restriction except those dictated by the patient's status.

Patient Education: Reassurance, American College of Obstetricians and Gynecologists Patient Education Pamphlet AP090 (*Early Pregnancy Loss:*

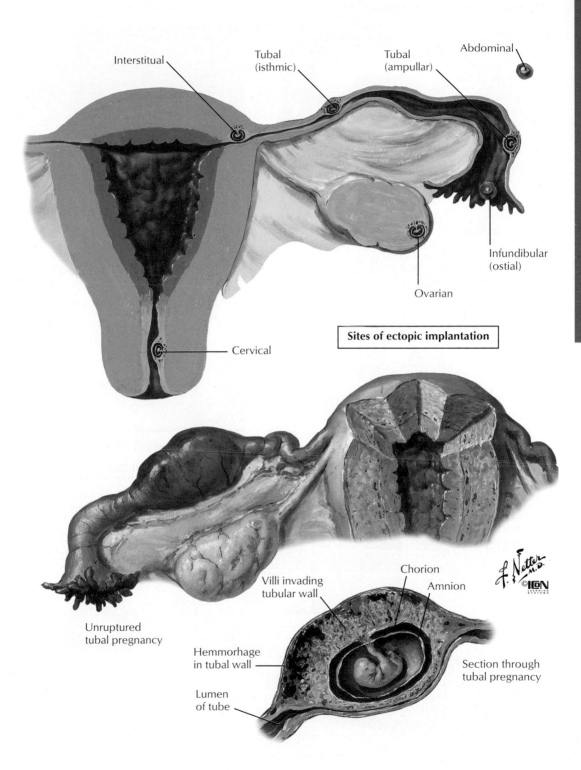

Interstitial

Tubal (isthmic)

Tubal (ampullar)

Abdominal

Infundibular (ostial)

Ovarian

Cervical

Sites of ectopic implantation

Unruptured tubal pregnancy

Villi invading tubular wall

Hemmorhage in tubal wall

Lumen of tube

Chorion

Amnion

Section through tubal pregnancy

Diagnosis of Ectopic Pregnancy

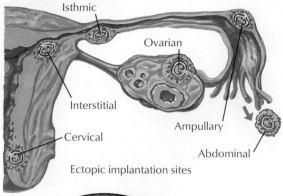

Isthmic

Ovarian

Interstitial

Cervical

Ampullary

Abdominal

Ectopic implantation sites

Laparoscopy may be used to confirm
diagnosis of ectopic pregnancy

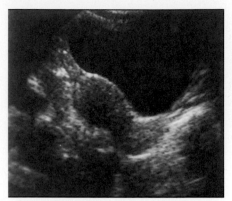

Sonogram of empty uterine cavity

Sonogram of gestational sac

JOHN A.CRAIG—AD
© ICN

Pregnancy monitoring with serial sonograms and β-HCG determinations

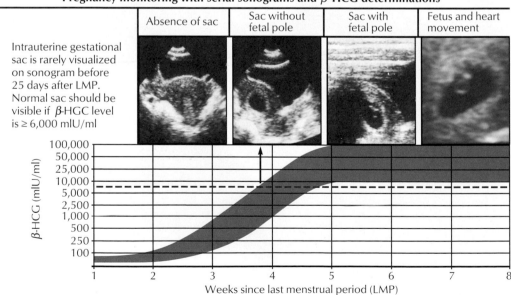

Absence of sac	Sac without fetal pole	Sac with fetal pole	Fetus and heart movement

Intrauterine gestational
sac is rarely visualized
on sonogram before
25 days after LMP.
Normal sac should be
visible if β-HGC level
is $\geq$ 6,000 mlU/ml

β-HCG (mlU/ml)

100,000
50,000
25,000
10,000
5,000
2,500
1,000
500
250
100

1   2   3   4   5   6   7   8

Weeks since last menstrual period (LMP)

Miscarriage, Ectopic Pregnancy, and Molar Pregnancy), AP077 *(Pelvic Inflammatory Disease [PID]),* American Society for Reproductive Medicine, *Ectopic Pregnancy: A Guide for Patients, 1996.*

Drug(s) of Choice

Methotrexate IM 50 mg/m^2 surface area with a maximum of 80 mg.

Contraindications: Methotrexate should not be used if the β-HCG level is greater than 15,000 mIU/mL, the adnexal mass is greater than 3 cm, or the patient's hemodynamic status is unstable. Patients with a history of active hepatic or renal disease, fetal cardiac activity demonstrated in the ectopic gestation, active ulcer disease, or significant alterations in blood count (white blood cell count <3,000, platelet count of <100,000) are not candidates for this therapy.

Precautions: A transient increase in abdominal symptoms is often encountered 48–72 hours after methotrexate therapy. Approximately 5%–10% of patients managed medically experience complications before medical therapy can be effective, necessitating surgical intervention.

Interactions: If patients are receiving methotrexate therapy, they should not take multivitamins with folic acid (eg, prenatal vitamins) because this counteracts the effects of the methotrexate.

FOLLOW-UP

Patient Monitoring: Follow-up assessment of serum β-HCG level to confirm a decline toward normal.

Prevention/Avoidance: Reduce modifiable risk factors, such as pelvic infections.

Possible Complications: Rupture of an ectopic pregnancy dooms the pregnancy and may result in catastrophic intraabdominal bleeding that jeopardizes the life of the mother. Maternal mortality from ectopic pregnancy has declined with earlier detection made possible by laboratory and ultrasonography diagnosis. Current statistics suggest a rate of 3.8 of 10,000 patients (varies with age and race—blacks have a 5-fold greater risk). Maternal death is most often associated with blood loss and delay in diagnosis.

Expected Outcome: With prompt diagnosis, the prognosis for the patient is good, although infertility rates are high (40%) and the likelihood of a successful pregnancy are reduced (50%). The prognosis for the current pregnancy is uniformly bad.

MISCELLANEOUS

Pregnancy Considerations: Poor outcomes for future pregnancy including increased risk of subsequent ectopic implantation and spontaneous pregnancy loss.

ICD-9-CM Codes: 633.1 (Tubal), 633.0 (Abdominal), 633.2 (Ovarian), 633.8 (Other site such as cervical or cornual).

REFERENCES

American College of Obstetricians and Gynecologists. *Medical Management of Tubal Pregnancy.* Washington, DC: ACOG; 1998. ACOG Practice Bulletin 3.

Ankum WM, Van der Veen F, Hamerlynck JVTH, Lammes FB. Suspected ectopic pregnancy: what to do when human chorionic gonadotropin levels are below the discrimination zone. *J Reprod Med* 1995;40:525.

Reich H, Freifeld ML, McGlynn F, Reich E. Laparoscopic treatment of tubal pregnancy. *Obstet Gynecol* 1987;69:275.

Russell JB. The etiology of ectopic pregnancy. *Clin Obstet Gynecol* 1987;30:181.

Shalev E, Yarom I, Bustan M, Weiner E, Ben-Shlomo I. Transvaginal sonography as the ultimate diagnostic tool for the management of ectopic pregnancy: experience with 840 cases. *Fertil Steril* 1998;69:62.

Stovall TG, Ling FW, Buster JE. Outpatient chemotherapy of unruptured ectopic pregnancy. *Fertil Steril* 1989;51:435.

ENDOMETRIOSIS

INTRODUCTION

Description: A benign but progressive condition characterized by endometrial glands and stroma found in locations other than the endometrium.

Prevalence: Five percent to fifteen percent of women, 20% of gynecologic laparotomies, 30%–50% of infertility patients.

Predominant Age: Third and forth decades of life, 5% diagnosed after menopause.

Genetics: Familial predisposition (polygenic or multifactorial inheritance pattern).

ETIOLOGY AND PATHOGENESIS

Causes: Endometriosis may arise by one of several proposed mechanisms—lymphatic spread, metaplasia of celomic epithelium or müllerian rests, seeding by retrograde menstruation, or direct hematogenous spread. Instances of presumed iatrogenic spread (surgical) have been reported. A role for an immunologic defect is debated, but remains to be conclusively established.

Risk Factors: Obstructive anomalies such as an unrecognized double uterus or a cervical and/or vaginal outflow-tract obstruction.

CLINICAL CHARACTERISTICS

Signs and Symptoms:

Asymptomatic (up to 30%)

Cyclic pelvic pain or dyspareunia (both worst 36–48 hours before menses), premenstrual and menstrual pain, dyschezia, midcycle (ovulatory) pain—often the pain reported by patients seems inversely proportional to the amount of disease; small implants seem to be exquisitely painful and large endometriomata may be asymptomatic

Infertility

Intermenstrual bleeding (15%–20%)

Anovulation (15%)

Intermittent constipation or diarrhea

Adnexal mass(es)

Uterine retroversion, scarring and nodularity of the posterior cul-de-sac

DIAGNOSTIC APPROACH

Differential Diagnosis:

Pelvic adhesive disease (secondary to pelvic infection, surgery)

Uterine fibroids

Gastrointestinal, urologic, or musculoskeletal problems

Corpus luteum cysts

Ovarian neoplasia

Adenocarcinoma of the large bowel (endometrial implants my be difficult to differentiate grossly from a primary neoplasm of the large bowel)

Associated Conditions: Infertility, nulliparity, pelvic pain, dyspareunia (deep thrust), uterine retroversion, premenstrual and menstrual pain, intermenstrual bleeding, and adenomyosis (20% of these patients).

Workup and Evaluation

Laboratory: No evaluation indicated (CA-125 is not useful for screening or follow-up).

Imaging: No imaging indicated, pelvic or transvaginal ultrasonography, or magnetic resonance imaging (MRI) may demonstrate endometriomas or signs of scarring (nonspecific).

Special Tests: None indicated.

Diagnostic Procedures: The ultimate diagnosis of endometriosis rests on direct inspection of the involved area (laparoscopy or laparotomy), supported by histologic confirmation.

Pathologic Findings

Endometriosis is characterized by endometrial glands and stroma found in locations other than the endometrium. Nests of endometrial glands and stroma may occur in many distant locations throughout the body, although they are most common in the pelvis (60% on the surfaces of the ovaries). Vulva implants occur in 1 in 500 patients with eneometriosis, generally at the site of an episiotomy or obstetric laceration. Evidence of old hemorrhage (hemosiderin-laden macrophages) is often present.

MANAGEMENT AND THERAPY

Nonpharmacologic

General Measures: Analgesics (nonsteroidal anti-inflammatory drugs), modification of periods (oral contraceptives), suppression of periods (gonadotropin-releasing hormone [GnRH] agonists, danazol sodium, oral progestins, long-acting progestins, continuous oral contraceptives).

Specific Measures: The selection of therapy depends on many factors—reliability of diagnosis, the extent of disease and symptoms, the patient's desire for fertility, and degree of involvement with other organs. Endometriomata of greater than 5 cm require surgical therapy. Surgical therapy may be conservative (resection of lesions) or definitive (hysterectomy, oophorectomy).

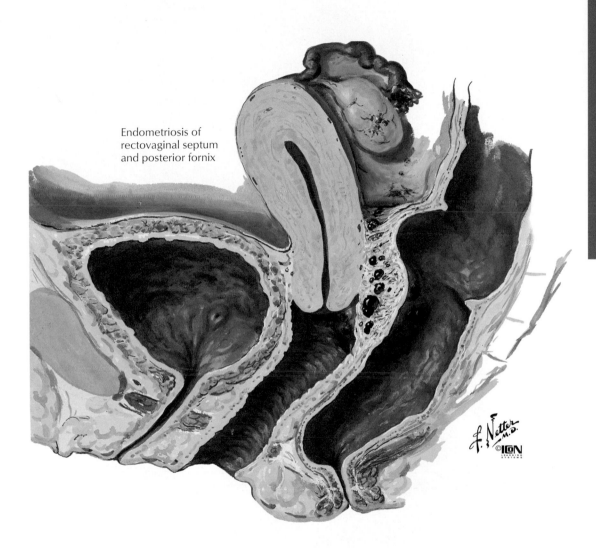

Endometriosis of
rectovaginal septum
and posterior fornix

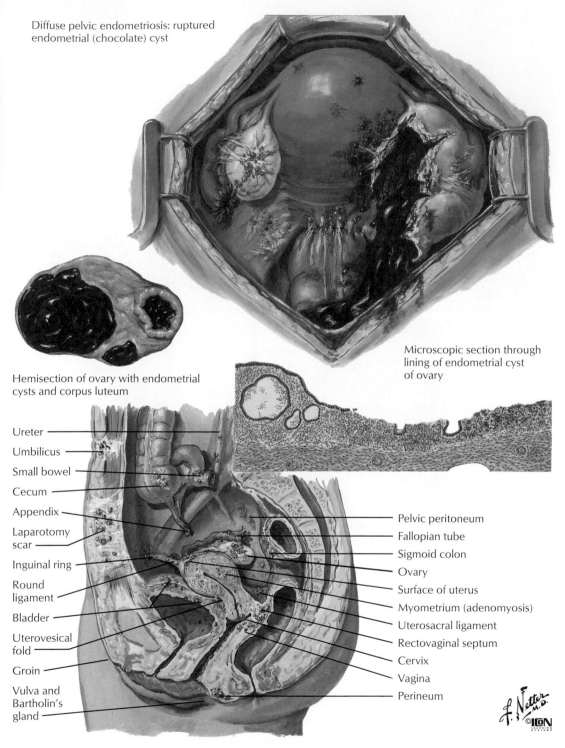

Diffuse pelvic endometriosis: ruptured endometrial (chocolate) cyst

Hemisection of ovary with endometrial cysts and corpus luteum

Microscopic section through lining of endometrial cyst of ovary

Ureter
Umbilicus
Small bowel
Cecum
Appendix
Laparotomy scar
Inguinal ring
Round ligament
Bladder
Uterovesical fold
Groin
Vulva and Bartholin's gland

Pelvic peritoneum
Fallopian tube
Sigmoid colon
Ovary
Surface of uterus
Myometrium (adenomyosis)
Uterosacral ligament
Rectovaginal septum
Cervix
Vagina
Perineum

Possible sites of distribution of endometriosis

Diet: No specific dietary changes indicated.

Activity: No restriction.

Patient Education: Reassurance, American College of Obstetricians and Gynecologists Patient Education Pamphlet AP013 (*Important Facts About Endometriosis*), AP002 (*Infertility: Causes and Treatments*).

Drug(s) of Choice

GnRH agonists for 6 months: leuprolide acetate (Lupron) 3.75 mg IM monthly; nafarelin acetate (Synarel) 200 μg intranasal in morning and in opposite nostril hs; goserelin acetate (Zoladex) 3.6 mg implant monthly.

Contraindications: Known or suspected pregnancy, breast-feeding, undiagnosed vaginal bleeding.

Precautions: A decrease in bone mass of 5%–7% during a 6-month course of therapy with GnRH agonists has been documented. This is believed to be reversible.

Add-Back Therapy: Progestins, low-dose estrogens, or both may be used to suppress bothersome side effects without reducing efficacy.

Alternative Drugs

Danazol sodium 200 mg PO qid for 6–9 months (80% of patients experience side effects, 10%–20% discontinue therapy because of them) or

Continuous combination oral contraceptives (monophasic formulation) taken daily for 6–9 months (if breakthrough bleeding occurs, the dose is doubled for 5 days) or

Medroxyprogesterone acetate 30 mg PO daily or 150 mg IM every 3 months for 6–9 months

FOLLOW-UP

Patient Monitoring: Any therapy must be reevaluated at no less than 6-month intervals. History and physical evaluations are usually sufficient.

Prevention/Avoidance: None.

Possible Complications: Pelvic scarring, chronic pelvic pain, erosion into bowel or urinary track resulting in hematochezia or hematuria.

Expected Outcome: Endometriosis is never considered to be "cured." Symptoms may be resolved and progression of the disease may be halted through medical or surgical therapy, although 5%–15% of patients have a recurrence after 1 year and 40%–50% have a recurrence by 5 years. The success of therapy and the risk of recurrence are proportional to the extent of the initial disease. Up to 40% of patients may eventually conceive with therapy. Endometriosis generally regresses after menopause (natural or hormonally induced).

MISCELLANEOUS

Pregnancy Considerations: No effect on pregnancy once pregnancy is achieved. Pregnancy may actually resolve symptoms of endometriosis and promote regression of implants in some patients.

ICD-9-CM Codes: 617.9 (Codes 617.0–617.8 used for specific sites).

REFERENCES

Barbieri RL. Etiology and epidemiology of endometriosis. *Am J Obstet Gynecol* 1990;162:565.

Cook AS, Rock JA. The role of laparoscopy in the treatment of endometriosis. *Fertil Steril* 1991;55:663.

Friedman AJ, Hornstein MD. Gonadotropin-releasing hormone agonist plus estrogen-progestin "add-back" therapy for endometriosis-related pelvic pain. *Fertil Steril* 1993;60:236.

Hughes EG, Fedorkow DM, Collins JA. A quantitative overview of controlled trials in endometriosis-associated infertility. *Fertil Steril* 1993;59:963.

Olive DL, Schwartz LB. Endometriosis. *N Engl J Med* 1993;328:1759.

Waller KG, Shaw RW. GnRH analogs in the treatment of endometriosis: long-term follow-up. *Fertil Steril* 1993;59:511.

Wright S, Valdes CT, Dunn RC, Franklin RR. Short-term Lupron or Danazol therapy for pelvic endometriosis. *Fertil Steril* 1995;63:504.

EPITHELIAL STROMAL OVARIAN TUMORS

INTRODUCTION

Description: The most common type of ovarian tumors (65% of ovarian tumors, 85% of ovarian malignancies), these are derived from the surface (celomic) epithelium and the ovarian stroma and include serous (20%–50%), mucinous (15%–25%), endometrioid (5%), clear cell (<5%), and Brenner (2%–3%) types.

Prevalence: One of three ovarian tumors and 10% of ovarian malignancies, 14.3 of 100,000 women.

Predominant Age: Benign tumors—age 20–29, malignant tumors—one half are in women older than 50.

Genetics: No genetic pattern.

ETIOLOGY AND PATHOGENESIS

Causes: Unknown.

Risk Factors: Family history, high-fat diet, advanced age, nulliparity, early menarche, late menopause, white race, higher economic status. Oral contraception, high parity, and breastfeeding reduce risk.

CLINICAL CHARACTERISTICS

Signs and Symptoms:
Asymptomatic
Weight loss
Increasing abdominal girth despite constant or reduced caloric intake
Ascites
Adnexal mass (multilocular or partly solid masses in patients older than 40 are likely to be malignant; the risk of a mass being malignant is 1 in 3 for women older than 45, versus <1% for women 20 to 45 years of age)
Vague lower abdominal discomfort

DIAGNOSTIC APPROACH

Differential Diagnosis:
Functional cyst (corpus luteum, follicular)
Endometriosis
Hydrosalpinx
Paratubal cyst
Appendiceal abscess
Ectopic pregnancy
Pedunculated leiomyomata
Pelvic or horseshoe kidney
Gastrointestinal malignancy (colon, stomach)

Associated Conditions: None. In patients with advanced malignant disease, bowel obstruction, ascites, and inanition are common.

Workup and Evaluation

Laboratory: As indicated before surgery. β-Human chorionic gonadotropin or α-fetoprotein levels may be elevated in some tumors. (The CA-125 level may be useful for monitoring disease response to treatment or progression but is not a good prognostic test. Only 80% of epithelial ovarian tumors express CA-125, and many benign and other malignant processes [lung, breast, and pancreas] may cause CA-125 to rise above normal.)

Imaging: Preoperative evaluation (CT or ultrasonography) for possible lymph node enlargement or intraabdominal spread is indicated for patients in whom malignancy is a significant possibility.

Special Tests: A frozen section histologic evaluation (intraoperative consultation) should be considered for any ovarian mass that appears suspicious for malignancy.

Diagnostic Procedures: History, physical examination, and imaging. Final diagnosis is established by histologic evaluation.

Pathologic Findings

Varies with cell type. Malignant epithelial tumors are more likely to be bilateral than are benign epithelial neoplasms.

MANAGEMENT AND THERAPY

Nonpharmacologic

General Measures: Evaluation, supportive therapy based on symptoms.

Specific Measures: Generally requires surgical exploration and extirpation. In benign disease or tumors of borderline malignant potential, the uterus and other ovary generally may be spared. Adjunctive chemotherapy (platinum-based and paclitaxel [Taxol]) or radiation therapy is often included, based on the location and stage of the disease. It currently is not recommended that a grossly normal opposite ovary be bisected to look for a contralateral mass.

Diet: No specific dietary changes indicated, except those imposed by advanced disease.

Activity: No restriction, except that imposed by advanced disease.

Patient Education: American College of Obstetricians and Gynecologists Patient Education Pamphlet AP096 (*Cancer of the Ovary*), AP075 (*Ovarian Cysts*).

Drug(s) of Choice

None, except as adjunctive or symptomatic therapy. Preoperative bowel cleansing (mechanical or

Epithelial Stromal Ovarian Tumors

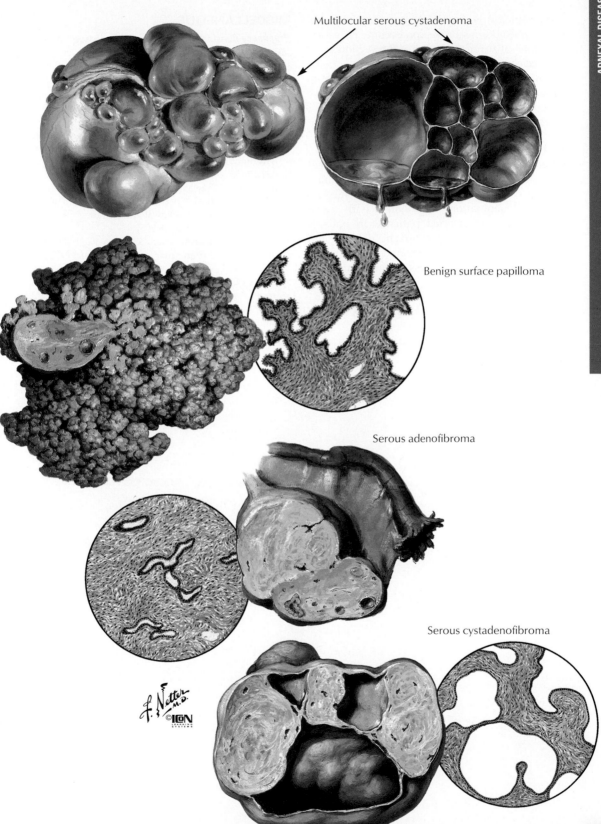

Multilocular serous cystadenoma

Benign surface papilloma

Serous adenofibroma

Serous cystadenofibroma

with antibiosis) is often recommended as a precaution should bowel resection become necessary at the time of surgical staging and resection.

Contraindications: See individual agents.

Precautions: Alkylating agents are associated with an increased risk of future leukemia (10% by 8 years after therapy).

Interactions: See individual agents.

FOLLOW-UP

Patient Monitoring: Careful follow-up for recurrent pelvic disease or enlargement of the remaining ovary (if any). This is generally performed by pelvic examination, augmented with ultrasonography in selected patients. In patients suspected of having recurrent disease and other selected patients, second-look surgery may be desirable to assess progress and discover occult disease.

Prevention/Avoidance: None.

Possible Complications: Spread and advancement of malignant tumors.

Expected Outcome: Generally good.

MISCELLANEOUS

Pregnancy Considerations: No effect on pregnancy.

ICD-9-CM Codes: Based on cause and type.

REFERENCES

American College of Obstetricians and Gynecologists. *Cancer of the Ovary.* Washington, DC: ACOG; 1990. ACOG Technical Bulletin 141.

American College of Obstetricians and Gynecologists. *Classification and Staging of Gynecologic Malignancies.* Washington, DC: ACOG; 1991. ACOG Technical Bulletin 155.

Bostwick DG, Tazelaar HD, Ballon SC, Hendrickson MR, Kempson RL. Ovarian epithelial tumors of borderline malignancy: clinical and pathologic study of 109 cases. *Cancer* 1986;58:2052.

Fleischer AC. Transabdominal and transvaginal sonography of ovarian masses. *Clin Obstet Gynecol* 1991;34:433.

Schwarts PE, Smith JP. Treatment of ovarian stromal tumors. *Am J Obstet Gynecol* 1976;125:402.

Scully RE. Sex cord-stromal, steroid cell, and germ cell tumors of the ovary. In: Sciarra JJ, ed. *Gynecology and Obstetrics.* Vol 4. Philadelphia, Pa: JB Lippincott, 1995;1:1.

GERM CELL TUMOR

INTRODUCTION

Description: The second most common type of ovarian tumor, these tumors contain cells that echo the three layers of embryonic tissue (ectoderm, mesoderm, and endoderm) or extraembryonic elements.

Prevalence: Second most frequent ovarian neoplasm (25% of tumors).

Predominant Age: Younger than 30, most common malignancy of those in their teens and 20s.

Genetics: No genetic pattern.

ETIOLOGY AND PATHOGENESIS

Causes: Unknown (may differentiate from primitive germ cells).

Risk Factors: None known.

CLINICAL CHARACTERISTICS

Signs Symptoms:
  Asymptomatic
  Ovarian enlargement (Ovarian masses in premenarchal girls are most often germ cell tumors.)

DIAGNOSTIC APPROACH

Differential Diagnosis:
  Benign adnexal masses (corpus luteum, follicular cyst)
  Endometriosis
  Hydrosalpinx
  Paratubal cyst
  Appendiceal abscess
  Ectopic pregnancy
  Pedunculated leiomyomata
  Pelvic or horseshoe kidney
  Nongynecologic pelvic masses

Associated Conditions: Varies with cell type.

Workup and Evaluation

Laboratory: As indicated before surgery. β-Human chorionic gonadotropin or α-fetoprotein may be elevated in some tumors (dysgerminoma, primary choriocarcinoma). (The CA-125 level may be useful for monitoring disease response to treatment or progression but is not a good prognostic test. Only 80% of epithelial ovarian tumors express CA-125 and many benign and other malignant tumors [lung, breast, and pancreas] may also cause CA-125 to rise above normal.)

Imaging: Preoperative evaluation (CT or ultrasonography) for possible lymph node enlargement or intraabdominal spread is indicated for patients in whom malignancy is a significant possibility.

Special Tests: None indicated.

Diagnostic Procedures: History, physical examination, imaging. Final diagnosis is established by histologic evaluation.

Pathologic Findings

Germ cell tumors include dysgerminoma (45% of malignant germ cell tumors), endodermal sinus tumors (10%), embryonal carcinoma, choriocarcinoma, teratomas (immature, mature, solid and cystic, struma ovarii, carcinoid) and mixed forms. Roughly one third of germ cell tumors in women younger than 21 are malignant.

MANAGEMENT AND THERAPY

Nonpharmacologic

General Measures: Evaluation, supportive therapy based on symptoms.

Specific Measures: Surgical exploration and resection (often with salvage of the ovary in the case of teratomas). Immature (malignant) teratomas are often treated with adjunctive chemotherapy (vincristine, actinomycin D, and cyclophosphamide); endodermal sinus tumors should all be treated with chemotherapy after surgical resection.

Diet: No specific dietary changes indicated, except those imposed by advanced disease.

Activity: No restriction, except that imposed by advanced disease.

Patient Education: American College of Obstetricians and Gynecologists Patient Education Pamphlet AP096 (*Cancer of the Ovary*), AP075 (*Ovarian Cysts*).

Drug(s) of Choice

  Vincristine (1.5 mg/m^2 IV weekly for 12 weeks), actinomycin D, and cyclophosphamide (0.5 mg of actinomycin D + 5 to 7 mg/kg/d cyclophosphamide, IV daily for 5 days every 4 weeks).

  Adjunctive or symptomatic therapy. Preoperative bowel cleansing (mechanical or with antibiosis) is often recommended as a precaution should bowel resection become necessary at the time of surgical staging and resection.

Contraindications: See individual agents.

Precautions: Alkylating agents are associated with an increased risk of future leukemia (10% by 8 years after therapy).

Interactions: See individual agents.

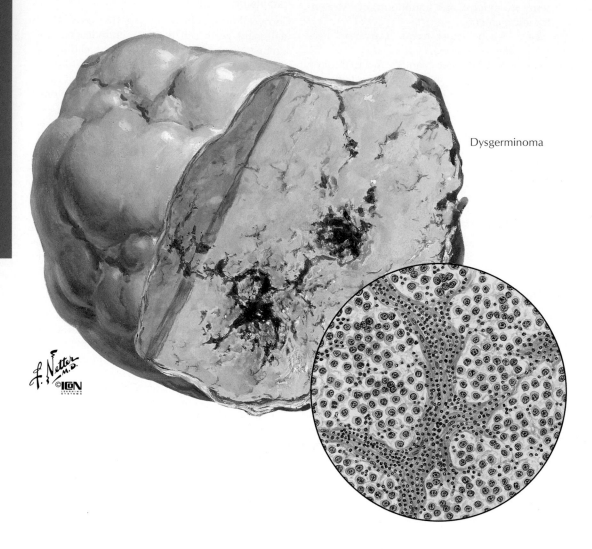

Dysgerminoma

Alternative Drugs

Chemotherapy for endodermal sinus tumors may alternately include actinomycin D, 5-fluorouracil, and cyclophosphamide.

FOLLOW-UP

Patient Monitoring: Careful follow-up for recurrent pelvic disease or enlargement of the remaining ovary (if any). This is generally performed by pelvic examination, augmented with ultrasonography in selected patients. In patients suspected of recurrent disease and other selected patients, second-look surgery may be desirable to assess progress and discover occult disease.

Prevention/Avoidance: None.

Possible Complications: Spread and advancement in the case of malignant tumors.

Expected Outcome: Generally good.

MISCELLANEOUS

Pregnancy Considerations: No effect on pregnancy.

ICD-9-CM **Codes:** Based on cause and type.

REFERENCES

American College of Obstetricians and Gynecologists. *Cancer of the Ovary.* Washington, DC: ACOG; 1990. ACOG Technical Bulletin 141.

American College of Obstetricians and Gynecologists. *Classification and Staging of Gynecologic Malignancies.* Washington, DC: ACOG; 1991. ACOG Technical Bulletin 155.

Creasman WT, Soper JT. Assessment of the contemporary management of germ cell malignancy. *Am J Obstet Gynecol* 1985;153:828.

Fleischer AC. Transabdominal and transvaginal sonography of ovarian masses. *Clin Obstet Gynecol* 1991;34:433.

Kurman RJ, Norris HJ. Malignant germ cell tumors of the ovary. *Hum Pathol* 1977;8:551.

Peccatori F, Bonazzi C, Chiari S, Landoni F, Colombo N, Mangioni C. Surgical management of malignant ovarian germ-cell tumors: 10 years' experience of 129 patients. *Obstet Gynecol* 1995;86:367.

GRANULOSA CELL TUMORS

INTRODUCTION

Description: A sex cord stromal tumor of the ovary made up of granulosa cells (sex cord) and stromal cells (thecal cells or fibroblasts). The tumor often secretes estrogen.

Prevalence: Six percent of ovarian neoplasms and the majority of hormonally active tumors.

Predominant Age: Any, 5% before puberty.

Genetics: No genetic pattern.

ETIOLOGY AND PATHOGENESIS

Causes: Unknown.

Risk Factors: None known.

CLINICAL CHARACTERISTICS

Signs and Symptoms:

Asymptomatic

Enlarging or ruptured adnexal mass (may present with acute pain and an acute abdomen with hemoperitoneum, 6%); 10%–15% are not palpable; tumors are bilateral in <2% of cases

Ascites (10%)

Precocious (pseudoprecocious) puberty in young children (5%) (granulosa tumors are responsible of 10% of precocious puberty cases)

Abnormal menstrual patterns, menorrhagia, amenorrhea

Postmenopausal bleeding

DIAGNOSTIC APPROACH

Differential Diagnosis:

Benign adnexal masses (corpus luteum, follicular cyst)

Endometriosis

Hydrosalpinx

Paratubal cyst

Appendiceal abscess

Pedunculated leiomyomata

Pelvic or horseshoe kidney

Nongynecologic pelvic masses

Hepatic, renal, or cardiac disease resulting in weight loss and ascites

Ectopic pregnancy (reproductive age women)

Gastrointestinal malignancy (colon, stomach)

Associated Conditions: Evidence of increased estrogen (eg, breast tenderness, menstrual disturbances, isosexual pseudoprecocity). Virilization rarely occurs.

Workup and Evaluation

Laboratory: As indicated before surgery. (Serum testing for tumor markers, such as CA-125, lipid-associated sialic acid, carcinoembryonic antigen, α-fetoprotein, and others, should be reserved for following the progress of patients with known malignancies and not for prognostic evaluation.)

Imaging: Preoperative evaluation (CT or ultrasonography) for possible lymph node enlargement or intraabdominal spread is indicated for patients in whom malignancy is a significant possibility.

Special Tests: None indicated.

Diagnostic Procedures: History, physical examination, and imaging. Final diagnosis is established by histologic evaluation.

Pathologic Findings

Derived from the sex cords of the ovary and the stroma of the developing gonad, these tumors have a predominance of granulosa cells. Classically, these tumors contain eosinophilic bodies surrounded by granulosa cells (Call-Exner bodies). Poorly differentiated tumors may be confused with adenocarcinomas (especially small cell carcinoma).

MANAGEMENT AND THERAPY

Nonpharmacologic

General Measures: Evaluation, supportive therapy based on symptoms.

Specific Measures: Surgical exploration and resection. Because <5% of these tumors are bilateral, conservative surgery is generally indicated for tumors at stage IA or lower. Chemotherapy (cisplatin, doxorubicin) and radiation have been used for recurrent disease.

Diet: No specific dietary changes indicated, except those imposed by advanced disease.

Activity: No restriction, except that imposed by advanced disease.

Patient Education: American College of Obstetricians and Gynecologists Patient Education Pamphlet AP096 (*Cancer of the Ovary*), AP075 (*Ovarian Cysts*).

Drug(s) of Choice

Adjunctive or symptomatic therapy. Preoperative bowel cleansing (mechanical or with antibiosis) is often recommended as a precaution should bowel resection become necessary at the time of surgical staging and resection.

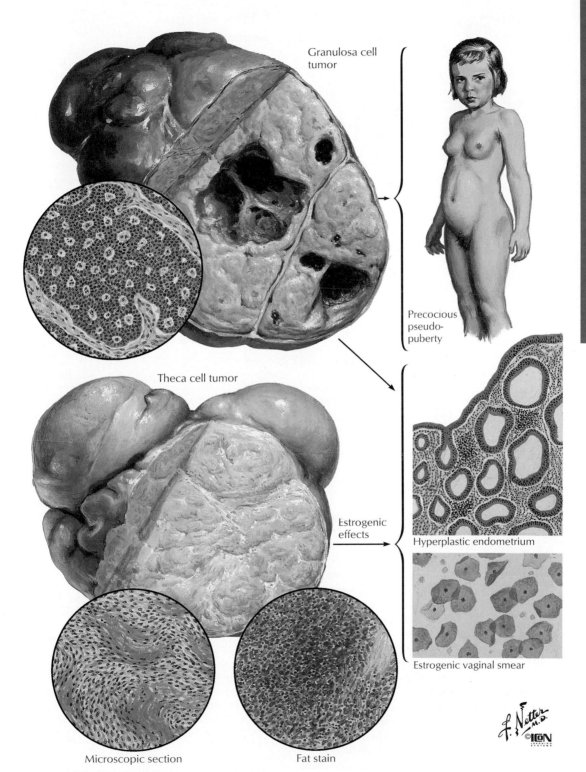

Granulosa cell tumor

Precocious pseudo-puberty

Theca cell tumor

Estrogenic effects

Hyperplastic endometrium

Estrogenic vaginal smear

Microscopic section

Fat stain

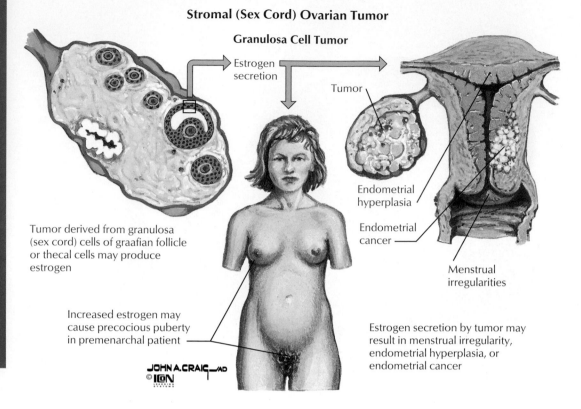

Stromal (Sex Cord) Ovarian Tumor

Granulosa Cell Tumor

Estrogen secretion

Tumor

Endometrial hyperplasia

Endometrial cancer

Menstrual irregularities

Tumor derived from granulosa (sex cord) cells of graafian follicle or thecal cells may produce estrogen

Increased estrogen may cause precocious puberty in premenarchal patient

Estrogen secretion by tumor may result in menstrual irregularity, endometrial hyperplasia, or endometrial cancer

JOHN A. CRAIG—AD
©ICN

Contraindications: See individual agents.

Precautions: Alkylating agents are associated with an increased risk of future leukemia (10% by 8 years after therapy).

Interactions: See individual agents.

Alternative Drugs

Chemotherapy with alternative use of actinomycin D, 5-fluorouracil, and cyclophosphamide.

FOLLOW-UP

Patient Monitoring: Careful follow-up for recurrent pelvic disease or enlargement of the remaining ovary (if any). This is generally performed by pelvic examination, augmented with ultrasonography in selected cases. In those suspected of having recurrent disease and other selected patients, second-look surgery may be desirable to assess progress and discover occult disease.

Prevention/Avoidance: None.

Possible Complications: Recurrences are frequent even 5 years after initial therapy. In 10% of patients the tumor is diagnosed when it ruptures, causing pain or intraperitoneal bleeding.

Expected Outcome: Prognosis does not correlate with the histologic pattern of the tumor: 90% of tumors found are stage I and the prognosis is good (90% 10-year survival); a poorer prognosis is found with tumors >15 cm that have ruptured or that have a high mitotic rate or aneuploidy.

MISCELLANEOUS

Pregnancy Considerations: No effect on pregnancy.

ICD-9-CM Codes: Specific to cell type and location.

REFERENCES

American College of Obstetricians and Gynecologists. *Cancer of the Ovary.* Washington, DC: ACOG; 1990. ACOG Technical Bulletin 141.

Bjorkholm E, Silfversward C. Prognostic factors in granulosa cell tumor. *Gynecol Oncol* 1981;11:261.

Columbo N, Sessa C, Landoni F, Sartori E, Percorelli S, Mangioni C. Cisplatin, vinblastine, and bleomycin, combination chemotherapy in metastatic granulosa cell tumor of the ovary. *Obstet Gynecol* 1986;67:265.

Lack EE, Perez-Atayde AR, Murthy AS, Goldstein DP, Crigler JF Jr, Vawter GF. Granulosa theca cell tumors in premenarcheal girls: a clinical and pathological study of 10 cases. *Cancer* 1981;48:1846.

Segal R, DePetrillo AD, Thomas G. Clinical review of adult granulosa cell tumors of the ovary. *Gynecol Oncol* 1995;56:338.

Swanson SA, Norris HJ, Kelsten ML, Wheeler JE. DNA content of juvenile granulosa tumors determined by flow cytometry. *Int J Gynecol Pathol* 1990;9:101.

HYDROSALPINX (CHRONIC PELVIC INFLAMMATORY DISEASE)

INTRODUCTION

Description: Recurrent or chronic adnexal infections may result in a cystic dilatation of the fallopian tube (hydrosalpinx), which may present as an adnexal mass.

Prevalence: Forty percent of female infertility is the result of tubal damage, including the most severe form, hydrosalpinx.

Predominant Age: 15–25.

Genetics: No genetic pattern.

ETIOLOGY AND PATHOGENESIS

Causes: Recurrent or chronic adnexal infection. This is the end stage condition of pyosalpinx.

Risk Factors: Early (age) sexual activity, multiple sexual partners, pelvic inflammatory disease, sexually transmitted diseases (*Chlamydia*, gonorrhea), uterine instrumentation (hysterosalpingography, IUCD placement, endometrial biopsy, dilation and curettage), and douching.

CLINICAL CHARACTERISTICS

Signs and Symptoms:
Asymptomatic (most common)
Vague lower abdominal pressure or chronic pelvic pain
Infertility
Unilateral or bilateral cystic masses (often elongated or sausage-shaped)

DIAGNOSTIC APPROACH

Differential Diagnosis:
Functional cysts (follicle, corpus luteum)
Epithelial tumors (cystic or solid)
Ovarian cysts
Paratubal or paraovarian cysts
Uterine leiomyomata
Ectopic pregnancy
Tubo-ovarian abscess
Endometrioma
Appendiceal abscess

Associated Conditions: Pelvic pain, infertility, and sexually transmissible infections.

Workup and Evaluation

Laboratory: Complete blood count or erythrocyte sedimentation rate if active infection is suspected. Screening for coexistent sexually transmissible diseases should be strongly considered.

Imaging: Ultrasonography (abdominal or transvaginal), CT or MRI may be used but are more expensive without providing greater specificity.

Special Tests: None indicated.

Diagnostic Procedures: History, physical examination, and ultrasonography.

Pathologic Findings

Chronic induration and inflammation with cystic dilation or the fallopian tube and flattening and atrophy of the epithelial lining. The fluid found is generally sterile.

MANAGEMENT AND THERAPY

Nonpharmacologic

General Measures: Evaluation, including screening for other sexually transmitted diseases.

Specific Measures: Generally requires surgical evaluation and therapy (laparoscopy or laparotomy).

Diet: No specific dietary changes indicated.

Activity: No restriction.

Patient Education: American College of Obstetricians and Gynecologists Patient Education Pamphlet AP077 (*Pelvic Inflammatory Disease*), AP009 (*How to Prevent Sexually Transmitted Diseases*), AP099 (*Pelvic Pain*), AP071 (*Gonorrhea and Chlamydia*), AP002 (*Infertility: Causes and Treatments*), AP020 (*Pain During Intercourse*).

Drug(s) of Choice

Broad-spectrum antibiotics if active infection is suspected. (Most hydrosalpinx are sterile and are the inactive end-stage disease.)

FOLLOW-UP

Patient Monitoring: Normal health maintenance, periodic surveillance for other sexually transmissible infections.

Prevention/Avoidance: Avoidance of sexually transmissible infections (barrier contraception, "safe sex"), screening for those at risk, and aggressive treatment.

Possible Complications: Chronic pelvic pain, infertility, increased risk of hysterectomy, and oophorectomy.

Expected Outcome: Surgical therapy (salpingectomy or salpingo-oophorectomy) is curative. Neosalpingostomy may be considered when fertility is to be maintained, but the success of this procedure is inversely proportional to the size of the hydrosalpinx and is generally less than 15%.

Hydrosalpinx (Chronic Pelvic Inflammatory Disease)

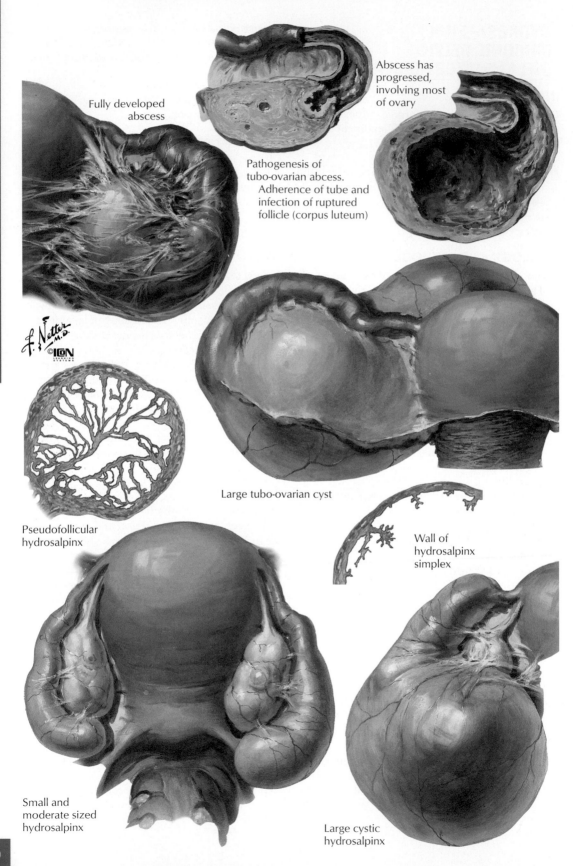

Fully developed abscess

Abscess has progressed, involving most of ovary

Pathogenesis of tubo-ovarian abcess. Adherence of tube and infection of ruptured follicle (corpus luteum)

Large tubo-ovarian cyst

Pseudofollicular hydrosalpinx

Wall of hydrosalpinx simplex

Small and moderate sized hydrosalpinx

Large cystic hydrosalpinx

MISCELLANEOUS

Pregnancy Considerations: Successful pregnancy is much less likely because of the increased risk of infertility and ectopic pregnancy.

***ICD-9-CM* Codes:** 614.1.

REFERENCES

American College of Obstetricians and Gynecologists. *Gonorrhea and Chlamydial Infections.* Washington, DC: ACOG; 1994. Technical Bulletin 190.

American College of Obstetricians and Gynecologists. *Chronic Pelvic Pain.* Washington, DC: ACOG; 1996. Technical Bulletin 223.

American College of Obstetricians and Gynecologists. *Antibiotics and Gynecologic Infections.* Washington, DC: ACOG; 1997. Technical Bulletin 237.

KRUKENBERG TUMOR

INTRODUCTION

Description: Metastatic tumor (generally from the gastrointestinal tract) that is characterized by large signet-ring cells. The most common site or origin is the stomach or large intestine.
Predominant Age: Postmenopausal.
Genetics: No genetic pattern.

ETIOLOGY AND PATHOGENESIS

Causes: Metastatic spread of carcinoma from the gastrointestinal tract (most commonly the stomach or colon). Metastatic breast cancer may appear similar histologically.
Risk Factors: None known.

CLINICAL CHARACTERISTICS

Signs and Symptoms:
Asymptomatic
Adnexal enlargement (bilateral solid adnexal masses in an older patient should always suggest the possibility of a gastrointestinal tract source)

DIAGNOSTIC APPROACH

Differential Diagnosis:
Benign adnexal masses (corpus luteum, follicular cyst)
Endometriosis
Hydrosalpinx
Paratubal cyst
Appendiceal abscess
Ectopic pregnancy
Pedunculated leiomyomata
Pelvic or horseshoe kidney
Nongynecologic pelvic masses
Breast cancer
Lung cancer
Associated Conditions: Gastrointestinal or breast malignancy.

Workup and Evaluation

Laboratory: As indicated before surgery.
Imaging: Preoperative evaluation (CT or ultrasonography) for possible lymph node enlargement or intraabdominal spread is indicated for patients in whom malignancy is a significant possibility. Radiographic evaluation of the gastrointestinal tract. Mammography as indicated based on differential diagnosis and routine screening needs.
Special Tests: None indicated.

Diagnostic Procedures: History, physical examination, and imaging. Final diagnosis is established by histologic evaluation.

Pathologic Findings

Nests of mucin-filled signet-ring cells in a cellular stroma.

MANAGEMENT AND THERAPY

Nonpharmacologic

General Measures: Evaluation, establishment of location of primary tumor (most often stomach or large intestine).
Specific Measures: Therapy of the original tumor.
Diet: No specific dietary changes indicated except those dictated by the original tumor and its therapy.
Activity: No restriction except those dictated by the original tumor and its therapy.
Patient Education: American College of Obstetricians and Gynecologists Patient Education Pamphlet AP096 (*Cancer of the Ovary*), AP075 (*Ovarian Cysts*).

Drug(s) of Choice

None (based on primary tumor and its therapy).

FOLLOW-UP

Patient Monitoring: Based on primary tumor.
Prevention/Avoidance: None.
Possible Complications: Progression and spread of the primary tumor is generally well underway when the ovarian sites are discovered.
Expected Outcome: Generally poor, with 5-year survival unlikely.

MISCELLANEOUS

Pregnancy Considerations: Does not directly threaten pregnancy except by the jeopardy caused to the mother.
ICD-9-CM Codes: 198.6.

REFERENCES

American College of Obstetricians and Gynecologists. *Cancer of the Ovary.* Washington, DC: ACOG; 1990. ACOG Technical Bulletin 141.
American College of Obstetricians and Gynecologists. *Classification and Staging of Gynecologic Malignancies.* Washington, DC: ACOG; 1991. ACOG Technical Bulletin 155.
Fleischer AC. Transabdominal and transvaginal sonography of ovarian masses. *Clin Obstet Gynecol* 1991;34:433.

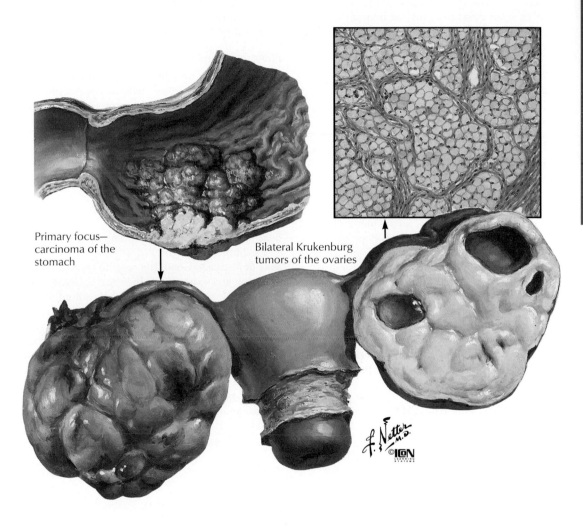

Primary focus—
carcinoma of the
stomach

Bilateral Krukenburg
tumors of the ovaries

MUCINOUS OVARIAN CYSTS

INTRODUCTION

Description: A group of benign and malignant epithelial tumors of the ovary that are characterized by the secretion of mucin. These tumors tend to be the largest types of ovarian masses encountered and may be 30 cm or greater in size.

Prevalence: Fifteen percent to twenty-five percent of ovarian cysts, 6%–10% of ovarian cancers. Although ovarian cysts are common in younger women, mucinous cysts account for about 50% of those that do occur in women older than 20 years.

Predominant Age: Reproductive (benign), 30–60 (malignant tumors).

Genetics: No genetic pattern.

ETIOLOGY AND PATHOGENESIS

Causes: Unknown. May represent a monomorphic endodermal differentiation of a teratoma or a tumor of müllerian origin.

Risk Factors: Family history, high-fat diet, advanced age, nulliparity, early menarche and late menopause, white race, higher economic status. Oral contraception, high parity, and breast-feeding reduce risk.

CLINICAL CHARACTERISTICS

Signs and Symptoms:
Asymptomatic
Vague lower abdominal symptoms
Adnexal mass (bilateral in 5% of benign and 10%–20% of malignant lesions) up to 50 cm in diameter (average 15–30 cm)

DIAGNOSTIC APPROACH

Differential Diagnosis:
Benign adnexal masses (corpus luteum, follicular cyst)
Endometriosis
Hydrosalpinx
Paratubal cyst
Appendiceal abscess
Ectopic pregnancy
Pedunculated leiomyomata
Pelvic or horseshoe kidney
Nongynecologic pelvic masses
Associated Conditions: Pseudomyxoma peritonei.

Workup and Evaluation

Laboratory: As indicated before surgery. (CA-125 levels may be useful for the monitoring of disease response to treatment or progression but is not a good prognostic test. Only 80% of epithelial ovarian tumors express CA-125, and many benign and other malignant processes [lung, breast, and pancreas] may also cause CA-125 to rise above normal.)

Imaging: No imaging indicated.

Special Tests: A frozen section histologic evaluation should be considered for any ovarian mass that appears suspicious for malignancy.

Diagnostic Procedures: History, physical examination, and imaging. Final diagnosis is established by histologic evaluation.

Pathologic Findings

Gross—smooth translucent cyst wall with infrequent papillary areas. Microscopic—epithelial cells filled with mucin that resemble cells of the endocervix or intestinal epithelium. Mucinous tumors have a higher chance of being of borderline malignant potential (grade 0) than do other epithelial tumors.

MANAGEMENT AND THERAPY

Nonpharmacologic

General Measures: Evaluation, supportive therapy based on symptoms.

Specific Measures: Generally require surgical exploration and extirpation. In benign disease or tumors of borderline malignant potential, the uterus and other ovary generally may be spared. Adjunctive chemotherapy (platinum-based and paclitaxel [Taxol]) or radiation therapy is often included, based on the location and stage of malignant disease.

Diet: No specific dietary changes indicated, except those imposed by advanced disease.

Activity: No restriction, except that imposed by advanced disease.

Patient Education: American College of Obstetricians and Gynecologists Patient Education Pamphlet AP096 (*Cancer of the Ovary*), AP075 (*Ovarian Cysts*).

Drug(s) of Choice

None, except as adjunctive or symptomatic therapy. Preoperative bowel cleansing (mechanical or with antibiosis) is often recommended as a precaution should bowel resection become necessary at the time of surgical staging and resection.

Contraindications: See individual agents.

Precautions: Alkylating agents are associated with an increased risk of future leukemia (10% by 8 years after therapy).

Interactions: See individual agents.

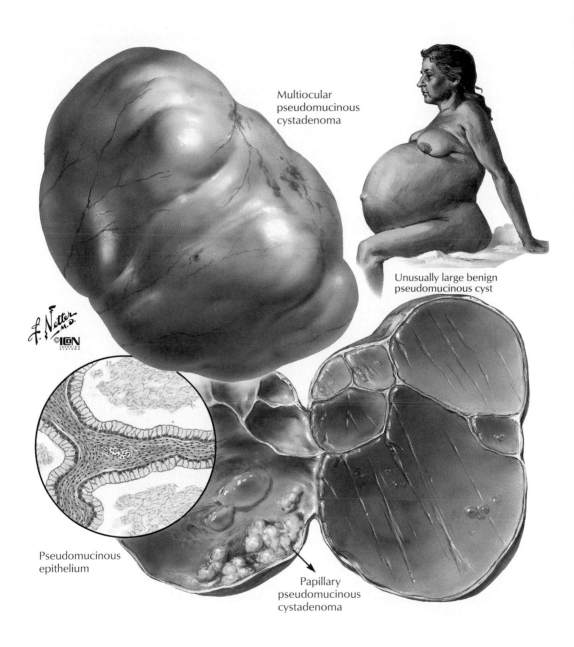

Multiocular
pseudomucinous
cystadenoma

Unusually large benign
pseudomucinous cyst

Pseudomucinous
epithelium

Papillary
pseudomucinous
cystadenoma

FOLLOW-UP

Patient Monitoring: Careful follow-up for recurrent pelvic disease or enlargement of the remaining ovary (if any). This is generally performed by pelvic examination, augmented with ultrasonography in selected patients. In those suspected of having recurrent disease and other selected patients, second-look surgery may be desirable to assess progress and discover occult disease.

Prevention/Avoidance: None.

Possible Complications: Perforation of the tumor capsule with rupture, which may lead to the seeding of the peritoneal cavity (pseudomyxoma peritonei, 2%–5% of patients).

Expected Outcome: Tumors with borderline malignant potential tend to grow slowly, and patients have prolonged survival with these tumors (40% 20-year survival with stage III disease). Of ovarian malignancies, mucinous cystadenocarcinoma has one of the best 5-year survival rates (40%).

MISCELLANEOUS

Pregnancy Considerations: No effect on pregnancy. More than 10% of tumors with borderline malignant potential are discovered during pregnancy.

ICD-9-CM **Codes:** Specific to cell type and location.

REFERENCES

American College of Obstetricians and Gynecologists. *Cancer of the Ovary.* Washington, DC: ACOG; 1990. ACOG Technical Bulletin 141.

American College of Obstetricians and Gynecologists. *Classification and Staging of Gynecologic Malignancies.* Washington, DC: ACOG; 1991. ACOG Technical Bulletin 155.

Carter J, Carson LF, Moradi MM, Adcock LA, Twiggs LB. Pseudomyxoma peritonei: a review. *Int J Gynecol Cancer* 1991;1:243.

Chaitin BA, Gershenson DM, Evans HL. Mucinous tumors of the ovary: a clinicopathologic study of 70 cases. *Cancer* 1985;55:1958.

Fleischer AC. Transabdominal and transvaginal sonography of ovarian masses. *Clin Obstet Gynecol* 1991;34:433.

Russell P. Surface epithelial-stromal tumors of the ovary. In: Kurman RJ, ed. *Blaustein's Pathology of the Female Genital Tract.* 4th ed. New York, NY: Springer-Verlag; 1994:724.

OVARIAN CANCER

INTRODUCTION

Description: A malignancy arising in the ovary, generally of epithelial origin. This represents the second most common malignancy of the genital tract (after endometrial cancer), but is the most common fatal gynecologic cancer.

Prevalence: Annually: 26,700 cases; 14,800 deaths. The lifetime risk of developing ovarian cancer is approximately 1 in 70.

Predominant Age: Postmenopausal, average 59, highest rate 60–64 years. Only one quarter of ovarian tumors in postmenopausal women are malignant.

Genetics: Family pattern recognized in a small percentage of cases. Possible association with abnormalities of the breast cancer (BRCA1 and BRCA2) gene. Hereditary ovarian cancers are rare but usually fatal; 95% of ovarian cancers are sporadic.

ETIOLOGY AND PATHOGENESIS

Causes: Unknown.

Risk Factors: Family history (greatest risk in those few women with an inheritable cancer syndrome, such as Lynch II), high-fat diet, advanced age, nulliparity, early menarche, late menopause, white race, higher economic status. More than 95% of patients with ovarian cancer have no risk factor. Oral contraception, high parity, and breast-feeding reduce risk.

CLINICAL CHARACTERISTICS

Signs and Symptoms:
Asymptomatic until late in the disease
Weight loss
Increasing abdominal girth despite constant or reduced caloric intake
Ascites
Adnexal mass (multilocular or partly solid masses in patients older than age 40 likely to be malignant; ovarian masses in premenarchial girls are most often germ cell tumors)
Vague lower abdominal discomfort (severe pain uncommon)

DIAGNOSTIC APPROACH

Differential Diagnosis:
Benign adnexal masses (corpus luteum, follicular cyst)
Nongynecologic pelvic masses
Hepatic, renal, or cardiac disease resulting in weight loss and ascites
Endometriosis
Hydrosalpinx
Ectopic pregnancy (reproductive age women)
Pedunculated leiomyomata
Pelvic or horseshoe kidney
Gastrointestinal malignancy

Associated Conditions: Breast cancer, endometrial cancer.

Workup and Evaluation

Laboratory: Serum testing for tumor markers, such as CA-125, lipid-associated sialic acid, carcinoembryonic antigen, α-fetoprotein, and others, should be reserved for following the progress of patients with known malignancies and not for prognostic evaluation.

Imaging: Ultrasonography, MRI, and CT are helpful in evaluating patients suspected of having ovarian cancer. (The normal postmenopausal ovary is typically 1.5–2 cm in size.)

Special Tests: A frozen section histologic evaluation (intraoperative consultation) should be considered for any ovarian mass that appears suspicious for malignancy. Flow cytometry may be of prognostic value.

Diagnostic Tests: History, physical examination, and imaging. Final diagnosis is established by histologic evaluation.

Pathologic Findings

More than 90% of ovarian cancer is of the epithelial cell type, thought to arise from pluripotential mesothelial cells of the visceral peritoneum of the ovarian capsule. Lymphatic spread occurs in roughly 20% of tumors that appear grossly confined to the ovary.

MANAGEMENT AND THERAPY

Nonpharmacologic

General Measures: Evaluation, supportive therapy based on symptoms.

Specific Measures: Ovarian cancer is a disease that requires surgical exploration and extirpation (including the uterus and contralateral ovary). Adjunctive chemotherapy (platinum-based and paclitaxel [Taxol]) or radiation therapy is often included based on the location and stage of the disease.

Diet: No changes except those imposed by advanced disease. Parenteral nutrition may be required before or after surgery in advanced disease.

Activity: No restriction, except that imposed by advanced disease.

Patient Education: Reassurance, American College of Obstetricians and Gynecologists Patient

Ovarian Cancer

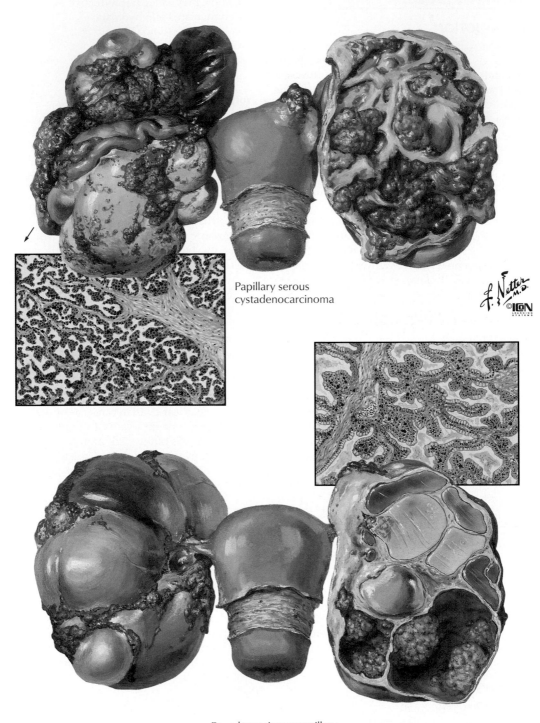

Papillary serous
cystadenocarcinoma

Pseudomucinous papillary
cystadenocarcinoma

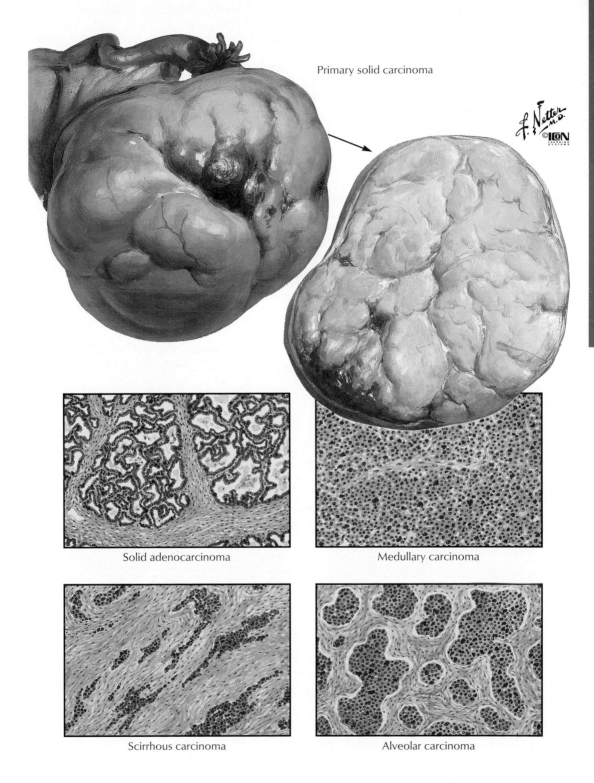

Primary solid carcinoma

Solid adenocarcinoma

Medullary carcinoma

Scirrhous carcinoma

Alveolar carcinoma

Education Pamphlet AP096 (*Cancer of the Ovary*), AP075 (*Ovarian Cysts*).

Drug(s) of Choice

None, except as adjunctive therapy. Preoperative bowel cleansing (mechanical or with antibiosis) is often recommended as a precaution should bowel resection become necessary at the time of surgical staging and resection.

Precautions: Alkylating agents are associated with an increased risk of future leukemia (10% by 8 years after therapy).

FOLLOW-UP

Patient Monitoring: As yet, there are no effective screening tools for the early detection of primary ovarian cancer. Ultrasonography, MRI, CT, and biochemical markers such as CA 125, which are useful for evaluating a suspicious mass or following the progress of treatment, are not of value for mass screening. In those suspected of having recurrent disease and other selected patients, second-look surgery may be desirable to assess progress and discover occult disease.

Prevention/Avoidance: For those few patients at truly high risk (familial cancer syndromes), prophylactic oophorectomy after childbearing is completed is preferable to any attempt at prolonged surveillance with current technology. Even this aggressive step does not preclude the development of "ovarian" cancer; up to 10% of ovarian cancers are found in women who have had bilateral oophorectomies.

Possible Complications: Ascites, pulmonary effusion, small bowel obstruction, disease progression, and death.

Expected Outcome: Ovarian cancer has the highest mortality of any gynecologic cancer, resulting in more deaths annually than cervical and endometrial cancer combined. If discovered early in the process and treated with aggressive surgical resection and adjunctive therapy, disease-free survival is possible. Survival is affected by stage, grade, cell type, and residual tumor after surgical resection. Survival (5-year) by stage: stage I 80%; stage II 60%; stage III 25%; stage IV 15%.

MISCELLANEOUS

ICD-9-CM **Codes:** Based on type and stage.

REFERENCES

American College of Obstetricians and Gynecologists. *Cancer of the Ovary.* Washington, DC: ACOG;1990. ACOG Technical Bulletin 141.

American College of Obstetricians and Gynecologists. *Classification and Staging of Gynecologic Malignancies.* Washington, DC: ACOG;1991. ACOG Technical Bulletin 155.

Averette HE, Nguyen HN. The role of prophylactic oophorectomy in cancer prevention. *Gynecol Oncol* 1994;55:S38.

Bell R, Petticrew M, Sheldon T. The performance of screening tests for ovarian cancer: results of a systematic review. *Br J Obstet Gynaecol* 1998;105:1136.

Boente MP, Godwin AK, Hogan WM. Screening, imaging and early diagnosis of ovarian cancer. *Clin Obstet Gynecol* 1994;37:377.

Lynch HT, Watson P, Conway T, Lynch J. Hereditary ovarian cancer: natural history, surveillance, management, and genetic counseling. *Hematol/Oncol Ann* 1994;2:107.

OVARIAN CYSTS

THE CHALLENGE

Description: A cystic growth within the ovary, generally arising from epithelial components and most often benign.

Scope of the Problem: Benign ovarian tumors are most frequently diagnosed at the time of routine examination and are asymptomatic. When symptoms do occur, they generally are either catastrophic (as when bleeding, rupture, or torsion occur) or indolent and nonspecific (such as a vague sense of pressure or fullness).

Objectives of Management: The most important objective of the management of an ovarian cyst is the timely diagnosis of its type and origin. Subsequent therapy and assessment of risk is based on the correctness of the diagnosis. For acutely symptomatic cysts, rapid evaluation and intervention may be necessary.

TACTICS

Relevant Pathophysiology: Approximately 90% of ovarian tumors encountered in younger women are benign and metabolically inactive. More than 75% of the benign adnexal masses are functional. Functional cysts are not true neoplasms, but rather are anatomic variants resulting from the normal function of the ovary. Follicular cysts occur when ovulation fails to take place, leaving the developing follicle to continue beyond its normal time. In a similar manner, the corpus luteum may persist, or through internal bleeding, enlarge and become symptomatic. Approximately 25% of ovarian enlargements in reproductive age women represent true neoplasia, with only approximately 10% being malignant. The largest group of benign ovarian tumors are those that arise from the epithelium of the ovary and its capsule. Despite the diversity of tumors with epithelial beginnings, the most common ovarian tumor in young reproductive age women is the cystic teratoma, or dermoid, which is germ cell in origin. These tumors are derived from primary germ cells and include tissues from all three embryonic germ layers (ectoderm, mesoderm, and endoderm).

Strategies: History and physical examination are generally sufficient to establish the presence of the mass. There are no laboratory tests that are of specific help in the global diagnosis of ovarian cysts. Laboratory investigations may support specific diagnoses. Ultrasonography, CT, and MRI are of limited value in evaluating asymptomatic masses in young patients. Exceptions to this are patients in whom clinical assessment is impractical or inadequate (eg, massive obesity) or those in whom malignancy is suspected. Serum testing for tumor markers, such as CA-125, lipid-associated sialic acid, carcinoembryonic antigen, α-fetoprotein, and others, should be reserved for following the progress of patients with known malignancies and not for prognostic evaluation.

Patient Education: Reassurance, American College of Obstetricians and Gynecologists Patient Education Pamphlet AP075 (*Ovarian Cysts*).

IMPLEMENTATION

Special Considerations: Some authors favor giving young patients with small, presumably benign, cystic masses ovulation suppression therapy, such as oral contraceptives, to hasten the process of regression. Regression rates of 65%–75% are often cited for this approach, but this strategy is largely a matter of personal choice because definitive studies are lacking. Physiologic ovarian enlargements, including follicular or corpus luteum cysts, should not be present if a patient is using oral contraceptives. For this reason, patients who are already using oral contraceptives and develop adnexal masses are more likely to have pathologic conditions that will not regress, increasing the possibility that eventual surgical exploration may be required. Perimenopausal and postmenopausal patients may still have benign processes as a cause of an adnexal mass, but the likelihood of a malignant process is much increased, altering management. In these patients, masses larger than 6 cm generally prompt surgical exploration and excision. The availability of transvaginal ultrasonography to measure and track masses has allowed smaller masses that once would have required exploration to be followed conservatively. As in younger patients, the size, shape, mobility, and consistency of the mass should be estimated. Irregular, immobile, or mixed character masses (solid and cystic) are more likely to be malignant and deserve immediate consultation with a surgeon for exploration. The final diagnosis of ovarian cancer must be made surgically.

REFERENCES

Fenoglio CM, Richart RM. Common epithelial ovarian tumors. In: Sciarra JJ, ed. *Gynecology and Obstetrics.* Vol 4. Philadelphia, Pa: JB Lippincott; 1989;30:1.

Fleischer AC. Transabdominal and transvaginal sonography of ovarian masses. *Clin Obstet Gynecol* 1991;34:433.

Petersen WF, Prevost EC, Edmunds FT, Hundley JM, Morriss FK. Benign cystic teratomas of the ovary. *Am J Obstet Gynecol* 1955;70:368.

Ovarian Cysts

Differential Diagnosis

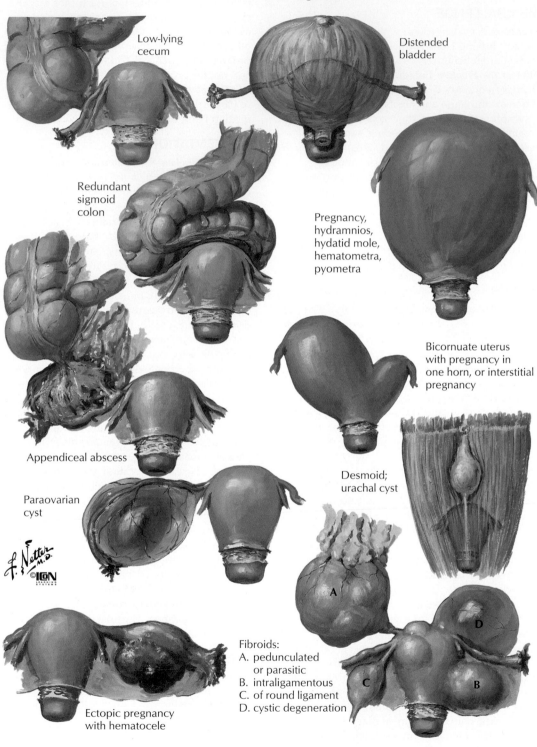

Low-lying cecum

Distended bladder

Redundant sigmoid colon

Pregnancy, hydramnios, hydatid mole, hematometra, pyometra

Bicornuate uterus with pregnancy in one horn, or interstitial pregnancy

Appendiceal abscess

Paraovarian cyst

Desmoid; urachal cyst

Ectopic pregnancy with hematocele

Fibroids:
A. pedunculated or parasitic
B. intraligamentous
C. of round ligament
D. cystic degeneration

OVARIAN FIBROMA

INTRODUCTION

Description: The most common benign ovarian tumor, this tumor is composed of stromal cells (fibroblasts). Although benign, these tumors are sometimes associated with ascites and hydrothorax (Meigs' syndrome, 1% of patients).

Prevalence: Four percent of all ovarian tumors, most common solid tumor.

Predominant Age: Any, most common in perimenopausal and menopausal women, average: 48, <10% younger than 30.

Genetics: No genetic pattern with the exception of Gorlin's syndrome.

ETIOLOGY AND PATHOGENESIS

Causes: Unknown.
Risk Factors: None known.

CLINICAL CHARACTERISTICS

Signs and Symptoms:
Asymptomatic (may grow to a large size without detection)
Adnexal mass (average size 6 cm, may weigh as much as 50 pounds)
Ascites (40% if the tumor is >10 cm)
Hydrothorax (Meigs' syndrome, regresses after removal of the tumor)
Estrogen secretion (when theca cells predominate)
Bilateral masses in <10% of patients

DIAGNOSTIC APPROACH

Differential Diagnosis:
Benign adnexal masses (corpus luteum, follicular cyst)
Endometriosis
Hydrosalpinx
Paratubal cyst
Appendiceal abscess
Ectopic pregnancy
Pedunculated leiomyomata
Pelvic or horseshoe kidney
Nongynecologic pelvic masses
Fibromatosis
Stromal hyperplasia
Fibrosarcoma

Associated Conditions: Ascites, hydrothorax, basal cell nevus syndrome (Gorlin's syndrome—early basal cell carcinomas, keratosis of the jaw, calcification of the dura, mesnetaric cysts, and bilateral ovarian fibromas).

Workup and Evaluation

Laboratory: As indicated before surgery.

Imaging: Preoperative evaluation (CT or ultrasonography) for possible lymph node enlargement or intraabdominal spread is indicated for patients in whom malignancy is a significant possibility.

Special Tests: None indicated.

Diagnostic Tests: History, physical examination, and imaging. Final diagnosis is established by histologic evaluation.

Pathologic Findings

These tumors contain fibroblasts and spindle cells and may grow to a large size without detection. The cut surface reveals hard, flat, chalky-white surfaces with a whorled appearance. Small cyst formation is relatively common.

MANAGEMENT AND THERAPY

Nonpharmacologic

General Measures: Evaluation, supportive therapy based on symptoms.

Specific Measures: Surgical exploration and resection is adequate. In older women, hysterectomy and removal of the contralateral ovary is generally performed. Fibromas of low malignant potential are rare.

Diet: No specific dietary changes indicated.

Activity: No restriction.

Patient Education: American College of Obstetricians and Gynecologists Patient Education Pamphlet AP096 (*Cancer of the Ovary*), AP075 (*Ovarian Cysts*).

Drug(s) of Choice

Adjunctive or symptomatic therapy.

FOLLOW-UP

Patient Monitoring: Normal health maintenance.

Prevention/Avoidance: None.

Possible Complications: Uncommon. Torsion or bleeding may occur. Fibromas of low malignant potential that are adherent or that are ruptured may recur.

Expected Outcome: Simple surgical excision is generally curative.

MISCELLANEOUS

Pregnancy Considerations: No effect on pregnancy. Hormonally active tumors (thecoma) may disrupt menstrual patterns and ovulation, leading to reduced fertility.

ICD-9-CM Codes: 220 (Benign neoplasm of ovary).

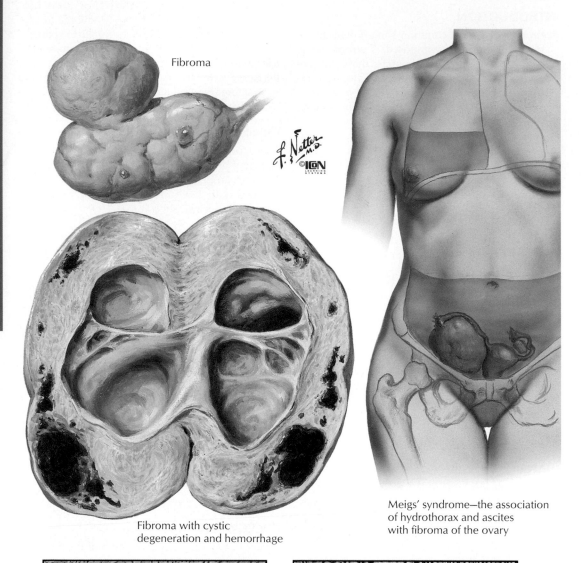

Fibroma

Fibroma with cystic
degeneration and hemorrhage

Meigs' syndrome—the association
of hydrothorax and ascites
with fibroma of the ovary

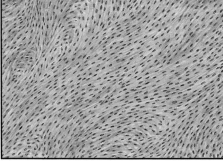

Fibroma

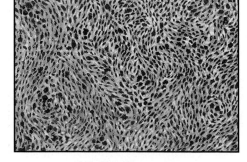

Spindle cell sarcoma

REFERENCES

American College of Obstetricians and Gynecologists. *Cancer of the Ovary.* Washington, DC: ACOG; 1990. ACOG Technical Bulletin 141.

American College of Obstetricians and Gynecologists. *Classification and Staging of Gynecologic Malignancies.* Washington, DC: ACOG; 1991. ACOG Technical Bulletin 155.

Burket RL, Rauh JL. Gorlin's syndrome. Ovarian fibromas at adolescence. *Obstet Gynecol* 1976;47:43s.

Fleischer AC. Transabdominal and transvaginal sonography of ovarian masses. *Clin Obstet Gynecol* 1991;34:433.

Meigs JV. Fibroma of the ovary with ascites and hydrothorax. Meigs' syndrome. *Am J Obstet Gynecol* 1954;67:962.

Young RH, Scully RE. Sex cord-stromal, steroid cell, and other ovarian tumors with endocrine, paraendocrine, and paraneoplastic manifestations. In: Kurman RJ, ed. *Blaustein's Pathology of the Female Genital Tract.* 4th ed. New York, NY: Springer-Verlag; 1994, 621.

ADNEXAL DISEASE

OVARIAN TORSION

INTRODUCTION

Description: The twisting of part or all of the adnexa on its mesentery, resulting in tissue ischemia and frank infarction. This usually involves the ovary, but may include the fallopian tube as well.

Prevalence: Uncommon; 2%–3% of gynecologic operative emergencies.

Predominant Age: Mid-20s.

Genetics: No genetic pattern.

ETIOLOGY AND PATHOGENESIS

Causes: Spontaneous twisting of the ovary on its mesentery, generally associated with ovarian enlargement (50%–60% have an ovarian tumor or cyst).

Risk Factors: Torsion of the adnexa is usually associated with the presence of an ovarian, tubal, or paratubal mass. Risk of torsion is higher during pregnancy or after ovulation induction.

CLINICAL CHARACTERISTICS

Signs and Symptoms:

Pain (generally abrupt, intense, and unilateral—the pain of adnexal torsion generally comes and goes with a periodicity that varies from hours to days or longer; this is in contrast to the variable pain caused by obstruction of the bowel, ureter, or common bile duct, which is more regular and frequent)

Nausea and vomiting (60%–70%)

Unilateral palpable (tender) mass (90% of patients)

DIAGNOSTIC APPROACH

Differential Diagnosis:

Ectopic pregnancy

Bleeding into an ovarian cyst

Ruptured corpus luteum

Adnexal abscess

Acute appendicitis

Small bowel obstruction

Associated Conditions: Adnexal mass.

Workup and Evaluation

Laboratory: Pregnancy test to evaluate the possibility of an ectopic pregnancy.

Imaging: Ultrasonography may demonstrate a cystic adnexal mass, but the acute character and intensity of symptoms usually encountered means that the diagnosis is most often made at the time of surgery.

Special Tests: None indicated.

Diagnostic Tests: History, physical examination, and imaging (if the patient's condition permits).

Pathologic Findings

Ischemia and infarction in ovarian or tubal tissues, other pathologic conditions based on a coexistent mass (50%–60% of patients have a mass).

MANAGEMENT AND THERAPY

Nonpharmacologic

General Measures: Evaluation, stabilization (when acute symptoms are present).

Specific Measures: Surgical exploration (conservative operative management may be possible in up to 75% of patients).

Diet: Nothing by mouth pending surgical exploration.

Activity: Bed rest.

Patient Education: American College of Obstetricians and Gynecologists Patient Education Pamphlet AP075 (*Ovarian Cysts*).

Drug(s) of Choice

Analgesics (based on patient condition).

Contraindications: No analgesics should be given until the diagnosis is established, and the patient's condition is stabilized.

FOLLOW-UP

Patient Monitoring: Normal health maintenance as follow-up.

Prevention/Avoidance: None.

Possible Complications: Complete loss of the involved ovary.

Expected Outcome: Part or all of the ovary may be salvaged in some patients if intervention takes place early enough in the process.

MISCELLANEOUS

Pregnancy Considerations: Twenty percent of cases occur during pregnancy.

ICD-9-CM Codes: 620.5.

REFERENCES

Bayer AI, Wiskind AK. Adnexal torsion: can the adnexa be saved? *Am J Obstet Gynecol* 1994;171:1506.

Bider D, Maschiach S, Dulitzky M, Kokia E, Lipitz S, Ben-Rafael Z. Clinical, surgical and pathologic findings of adnexal torsion in pregnant and nonpregnant women. *Surg Gynecol Obstet* 1991;173:363.

Gordon JD, Hopkins KL, Jeffrey RB, Giudice LC. Adnexal torsion: color Doppler diagnosis and laparoscopic treatment. *Fertil Steril* 1994;61:383.

Hibbard LT. Adnexal torsion. *Am J Obstet Gynecol* 1985;152:456.

Nichols DH, Julian PJ. Torsion of the adnexa. *Clin Obstet Gynecol* 1985;28:375.

Ovarian Torsion

Oelsner G, Bider D, Goldenberg M, Admon D, Mashiach S. Long-term follow-up of the twisted ischemic adnexa managed by detorsion. *Fertil Steril* 1993;60:976.

Zweizig S, Perron J, Grubb D, Mishell DR Jr. Conservative management of adnexal torsion. *Am J Obstet Gynecol* 1993;168:1791.

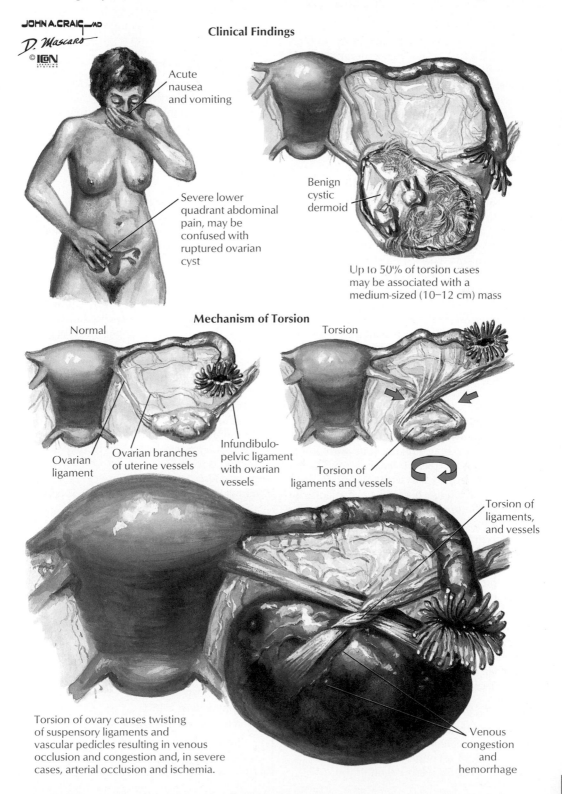

JOHN A. CRAIG—AD
D. Mascaro
© IGN

Clinical Findings

Acute nausea and vomiting

Severe lower quadrant abdominal pain, may be confused with ruptured ovarian cyst

Benign cystic dermoid

Up to 50% of torsion cases may be associated with a medium-sized (10–12 cm) mass

Mechanism of Torsion

Normal

Torsion

Ovarian ligament

Ovarian branches of uterine vessels

Infundibulo-pelvic ligament with ovarian vessels

Torsion of ligaments and vessels

Torsion of ligaments, and vessels

Torsion of ovary causes twisting of suspensory ligaments and vascular pedicles resulting in venous occlusion and congestion and, in severe cases, arterial occlusion and ischemia.

Venous congestion and hemorrhage

PELVIC INFLAMMATORY DISEASE

INTRODUCTION

Description: A serious, diffuse, frequently multiorganism infection of the pelvic organs that results in significant morbidity.

Prevalence: One percent to three percent of women; most common gynecologic reason for emergency visits for women aged 15–44.

Predominant Age: 16 to 25; 85% of cases found in sexually active women of menstrual age.

Genetics: No genetic pattern.

ETIOLOGY AND PATHOGENESIS

Causes: In roughly one third of cases, the causative organism is *Neisseria gonorrhoeae* alone. One third of cases involve infection with *N gonorrhoeae* and additional "mixed" infections with other organisms. The last third of infections are due to mixed aerobic and anaerobic bacteria, including respiratory pathogens such as *Haemophilus influenzae, Streptococcus pneumoniae,* and *Streptococcus pyogenes* found in up to 5% of patients. Polymicrobial infections are present in more than 40% of patients with laparoscopically proven salpingitis, with one study reporting an average of 6.8 bacterial types per patient. Only approximately 15% of women with cervical *N gonorrhoeae* infections develop acute pelvic infections. Orgasmic uterine contractions or the attachment of *N gonorrhoeae* to sperm may provide transportation to the upper genital tract. *Chlamydia* is involved in roughly 20% of patients, with this rate rising to roughly 40% among hospitalized patients. Infection of the upper genital tract by *Chlamydia* causes a milder form of salpingitis with more insidious symptoms.

Risk Factors: Multiple sexual partners, uterine or cervical instrumentation, douching. Because many of the anaerobic bacteria found in mixed infections mimic those found in the vagina of patients with bacterial vaginosis, bacterial vaginosis is considered a risk factor for the development of pelvic infections. Fifteen percent of cases occur after instrumentation such as endometrial biopsy, hysterosalpingography, IUCD placement, or the like.

CLINICAL CHARACTERISTICS

Signs and Symptoms (see below):

Pelvic pain and tenderness (100%), muscular guarding, or rebound tenderness

Fever (up to 39.5°C, 40%) or chills

Elevated white blood cell count

Irregular vaginal bleeding or discharge

Tachycardia, nausea, and vomiting

Purulent cervical discharge is often demonstrated (should be sampled for Gram's staining and culture)

DIAGNOSTIC APPROACH

Differential Diagnosis:

Ectopic pregnancy

Adnexal accident (torsion, bleeding)

Appendicitis

Endometriosis

Cholecystitis

Enteritis

Septic incomplete abortion

Diverticular abscess

Associated Conditions: Tubal factor infertility, ectopic pregnancy, and chronic abdominal pain.

Workup and Evaluation

Laboratory: Complete blood count, including differential, white blood cell count, and erythrocyte sedimentation rate. Cervical culture (even though there is only a 50% correlation between cervical culture and upper tract organisms) and Gram's staining.

Imaging: Ultrasonography may demonstrate free fluid in the posterior cul-de-sac (supportive, but not diagnostic).

Special Tests: Confirmation by laparoscopy should be considered for any patient who does not respond in a timely manner or for whom the diagnosis is uncertain. In 35% of patients no infection is found.

Diagnostic Tests: History, physical examination and ultrasonography. Diagnostic criteria are shown in the following box.

Diagnostic Criteria for Pelvic Inflammatory Disease
Must have all three:
Abdominal tenderness
Adnexal tenderness
Cervical tenderness
Must have at least one:
Positive Gram's stain
Temperature >38°C
White blood cell count >10,000
Pus on culdocentesis or laparoscopy
Tubo-ovarian abscess

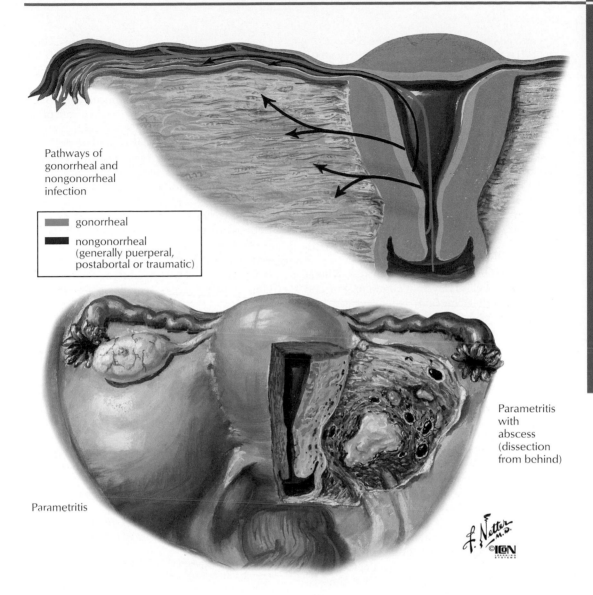

Pathways of gonorrheal and nongonorrheal infection

gonorrheal

nongonorrheal (generally puerperal, postabortal or traumatic)

Parametritis

Parametritis with abscess (dissection from behind)

Pathologic Findings

Inflammation of the fallopian tubes, ovaries, and surrounding peritoneal surfaces.

MANAGEMENT AND THERAPY

Nonpharmacologic

General Measures: Rapid evaluation, cervical cultures, supportive therapy (fluids, analgesics, and antipyretics).

Specific Measures: Aggressive antibiotic therapy. For some, hysterectomy may be required. Rupture of a tubo-ovarian abscess, with subsequent septic shock, may be life threatening.

Diet: No specific dietary changes indicated.

Activity: Pelvic rest. Ambulatory care is possible with early mild infections; hospitalization may be required.

Patient Education: American College of Obstetricians and Gynecologists Patient Education Pamphlet AP077 (*Pelvic Inflammatory Disease*), AP009 (*How to Prevent Sexually Transmitted Diseases*), AP099 (*Pelvic Pain*), AP071 (*Gonorrhea and Chlamydia*), AP002 (*Infertility: Causes and Treatments*), AP020 (*Pain During Intercourse*).

Drug(s) of Choice

Ambulatory care—cefoxitin (2 g IM) plus probenecid (1 g PO) combined with a 14-day course of doxycycline (100 mg, bid) or a combination of ceftriaxone (250 mg IM) plus the 14-day course of doxycycline

Hospitalized patients—cefoxitin (2 g IV q6h) or cefotetan (2 g IV q12h) with doxycycline (100 mg q12h PO or IV) is recommended

For mixed infections, clindamycin (900 mg IV q8h) plus an aminoglycoside such as gentamicin (2 mg/kg loading doses, then 1.5 mg/kg q8h) will give better protection

After discharge—doxycycline (100 mg PO bid) or clindamycin (450 mg qid) for 14 days.

Contraindications: See individual agents.
Precautions: See individual agents.
Interactions: See individual agents.

Alternative Drugs

Ofloxacin (400 mg PO bid for 14 days) combined with either oral clindamycin (450 mg qid) or oral metronidazole (500 mg bid) has also been proposed. Augmentin (500 mg tid for 10 days) may also be used with similar results. Excellent results have been reported with the combination of clindamycin and aztreonam (2 g IM q8h). Piperacillin (4 g) combined with tazobactam (500 mg) given IV q8h may also be used, but has given cure rates of only 90% (5% improved).

FOLLOW-UP

Patient Monitoring: Hospitalized care is indicated when differential diagnosis includes ectopic pregnancy or appendicitis, human immunodeficiency virus-infected patients, immunosuppressed patients, IUCD use, nulliparity, paralytic ileus, peritonitis or toxicity, pregnancy, previous treatment failure, significant gastrointestinal symptoms, significant morbidity, temperature >39°C, tubo-ovarian abscess, uncertain or complicated differential diagnosis, unreliable patient, or white blood cell count >20,000 or <4,000.

Prevention/Avoidance: Prevention of these sequelae is based on prevention of infection (barrier contraception, "safe sex"), screening for those at risk, and aggressive treatment. As with most sexually transmitted diseases, the partners of patients with pelvic inflammatory disease should be screened for gonococcal, chlamydial, or human immunodeficiency virus infections and treated accordingly.

Possible Complications: Pelvic inflammatory disease leads to tubal factor infertility, ectopic pregnancy, and chronic abdominal pain in a high percentage of patients. The risk of infertility roughly doubles with each subsequent episode, resulting in a 40% rate of infertility after only three episodes. Women with documented salpingitis have a 4-fold increase in their rate of ectopic pregnancy, and 5%–15% of women require surgery because of damage caused by pelvic inflammatory disease. Peritoneal involvement may spread to include perihepatitis (Fitz-Hugh–Curtis syndrome). Rupture of a tubo-ovarian abscess, with subsequent septic shock, may be life threatening. Death from pelvic infections or their complications (for women aged 15–45) is reported to be 0.29 of 100,000.

Expected Outcome: Early, aggressive therapy is generally associated with resolution, but the possibility of recurrence or sequelae is significant.

MISCELLANEOUS

Pregnancy Considerations: Often associated with reduced fertility and an increased risk of ectopic pregnancy. Once pregnancy is established, the risk of new infection is reduced because of obstruction of the upper genital tract by the gestation. Scarring from previous infections may cause pain when stretched by the enlarging uterus.

ICD-9-CM Codes: 614.3 (others based on chronicity, structures involved, and relation to pregnancy).

REFERENCES

Dodson MG. Antibiotic regimens for treating acute pelvic inflammatory disease: an evaluation. *J Reprod Med* 1994;39:285.

Hager WE, Eschenbach DA, Spence MR, Sweet RL. Criteria for diagnosis and grading of salpingitis. *Obstet Gynecol* 1983;61:113.

Jacobson LJ. Differential diagnosis of acute pelvic inflammatory disease. *Am J Obstet Gynecol* 1980;138:1006.

Ledger WJ. Laparoscopy in the diagnosis and management of patients with suspected salpingo-oophoritis. *Am J Obstet Gynecol* 1980;138:1012.

Pastorek JG 2nd, Cole C, Aldridge KE, Crapanzano JC. Aztreonam plus clindamycin as therapy for pelvic infections in women. *Am J Med* 1985;78(suppl 2A):47.

Tapp A, Wise B, Cardozo L. Efficacy and safety of piperacillin/tazobactam in gynecologic infections. *J Antimicrob Chemother* 1993;suppl B:61.

Washington AE, Cates W, Zaidi AA. Hospitalization for pelvic inflammatory disease. *JAMA* 1984;25:2529.

PSEUDOMYXOMA PERITONEI

INTRODUCTION

Description: The intraperitoneal spread of a mucin-secreting tumor (either a mucinous cystadenoma or carcinoma), which results in recurrent abdominal masses, often massive ascites, and multiple bowel obstructions. Frequently, this tumor may begin in the appendix.

Prevalence: Two of 10,000 laparotomies, 2%–5% of ovarian mucinous tumors (16% in mucinous cystadenocarcinomas).

Predominant Age: Middle to late reproductive.

Genetics: No genetic pattern.

ETIOLOGY AND PATHOGENESIS

Causes: Spread, rupture, spill, or leakage of a primary appendiceal tumor or other gastrointestinal or ovarian tumor. Recent histologic studies suggest that in the majority of patients the appendix is the primary tumor source. In rare cases, metaplasia by the cells of the peritoneal surface may account for this tumor.

Risk Factors: Rupture or leakage of an ovarian mucinous tumor at the time of surgical resection. (This role has been debated in recent literature.)

CLINICAL CHARACTERISTICS

Signs and Symptoms:

Accumulation of large amounts of mucinous material in the peritoneal cavity

Recurrent bowel obstruction

Implants of tumor on the omentum, undersurface of the diaphragm, pelvis, right retrohepatic space, left abdominal gutter, and ligament of Treitz (the peritoneal surface of the bowel is generally spared [in contrast to carcinoma]; metastasis outside the peritoneal cavity does not occur.)

DIAGNOSTIC APPROACH

Differential Diagnosis:

Disseminated ovarian cancer

Metastatic colon cancer

Disseminated leiomyomata

Ascites

Associated Conditions: Gastrointestinal tumors, bowel obstruction.

Workup and Evaluation

Laboratory: As indicated before surgery. (Serum testing for tumor markers, such as CA-125, lipid-associated sialic acid, carcinoembryonic antigen, α-fetoprotein, and others, should be reserved for following the progress of patients with known malignancies and not for prognostic evaluation.)

Imaging: Ultrasonography or CT may be helpful in determining the extent of disease.

Special Tests: None indicated.

Diagnostic Tests: History, physical examination, and imaging. Final diagnosis is established by histologic evaluation.

Pathologic Findings

Perforation of the capsule of a mucinous tumor with rupture and seeding of the peritoneal cavity. Most often associated with malignant tumors, although benign mucinous neoplasms may perforate and result in pseudomyxoma peritonei as well. Tumors of the ovary and appendix may be synchronous, making the determination of origin difficult or impossible.

MANAGEMENT AND THERAPY

Nonpharmacologic

General Measures: Evaluation, supportive therapy based on symptoms.

Specific Measures: Surgical exploration and extirpation. Extensive bowel resection is often required because of diffuse peritoneal implants of tumor.

Diet: No specific dietary changes indicated, except those imposed by advanced disease.

Activity: No restriction, except that imposed by advanced disease.

Patient Education: Reassurance, American College of Obstetricians and Gynecologists Patient Education Pamphlet AP075 (*Ovarian Cysts*), AP096 (*Cancer of the Ovary*), AP080 (*Preparing for Surgery*).

Drug(s) of Choice

None, except as adjunctive or symptomatic therapy. Chemotherapy (systemic or intraperitoneal alkylating agents) and mucolytic agents have not been shown to be effective. Preoperative bowel cleansing (mechanical or with antibiosis) is often recommended as a precaution should bowel resection become necessary at the time of surgical staging and resection.

Precautions: Alkylating agents are associated with an increased risk of future leukemia (10% by 8 years after therapy).

FOLLOW-UP

Patient Monitoring: Careful follow-up for recurrent pelvic disease or enlargement of the remaining ovary (if any). This is generally performed by

ADNEXAL DISEASE

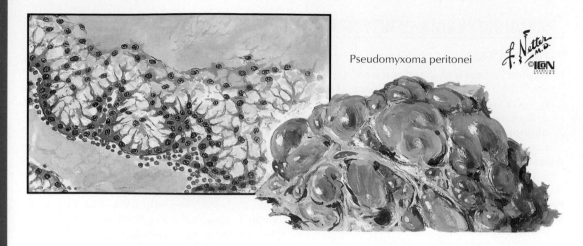

Pseudomyxoma peritonei

pelvic examination, augmented with ultrasonography in selected patients.

Prevention/Avoidance: Care in the handling and surgical removal of ovarian masses.

Possible Complications: Generally follows an indolent course with progressive bowel dysfunction, intercurrent infection, inanition, and death.

Expected Outcome: The prognosis is better for patient when the tumor arises from adenomas (appendiceal or ovarian) than if it comes from a carcinoma.

MISCELLANEOUS

Pregnancy Considerations: No effect on pregnancy.
ICD-9-CM Codes: 197.6.

REFERENCES

American College of Obstetricians and Gynecologists. *Cancer of the Ovary.* Washington, DC: ACOG; 1990. ACOG Technical Bulletin 141.

Amortegui AJ. Ovarian tumors of low malignant potential (atypically proliferating ovarian tumors) In: Sciarra JJ, ed. *Gynecology and Obstetrics.* Vol 4. Philadelphia, Pa: JB Lippincott; 1996;29:20.

Jones DH. Pseudomyxoma peritonei. *Br J Clin Pract* 1965;19:675.

Ronnett BM, Kurman RJ, Zahn CM, et al. Pseudomyxoma peritonei in women: a clinicopathologic analysis of 30 cases with emphasis on site of origin, prognosis, and relationship to ovarian mucinous tumors of low malignant potential. *Hum Pathol* 1995;26:509.

Rutgers JL, Baergen RN. Mucin histochemistry of ovarian borderline tumors of mucinous and mixed-epithelial types. *Mod Pathol* 1994;7:825.

Wertheim I, Fleischhacker D, McLachlin CM, Rice LW, Berkowitz RS, Goff BA. Pseudomyxoma peritonei: a review of 23 cases. *Obstet Gynecol* 1994;84:17.

SEROUS OVARIAN CYSTS

INTRODUCTION

Description: A group of benign and malignant epithelial tumors of the ovary that are characterized as serous cells. These tumors are the most commonly encountered epithelial ovarian tumors. When malignant, these tumors tend to be high grade and virulent.

Prevalence: Twenty percent of all benign ovarian neoplasms.

Predominant Age: Reproductive.

Genetics: No genetic pattern.

ETIOLOGY AND PATHOGENESIS

Causes: Unknown.

Risk Factors: Family history, high-fat diet, advanced age, nulliparity, early menarche and late menopause, white race, higher economic status. Oral contraception, high parity, and breast-feeding reduce risk.

CLINICAL CHARACTERISTICS

Signs and Symptoms:

Asymptomatic

Vague lower abdominal symptoms

Adnexal mass (bilateral in 10% of benign and in 33%–66% of malignant lesions), cystic and filled with a clear serous fluid (Benign tumors tend to be unilocular and smooth; malignant tumors are more often multilocular with papillary projections over much of the surface.)

DIAGNOSTIC APPROACH

Differential Diagnosis:

Benign adnexal masses (corpus luteum, follicular cyst)

Endometriosis

Hydrosalpinx

Paratubal cyst

Appendiceal abscess

Paratubal cyst

Ectopic pregnancy

Pedunculated leiomyomata

Pelvic or horseshoe kidney

Nongynecologic pelvic masses

Associated Conditions: None.

Workup and Evaluation

Laboratory: As indicated before surgery. (CA-125 levels may be useful for the monitoring of disease response to treatment or progression but is not a good prognostic test. Only 80% of epithelial ovarian tumors express CA-125, and many benign and other malignant processes [lung, breast, and pancreas] may also cause CA-125 to rise above normal.)

Imaging: No imaging indicated.

Special Tests: A frozen section histologic evaluation should be considered for any ovarian mass that appears suspicious for malignancy.

Diagnostic Tests: History, physical examination, and imaging. Final diagnosis is established by histologic evaluation.

Pathologic Findings

Serous tumors are more likely to be found with poorer differentiation and are more likely to be discovered late in the disease process. Papillary surface carcinomas of the ovary are most likely to be serous in type. The diagnosis is made based on the histologic analysis of the cyst wall and not on the character of the cyst fluid.

MANAGEMENT AND THERAPY

Nonpharmacologic

General Measures: Evaluation, supportive therapy based on symptoms.

Specific Measures: Generally require surgical exploration and extirpation. In benign disease or tumors of borderline malignant potential, the uterus and other ovary generally may be spared. Adjunctive chemotherapy (platinum-based and paclitaxel [Taxol]) or radiation therapy is often included based on the location and stage of the disease.

Diet: No specific dietary changes indicated, except those imposed by advanced disease.

Activity: No restriction, except that imposed by advanced disease.

Patient Education: American College of Obstetricians and Gynecologists Patient Education Pamphlet AP096 (*Cancer of the Ovary*), AP075 (*Ovarian Cysts*).

Drug(s) of Choice

None, except as adjunctive or symptomatic therapy. Preoperative bowel cleansing (mechanical or with antibiosis) is often recommended as a precaution should bowel resection become necessary at the time of surgical staging and resection.

Precautions: Alkylating agents are associated with an increased risk of future leukemia (10% by 8 years after therapy).

FOLLOW-UP

Patient Monitoring: Careful follow-up for recurrent pelvic disease or enlargement of the remaining ovary (if any). This is generally performed by

Serous Ovarian Cysts

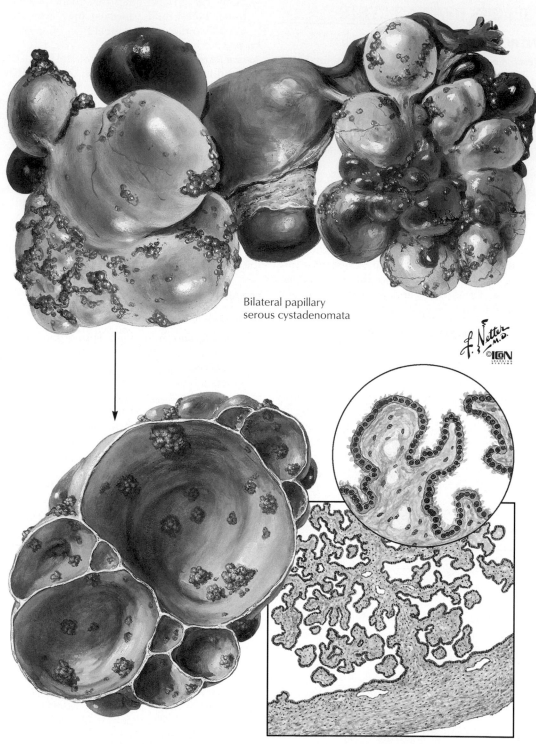

Bilateral papillary
serous cystadenomata

Hemisection showing
internal papillary excrescences

Branching architecture
of papillary growth

pelvic examination, augmented with ultrasonography in selected patients. In those suspected of having recurrent disease and other selected patients, second look surgery may be desirable to assess progress and discover occult disease.

Prevention/Avoidance: None.

Possible Complications: Torsion, hemorrhage, progression, and spread of malignant disease.

Expected Outcome: Generally good for benign tumors; the prognosis for malignant tumors is based on stage. Overall, 5-year survival for malignant serous carcinomas is roughly 20%. Seventy-five percent of malignant serous carcinomas are at an advanced stage at the time of diagnosis.

MISCELLANEOUS

Pregnancy Considerations: No effect on pregnancy.

ICD-9-CM Codes: Specific to cell type and location.

REFERENCES

American College of Obstetricians and Gynecologists. *Cancer of the Ovary.* Washington, DC: ACOG; 1990. ACOG Technical Bulletin 141.

American College of Obstetricians and Gynecologists. *Classification and Staging of Gynecologic Malignancies.* Washington, DC: ACOG; 1991. ACOG Technical Bulletin 155.

Fenoglio CM, Richart RM. Common epithelial ovarian tumors. In: Sciarra JJ, ed. *Gynecology and Obstetrics.* Vol 4. Philadelphia, Pa: JB Lippincott; 1989;30:24.

Fromm GL, Gershenson DM, Silva EG. Papillary serous carcinoma of the peritoneum. *Obstet Gynecol* 1990;75:89.

Fromm GL, Silva EG. Metastatic serous ovarian tumors of low malignant potential. *Cancer* 1990;65:578.

Fleischer AC. Transabdominal and transvaginal sonography of ovarian masses. *Clin Obstet Gynecol* 1991; 34:433.

SERTOLI-LYDIG CELL TUMOR

INTRODUCTION

Description: A rare sex cord tumor of the ovary that carries male elements and may be associated with virilization. Tumors vary in size but generally are 5–15 cm in diameter.

Prevalence: Very rare (<0.5% of ovarian tumors).

Predominant Age: Older than 30 (70%), <10% older than 50.

Genetics: No genetic pattern.

ETIOLOGY AND PATHOGENESIS

Causes: Unknown.

Risk Factors: None known.

CLINICAL CHARACTERISTICS

Signs and Symptoms:
 Asymptomatic
 Adnexal enlargement (1.5% bilateral)
 Abdominal swelling or pain
 Ascites (4%)
 Oligomenorrhea or amenorrhea
 Loss of female secondary sex characteristics
  (breast atrophy, loss of body contours)
 Virilization or masculinization (one third
  of patients) (acne, hirsutism, temporal
  balding, deepening of voice, clitoral
  enlargement)

DIAGNOSTIC APPROACH

Differential Diagnosis:
 Adrenal virilizing tumors
 Benign adnexal masses (corpus luteum, follic-
  ular cyst)
 Endometriosis
 Hydrosalpinx
 Paratubal cyst
 Appendiceal abscess
 Ectopic pregnancy
 Pedunculated leiomyomata
 Pelvic or horseshoe kidney
 Nongynecologic pelvic masses

Associated Conditions: Virilization, hirsutism, clitoral enlargement.

Workup and Evaluation

Laboratory: As indicated before surgery. Plasma levels of testosterone, androstenedione, and other androgens may be elevated; urinary 17-ketosteroid values are usually normal. (Androgen secretion by the tumor may result in erythrocytosis.) Laboratory studies cannot reliably differentiate between virilization caused by adrenal tumors and virilization caused by ovarian sources.

Imaging: Preoperative evaluation (CT or ultrasonography) for possible lymph node enlargement or intraabdominal spread is indicated for patients in whom malignancy is a significant possibility.

Special Tests: None indicated.

Diagnostic Tests: History, physical examination, and imaging. Final diagnosis is established by histologic evaluation.

Pathologic Findings

Variable gross appearance. Sex cord (Sertoli) cells and stromal (Leydig) cells are present in varying proportion, but tubular patterns predominate. Individual cells may appear immature. Lipochrome pigments (crystalloids of Reinke) are present in 20% of tumors. These tumors may be hard to differentiate from granulosa cell tumors and may mimic endometrioid or Krukenberg tumors. Eighty percent of tumors are stage IA at discovery.

MANAGEMENT AND THERAPY

Nonpharmacologic

General Measures: Evaluation, supportive therapy based on symptoms.

Specific Measures: Surgical exploration and resection. Young patients with stage 1A disease may be treated with unilateral salpingo-oophorectomy. Undifferentiated tumors or advanced stage disease requires more aggressive surgical resection and may be treated with adjunctive chemotherapy (vincristine, actinomycin D, and cyclophosphamide) or radiation.

Diet: No specific dietary changes indicated.

Activity: No restriction.

Patient Education: American College of Obstetricians and Gynecologists Patient Education Pamphlet AP096 (*Cancer of the Ovary*), AP075 (*Ovarian Cysts*).

Drug(s) of Choice

Vincristine (1.5 mg/m² IV weekly for 12 weeks), actinomycin D, and cyclophosphamide (0.5 mg of actinomycin D + 5–7 mg/kg/d of cyclophosphamide, IV daily for 5 days every 4 weeks). Adjunctive or symptomatic therapy as required.

Precautions: Alkylating agents are associated with an increased risk of future leukemia (10% by 8 years after therapy).

FOLLOW-UP

Patient Monitoring: Careful follow-up and normal health maintenance.

Prevention/Avoidance: None.

Possible Complications: Disease progression or spread (<20%). In advanced stage disease, recurrence within 1 year in two thirds of patients.

Expected Outcome: These tumors behave as low-grade malignancies and have 5-year survivals of 70%–90%. Survival is poorer for higher stage and poorly differentiated tumors. Menses may be anticipated to return approximately 4 weeks after removal of the tumor. Excessive hair often regresses but does not disappear; clitoral enlargement and voice changes (if present) are unlikely to reverse.

MISCELLANEOUS

Pregnancy Considerations: Pregnancy unlikely in the presence of these tumors. No direct effect on the pregnancy, should they coexist. (Hormonal effects on the fetus could be postulated, but tumors with significant hormonal function generally preclude pregnancy.)

ICD-9-CM **Codes:** Based on location and tumor character.

REFERENCES

American College of Obstetricians and Gynecologists. *Cancer of the Ovary.* Washington, DC: ACOG; 1990. ACOG Technical Bulletin 141.

American College of Obstetricians and Gynecologists. *Classification and Staging of Gynecologic Malignancies.* Washington, DC: ACOG; 1991. ACOG Technical Bulletin 155.

Fleischer AC. Transabdominal and transvaginal sonography of ovarian masses. *Clin Obstet Gynecol* 1991;34:433.

Young RH, Scully RE. Ovarian Sertoli-Leydig cell tumors: a clinicopathological analysis of 207 cases. *Am J Surg Pathol* 1985;9:543.

Young RH, Scully RE. Sex cord-stromal, steroid cell, and other ovarian tumors with endocrine, paraendocrine, and paraneoplastic manifestations. In: Kurman RJ, ed. *Blaustein's Pathology of the Female Genital Tract.* 4th ed. New York, NY: Springer-Verlag; 1994:626.

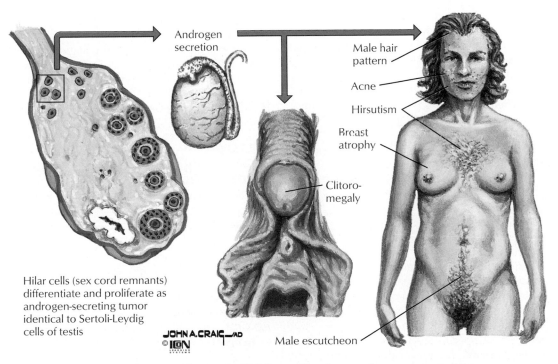

Androgen secretion

Male hair pattern

Acne

Hirsutism

Breast atrophy

Clitoro-megaly

Hilar cells (sex cord remnants) differentiate and proliferate as androgen-secreting tumor identical to Sertoli-Leydig cells of testis

JOHN A.CRAIG—AD
©ICON

Male escutcheon

Excessive androgen production results in loss of female secondary sex characteristics

ADNEXAL DISEASE

TRANSITIONAL CELL (BRENNER) TUMOR

INTRODUCTION

Description: An epithelial tumor that is made up of cells that resemble urothelium and Walthard's cell nests, intermixed with the ovarian stroma. Most are benign.

Prevalence: One percent to three percent of ovarian tumors.

Predominant Age: 40–80, average 50.

Genetics: No genetic pattern.

ETIOLOGY AND PATHOGENESIS

Causes: Unknown. Most are derived from ovarian surface epithelium that undergoes metaplasia to form the typical urothelial-like components.

Risk Factors: None known.

CLINICAL CHARACTERISTICS

Signs and Symptoms:

Asymptomatic (often an incidental finding after oophorectomy)

Adnexal mass, generally solid, most smaller than 2 cm, bilateral in 6% (unilateral lesions are more common in the left ovary)

Abdominal pain and swelling, with abnormal uterine bleeding (20%) if malignant disease (malignant masses are more likely to be large [10–30 cm] and contain cystic areas; when the ovary is paplably enlarged, the risk of malignancy is approximately 5%)

DIAGNOSTIC APPROACH

Differential Diagnosis:

Thecoma (fibroma)

Stromal and germ cell tumors

Endometrioma

Benign cystic teratoma

Serous or mucinous cystadenoma

Metastatic tumors

Pedunculated leiomyomata

Associated Conditions: Malignant tumors are associated with endometrial hyperplasia.

Workup and Evaluation

Laboratory: No specific evaluation indicated.

Imaging: No imaging indicated. Ultrasonography may be used to differentiate solid and cystic adnexal masses but does not establish the diagnosis.

Special Tests: None indicated.

Diagnostic Tests: Histopathologic evaluation.

Pathologic Findings

Cells that resemble transitional epithelium of the bladder and Walthard's cells of the ovary with abundant stroma. The cut surface of the tumor is generally whorled or lobulated. The nests of cells often demonstrate nuclei with obvious nucleoli containing longitudinal grooves, which gives them a "coffee-bean" appearance. Atypia and mitoses are rare. Occasionally, small transitional cell tumors may be found in the walls of otherwise typical mucinous cystademonas. Atypical or malignant forms may be associated with similar bladder tumors.

MANAGEMENT AND THERAPY

Nonpharmacologic

General Measures: Evaluation and diagnosis.

Specific Measures: Simple surgical excision. When changes associated with borderline malignant potential are present, bilateral oophorectomy with hysterectomy is sufficient, and unilateral oophorectomy may be considered in younger patients.

Diet: No specific dietary changes indicated.

Activity: No restriction.

Patient Education: Reassurance, American College of Obstetricians and Gynecologists Patient Education Pamphlet AP075 (*Ovarian Cysts*), AP096 (*Cancer of the Ovary*).

Drug(s) of Choice

None.

FOLLOW-UP

Patient Monitoring: Normal health maintenance.

Prevention/Avoidance: None.

Possible Complications: The rare malignant form has a poor prognosis despite surgical therapy. Chemotherapy has not been proven to be effective.

Expected Outcome: Most Brenner tumors are benign and are cured by simple oophorectomy.

MISCELLANEOUS

Pregnancy Considerations: No effect on pregnancy.

ICD-9-CM Codes: 220, 236.2 (Borderline or proliferative), 183.0 (Malignant).

REFERENCES

Austin RM, Norris HJ. Malignant Brenner tumors and transitional cell carcinoma of the ovary. *Int J Gynecol Pathol* 1987;6:29.

Miles PA, Norris HJ. Proliferative and malignant Brenner tumors of the ovary. *Cancer* 1972;30:174.

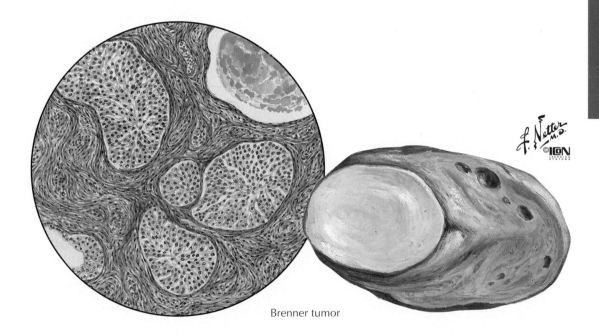

Brenner tumor

Roth LM, Czernobilsky B. Ovarian Brenner tumors. II: Malignant. *Cancer* 1985;56:592.

Roth LM, Dallenbach-Hellweg G, Czernobilsky B. Ovarian Brenner tumors. I: Metaplastic, proliferating and of low malignant potential. *Cancer* 1985;56:582.

Roth LM, Gershell DJ, Ulbright TM. Ovarian Brenner tumors and transitional cell carcinoma: recent developments. *Int J Gynecol Pathol* 1993;12:128.

Russell P. Surface epithelial-stromal tumors of the ovary. In: Kurman RJ, ed. *Blaustein's Pathology of the Female Genital Tract.* 4th ed. New York, NY: Springer-Verlag; 1994, 762.

Silverberg SG. Brenner tumor of the ovary. A clinico-pathologic study of 60 tumors in 54 women. *Cancer* 1971;28:588.

Breast Diseases and Conditions

BREAST: ACCESSORY NIPPLES

INTRODUCTION

Description: Supernumerary nipples found along defined developmental lines known as the "milk lines."

Prevalence: Seen in 0.22%–2.5% of women.

Predominant Age: Congenital in origin.

Genetics: No genetic pattern.

ETIOLOGY AND PATHOGENESIS

Causes: Developmental abnormality.

Risk Factors: More common in males and in blacks.

CLINICAL CHARACTERISTICS

Signs and Symptoms:

Asymptomatic

Most commonly found below a normal left breast. Patients with one or more extra nipples (polythelia) are more common than those with true accessory breasts (polymastia).

DIAGNOSTIC APPROACH

Differential Diagnosis:

Skin papilloma

Nevis

Associated Conditions: Polymastia, duplicate renal arteries.

Workup and Evaluation

Laboratory: No evaluation indicated.

Imaging: No imaging indicated.

Special Tests: None indicated.

Diagnostic Procedures: History, physical examination.

Pathologic Findings

None.

MANAGEMENT AND THERAPY

Nonpharmacologic

General Measures: Evaluation and reassurance.

Specific Measures: None.

Diet: No specific dietary changes indicated.

Activity: No restriction.

Patient Education: Reassurance, instruction on monthly breast self-examination, American College of Obstetricians and Gynecologists Patient Education Pamphlet AP026 (*Detecting and Treating Breast Problems*).

Drug(s) of Choice

None.

FOLLOW-UP

Patient Monitoring: Normal health maintenance.

Prevention/Avoidance: None.

MISCELLANEOUS

Pregnancy Considerations: No effect on pregnancy, although occasionally accessory nipples undergo hypertrophy during pregnancy.

ICD-9-CM Codes: 757.6.

REFERENCES

American College of Obstetricians and Gynecologists. *Nonmalignant Conditions of the Breast.* Washington, DC: ACOG; 1991. ACOG Technical Bulletin 156.

Sapira JD. *The Art and Science of Bedside Diagnosis.* Baltimore, Md: Williams & Wilkins; 1990:239.

Smith RP. *Gynecology in Primary Care.* Baltimore, Md: Williams & Wilkins; 1997:319.

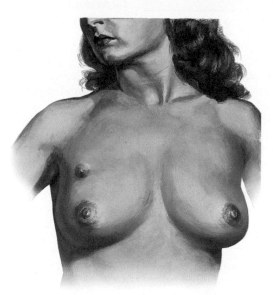

Polythelia

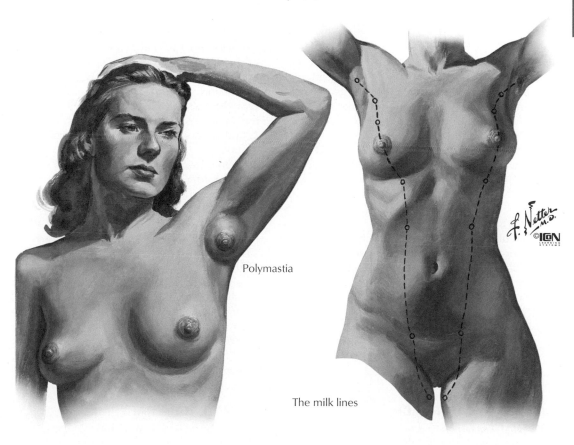

Polymastia

The milk lines

BREAST: CANCER

INTRODUCTION

Description: Malignant neoplasm of the breast classified by cell type, location and degree of invasion. Breast cancer is the most common malignancy of women, accounting for almost one third of all women's malignancies. Breast cancer accounts for approximately 18% of cancer deaths and results in about the same number of deaths per year as auto accidents.

Prevalence: Lifetime risk of 1 in 10, 185,000 new cases, 48,000 deaths annually. Roughly one new case of breast cancer is diagnosed every 3 minutes and every 11 minutes there is a breast cancer death.

Predominant Age: Of all breast cancer, 85% occurs after 40 and 75% after 50.

Genetics: Women with BRCA-1 mutations have a 60% lifetime risk of breast cancer. Only 20% of breast cancer patients have a family history of breast cancer.

ETIOLOGY AND PATHOGENESIS

Causes: Unknown.

Risk Factors: First-degree relative with breast cancer (relative risk [RR] = 2.3, RR = 10.5 with bilateral disease), moderate alcohol use (>3–5 drinks/day, RR = 1.41), early menarche, late menopause, nulliparity or late first pregnancy (>30 years), prior history of breast cancer (5%/yr), estrogen use (RR = 1.12). Only 21% of patients with breast cancer aged 30 to 54 years are identified by risk factors.

CLINICAL CHARACTERISTICS

Signs and Symptoms:
Palpable mass (55%), 60% located in the upper outer quadrant of the breast
Abnormal mammogram without a palpable mass (35%)
Skin change—color or dimpling (*peau d'orange*)
Nipple retraction (nipple discharge [bloody or otherwise], skin changes, or ulceration are late occurrences and portend a bad prognosis)
Axillary mass

DIAGNOSTIC APPROACH

Differential Diagnosis:
Benign breast disease (abscess, fat necrosis, fibrocystic disease, fibroadenomas).

Associated Conditions: Metastatic spread to other organs (bone, brain, and ovaries).

Workup and Evaluation

Laboratory: Complete blood count and assessment of liver and bone enzymes once diagnosis is made.

Imaging: Mammography (detects 80% of all tumors), ultrasonography (may help to differentiate between solid and cystic masses), bone scan, and chest radiograph after diagnosis is established.

Special Tests: Fine needle aspiration (FNA) of cells from a breast mass can provide histologic confirmation of malignancy and help direct definitive therapy.

Diagnostic Procedures: One quarter of all breast cancers are found during routine examination. Excisional biopsy with or without radiographic control provides the only definitive diagnosis.

Pathologic Findings

Based on cell type. At the time of diagnosis, 70% of breast cancers show signs of invasion.

MANAGEMENT AND THERAPY

Nonpharmacologic

General Measures: Evaluation and staging. If surgical treatment affects pectoralis muscles, physical or occupational therapy may speed return to function.

Specific Measures: Surgical resection with or without adjunctive chemotherapy.

Diet: Moderation in alcohol use recommended to reduce risk.

Activity: No restriction.

Patient Education: Instruction on monthly breast self-examination, American College of Obstetricians and Gynecologists Patient Education Pamphlet AP026 (*Detecting and Treating Breast Problems*), AP076 (*Mammography*).

Drug(s) of Choice

Adjuvant chemotherapy considered for stage I and II disease (cyclophosphamide, methotrexate, fluorouracil, anthracyclines, or taxanes, single agent or in combination).

Contraindications: Strict guidelines for hepatic and renal function before chemotherapy.

Precautions: Increased risk of infection during chemotherapy.

ALTERNATIVE THERAPY

Adjunctive or palliative radiation therapy is often recommended. Agents that suppress cancer growth by interfering with surface proteins that are involved with cell division are now under development. An example of this approach is trastuzumab (Herceptin), approved by the Food and Drug Administration (FDA) in 1998.

A large number of studies suggest that estrogen therapy (for other indications) may actually reduce the mortality of patients who are being treated for breast cancer.

FOLLOW-UP

Patient Monitoring: Watch for recurrence (60% risk in first 5 years).

Prevention/Avoidance: Reduced dietary fat and alcohol have been suggested but are unproven. Prophylactic use of tamoxifen is under study and was approved by the FDA late in 1998 for use in high-risk women. Routine mammography.

Possible Complications: Postoperative lymphedema, seroma, wound infections, or breakdown. Chemotherapy associated with nausea, vomiting, alopecia, leukopenia, stomatitis, fatigue, and infections. Tamoxifen therapy associated with hot flashes, menstrual irregularity, endometrial hyperplasia, or carcinoma. Radiation therapy associated with fibrosis and scarring, brachial neuropathy, and pulmonary fibrosis.

Expected Outcome: Breast cancer disseminates by vascular and lymphatic routes, in addition to direct infiltration. There is also a growing trend to view breast cancer as a multifocal disease. Breast cancer survival depends less on cell type than it does on the size of the tumor and stage of disease. Ten-year survival based on stage: stage I 95%; stage II 40%; stage III 15%; stage IV (metastatic), 0%.

MISCELLANEOUS

Pregnancy Considerations: Breast cancer occurs infrequently during pregnancy, accounting for only 2%–3% of all cancers: No effect on pregnancy. Pregnancy often results in a delay in diagnosis but does not appreciably affect clinical course.

ICD-9-CM Codes: 174.

Clinical Signs of Cancer

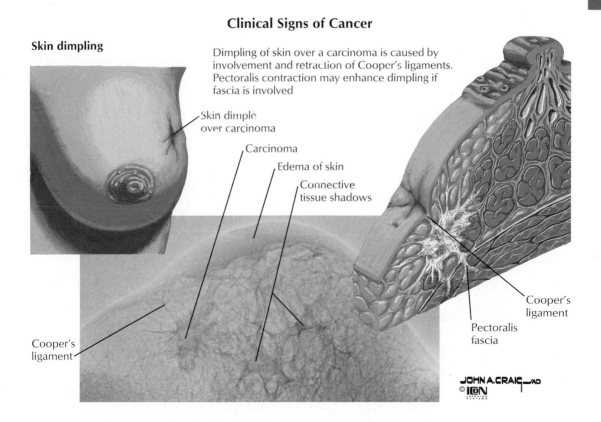

Skin dimpling

Dimpling of skin over a carcinoma is caused by involvement and retraction of Cooper's ligaments. Pectoralis contraction may enhance dimpling if fascia is involved

Skin dimple over carcinoma

Carcinoma

Edema of skin

Connective tissue shadows

Cooper's ligament

Cooper's ligament

Pectoralis fascia

JOHN A. CRAIG—AD
©ICON

Needle Biopsy

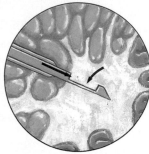

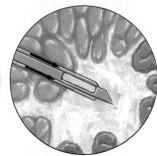

Disposable
biopsy needle

Cannula

Obturator

Lesion

1. Closed needle assembly is
advanced to edge of lesion

2. Obturator tip is advanced
into lesion. Tissue prolapses
into open specimen notch

3. Cannula is advanced over
obturator, entrapping tissue
specimen within notch. Needle
is withdrawn

Vascular signs

Skin edema

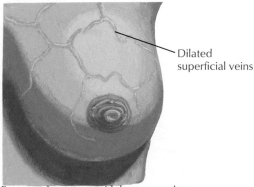

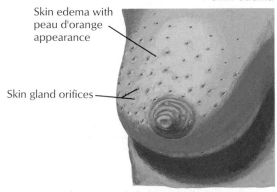

Dilated
superficial veins

Skin edema with
peau d'orange
appearance

Skin gland orifices

Fast-growing tumor with large vascular
demand may cause dilatation of superficial
veins, creating prominent vascular pattern
over breast

Involvement and obstruction of subcutaneous
lymphatics by tumor result in lymphatic dilatation
and lymph accumulation in the skin. Resultant
edema creates "orange peel" appearance due to
prominence of skin gland orifices

REFERENCES

American College of Obstetricians and Gynecologists. *Carcinoma of the Breast.* Washington, DC: ACOG; 1991. ACOG Technical Bulletin 158.

Breast cancer screening guidelines agreed on by AMA, other medically related organizations [medical news and perspectives]. *JAMA* 1989;262:1155.

Butler JA, Vargas HI, Worthen N, Wilson SE. Accuracy of combined clinical-mammographic-cytologic diagnosis of dominant breast masses: a prospective study. *Arch Surg* 1990;125:893.

Fletcher SW, Black W, Harris R, Rimer BK, Shapiro S. *Report of the International Workshop on Screening for Breast Cancer.* Bethesda, Md: National Cancer Institute; 1993.

Harris JR, Lippman ME, Veronesi U, Willett W. Breast cancer. *N Engl J Med* 1992;327:319, 390, 473.

Marchant DJ, Sutton SM. Use of mammography—United States 1990. *MMWR Morb Mortal Wkly Rep* 1990;39:621.

BREAST: CYSTS

THE CHALLENGE

Cystic breast masses are frequently encountered in the clinical care of women. Sorting out those that represent a threat from those that may be followed conservatively is the challenge posed by the presence of breast cysts.

Scope of the Problem: Some authors estimate that cysts form in the breasts of roughly 50% of women during their reproductive years. Roughly one in four women require medical attention for some form of breast problem; often this takes the form of a palpable mass. The most common cause of a palpable breast cyst is fibrocystic change, which is estimated to be found in one third to three quarters of all women. Dilation of ducts and complications of breast-feeding (galactoceles, abscess) may also cause cysts.

Objectives: To appropriately diagnose and treat patients with a cystic breast, to allay fear and protect health.

TACTICS

Relevant Pathophysiology: The pathogenesis is not clear for the most common types of cystic change (those associated with fibrocystic change). Cyclic changes in hormones induce stromal and epithelial changes that may lead to fibrosis and cyst formation. Cysts may be single or be found in clusters, with some up to 4 cm in diameter. Small cysts have a firm character and are filled with clear fluid, giving the cyst a bluish cast. Larger cysts may have a brown color resulting from hemorrhage into the cyst. Inspissated secretions or milk may form a cystic dilation of ducts (galactocele, ductal ectasia) that may be palpable as a cystic mass. Variable degrees of fibrosis and inflammation may be seen in the surrounding stroma. (Leakage of cyst fluid into the surrounding tissue induces an inflammatory response that may alter physical findings and imitate cancer.) The microscopic findings associated with breast cysts depend on the pathophysiologic changes involved.

Strategies: The diagnosis and management of cystic masses in the breast are based on history, physical examination, and aspiration, with the occasional adjunctive use of mammography and ultrasonography. (Ultrasonography is useful in differentiating solid and cystic breast masses, but it has limited spatial resolution and cannot be used to differentiate benign and malignant tissues.) Needle aspiration with a 22- to 25-gauge needle may be both diagnostic and therapeutic. If the cyst disappears completely and does not reform by a 1-month follow-up examination, no further therapy is required. Fluid aspirated from patients with fibrocystic changes is customarily straw colored. Fluid that is dark brown or green occurs in cysts that have been present for a long time, but is also innocuous. Bloody fluid requires further evaluation. Cytologic evaluation of the fluid obtained is of little value. After aspiration of a cyst, the patient should be rechecked in 2–4 weeks. Recurrence of the cyst or the presence of a palpable mass should prompt additional evaluation, such as FNA or open biopsy.

Patient Education: Instruction on monthly breast self-examination, American College of Obstetricians and Gynecologists Patient Education Pamphlet AP026 (*Detecting and Treating Breast Problems*), AP076 (*Mammography*).

IMPLEMENTATION

Special Considerations: Whereas most cystic changes in the breast are not associated with malignancy and are not premalignant, the presence of atypia in any of the cellular components requires special attention because this is associated with a roughly 5-fold increased risk for malignancy. In women older than 35, mammography before aspiration should be considered because of the increased incidence of malignancy. Once aspiration has been attempted, mammography should be delayed several weeks because of artifactual changes induced by the manipulation, making mammograms difficult to interpret. Patients with a history of multiple cysts or diffuse fibrocystic change or a strong family history of breast disease should have close follow-up, including mammography, to delve for other occult lesions.

REFERENCES

American College of Obstetricians and Gynecologists. *Nonmalignant Conditions of the Breast.* Washington, DC: ACOG; 1991. ACOG Technical Bulletin 156.

Donegan WL. Evaluation of a palpable breast mass. *N Engl J Med* 1992;327:937.

Ferguson CM, Powel RW. Breast masses in young women. *Arch Surg* 1989;124:1338.

Seltzer MH, Skiles MS. Disease of the breast in young women. *Surg Gynecol Obstet* 1980;150:360.

Smith RP. *Gynecology in Primary Care.* Baltimore, Md: Williams & Wilkins; 1997:319.

Smith RP, Ling FW. *Procedures in Women's Health.* Baltimore, Md: Williams & Wilkins; 1997:37.

Aspiration

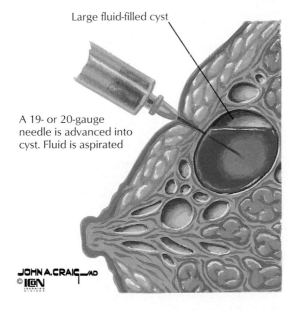

Large fluid-filled cyst

A 19- or 20-gauge
needle is advanced into
cyst. Fluid is aspirated

JOHN A. CRAIG—MD
© ICN

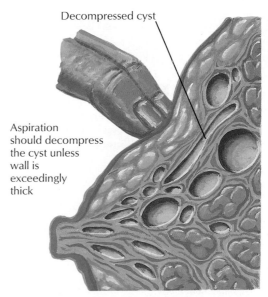

Decompressed cyst

Aspiration
should decompress
the cyst unless
wall is
exceedingly
thick

BREAST: DUCT ECTASIA

INTRODUCTION

Description: Dilation of the ducts of the breast with inspissation of normal secretions, arising from chronic intraductal and periductal inflammation.

Prevalence: Relatively common in asymptomatic form.

Predominant Age: Older than 50.

Genetics: No genetic pattern.

ETIOLOGY AND PATHOGENESIS

Causes: Chronic intraductal and periductal inflammation.

Risk Factors: Mastitis, breast abscess.

CLINICAL CHARACTERISTICS

Signs and Symptoms:
- Thick gray to black nipple discharge
- Pain and nipple tenderness
- Thickening often present; may be difficult to distinguish from cancer (firm, rounded and fixed, with skin retraction)
- Nipple retraction common (ductal ectasia is the most common cause of an acquired nipple inversion)

DIAGNOSTIC APPROACH

Differential Diagnosis:
- Galactocele
- Lipoma
- Fibrocystic change
- Fibroadenoma
- Breast abscess

Associated Conditions: Mastitis, galactocele, and nipple discharge.

Workup and Evaluation

Laboratory: No evaluation indicated.

Imaging: No imaging indicated.

Special Tests: None indicated.

Diagnostic Procedures: History and physical examination; biopsy confirms the diagnosis. (The characteristic discharge may easily be demonstrated during clinical examination.)

Pathologic Findings

Dilation of the ducts with atrophy of the epithelium, thickening of the underlying wall, and inflammatory reaction in the duct wall and surrounding tissue.

MANAGEMENT AND THERAPY

Nonpharmacologic

General Measures: Evaluation and reassurance.

Specific Measures: No further therapy is needed unless warranted by the patient's symptoms. When therapy is required, surgical excision with a cone of tissue surrounding the duct is curative.

Diet: No specific dietary changes indicated.

Activity: No restriction.

Patient Education: Instruction on monthly breast self-examination, American College of Obstetricians and Gynecologists Patient Education Pamphlet AP026 (*Detecting and Treating Breast Problems*), AP076 (*Mammography*).

Drug(s) of Choice

None.

FOLLOW-UP

Patient Monitoring: Normal health maintenance.

Prevention/Avoidance: None.

Possible Complications: Secondary infection and abscess formation.

Expected Outcome: Gradual resolution of symptoms, complete resolution with surgical excision.

MISCELLANEOUS

Pregnancy Considerations: No effect on pregnancy.

ICD-9-CM Codes: 610.4.

REFERENCES

American College of Obstetricians and Gynecologists. *Nonmalignant Conditions of the Breast.* Washington, DC: ACOG; 1991. ACOG Technical Bulletin 156.

Seltzer MH, Skiles MS. Disease of the breast in young women. *Surg Gynecol Obstet* 1980;150:360.

Smith RP. *Gynecology in Primary Care.* Baltimore, Md: Williams & Wilkins; 1997:319.

Mammary Duct Ectasia

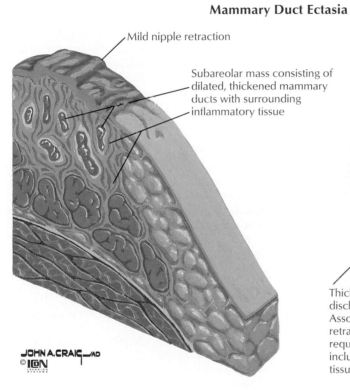

Mild nipple retraction

Subareolar mass consisting of dilated, thickened mammary ducts with surrounding inflammatory tissue

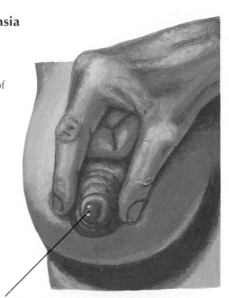

JOHN A.CRAIG—AD
© ICN

Thick, sticky, green to greenish-black discharge suggests mammary duct ectasia. Associated subareolar mass and/or nipple retraction may also be present. Treatment requires major mammary duct excision, including the surrounding inflammatory tissue

BREAST: FAT NECROSIS

INTRODUCTION

Description: Trauma to the breast may result in necrosis of fatty tissues leading to an ill-defined mass that can mimic cancer.

Prevalence: Uncommon.

Predominant Age: Reproductive.

Genetics: No genetic pattern.

ETIOLOGY AND PATHOGENESIS

Causes: Fat necrosis is most often the result of trauma, although the causative event cannot be identified (or recalled) in roughly one half of patients. May also follow surgical intervention in the breast, such as biopsy or augmentation.

Risk Factors: Trauma to the breast.

CLINICAL CHARACTERISTICS

Signs and Symptoms:

Solitary, irregular, ill-defined, tender mass that is easily confused with cancer

Skin retraction sometimes present

Fine, stippled calcification and stellate or infiltrative fibrosis often seen on mammograms

DIAGNOSTIC APPROACH

Differential Diagnosis:

Cancer

Lipoma

Associated Conditions: Mastalgia.

Workup and Evaluation

Laboratory: No evaluation indicated.

Imaging: Mammography findings mimic cancer.

Special Tests: Open biopsy often required to establish the diagnosis.

Diagnostic Procedures: Even with a history of trauma, the commonality of findings between fat necrosis and cancer with physical examination, mammography, and ultrasonography generally mandates further evaluation and biopsy.

Pathologic Findings

Diffuse changes consistent with necrosis and fibrosis of tissue. Hemorrhage and cystic spaces are common. Calcification of older lesions may occur. Histiocytic foam cells with mitotic figures and pleomorphism are common.

MANAGEMENT AND THERAPY

Nonpharmacologic

General Measures: Evaluation.

Specific Measures: Excisional biopsy.

Diet: No specific dietary changes indicated.

Activity: No restriction.

Patient Education: Instruction on monthly breast self-examination, American College of Obstetricians and Gynecologists Patient Education Pamphlet AP026 (*Detecting and Treating Breast Problems*), AP076 (*Mammography*).

Drug(s) of Choice

None.

FOLLOW-UP

Patient Monitoring: Normal health maintenance, periodic mammography screening.

Prevention/Avoidance: Minimize the risk of trauma.

Possible Complications: An occult malignancy may be missed if a mass is presumed to be fat necrosis without tissue evaluation for confirmation.

Expected Outcome: With excision, complete resolution.

MISCELLANEOUS

Pregnancy Considerations: No effect on pregnancy.

ICD-9-CM Codes: 611.3.

REFERENCES

American College of Obstetricians and Gynecologists. *Nonmalignant Conditions of the Breast.* Washington, DC: ACOG; 1991. ACOG Technical Bulletin 156.

Seltzer MH, Skiles MS. Disease of the breast in young women. *Surg Gynecol Obstet* 1980;150:360.

Smith RP. *Gynecology in Primary Care.* Baltimore, Md: Williams & Wilkins; 1997:319.

Fat Necrosis of Breast

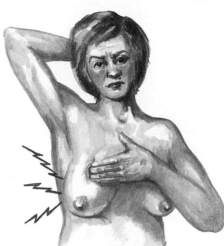

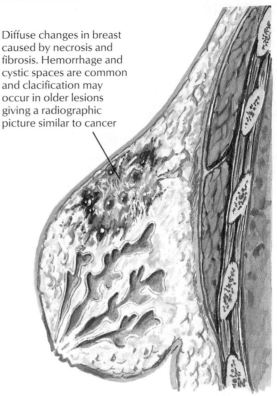

Diffuse changes in breast caused by necrosis and fibrosis. Hemorrhage and cystic spaces are common and clacification may occur in older lesions giving a radiographic picture similar to cancer

Trauma to breast may result in fat necrosis, an ill defined irregular tender mass that may be confused with cancer both clinically and radiographically

JOHN A. CRAIG—AD

D. Mascaro

©ICON

Excision Biopsy for Fat Necrosis

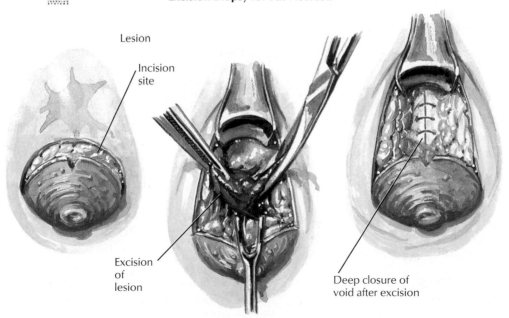

Lesion

Incision site

Excision of lesion

Deep closure of void after excision

Excisional biopsy indicated to confirm diagnosis and rule out cancer

BREAST: FIBROADENOMA

INTRODUCTION

Description: Fibroadenomas are the second most common form of breast disease, and the most common breast mass.

Prevalence: Two percent to three percent of women (some state as many as 25% of all women).

Predominant Age: 21–25, most younger than 30.

Genetics: No genetic pattern.

ETIOLOGY AND PATHOGENESIS

Causes: Unknown.

Risk Factors: Twice as common in blacks (30% of breast complaints), patients with high hormone states (adolescence, pregnancy), and patients receiving unopposed estrogen therapy.

CLINICAL CHARACTERISTICS

Signs and Symptoms:

Firm, painless, mobile, rubbery, solitary breast mass (may grow rapidly during adolescence or in high-estrogen states [pregnancy, estrogen therapy])

Generally discovered incidentally or during breast self-examination and average 2-3 cm in diameter. Fibroadenomas may grow to as large as 6–10 cm.

Multiple fibroadenomas in 15%–20% of patients; bilateral in 10%–20% of patients

Generally undergo no cyclic change

DIAGNOSTIC APPROACH

Differential Diagnosis:

Fibrocystic change

Solitary cyst

Associated Conditions: None.

Workup and Evaluation

Laboratory: No evaluation indicated.

Imaging: Mammography is generally avoided, but can be diagnostic if needed. Breast ultrasonography can distinguish between solid and cystic masses although it is often not required.

Special Tests: FNA of the mass may be performed in the office.

Diagnostic Procedures: History and physical examination.

Pathologic Findings

Centrifugal nodule with sharply circumscribed, fleshy, and homogeneous character, usually spherical or ovoid in shape. Pink or tan-white fibrous whorls bulge from the surface when cut. Hemorrhagic infarcts are common.

MANAGEMENT AND THERAPY

Nonpharmacologic

General Measures: Reassurance and observation may be sufficient for small, asymptomatic tumors.

Specific Measures: Primary therapy is surgical excision, although tamoxifen and danazol have been used.

Diet: No specific dietary changes indicated.

Activity: No restriction.

Patient Education: Instruction on monthly breast self-examination, American College of Obstetricians and Gynecologists Patient Education Pamphlet AP026 (*Detecting and Treating Breast Problems*), AP076 (*Mammography*).

Drug(s) of Choice

Danazol sodium 50–200 mg PO bid (therapy should start during menstruation or pregnancy must be ruled out). Side effects may be significant and recurrence is likely after therapy is discontinued.

Contraindications: Danazol sodium is contraindicated in pregnancy (category X drug). It may also worsen epilepsy, migraine headaches, and cardiac or renal function.

Interactions: Danazol sodium may prolong prothrombin time in patients receiving warfarin.

Alternative Drugs

Tamoxifen has been advocated in some studies.

FOLLOW-UP

Patient Monitoring: Normal health maintenance.

Prevention/Avoidance: Combination oral contraceptives provide some protection when taken for more than 1 year.

Possible Complications: Hemorrhage into the fibroadenoma may result in pain or rapid growth of the tumor. Malignant change is extremely rare.

Expected Outcome: Lesions tend to grow over time without treatment. Prognosis with surgical excision is excellent and fair with medical therapy. After menopause fibroadenomas tend to regress and become hyalinized, but may remain unchanged or grow with estrogen replacement therapy.

MISCELLANEOUS

Pregnancy Considerations: No effect on pregnancy; fibroadenomas may grow rapidly during pregnancy.

ICD-9-CM Codes: 217.

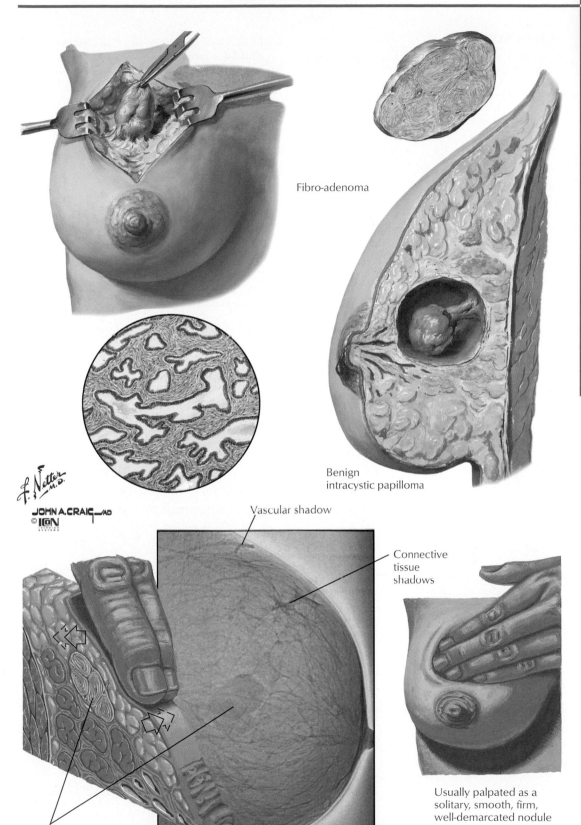

Fibro-adenoma

Benign
intracystic papilloma

Vascular shadow

Connective
tissue
shadows

Fibroadenoma

Usually palpated as a
solitary, smooth, firm,
well-demarcated nodule

REFERENCES

American College of Obstetricians and Gynecologists. *Nonmalignant Conditions of the Breast.* Washington, DC: ACOG; 1991. ACOG Technical Bulletin 156.

Seltzer MH, Skiles MS. Disease of the breast in young women. *Surg Gynecol Obstet* 1980;150:360.

Smith RP. *Gynecology in Primary Care.* Baltimore, Md: Williams & Wilkins; 1997:319.

Yoshida Y, Takaoka M, Fukumoto M. Carcinoma arising in fibroadenoma: case report and review of the world literature. *J Surg Oncol* 1985;29:132.

BREAST: FIBROCYSTIC BREAST CHANGE

INTRODUCTION

Description: Stromal and ductal proliferation that results in cyst formation, diffuse thickening, cyclic pain, and tenderness. The term *fibrocystic change* encompasses a multitude of different processes and older terms, including *fibrocystic disease*. It is the most common of all benign breast conditions, accounting for its linguistic demotion to *change* from the designation *disease*.

Prevalence: Sixty percent to seventy-five percent of all women.

Predominant Age: Most common 30 and 50, 10% of women younger than 21.

Genetics: A family history of fibrocystic change is often present, but causality is difficult to establish.

ETIOLOGY AND PATHOGENESIS

Causes: The cause or causes of fibrocystic change are unknown, but it is postulated to arise from an exaggerated response to hormones. A role for progesterone has been suggested based on the common occurrence of premenstrual breast swelling and tenderness. Other proposed sources for fibrocystic changes are altered ratios of estrogen and progesterone or an increased rate of prolactin secretion, but none of these has been conclusively established.

Risk Factors: Methylxanthine intake has been proposed, but hard data are lacking. There is no evidence that oral contraceptives increase the risk of these changes.

CLINICAL CHARACTERISTICS

Signs and Symptoms:
Asymptomatic (50%)
Cyclic, diffuse, bilateral pain and engorgement, with the worst symptoms occurring just before menses (the pain associated with fibrocystic change often radiates to the shoulders or upper arms)
Multiple cysts and nodules intermixed with scattered bilateral nodularity typical, ropy thickening, especially in the upper outer quadrants of the breast

DIAGNOSTIC APPROACH

Differential Diagnosis:
Fibroadenoma
Carcinoma
Fat necrosis
Lipoma
Associated Conditions: Mastalgia, fibroadenoma.

Workup and Evaluation

Laboratory: No evaluation indicated.

Imaging: Mammography may be used to assist with the diagnosis or to provide a base line, but it is not necessary for diagnosis. Mammography is more difficult in the younger women who predominately have these complaints.

Special Tests: If the patient has a cystic breast mass, needle aspiration with a 22- to 25-gauge needle may be both diagnostic and therapeutic.

Diagnostic Procedures: Diagnosis is based on symptoms and physical findings rather than histologic evaluation.

Pathologic Findings

Fibrocystic changes appear in three steps: (1) proliferation of stroma, especially in the upper outer quadrants of the breast is seen; (2) proliferation of the ducts and alveolar cells occurs, adenosis ensues, and cysts are formed; and (3) larger cysts are found and pain generally decreases. Proliferative changes may be extensive (although usually benign) in any of the involved tissues.

MANAGEMENT AND THERAPY

Nonpharmacologic

General Measures: Mechanical support (a well-fitting brassiere worn day and night), analgesics, and reassurance. Cold compresses or ice may be helpful for acute exacerbations.

Specific Measures: Diuretics (such as spironolactone or hydrochlorothiazide given before menstrual periods), for severe symptoms, danazol, bromocriptine, tamoxifen, or gonadotropin-releasing hormone (GnRH) agonists may be needed. Rarely, patients with intractable pain refractory to medical management may require subcutaneous mastectomy.

Diet: Reduction in methylxanthine intake is often beneficial. Premenstrual restriction of salt or fluids is useful for selected patients. The role of vitamins A and E is unknown.

Activity: No restriction. To reduce discomfort, good breast support is recommended during vigorous activity.

Patient Education: Instruction on monthly breast self-examination, American College of Obstetricians and Gynecologists Patient Education Pamphlet AP026 (*Detecting and Treating Breast Problems*), AP076 (*Mammography*).

Drug(s) of Choice

Combination oral contraceptives (70%–90% success).

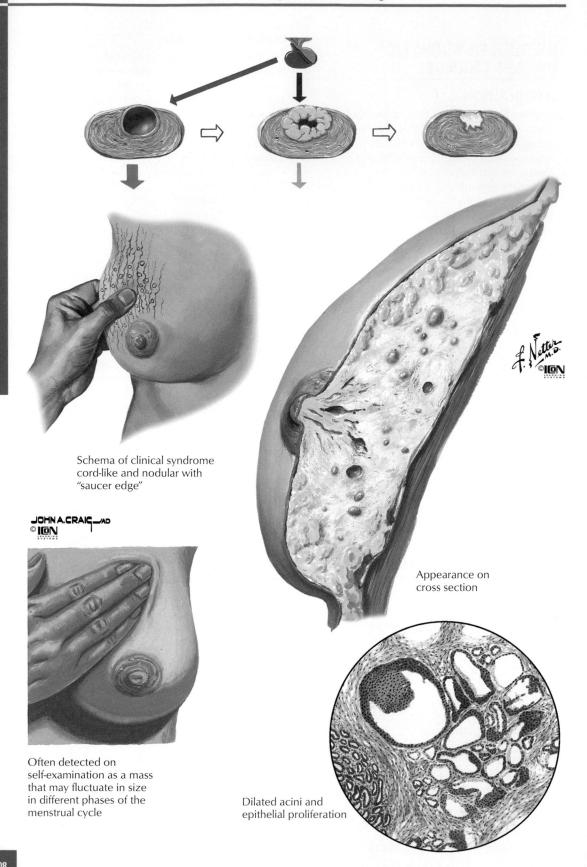

Schema of clinical syndrome
cord-like and nodular with
"saucer edge"

Appearance on
cross section

Often detected on
self-examination as a mass
that may fluctuate in size
in different phases of the
menstrual cycle

Dilated acini and
epithelial proliferation

Spironolactone 50 mg PO bid given 7–10 days before periods).

Danazol sodium 200 mg PO bid (therapy should start during menstruation or pregnancy must be ruled out); side effects may be significant and recurrence is likely after therapy is discontinued.

Bromocriptine 2.5 mg PO qd (with food), may be increased after 3–7 days if needed.

Contraindications: Spironolactone is contraindicated in the presence of anuria, renal insufficiency, or hyperkalemia. Danazol sodium is contraindicated in pregnancy (category X). It may also worsen epilepsy, migraine headaches, and cardiac or renal function. Bromocriptine is contraindicated in patients with uncontrolled hypertension or in those known to be sensitive to ergot alkaloids.

Precautions: Diuretics must be used with care to avoid fluid and electrolyte disturbances. Bromocriptine may cause hypotension during the first several days of therapy. Care should also be exercised with patients who have compromised hepatic or renal function.

Interactions: Spironolactone enhances the action of other diuretics and increases digoxin levels. Danazol sodium may prolong prothrombin time in patients receiving warfarin.

Alternative Drugs

Hydrochlorothiazide 25 mg PO qhs for 7–10 days before menses. GnRH agonists (Lupron 3.75 mg IM monthly for no more than 6 months).

FOLLOW-UP

Patient Monitoring: Patients with mastalgia but no dominant mass may be safely rechecked at a different portion of the next menstrual cycle.

After aspiration of a cyst (yielding clear fluid and complete loss of the mass), the patient should be rechecked in 2–4 weeks. Recurrence of the cyst or the presence of a palpable mass should prompt additional evaluation, such as FNA or open biopsy.

Prevention/Avoidance: None.

Possible Complications: When atypia is found in hyperplastic ducts or apocrine cells, there is a 5-fold increase in the risk of development of carcinoma in the future.

Expected Outcome: Symptomatic relief can generally be achieved with a combination of diet changes, analgesics, and specific medications. The underlying pathologic features remain unchanged or progress.

MISCELLANEOUS

Pregnancy Considerations: No effect on pregnancy. The hormonal changes of pregnancy may worsen symptoms.

ICD-9-CM Codes: 610.1.

REFERENCES

American College of Obstetricians and Gynecologists. *Nonmalignant Conditions of the Breast.* Washington, DC: ACOG; 1991. ACOG Technical Bulletin 156.

Boyle CA, Berkowitz GS, LiVolsi VA, et al. Caffeine consumption and fibrocystic breast disease: A case control epidemiologic study. *J Natl Cancer Inst* 1984;72:1015.

Donegan WL. Evaluation of a palpable breast mass. *N Engl J Med* 1992;327:937.

Ferguson CM, Powel RW. Breast masses in young women. *Arch Surg* 1989;124:1338.

Seltzer MH, Skiles MS. Disease of the breast in young women. *Surg Gynecol Obstet* 1980;150:360.

Smith RP. *Gynecology in Primary Care.* Baltimore, Md: Williams & Wilkins; 1997:319.

BREAST: GALACTOCELE

INTRODUCTION

Description: Cystic dilatation of a duct or ducts, with inspissated milk and desquamated epithelial cells, that may become infected, resulting in acute mastitis or an abscess.
Prevalence: Common in asymptomatic form.
Predominant Age: Reproductive.
Genetics: No genetic pattern.

ETIOLOGY AND PATHOGENESIS

Causes: Ductal obstruction and inflammation during or soon after lactation may lead to cystic dilatation of a duct or ducts and the subsequent development of a galactocele. Galactocele is generally associated with nursing, but may on rare occasions be associated with galactorrhea or oral contraceptive use.
Risk Factors: Nursing, mastitis, galactorrhea, and abrupt weaning.

CLINICAL CHARACTERISTICS

Signs and Symptoms:
    Painless mass palpable in the central portion of the breast

DIAGNOSTIC APPROACH

Differential Diagnosis:
    Duct ectasia
    Lipoma
    Fibrocystic change
    Fibroadenoma
    Breast abscess
Associated Conditions: Mastitis, ductal ectasia, and nipple discharge.

Workup and Evaluation

Laboratory: No evaluation indicated.
Imaging: No imaging indicated.
Special Tests: Aspiration produces thick, creamy material.
Diagnostic Procedures: History and physical examination, needle aspiration.

Pathologic Findings

Cystic dilation of ducts with milky white material made of lipid-rich foam cells and ductal epithelial cells, granular eosinophilic secretions, and lipids.

MANAGEMENT AND THERAPY

Nonpharmacologic

General Measures: Evaluation and reassurance.
Specific Measures: No specific therapy is required for a galactocele, and the mass will subside in a few weeks. When uncomplicated by infection, needle aspiration or drainage by gentle pressure is diagnostic and decompression is curative. Excision may be required for recurrences.
Diet: No specific dietary changes indicated.
Activity: No restriction.
Patient Education: Instruction on monthly breast self-examination, American College of Obstetricians and Gynecologists Patient Education Pamphlet AP026 (*Detecting and Treating Breast Problems*), AP029 (*Breast-Feeding Your Baby*), AP076 (*Mammography*).

Drug(s) of Choice

None.

FOLLOW-UP

Patient Monitoring: Normal health maintenance.
Prevention/Avoidance: None.
Possible Complications: Secondary infection and abscess formation.
Expected Outcome: The mass will subside in a few weeks with no therapy.

MISCELLANEOUS

Pregnancy Considerations: No effect on pregnancy.
ICD-9-CM Codes: 611.5.

REFERENCES

American College of Obstetricians and Gynecologists. *Nonmalignant Conditions of the Breast.* Washington, DC: ACOG; 1991. ACOG Technical Bulletin 156.
Seltzer MH, Skiles MS. Disease of the breast in young women. *Surg Gynecol Obstet* 1980;150:360.
Smith RP. *Gynecology in Primary Care.* Baltimore, Md: Williams & Wilkins; 1997:319.
Winker JM. Galactocele of the breast. *Am J Surg* 1964;108:357.

Galactocele

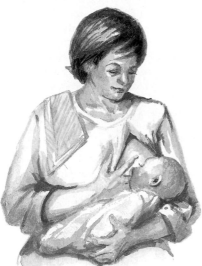

Galactocele results from cystic dilation of mammary duct or ducts filled with inspissated milk and desquamated epithelial cells

Ductal obstruction resulting in galactocele formation usually occurs during or soon after lactation or abrupt weaning

JOHN A.CRAIG—AD
D. Mascaro
©ICN

Normal duct

Clinical Findings

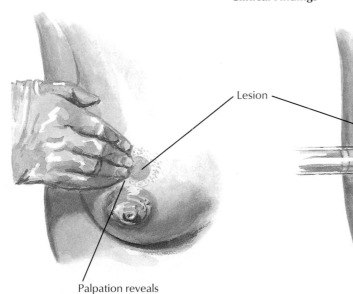

Lesion

Palpation reveals centrally located non-tender mass

Aspiration of breast yields creamlike contents of galactocele and confirms diagnosis

BREAST: INTRADUCTAL PAPILLOMA

INTRODUCTION

Description: Polypoid fibrovascular tumors, covered by benign ductal epithelium that arise in the ducts of the breast.

Prevalence: Found in 0.4% of the general population and up to 20% of women older than 70.

Predominant Age: Median 40, most common just before menopause.

Genetics: No genetic pattern.

ETIOLOGY AND PATHOGENESIS

Causes: Unknown.

Risk Factors: None known.

CLINICAL CHARACTERISTICS

Signs and Symptoms:

Spontaneous, intermittent, bloody, serous, or cloudy unilateral nipple discharge (roughly 50%–75% of patients), varying from a few drops to a few milliliters of fluid (Serosanguineous or bloody nipple discharge is associated with malignancy in between 7% and 17% of cases, but the color or clarity of the fluid cannot diagnose or rule out carcinoma)

Sense of fullness below the nipple, relieved by passage of discharge

Mass rare—tumors from 2 to 5 mm in diameter typically are not palpable

DIAGNOSTIC APPROACH

Differential Diagnosis:

Breast cancer

Galactocele

Ductal ectasia

Fibrocystic change

Associated Conditions: Fibrocystic change, fibroadenoma.

Workup and Evaluation

Laboratory: No evaluation indicated.

Imaging: Ductogram or galactogram is diagnostic.

Special Tests: Cytologic evaluation of the nipple discharge is associated with a false-negative rate of almost 20%, and is therefore of little value.

Diagnostic Procedures: History, physical examination, and excisional biopsy.

Pathologic Findings

A pedunculated proliferation of duct epithelium that generally arises within 1 cm of the areola and rarely is greater than 5 mm in size. The associated duct is generally dilated. The epithelium is friable with a delicate villus structure made up of fibrovascular tissue covered by epithelial cells. Intraductal papilloma be difficult to differentiate from papillary carcinoma, especially on frozen section.

MANAGEMENT AND THERAPY

Nonpharmacologic

General Measures: Evaluation and reassurance.

Specific Measures: Intraductal papillomas are most often benign, but the similarity of symptoms to those of a carcinoma and a sometimes confusing histologic picture mandate excisional biopsy for most patients.

Diet: No specific dietary changes indicated.

Activity: No restriction.

Patient Education: Instruction on monthly breast self-examination, American College of Obstetricians and Gynecologists Patient Education Pamphlet AP026 (*Detecting and Treating Breast Problems*), AP076 (*Mammography*).

Drug(s) of Choice

None.

FOLLOW-UP

Patient Monitoring: Normal health maintenance.

Prevention/Avoidance: None.

Possible Complications: Atypia of the epithelial cells may occur and increases the possibility of malignancy.

Expected Outcome: Surgical excision is both diagnostic and therapeutic.

MISCELLANEOUS

Pregnancy Considerations: No effect on pregnancy.

ICD-9-CM Codes: 611.9.

REFERENCES

American College of Obstetricians and Gynecologists. *Nonmalignant Conditions of the Breast.* Washington, DC: ACOG; 1991. ACOG Technical Bulletin 156.

Devitt JE. Benign disorders of the breast in older women. *Surg Gynecol Obstet* 1986;162:340.

Smith RP. *Gynecology in Primary Care.* Baltimore, Md: Williams & Wilkins; 1997:319.

Stehman FB. Benign neoplasms of the breast. In Hindle WH, ed. *Breast Disease for Gynecologists.* Baltimore, Md: Williams & Wilkins; 1990:168.

Solitary Intraductal Papilloma

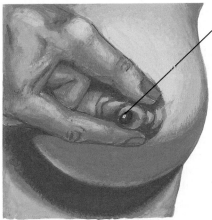

Blood-tinged or brownish
nipple discharge suggests
intraductal papilloma

Single large
papilloma located
within a dilated
mammary duct

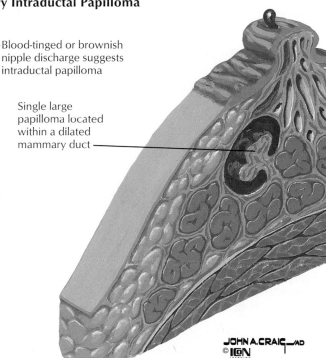

Palpation will often reveal a mass
near the nipple. Duct opening can
be cannulated with a fine probe,
and only involved duct
need be excised

JOHN A.CRAIG—AD
© ICON
LEARNING
SYSTEMS

BREAST: MONDOR'S DISEASE

INTRODUCTION

Description: Mondor's disease, or superficial angiitis, is a superficial thrombophlebitis of the breast.
Prevalence: Uncommon.
Predominant Age: 30–60.
Genetics: No genetic pattern.

ETIOLOGY AND PATHOGENESIS

Causes: Phlebitis is most often linked to recent pregnancy, trauma, or operative procedures, but may occur spontaneously. It most often involves the thoracoepigastric veins of the breast.
Risk Factors: Pregnancy, trauma, or operative procedures.

CLINICAL CHARACTERISTICS

Signs and Symptoms:
Pain (acute, generally upper, outer quadrant)
Dimpling of the skin or a distinct cord with erythematous margins
Shallow groove seen extending upward toward the axilla when the arm is raised

DIAGNOSTIC APPROACH

Differential Diagnosis:
Breast abscess
Duct ectasia
Carcinoma
Mastitis
Fat necrosis
Scarring from previous surgery (biopsy, augmentation, or reduction)
Associated Conditions: Mastitis.

Workup and Evaluation

Laboratory: No evaluation indicated.
Imaging: Mammography may be required to rule out other processes, but the diagnosis is generally established by examination and history.
Special Tests: In some patients, biopsy may be required to establish the diagnosis.
Diagnostic Procedures: History and physical examination. (Accentuation of dimpling, or the formation of a groove over the affected vein, often occurs when the ipsilateral arm is raised during physical examination.)

Pathologic Findings

Thrombophlebitis of the superficial veins.

MANAGEMENT AND THERAPY

Nonpharmacologic

General Measures: Evaluation and reassurance, symptomatic therapy.
Specific Measures: Analgesics and heat reduces symptoms. The condition generally resolves in 2–3 weeks, but it may take 6 weeks or longer.
Diet: No specific dietary changes indicated.
Activity: No restriction. Good support improves comfort during vigorous activity.
Patient Education: Instruction on monthly breast self-examination, American College of Obstetricians and Gynecologists Patient Education Pamphlet AP026 (*Detecting and Treating Breast Problems*), AP029 (*Breast-Feeding Your Baby*), AP076 (*Mammography*).

Drug(s) of Choice

Nonsteroidal antiinflammatory agents. (Antibiotics and anticoagulants have little effect on the course of the disease and are not indicated.)

FOLLOW-UP

Patient Monitoring: Normal health maintenance.
Prevention/Avoidance: Avoidance of breast trauma.
Possible Complications: Unlikely.
Expected Outcome: Mondor's disease is self-limited, although full resolution may take 8–10 weeks.

MISCELLANEOUS

Pregnancy Considerations: No effect on pregnancy.
ICD-9-CM Codes: 451.89.

REFERENCES

American College of Obstetricians and Gynecologists. *Nonmalignant Conditions of the Breast.* Washington, DC: ACOG; 1991. ACOG Technical Bulletin 156.
Camiel MR. Mondor's disease in the breast. *Am J Obstet Gynecol* 1985;152:879.
Drukker BH. The diagnosis and management of breast disease. In: Sciarra JJ, ed. *Gynecology and Obstetrics.* Vol 1. Philadelphia, Pa: JB Lippincott; 1993;26:10.
Duff P. Mondor's disease in pregnancy. *Obstet Gynecol* 1981;58:117.
Haagensen CD. Thrombophlebitis of the superficial veins of the breast (Mondor's disease). In: Haagensen CD, ed. *Disease of the Breast.* Philadelphia, Pa: WB Saunders, 1986:379.
Hindle WH. *Breast Disease for Gynecologists.* East Norwalk, Conn: Appleton & Lange; 1990:154, 199.
Seltzer MH, Skiles MS. Disease of the breast in young women. *Surg Gynecol Obstet* 1980;150:360.

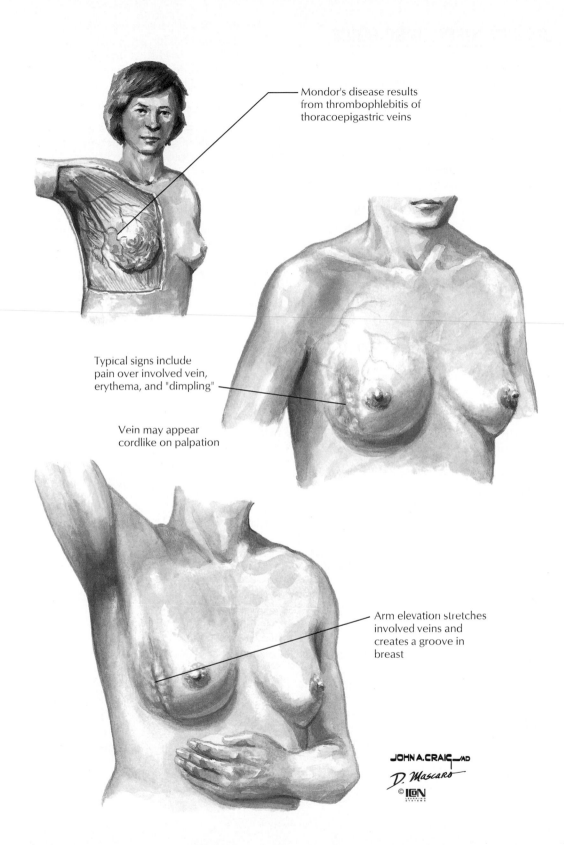

Mondor's disease results
from thrombophlebitis of
thoracoepigastric veins

Typical signs include
pain over involved vein,
erythema, and "dimpling"

Vein may appear
cordlike on palpation

Arm elevation stretches
involved veins and
creates a groove in
breast

JOHN A. CRAIG—MD

D. Mascaro

©ICN

BREAST: NIPPLE DISCHARGE

INTRODUCTION

Description: A distressing symptom that accounts for roughly 5% of breast complaints.

Prevalence: Three percent to five percent of breast problems, 5% of nonlactating women, >50% of women can express secretions.

Predominant Age: Reproductive (based on pathophysiologic changes).

Genetics: No genetic pattern.

ETIOLOGY AND PATHOGENESIS

Causes: Based on underlying pathophysiologic changes.

Risk Factors: See individual pathologic conditions.

CLINICAL CHARACTERISTICS

Signs and Symptoms:

Spontaneous, continuous, or intermittent release of fluid from one or both breasts that may be milky, bloody, serous, serosanguinous, or cloudy (most physiologic discharge is white or green, clear, or yellow; serosanguineous or bloody nipple discharge is associated with malignancy in between 7% and 17% of cases, but the color or clarity of the fluid cannot diagnose or rule out carcinoma)

DIAGNOSTIC APPROACH

Differential Diagnosis:

Breast cancer

Intraductal papilloma

Galactocele

Ductal ectasia (associated with burning, itching, or local discomfort in older patients)

Fibrocystic change

Mastitis

Associated Conditions: Fibrocystic change, fibroadenoma.

Workup and Evaluation

Laboratory: Cytologic evaluation of the nipple discharge is associated with a false-negative rate of almost 20% and is therefore of little value. A simple fat stain of the discharge confirms the physiologic character of the discharge (milk).

Imaging: Ductogram or galactogram may be diagnostic; mammography may be of assistance in evaluation

Special Tests: Surgical excision of the involved duct may be required for diagnosis and treatment.

Roughly 25% of patients who undergo operations are found to have a malignancy.

Diagnostic Procedures: History and physical examination often differentiates between physiologic discharge and breast disease.

Pathologic Findings

Based on the pathophysiologic condition involved. Multiple papillomas or atypia suggest an increased risk for cancer.

MANAGEMENT AND THERAPY

Nonpharmacologic

General Measures: Evaluation and reassurance.

Specific Measures: Surgical excision of the affected duct or other pathologic process.

Diet: No specific dietary changes indicated.

Activity: No restriction.

Patient Education: Instruction on monthly breast self-examination, American College of Obstetricians and Gynecologists Patient Education Pamphlet AP026 (*Detecting and Treating Breast Problems*), AP076 (*Mammography*).

Drug(s) of Choice

None.

FOLLOW-UP

Patient Monitoring: Normal health maintenance.

Prevention/Avoidance: None.

Possible Complications: Failure to consider the possibility of significant disease may result in delay of diagnosis and treatment.

Expected Outcome: Surgical excision of the involved duct may be required for diagnosis and treatment.

MISCELLANEOUS

Pregnancy Considerations: No effect on pregnancy.

ICD-9-CM Codes: 611.79.

REFERENCES

American College of Obstetricians and Gynecologists. *Nonmalignant Conditions of the Breast*. Washington, DC: ACOG; 1991. ACOG Technical Bulletin 156.

Devitt JE. Benign disorders of the breast in older women. *Surg Gynecol Obstet* 1986;162:340.

Isaacs JH. Other nipple discharge. *Clin Obstet Gynecol* 1994;37:898.

Seltzer MH, Skiles MS. Disease of the breast in young women. *Surg Gynecol Obstet* 1980;150:360.

Smith RP. *Gynecology in Primary Care*. Baltimore, Md: Williams & Wilkins; 1997:319.

Clinical Considerations

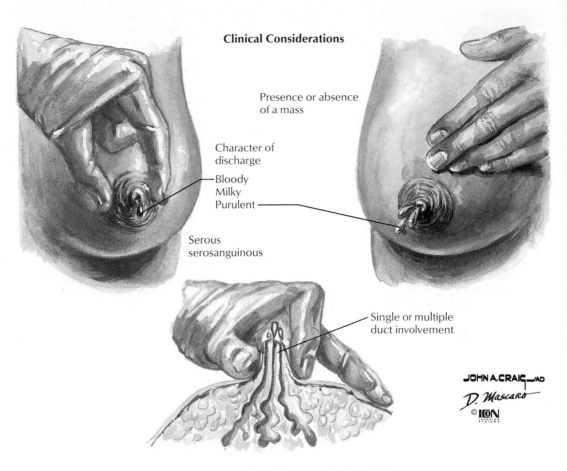

Presence or absence
of a mass

Character of
discharge
Bloody
Milky
Purulent

Serous
serosanguinous

Single or multiple
duct involvement

JOHN A. CRAIG—AD
D. Mascaro
© ICON

Management Algorithm For Nipple Discharge

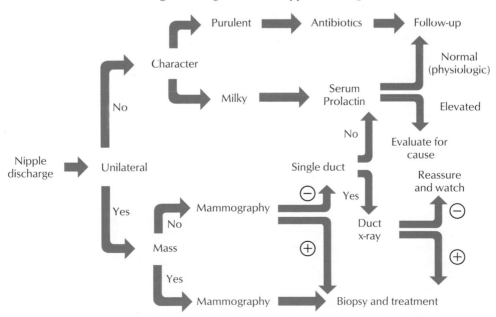

Nipple discharge → Unilateral

Character → Purulent → Antibiotics → Follow-up

Character → Milky → Serum Prolactin → Normal (physiologic) / Elevated → Evaluate for cause

Serum Prolactin → No → Single duct → Yes / No → Duct x-ray

Unilateral → No → Character

Unilateral → Yes → Mass

Mass → No → Mammography → ⊖ / ⊕

Mass → Yes → Mammography → Biopsy and treatment

Duct x-ray → ⊖ → Reassure and watch

Duct x-ray → ⊕ → Biopsy and treatment

BREAST: PAIN (MASTODYNIA, MASTALGIA)

INTRODUCTION

Description: Mastalgia is the nonspecific term used for breast pain of any etiology.

Prevalence: Most women experience breast pain at some point in their lives (may be transient).

Predominant Age: Reproductive.

Genetics: No genetic pattern.

ETIOLOGY AND PATHOGENESIS

Causes: Fibrocystic change. Rapid hormonal change (especially a change that involves a rise in estrogen levels, such as starting birth control pills or hormone replacement or pregnancy). In the absence of obvious pathologic changes, mastalgia has been attributed to caffeine consumption and high-fat diets, but hard data are lacking. Nongynecologic causes—dorsal radiculitis or inflammatory changes in the costochondral junction (Tietze's syndrome), sclerosing adenosis, chest wall muscle spasms, costochondritis, neuritis, fibromyalgia, and referred pain.

Risk Factors: Pregnancy, hormone therapy. Caffeine consumption and high-fat diets have been suggested but remain unconfirmed causes.

CLINICAL CHARACTERISTICS

Signs and Symptoms:

Diffuse breast pain, often with radiation to the shoulders or upper arms, which may or may not be related to the menstrual cycle
Unilateral or localized pain suggests a pathologic process

DIAGNOSTIC APPROACH

Differential Diagnosis:

Fibrocystic change (most commonly present as cyclic, diffuse, bilateral pain and engorgement, with the worst symptoms occurring just before menses)
Mastitis or breast abscess
Trauma
Chest wall abnormalities (herpes zoster, costochondritis, radicular pain)
Breast cancer (breast pain is a presenting complaint in less than 10% of patients with breast cancer)

Associated Conditions: Fibrocystic change, fibroadenoma, and mastitis.

Workup and Evaluation

Laboratory: No evaluation indicated.

Imaging: Mammography may be indicated for other reasons but seldom directly assists in the evaluation of mastalgia.

Special Tests: None indicated.

Diagnostic Procedures: History and physical examination. The presence of scattered bilateral nodularity suggests fibrocystic change.

Pathologic Findings

Based on pathophysiologic changes present.

MANAGEMENT AND THERAPY

Nonpharmacologic

General Measures: Analgesics, mechanical support (a well-fitting brassiere worn day and night), local heat, reassurance.

Specific Measures: Caffeine restriction, medical treatment of underlying pathophysiologic changes (eg, fibrocystic change).

Diet: A reduction in methylxanthine intake is often beneficial. Premenstrual restriction of salt or fluids is recommended for selected patients. The role of vitamins A and E is unknown.

Activity: No restriction. To reduce discomfort, good breast support is recommended during vigorous activity.

Patient Education: Instruction on monthly breast self-examination, American College of Obstetricians and Gynecologists Patient Education Pamphlet AP026 (*Detecting and Treating Breast Problems*), AP076 (*Mammography*).

Drug(s) of Choice

Combination oral contraceptives (70%–90% success)
Spironolactone 50 mg PO bid given 7–10 days before periods
Danazol sodium 200 mg PO bid (therapy should start during menstruation or pregnancy must be ruled out); side effects may be significant and recurrence is likely after therapy is discontinued
Bromocriptine 2.5 mg PO qd (with food), may be increased after 3–7 days if needed

Contraindications: Spironolactone is contraindicated in the presence of anuria, renal insufficiency, or hyperkalemia. Danazol sodium is contraindicated in pregnancy (category X). It may also worsen epilepsy, migraine headaches, and cardiac or renal function. Bromocriptine is contraindicated in patients with uncontrolled hypertension or in patients known to be sensitive to ergot alkaloids.

Precautions: Diuretics must be used with care to avoid fluid and electrolyte disturbances.

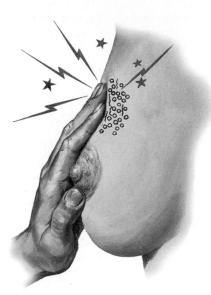

Schema of
clinical syndrome:
tender, granular swelling

Chronic cystic mastitis

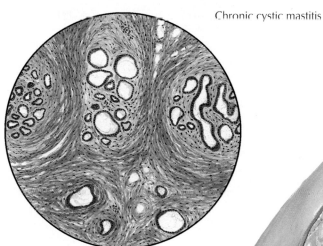

Microscopic aspect
(stunted lobules in proliferating
fibrous stroma)

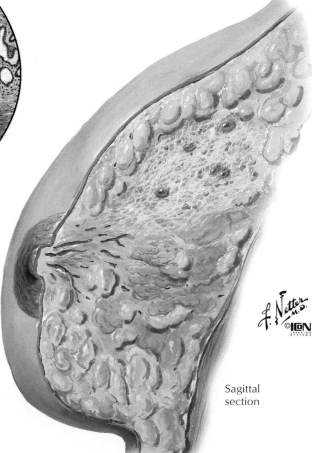

Sagittal
section

Bromocriptine may cause hypotension during the first several days of therapy. Care should also be exercised with patients who have compromised hepatic or renal function.

Interactions: Spironolactone enhances the action of other diuretics and increases digoxin levels. Danazol sodium may prolong prothrombin time in patients receiving warfarin.

Alternative Drugs

Hydrochlorothiazide 25 mg PO qhs for 7–10 days before menses.

Gonadotropin-releasing hormone agonists (leuprolide acetate [Lupron] 3.75 mg IM monthly for no more than 6 months).

FOLLOW-UP

Patient Monitoring: Patients with mastalgia but no dominant mass may be safely rechecked at a different portion of the next menstrual cycle.

Prevention/Avoidance: None.

Expected Outcome: Symptomatic relief can generally be achieved with a combination of diet changes, analgesics, and specific medications.

MISCELLANEOUS

Pregnancy Considerations: No effect on pregnancy, although pregnancy may induce mastalgia.

ICD-9-CM **Codes:** 611.71.

REFERENCES

American College of Obstetricians and Gynecologists. *Nonmalignant Conditions of the Breast.* Washington, DC: ACOG; 1991. ACOG Technical Bulletin 156.

Boyle CA, Berkowitz GS, LiVolsi VA, et al. Caffeine consumption and fibrocystic breast disease: A case control epidemiologic study. *J Natl Cancer Inst* 1984; 72:1015.

Ferguson CM, Powel RW. Breast masses in young women. *Arch Surg* 1989;124:1338.

Seltzer MH, Skiles MS. Disease of the breast in young women. *Surg Gynecol Obstet* 1980;150:360.

Smith RP. *Gynecology in Primary Care.* Baltimore, Md: Williams & Wilkins; 1997:319.

BREAST: POSTPARTUM ENGORGEMENT

INTRODUCTION

Description: Tender, swollen, hard breasts caused by accumulation of milk in the postpartum period or during weaning.

Prevalence: Common.

Predominant Age: Reproductive, 3–4 days after delivery.

Genetics: No genetic pattern.

ETIOLOGY AND PATHOGENESIS

Causes: Increased milk production relative to use. Generally occurs 3–4 days after delivery when milk first comes in or during weaning.

Risk Factors: High fluid intake, infrequent nursing, poor suckling by the infant, abrupt cessation of nursing.

CLINICAL CHARACTERISTICS

Signs and Symptoms:
Warm, hard, sore breasts with no fever or erythema

DIAGNOSTIC APPROACH

Differential Diagnosis:
Mastitis
Blocked (plugged) duct

Associated Conditions: Mastitis.

Workup and Evaluation

Laboratory: No evaluation indicated.

Imaging: No imaging indicated.

Special Tests: None indicated.

Diagnostic Procedures: History and physical examination.

Pathologic Findings

Firm, tender breasts without skin change, fever, or inflammation.

MANAGEMENT AND THERAPY

Nonpharmacologic

General Measures: Mild fluid restriction, analgesics, ice packs, support (well-fitting brassiere). The use of cabbage leaves (applied to the breast) has been advocated, but objective studies are lacking.

Specific Measures: More frequent nursing (if breast-feeding is to continue), firm binding.

Diet: Mild fluid restriction. If nursing is to continue, adequate calories (additional 200 kcal/d) and protein are required.

Activity: No restriction.

Patient Education: Reassurance, support, specific suggestions, American College of Obstetricians and Gynecologists Patient Education Pamphlet AP029 (*Breast-Feeding Your Baby*).

Drug(s) of Choice

Analgesics. Medication to suppress lactation has little value and recommendations for its use have been withdrawn.

FOLLOW-UP

Patient Monitoring: Normal health maintenance; watch for possible infection.

Prevention/Avoidance: Gradual weaning reduces engorgement.

Possible Complications: Ductal obstruction and ectasia (uncommon).

Expected Outcome: Generally resolves in 24–48 hours.

MISCELLANEOUS

ICD-9-CM Codes: 676.2.

REFERENCES

Morgans D. Bromocriptine and postpartum lactation suppression. *Br J Obstet Gynaecol* 1995;102:851.

Riordan J, Auerback K. *Pocket Guide to Breast-Feeding and Human Lactation.* Sudbury, Mass: Jones and Bartlett; 1997.

Seltzer MH, Skiles MS. Disease of the breast in young women. *Surg Gynecol Obstet* 1980;150:360.

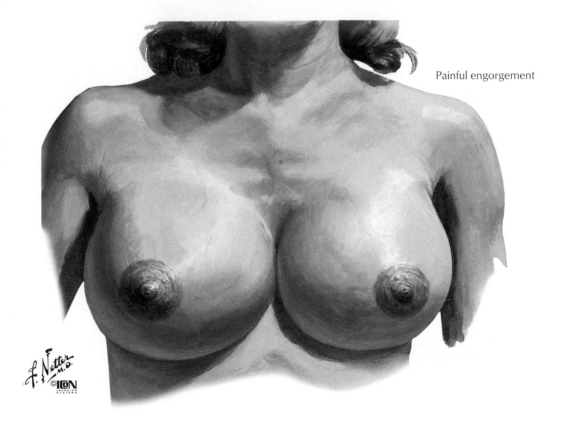

Painful engorgement

BREAST-FEEDING (LACTATION)

THE CHALLENGE

To assist patients in successfully nursing their infant(s).

Scope of the Problem: Sixty percent of new mothers breast-feed in the early postpartum period.

Objectives of Management: Encourage nursing as feeding strategy, assist patients to prepare for nursing and to deal with problems if they occur.

TACTICS

Relevant Pathophysiology: Breast-fed infants have fewer respiratory, gastrointestinal, and ear (otitis media) infections and fewer allergies. Breast milk is more easily digested, better absorbed, and less constipating. Breast-feeding hastens uterine involution. Stimulation of the areola causes the secretion of oxytocin, which is responsible for the letdown reflex and ductal contraction that expels the milk. Suckling stimulates further milk production. Milk production is often not well established until day 3 of nursing. Patients should maintain adequate fluid intake and an increase of approximately 200 kcal/d in dietary intake. Prenatal vitamin supplementation should be continued. Blocked ducts and mastitis are the most common complications. Mastitis mimics blocked ducts (sore, firm lump or lumps) with the addition of erythema and fever. Warm, moist packs; analgesics; and antibiotics that are effective against *Staphylococcus aureus* are appropriate therapies. Infection comes from the infant's nose and mouth. Other sources of fever must also be considered (endometritis).

Strategies: Preparation for nursing—encourage breast-feeding, discuss plans early, address issues such as work and weaning, discuss the role of supplementation, and introduce techniques. Preparation of the nipples in advance is not required. Nursing—initially the infant should nurse at least nine times in 24 hours to encourage milk production. Once milk production is established, the infant should dictate frequency and duration of nursing—six or more wet diapers per day and a weight gain of approximately 1 oz/d indicate adequate feeding. The breasts should be hard before and soft after nursing. Weaning—introduce the bottle by 3–4 weeks as an occasional supplement (may use pumped breast milk). Complete weaning may be done either gradually (substituting bottles for some feedings) or abruptly. If engorgement occurs, analgesia, ice, and compressive binding provides the greatest relief. Medication to suppress lactation is generally not effective.

Patient Education: Reassurance, support, specific suggestions, American College of Obstetricians and Gynecologists Patient Education Pamphlet AP029 (*Breast-Feeding Your Baby*).

IMPLEMENTATION

Special Considerations: Breast-feeding is contraindicated in patients with human immunodeficiency virus, cytomegalovirus, and hepatitis B virus infections. Substances of abuse pass to breast milk, as do some medications. Breast-fed infants often lose weight in the first few days and do not regain birth weight until as late as day 10. Growth spurts often occur at about 10 days, 6 weeks, 3 months, and 4–6 months. If the infant fails to thrive, support and evaluation are in order. Care must be taken to wash the hands well (and any other equipment used) before breast-feeding or breast manipulation. The nipples and the infant's face should also be clean before each feeding. Fresh breast milk may be safely kept for 6–10 hours at room temperature or 72 hours under refrigeration. Breast milk may also be frozen and kept for 6 months in a home freezer or 12 months at −20°C. Thawed breast milk should be used within 24 hours and may not be refrozen. Breast milk should never be warmed in a microwave oven. The volume of milk required for each feeding varies widely but is normally between 2 and 5 oz for newborns, 4–6 oz for infants 2–4 months of age, and 5–7 oz for babies 4–6 months old. One study found that 65% of women with augmentation mammoplasty have lactation insufficiency.

REFERENCES

Bumsted JR, Riddick DH. The breast during pregnancy and lactation. In: Sciarra JJ, ed. *Gynecology and Obstetrics*. Vol 5. Philadelphia, Pa: JB Lippincott; 1990;31:1.

Hurst NM. Lactation after augmentation mammoplasty. *Obstet Gynecol* 1996;135:30.

Newton ER. *Lactation and Its Disorders*. In: Mitchell GW Jr, Bassett LW, eds. *The Female Breast and Its Disorders*. Baltimore, Md: Williams & Wilkins; 1990:45.

Shadigian E, Van Bonn P, Cook M. Management of breast-feeding. *Female Patient* 1998;23(6):47.

Short RV. Breast feeding. *Sci Am* 1984;205:35.

Ziegler JB. Breast feeding and HIV. *Lancet* 1993;342:1438.

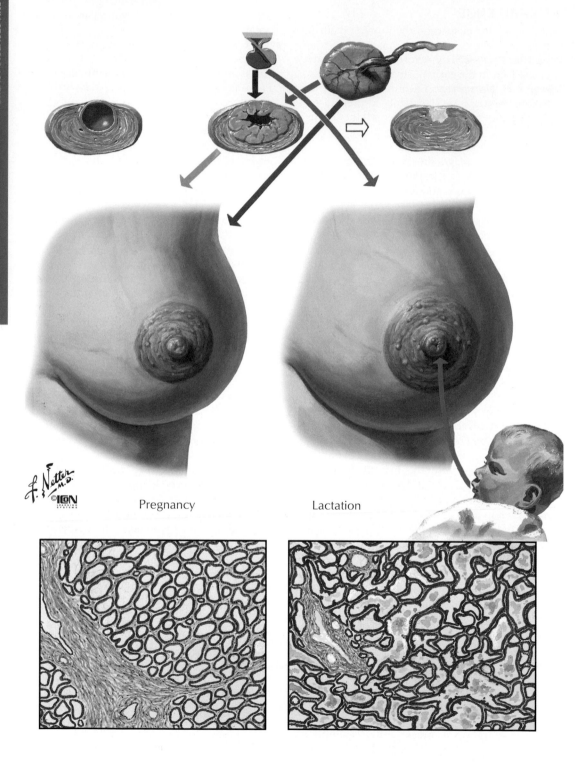

Pregnancy

Lactation

GALACTORRHEA

INTRODUCTION

Description: Spontaneous, bilateral nipple discharge (milky fluid only).

Prevalence: Uncommon but reports vary from 1% to 30%, depending on the population studied.

Predominant Age: Reproductive.

Genetics: No genetic pattern.

ETIOLOGY AND PATHOGENESIS

Causes: Pituitary adenoma, disruptions in thyroid or prolactin hormone levels, pharmacologic (most often those drugs that affect dopamine or serotonin), autoimmune disease (sarcoid, lupus), Cushing's disease, herpes zoster, chest wall/breast stimulation or irritation, physiologic changes during pregnancy or after childbirth and/or nursing.

Risk Factors: None known.

CLINICAL CHARACTERISTICS

Signs and Symptoms:

Bilateral, spontaneous milky discharge from both breasts

Often symptoms of underlying pathologic condition (eg, hypothyroidism, Cushing's disease, or pituitary enlargement)

Amenorrhea common

DIAGNOSTIC APPROACH

Differential Diagnosis:

Pregnancy

Breast cancer

Chronic nipple stimulation

Hypothyroidism

Sarcoidosis

Lupus

Cirrhosis or hepatic disease

Associated Conditions: One third of patients with an elevated prolactin level experience amenorrhea or infertility. Prolonged amenorrhea is associated with an increased risk of osteoporosis.

Workup and Evaluation

Laboratory: Pregnancy should always be considered if menses are absent. There is a poor correlation between serum prolactin levels and the size or delectability of a pituitary lesion.

Imaging: Computed tomography or magnetic resonance imagine (preferred) frequently indicated.

Special Tests: Testing of visual fields may be indicated.

Pathologic Findings

None.

MANAGEMENT AND THERAPY

Nonpharmacologic

General Measures: When prolactin levels are low and a coned-down view of the sella turcica is normal, observation alone may be sufficient. If observation is chosen, periodic reevaluation is required to check for the emergence of slow-growing tumors.

Specific Measures: Treatment with bromocriptine is recommended for patients who desire pregnancy or for those with distressing degrees of galactorrhea or to suppress intermediate-sized pituitary tumors. Rapidly growing tumors, tumors that are large at the time of discovery, or those that do not respond to bromocriptine therapy may require surgical therapy.

Diet: No specific dietary changes indicated.

Activity: No restriction.

Patient Education: Reassurance, discuss treatment options, American College of Obstetricians and Gynecologists Patient Education Pamphlet AP102 (*Infertility*), AP029 (*Breast-Feeding Your Baby*).

Drug(s) of Choice

If the prolactin level is elevated—bromocriptine (Parlodel) 2.5 mg daily increased gradually to tid.

Contraindications: Uncontrolled hypertension, pregnancy.

Precautions: With medical therapy—nausea, orthostatic hypotension, drowsiness, or syncope, hypertension or seizures.

Interactions: Medical therapy may interact with phenothiazines or butyrophenones.

Alternative Drugs

Intravaginal bromocriptine.

Dopamine agonists (Cabergoline) may become available.

FOLLOW-UP

Patient Monitoring: Normal health maintenance. If a pituitary adenoma is present, periodic assessment of visual fields should be considered.

Prevention/Avoidance: None.

Possible Complications: Visual field loss, symptoms may return after medication is discontinued.

Expected Outcome: Generally good depending on cause. Prolactin levels should be measured every 6–12 months and visual fields reassessed

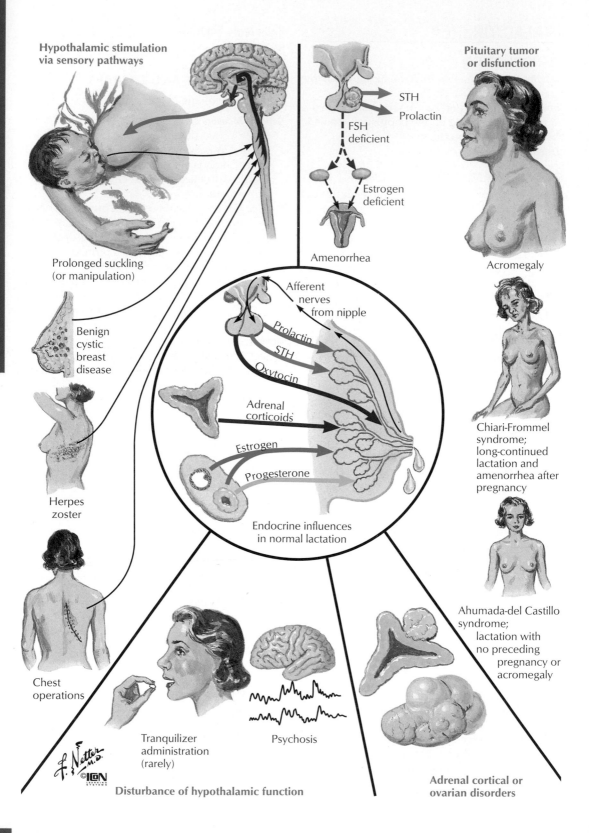

Hypothalamic stimulation via sensory pathways

Prolonged suckling (or manipulation)

Benign cystic breast disease

Herpes zoster

Chest operations

STH

Prolactin

FSH deficient

Estrogen deficient

Amenorrhea

Pituitary tumor or disfunction

Acromegaly

Chiari-Frommel syndrome; long-continued lactation and amenorrhea after pregnancy

Ahumada-del Castillo syndrome; lactation with no preceding pregnancy or acromegaly

Afferent nerves from nipple

Prolactin

STH

Oxytocin

Adrenal corticoids

Estrogen

Progesterone

Endocrine influences in normal lactation

Tranquilizer administration (rarely)

Psychosis

Disturbance of hypothalamic function

Adrenal cortical or ovarian disorders

yearly. The pituitary should be reevaluated every 2–5 years, based on initial diagnosis.

MISCELLANEOUS

Pregnancy Considerations: No effect on pregnancy, although pregnancy may cause adenomas to grow rapidly.

***ICD-9-CM* Codes:** 611.6, 626.0 (Amenorrhea), 676.6 (Galactorrhea) should only be used in conjunction with pregnancy and nursing.

REFERENCES

American College of Obstetricians and Gynecologists. *Amenorrhea*. Washington, DC: ACOG; 1989. Technical Bulletin 128.

Chang RJ, Keye WR, Young JR, Wilson CB, Jaffe RB. Detection, evaluation, and treatment of pituitary microadenomas in patients with galactorrhea and amenorrhea. *Am J Obstet Gynecol* 1977;128:356.

Schlechte J, Dolan K, Sherman B, Chapter F, Luciano A. The natural history of untreated hyperprolactinemia: a prospective analysis. *J Clin Endocrinol Metab* 1989;68:412.

Smith RP. *Gynecology in Primary Care.* Baltimore, Md: Williams & Wilkins; 1997:405.

Speroff L, Glass RH, Kase NG. *Clinical Gynecologic Endocrinology and Infertility.* 5th ed. Baltimore, Md: Williams & Wilkins; 1994:404, 555.

MAMMOGRAPHY

THE CHALLENGE

To improve the use of breast imaging to detect occult disease.

Scope of the Problem: Widespread use of mammography has been credited with reducing the mortality rate from breast cancer by up to 30%. Unfortunately, not all women receive appropriate screening on a regular basis. One study indicated that only 39% of women aged 50–59 and 36% of women aged 60–69 had had a mammogram in the preceding year. In another study, only 24% of women older than 65 followed the current recommendations for annual examinations. It has been estimated that breast cancer mortality could be reduced by as much as one half if all women older than 40 received annual screening. In one study, 6 cancers per 1000 screening mammograms were found, and 3 additional cancers per 1000 annual repeat studies were detected.

Objectives: To appropriately use mammography for the evaluation of breast complaints and to improve compliance with screening guidelines.

TACTICS

Relevant Pathophysiology: Mammography is the best mode of screening for early lesions currently available. Mammography localizes, documents, objectifies, and identifies other occult pathologic changes. Roughly 85% of breast cancers found by mammography are early stage lesions versus 54%–70% found by physicians and 38%–64% of tumors found by the patient herself during breast self-examination. Roughly 35% of breast cancers are found by an abnormal mammogram, without a palpable mass present. Mammography can identify small lesions (1–2 mm), calcifications, or other changes suspicious for malignancy roughly 2 years before a lesion is clinically palpable. Ten-year disease-free survival for patients with these lesions is 90%–95%. The average lesion found on breast self-examination is 2.5 cm, and half of these patients have nodal involvement. For these patients, 10-year survival falls to between 50% and 70%. Over one third of occult breast cancers have calcifications, making the otherwise undetected tumors visible through mammography.

Strategies: The American Cancer Society guidelines for mammographic screening are the following:

Baseline study between ages 35 and 40.

Mammography every 1–2 years from age 40 to 49.

Annual mammogram from age 50 on. (When the patient has a first-degree relative with premenopausal breast cancer, screening should begin roughly 5 years before the age at which the relative's cancer was diagnosed.)

Patient Education: Instruction on need for and timing of mammography, American College of Obstetricians and Gynecologists Patient Education Pamphlet AP026 (*Detecting and Treating Breast Problems*), AP076 (*Mammography*).

IMPLEMENTATION

Special Considerations: Mammography in younger women is more difficult to interpret than in older women because of the greater tissue density present during the reproductive years. Whereas the increasing ability to diagnose cancer in older women parallels their increasing risk, breast cancers in younger women are more easily missed. This diagnostic difficulty and the relatively higher rate of false-positive studies that necessitate further evaluation have raised questions about routine screening of women younger than 50. The finding of clusters of calcification that often are associated with cancer is nonspecific. Seventy-five percent of calcification clusters found on mammography are due to benign disease. Overall, mammography is approximately 85% accurate in diagnosing malignancy, with a 10%–15% false-negative rate. For this reason, it provides an adjunct to clinical impressions and the definitive procedure of biopsy, but does not replace them. Roughly, 10% of mammographic studies require additional views. Between 1% and 2% of screening studies necessitate histologic evaluation to establish a diagnosis. Mammographic radiation exposure is minimal (less than 1 rad). Based on this level of exposure, mammography might induce up to 5 new lifetime cancers for every 1 million women of age 40–44 screened and less than 1 per 1 million for women aged 60–64 (background risk is 115 and 292 for these age groups, respectively). Therefore, the risk of death caused by radiation exposure is roughly equivalent to the risk of death encountered by driving a car 220 miles, riding a bicycle for 10 miles, or smoking 1.5 cigarettes.

REFERENCES

American College of Obstetricians and Gynecologists. *Carcinoma of the Breast*. Washington, DC: ACOG; 1991. ACOG Technical Bulletin 158.

Mammography

Fletcher SW, Black W, Harris R, Rimer BK, Shapiro S. *Report of the International Workshop on Screening for Breast Cancer*. Bethesda, MD: National Cancer Institute; 1993.

Breast cancer screening guidelines agreed on by AMA, other medically related organizations [medical news and perspectives]. *JAMA* 1989;262:1155.

Position for craniocaudad projection

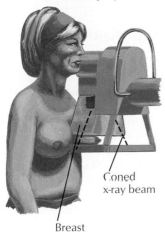

Usually two exposures at right angles (craniocaudad and lateral) are made of each breast

When additional breast and rib detail is needed, a mediolateral exposure is also made

Position for lateral projection

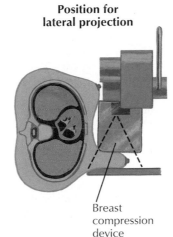

Position for mediolateral projection

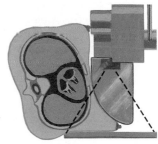

Coned x-ray beam

Breast compression device

JOHN A. CRAIG—AD
© ICON
LEARNING
SYSTEMS

Breast compression device

Translucent fatty tissue

Connective tissue shadows

Prominent ducts and glandular elements

Vascular shadows

Rib detail shown in this projection

Connective tissue shadows

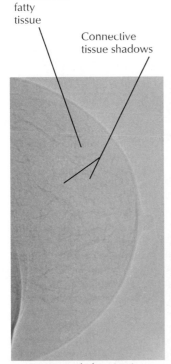

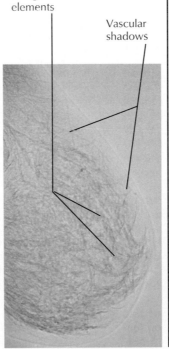

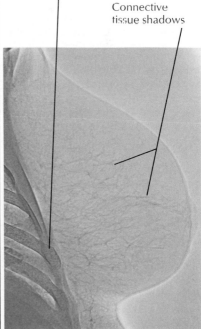

Craniocaudad projection of normal fatty breast

Lateral projection of normal dense glandular breast

Mediolateral projection of normal breast

MASTITIS (LACTATIONAL)

INTRODUCTION

Description: An infection of one or more ductal complexes of the breast, generally associated with breast-feeding, and potentially causing significant morbidity if not recognized and treated aggressively.

Prevalence: Two percent to three percent of nursing women after delivery.

Predominant Age: Reproductive, 2–4 weeks after delivery.

Genetics: No genetic pattern.

ETIOLOGY AND PATHOGENESIS

Causes: Infection comes from organisms carried in the nose and mouth of the nursing infant, most commonly *Staphylococcus aureus* and *Streptococcus* species. Common agents include β-hemolytic streptococci, *Haemophilus influenzae*, *Haemophilus parainfluenzae*, *Escherichia coli*, and *Klebsiella pneumoniae*.

Risk Factors: Diabetes, steroid use, heavy cigarette smoking, and retracted (inverted) nipples.

CLINICAL CHARACTERISTICS

Signs and Symptoms:
   Firm, sore, red, and tender portion of the breast, most commonly in the upper outer quadrant
   High fever, tachycardia, headaches, anorexia, and malaise
   Axillary nodes tender or enlarged
   In nonnursing patients, a palpable, recurrent mass, accompanied by a multicolored discharge from the nipple or adjacent to a Montgomery's follicle

DIAGNOSTIC APPROACH

Differential Diagnosis:
   Breast abscess
   Blocked (plugged) duct
   Breast engorgement
   Galactocele

Associated Conditions: Breast engorgement.

Workup and Evaluation

Laboratory: A complete blood count documents an elevated white blood cell count but is not required for diagnosis. A culture of the mother's milk and the infant's nose and mouth may be helpful, but are not required.

Imaging: No imaging indicated.

Special Tests: None indicated.

Diagnostic Procedures: History and physical examination combined with knowledge of the condition of the breast at or before delivery.

Pathologic Findings

Swelling and obstruction of the involved ducts with inflammation. When present in nonpregnant and postmenopausal women, it may be accompanied by squamous metaplasia. When well established, ductal thickening may lead to nipple retraction.

MANAGEMENT AND THERAPY

Nonpharmacologic

General Measures: Mild fluid restriction, analgesics, ice packs, and support (well fitting brassiere).

Specific Measures: Prompt and aggressive antibiotic therapy is indicated. Nursing from the opposite side, pumping or expression of the involved breast. If tenderness or fever do not decrease promptly, abscess must be suspected and prompt surgical drainage, usually under general anesthesia, is required.

Diet: No specific dietary changes indicated.

Activity: No restriction.

Patient Education: Reassurance, support, specific suggestions, American College of Obstetricians and Gynecologists Patient Education Pamphlet AP029 (*Breast-Feeding Your Baby*).

Drug(s) of Choice

Penicillin G or erythromycin (250–500 mg PO qid, erythromycin ethylsuccinate [EES] 400 mg PO qid) for 10 days. First-generation oral cephalosporins (cephalexin 500 mg PO bid, cefaclor 250 mg PO tid, or amoxicillin/clavulanate [Augmentin] 250 mg PO tid) may also be used. The level of erythromycin achieved in milk is very high.

Contraindications: Known or suspected allergy.

Precautions: If response to therapy is not prompt, surgical drainage is required.

Alternative Drugs

Dicloxacillin may be required for penicillin-resistant strains or severe infections.

FOLLOW-UP

Patient Monitoring: Normal health maintenance. Watch for development of an abscess.

Prevention/Avoidance: Attention to normal hygiene practices during nursing (avoid drying agents). Avoid cracking or fissuring of nipples. Use of breast or nipple shield when cracked nipples are present.

Possible Complications: Progression of infection, abscess formation, scarring, squamous metaplasia, ductal ectasia. Abscesses may form even while a patient is receiving antibiotic therapy.

Expected Outcome: Generally good with aggressive therapy.

MISCELLANEOUS

Pregnancy Considerations: No effect on pregnancy.
***ICD-9-CM* Codes:** 675.2.

REFERENCES

Riordan J, Auerback K. *Pocket Guide to Breast-Feeding and Human Lactation.* Sudbury, Mass: Jones and Bartlett; 1997.

Stehman FB. Infections and inflammations of the breast. In Hindle WH, ed. *Breast Disease for Gynecologists.* East Norwalk, Conn: Appleton & Lange; 1990:151.

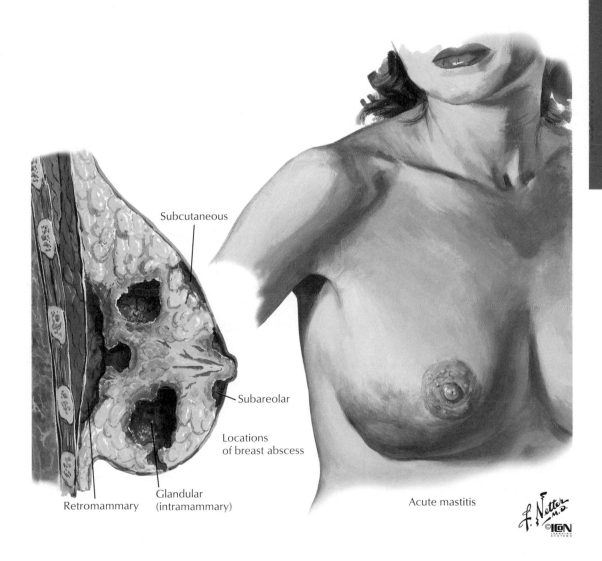

Subcutaneous

Subareolar

Locations
of breast abscess

Retromammary

Glandular
(intramammary)

Acute mastitis

PAGET'S DISEASE OF THE BREAST

INTRODUCTION

Description: A malignant process that involves the nipple and areola. Rarely, it may also involve the skin of the vulva.

Prevalence: Two percent of breast cancers.

Predominant Age: Menopausal and perimenopausal.

Genetics: No genetic pattern.

ETIOLOGY AND PATHOGENESIS

Causes: Thought to arise in the dermoepidermal junction from multipotent cells that can differentiate into either glandular or squamous cells.

Risk Factors: None known.

CLINICAL CHARACTERISTICS

Signs and Symptoms:

Pruritic, red, eczematoid skin lesion, often associated with bleeding and crusting

Almost always associated with infiltrating or intraductal carcinoma in deeper parts of the breast

DIAGNOSTIC APPROACH

Differential Diagnosis:

Eczema of the nipple

Inflammatory breast cancer

Chronic nipple irritation (jogger's nipples)

Associated Conditions: Infiltrating or intraductal carcinoma.

Workup and Evaluation

Laboratory: No evaluation indicated.

Imaging: Mammography to detect deeper lesions and lesions in the contralateral breast.

Special Tests: A touch smear obtained by softening the crust with saline and gently scraping the surface often demonstrates the characteristic Paget's cells.

Diagnostic Procedures: History, physical examination, and biopsy.

Pathologic Findings

Dermal infiltrates of large neoplastic cells (Paget's cells). These cells have abundant clear cytoplasm with mucin and irregular prominent nucleoli. Most often, these cells arise from infiltrating ductal carcinoma.

MANAGEMENT AND THERAPY

Nonpharmacologic

General Measures: Evaluation, mammography.

Specific Measures: Therapy is focused on treatment of the underlying malignancy.

Diet: No specific dietary changes indicated.

Activity: No restriction.

Patient Education: Instruction on monthly breast self-examination, American College of Obstetricians and Gynecologists Patient Education Pamphlet AP026 (*Detecting and Treating Breast Problems*), AP076 (*Mammography*).

Drug(s) of Choice

None. Adjunctive chemotherapy is often recommended based on cell type and stage.

FOLLOW-UP

Patient Monitoring: Increased surveillance for recurrence or the development of tumors in the contralateral breast.

Prevention/Avoidance: None.

Possible Complications: Progression and spread of the underlying malignancy. Local skin erosion with bleeding and discharge.

Expected Outcome: Local recurrence is common.

MISCELLANEOUS

Pregnancy Considerations: Generally not a consideration. No direct effect on pregnancy.

ICD-9-CM Codes: Based on location and severity of disease.

REFERENCES

American College of Obstetricians and Gynecologists. *Nonmalignant Conditions of the Breast.* Washington, DC: ACOG; 1991. ACOG Technical Bulletin 156.

Isaacs JH. Office surgery of breast lesions. In: Hindle WH, ed. *Breast Disease for Gynecologists.* East Norwalk, Conn: Appleton & Lange; 1990:262.

Navin J. Pathology and fine needle aspiration cytology of the breast. In: Hindle WH, ed. *Breast Disease for Gynecologists.* East Norwalk, Conn: Appleton & Lange; 1990:185.

Ramzy I. Pathology of malignant neoplasms. In: Mitchell GW Jr, Bassett LW, eds. *The Female Breast and Its Disorders.* Baltimore, Md: Williams & Wilkins; 1990:108.

Smith RP. *Gynecology in Primary Care.* Baltimore, Md: Williams & Wilkins; 1997:319.

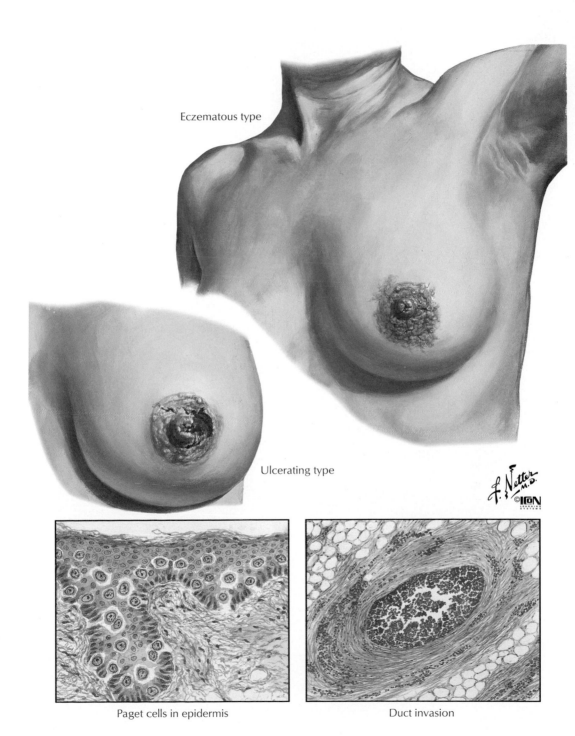

Eczematous type

Ulcerating type

Paget cells in epidermis

Duct invasion

Genetic and Endocrine Conditions

ABORTION: RECURRENT

INTRODUCTION

Description: When a woman has had two consecutive or three total first-trimester spontaneous pregnancy losses.

Prevalence: Found in 0.4%–0.8% of women.

Predominant Age: Reproductive.

Genetics: No genetic pattern.

ETIOLOGY AND PATHOGENESIS

Causes: Chromosomal abnormalities. When the losses occur early in gestation, there is a greater likelihood that a chromosomal abnormality is the cause, whereas for later abortions, a maternal cause such as a uterine anomaly is more likely. Although most chromosomal abnormalities result from disorders of meiosis in gamete formation or in mitosis after fertilization, 5% of couples who experience recurrent abortion have a detectable parental chromosomal abnormality, surgically correctable uterine abnormalities, an incompetent cervix, or intrauterine synechiae. Uterine anomalies are found in 15%– 25% of women with recurrent abortion. The possibility of immunologic factors as a cause of recurrent losses should also be evaluated (eg, lupus anticoagulant). Two thirds of recurrent abortions occur after 12 weeks gestation, which suggests maternal or environmental factors play a large role in this process.

Risk Factors: Those associated with spontaneous abortion, including increasing maternal and paternal age and autoimmune disorders.

CLINICAL CHARACTERISTICS

Signs and Symptoms:

Two consecutive or three total first-trimester spontaneous pregnancy losses.

DIAGNOSTIC APPROACH

Differential Diagnosis:

Uterine anomalies (fibroids, incompetent cervix, intrauterine synechiae, developmental abnormalities such as a septum or duplication)

Chromosomal abnormality (maternal or paternal, maternal more likely)

Immunologic causes (such as lupus anticoagulant)

Endocrinopathy (such as hypothyroidism)

Associated Conditions: None.

Workup and Evaluation

Laboratory: Screening for immunologic or endocrine abnormality as indicated.

Imaging: Ultrasonography of the pelvis or hysterosalpingography may be of assistance when a uterine anomaly is suspected.

Special Tests: Karyotyping of both parents is recommended when recurrent early abortions have occurred. Karyotyping of the abortus may be helpful but requires fresh tissue, specialized transport media, and laboratory capabilities.

Diagnostic Procedures: Hysteroscopy may be of limited value (indicated only when a uterine factor is strongly considered).

Pathologic Findings

None.

MANAGEMENT AND THERAPY

Nonpharmacologic

General Measures: Support and evaluation.

Specific Measures: Those with parental chromosomal anomalies may be offered donor oocytes or artificial insemination with donor sperm. Uterine anomalies or submucous fibroids may be treated, although care must be taken to recognize the possibility of continued failure for other reasons and the possible impact of future delivery options.

Diet: No specific dietary changes indicated.

Activity: No restriction.

Patient Education: Reassurance, American College of Obstetricians and Gynecologists Patient Education Pamphlet AP100 (*Repeated Miscarriage*), AP002 (*Infertility: Causes and Treatments*), AP090 (*Early Pregnancy Loss: Miscarriage, Ectopic Pregnancy, and Molar Pregnancy*).

Drug(s) of Choice

None. Progesterone and thyroid supplements have not been shown to reduce the risk of pregnancy loss. When immunologic factors are present the use of low-dose aspirin and subcutaneous heparin (5000 units twice daily) has reduced the rate of subsequent loss.

FOLLOW-UP

Patient Monitoring: Normal health maintenance.

Prevention/Avoidance: None.

Expected Outcome: Based on underlying pathologic condition.

MISCELLANEOUS

ICD-9-CM Codes: 646.3.

REFERENCES

American College of Obstetricians and Gynecologists. *Early Pregnancy Loss*. Washington, DC: ACOG; 1995. ACOG Technical Bulletin 212.

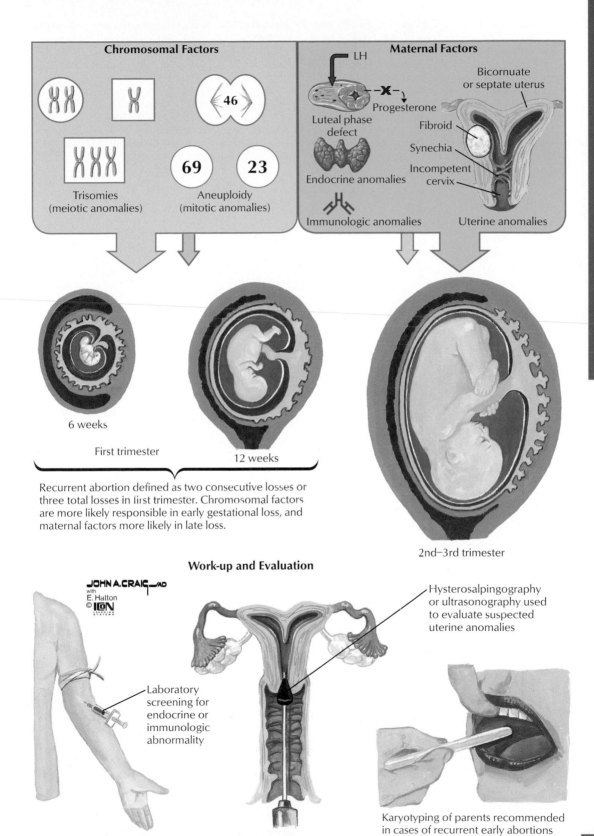

Chromosomal Factors

46

Trisomies
(meiotic anomalies)

69   **23**

Aneuploidy
(mitotic anomalies)

Maternal Factors

LH

Progesterone

Luteal phase
defect

Endocrine anomalies

Immunologic anomalies

Bicornuate
or septate uterus

Fibroid

Synechia

Incompetent
cervix

Uterine anomalies

6 weeks

First trimester

12 weeks

Recurrent abortion defined as two consecutive losses or
three total losses in first trimester. Chromosomal factors
are more likely responsible in early gestational loss, and
maternal factors more likely in late loss.

2nd–3rd trimester

Work-up and Evaluation

JOHN A.CRAIG__AD
with
E. Hatton
© ICN
LEARNING
SYSTEMS

Laboratory
screening for
endocrine or
immunologic
abnormality

Hysterosalpingography
or ultrasonography used
to evaluate suspected
uterine anomalies

Karyotyping of parents recommended
in cases of recurrent early abortions

GENETIC AND ENDOCRINE CONDITIONS

Backos M, Rai R, Baxter N, Chilcott IT, Cohen H, Regan L. Pregnancy complications in women with recurrent miscarriage associated with antiphospholipid antibodies treated with low dose aspirin and heparin. *Br J Obstet Gynaecol* 1999;106:102.

Byrne JLB, Ward K. Genetic factors in recurrent abortion. *Clin Obstet Gynecol* 1994;37:693.

Harger JH, Archer DF, Marchese SG, Muracca-Clemens M, Garver KL. Etiology of recurrent pregnancy losses and outcome of subsequent pregnancies. *Obstet Gynecol* 1983;62:574.

Hatasaka HH. Recurrent miscarriage: epidemiologic factors, definitions, and incidence. *Clin Obstet Gynecol* 1994;37:625.

Rai R, Cohen H, Dave M, Regan L. Randomized controlled trial of aspirin and aspirin plus heparin in pregnant women with recurrent miscarriage associated with phospholipid antibodies (or antiphospholipid antibodies). *BMJ* 1997;314:253.

Scott JR. Recurrent miscarriage: overview and recommendations. *Clin Obstet Gynecol* 1994;37:768.

Smith RP. *Gynecology in Primary Care.* Baltimore, Md: Williams & Wilkins; 1997:99.

AMENORRHEA: PRIMARY

INTRODUCTION

Description: The absence of normal menstruation in a patient without previously established cycles.

Prevalence: Uncommon.

Predominant Age: Mid to late teens.

Genetics: One third caused by chromosomal abnormalities such as 45,XO, 46,XY gonadal dysgenesis or 46,XX q5 X long-arm deletion.

ETIOLOGY AND PATHOGENESIS

Causes: Gonadal abnormalities (60% of patients)—autoimmune ovarian failure (Blizzard syndrome), gonadal dysgenesis, pure gonadal dysgenesis, 45,XO (Turner's syndrome), 46,XY gonadal dysgenesis (Swyer syndrome), 46,XX q5 X chromosome long-arm deletion, mixed or mosaic, follicular depletion, autoimmune disease, infection (eg, mumps), infiltrative disease processes (eg, tuberculosis, galactosemia), iatrogenic ovarian failure (eg, alkylating chemotherapy, irradiation), ovarian insensitivity syndrome (Savage's syndrome), 17α-hydroxylase deficiency, chronic anovulation of pubertal onset. Extragonadal anomalies (40%)—congenital absence of uterus and vagina (15%) (müllerian agenesis), constitutional delay, imperforate hymen, male pseudohermaphroditism (testicular feminization syndrome), pituitary-hypothalamic dysfunction, transverse vaginal septum.

Risk Factors: None known.

CLINICAL CHARACTERISTICS

Signs and Symptoms:

No period by age 14 with no secondary sex changes

No period by age 16 regardless of secondary sex changes

No period by 2 years after the start of secondary sex changes

Evaluation should not be delayed anytime there is the suggestion of a chromosomal abnormality or an obstructed genital tract.

DIAGNOSTIC APPROACH

Differential Diagnosis:

Pregnancy before first cycle

Obstructed outflow tract (making menstruation cryptic)

Gonadal dysgenesis

Uterine agenesis

Androgen insensitivity syndrome

Mayer-Rokitansky-Küster-Hauser syndrome

Associated Conditions: Infertility, abnormal stature (short or tall), and cardiac changes in some congenital syndromes, hypertension and hypokalemic alkalosis in 17α-hydroxylase deficiency, virilization, or hirsutism, and cyclic pelvic pain with outflow obstruction. Renal and skeletal abnormalities may also occur. Prolonged amenorrhea is associated with an increased risk of osteoporosis.

Workup and Evaluation

Laboratory: The development of sexual hair or breasts provide an outward sign of androgen and estrogen production respectively.

Imaging: Based on conditions being considered.

Special Tests: Based on conditions being considered.

Diagnostic Procedures: Laparoscopy to evaluate internal organs and gonads may be required.

Pathologic Findings

None.

MANAGEMENT AND THERAPY

Nonpharmacologic

General Measures: Determination of underlying cause(s).

Specific Measures: Based on the diagnosis and specific needs of the patient.

Diet: No specific dietary changes indicated.

Activity: No restriction.

Patient Education: Reassurance, American College of Obstetricians and Gynecologists Patient Education Pamphlet AP049 (*Menstruation*) or AP041 (*Growing Up* [for ages 9–14]).

Drug(s) of Choice

Based on underlying cause. Hormone replacement may be required or desirable for many patients.

FOLLOW-UP

Patient Monitoring: Normal health maintenance.

Prevention/Avoidance: None.

Possible Complications: Risk of gonadal malignancy is increased if a Y chromosome is present. Risk of osteoporosis if the patient is hypoestrogenic and does not receive replacement therapy. Extensive damage to the upper tract may occur if obstruction is not corrected.

Expected Outcome: Menstruation and fertility may be restored for many of these patients if there are no structural or chromosomal conditions that preclude the possibility (uterine agenesis,

GENETIC AND ENDOCRINE CONDITIONS

Neuroendocrine Regulation of Menstrual Cycle

Hypothalamic regulation of pituitary gonadotrophin production and release

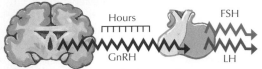

Pulsed release of GnRH by hypothalamus (1 pulse/1–2 hr) permits anterior pituitary production and release of FSH and LH (normal)

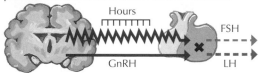

Continuous, excessive, absent, or more frequent GnRH release inhibits FSH and LH production and release (downloading)

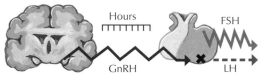

Decreased pulsed release of GnRH decreases LH secretion but increases FSH secretion (slow-pulsing model)

Ovarian feedback modulation of pituitary gonadotropin production and release

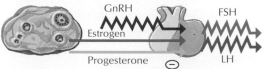

Presence of pulsed GnRH and low estrogen and progesterone levels result in increased levels of pulsed LH and FSH (negative feedback)

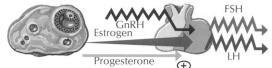

Presence of pulsed GnRH, rapidly increasing levels of estrogen, and small amounts of progesterone result in high pulsed LH and moderately increased pulsed FSH levels (positive feedback)

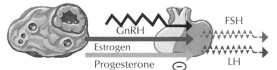

Presence of pulsed GnRH and high levels of estrogen and progesterone result in decreased LH and FSH levels (negative feedback)

Correlation of serum gonadotrophic and ovarian hormone levels and feedback mechanisms

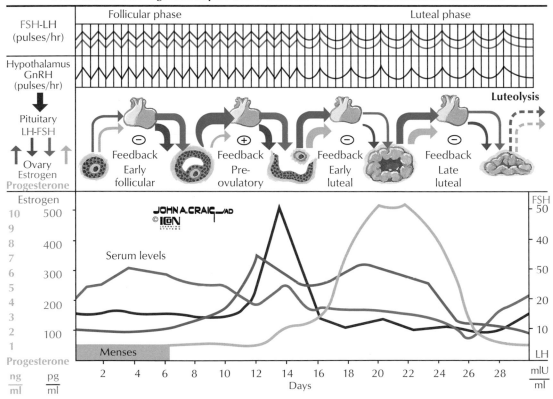

JOHN A. CRAIG—AD
©ICON
LEARNING SYSTEMS

androgen insensitivity syndrome, gonadal dysgenesis).

MISCELLANEOUS

Pregnancy Considerations: Infertility common. If pregnancy is achieved, there are no effects except those imposed by underlying cause.

ICD-9-CM **Codes:** 626.0.

REFERENCES

American College of Obstetricians and Gynecologists. *Amenorrhea.* Washington, DC: ACOG; 1989. Technical Bulletin 128.

Smith RP. *Gynecology in Primary Care.* Baltimore, Md: Williams & Wilkins; 1997:405.

Speroff L, Glass RH, Kase NG. *Clinical Gynecologic Endocrinology and Infertility.* 5th ed. Baltimore, Md: Williams & Wilkins; 1994:401.

AMENORRHEA: SECONDARY

INTRODUCTION

Description: The absence of normal menstruation in a patient with previously established cycles.
Prevalence: Common.
Predominant Age: Reproductive (menarche to menopause).
Genetics: No genetic pattern.

ETIOLOGY AND PATHOGENESIS

Causes: Most common—pregnancy. Other causes—end organ: Asherman's syndrome, outflow obstruction; ovarian: menopause, Savage's syndrome, toxin exposure, surgery, autoimmune disease; central, behavioral, and others: anorexia, obesity, athletics (overtraining), drugs/medications, nutritional deprivation, psychogenic (stress); medical: adenoma, craniopharyngioma, Sheehan's syndrome, tuberculosis, sarcoid, empty sella syndrome; virilizing syndromes: polycystic ovarian disease, adrenal hyperplasia, virilizing tumors.
Risk Factors: Unprotected intercourse, exposure to toxins, radiation, or surgery, overtraining, eating disorders, psychosocial stress.

CLINICAL CHARACTERISTICS

Signs and Symptoms:
Absent menstruation—may be associated with symptoms that suggest the cause

DIAGNOSTIC APPROACH

Differential Diagnosis:
Pregnancy
Menopause (natural or premature)
Exogenous hormone use
Virilization
Metabolically active ovarian tumor
Lactational amenorrhea
Associated Conditions: Endometrial hyperplasia, osteoporosis in hypoestrogenic states.

Workup and Evaluation

Laboratory: A pregnancy test is always indicated.
Imaging: Based on conditions being considered.
Special Tests: Women who have ovarian failure below age 30 should have a karyotype performed.
Diagnostic Procedures: Based on conditions being considered.

Pathologic Findings

None.

MANAGEMENT AND THERAPY

Nonpharmacologic

General Measures: Determination of underlying cause(s). If a pathologic condition has been ruled out and pregnancy is not desired, reassurance only. Evaluation should not be delayed any time there is the suggestion of an abnormality or pregnancy.
Specific Measures: Periodic (every 3–6 months) progestin withdrawal to prevent endometrial hyperplasia and to reevaluate status. Specific therapy is based on the underlying cause (such as estrogen/progestin replacement for menopause). Treatment is focused on restoring or inducing ovulation if pregnancy is desired.
Diet: No specific dietary changes indicated.
Activity: No restriction.
Patient Education: Reassurance, American College of Obstetricians and Gynecologists Patient Education Pamphlet AP049 (*Menstruation*) or AP047 (*The Menopause Years*) or AB008 (Menopause packet with 3 titles).

Drug(s) of Choice

Based on diagnosis (eg, thyroid replacement for hypothyroidism, estrogen and progestin therapy for ovarian failure, periodic progestin therapy [oral or transvaginal] or ovulation induction for anovulation).
Contraindications: All medical interventions are contraindicated until pregnancy has been ruled out.

FOLLOW-UP

Patient Monitoring: Normal health maintenance. Watch for changing status or intercurrent pregnancy.
Prevention/Avoidance: None (contraception).
Possible Complications: Endometrial hyperplasia with continued estrogen (unopposed) exposure.
Expected Outcome: Most causes of secondary amenorrhea may be successfully treated with return of menstruation.

MISCELLANEOUS

Pregnancy Considerations: Pregnancy must be ruled out.
ICD-9-CM Codes: 626.0.

REFERENCES

American College of Obstetricians and Gynecologists. *Amenorrhea.* Washington, DC: ACOG; 1989. Technical Bulletin 128.
Smith RP. *Gynecology in Primary Care.* Baltimore, Md: Williams & Wilkins; 1997:405.
Speroff L, Glass RH, Kase NG. *Clinical Gynecologic Endocrinology and Infertility.* 5th ed. Baltimore, Md: Williams & Wilkins; 1994:401.

Causes of Ovulatory Dysfunction

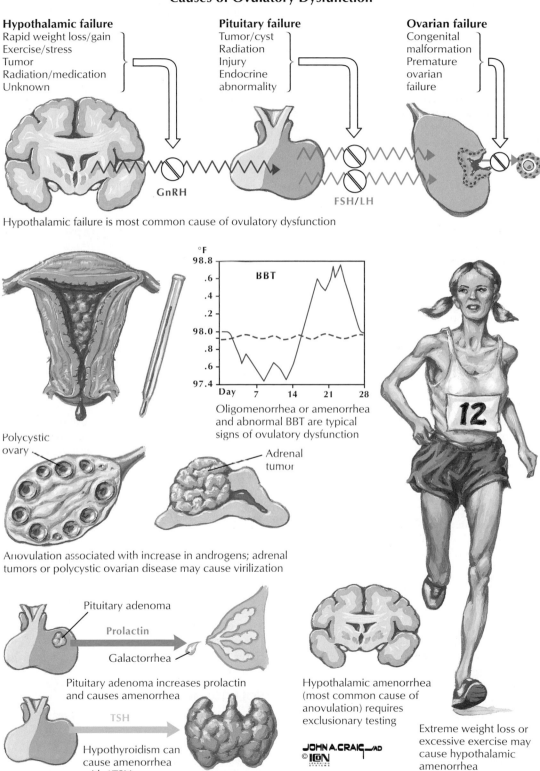

Hypothalamic failure
Rapid weight loss/gain
Exercise/stress
Tumor
Radiation/medication
Unknown

Pituitary failure
Tumor/cyst
Radiation
Injury
Endocrine
abnormality

Ovarian failure
Congenital
malformation
Premature
ovarian
failure

GnRH

FSH/LH

Hypothalamic failure is most common cause of ovulatory dysfunction

°F
98.8
.6
.4
.2
98.0
.8
.6
97.4
BBT
Day   7   14   21   28

Oligomenorrhea or amenorrhea
and abnormal BBT are typical
signs of ovulatory dysfunction

Polycystic
ovary

Adrenal
tumor

Anovulation associated with increase in androgens; adrenal
tumors or polycystic ovarian disease may cause virilization

Pituitary adenoma

Prolactin

Galactorrhea

Pituitary adenoma increases prolactin
and causes amenorrhea

TSH

Hypothyroidism can
cause amenorrhea
with ↑TSH

Hypothalamic amenorrhea
(most common cause of
anovulation) requires
exclusionary testing

JOHN A.CRAIG—AD
©ICON

Extreme weight loss or
excessive exercise may
cause hypothalamic
amenorrhea

ANDROGEN INSENSITIVITY SYNDROME

INTRODUCTION

Description: These patients have a normal male karyotype but a genetic alteration that results in somatic cells that cannot recognize or respond to testosterone.

Prevalence: Uncommon, 10% of patients with primary amenorrhea (third most common cause).

Predominant Age: Generally discovered in middle to late teens.

Genetics: Absence of an X-chromosome gene that encodes for cytoplasmic or nuclear testosterone receptor protein, X-linked recessive.

ETIOLOGY AND PATHOGENESIS

Causes: Testosterone and gonadotropin levels are essentially normal (there may be a slight increase in luteinizing hormone [LH]), but the testosterone is biologically ineffective because of the body's inability to use it. Consequently, masculinization does not take place, and the normal production of müllerian inhibiting factor results in regression of the upper genital tract and a blind vaginal pouch.

Risk Factors: None known.

CLINICAL CHARACTERISTICS

Signs and Symptoms:

Amenorrhea

Tall stature

Normal breast development with immature nipples and hypopigmented areolae

Short or absent blind vaginal pouch

Scant or no pubic or axillary hair

Gonads (testes) may be palpable in the inguinal canal or labioscrotal folds

Inguinal hernia (50%)

DIAGNOSTIC APPROACH

Differential Diagnosis:

Pregnancy before first cycle

Obstructed outflow tract (making menstruation cryptic)

Gonadal dysgenesis

Uterine agenesis

Complete lack of müllerian development (Mayer-Rokitansky-Küster-Hauser syndrome)

Associated Conditions: Infertility, amenorrhea, mildly impaired visual-spatial ability, horseshoe kidney.

Workup and Evaluation

Laboratory: Measurement of gonadotropins, estrogen, and testosterone (not required for diagnosis).

Imaging: Ultrasonography may be used to confirm the absence of the uterus, although it is not required for diagnosis.

Special Tests: Chromosomal analysis confirms the diagnosis.

Diagnostic Procedures: History and physical examination should provide the suggestion, confirmed by chromosomal analysis.

Pathologic Findings

The presence of testicular tissue in the labioscrotal folds.

MANAGEMENT AND THERAPY

Nonpharmacologic

General Measures: Evaluation and reassurance.

Specific Measures: Surgical extirpation of the gonads must be performed because of a 25%–30% risk of malignant gonadal tumor formation. This should not be performed until complete breast development has occurred and there has been epiphyseal closure (age 18). Genetic counseling should be offered to siblings.

Diet: No specific dietary changes indicated.

Activity: No restriction.

Patient Education: Frank discussion about the syndrome and its effects (infertility and amenorrhea). Patients should be informed that they carry an abnormal sex chromosome without mentioning the Y chromosome specifically because of the "male" connotations this carries. In addition, the term *gonads* should be used rather than *testes* when discussing the need for removal.

Drug(s) of Choice

None. (Estrogen replacement therapy is generally not necessary after removal of the gonads; the insensitivity of the peripheral tissues to the effects of circulating androgens results in unopposed estrogen effects from the low levels of estrogen that come from adrenal and peripheral conversion sources.)

FOLLOW-UP

Patient Monitoring: Normal health maintenance once the diagnosis is established and the gonads are removed (at the appropriate time).

Prevention/Avoidance: None.

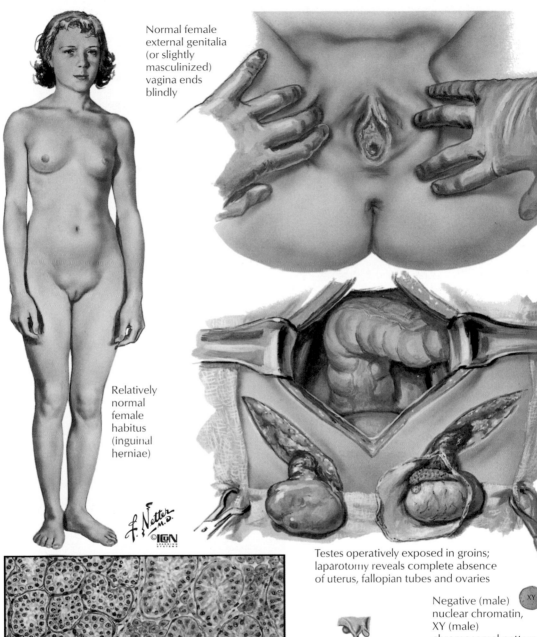

Normal female external genitalia (or slightly masculinized) vagina ends blindly

Relatively normal female habitus (inguinal herniae)

Testes operatively exposed in groins; laparotomy reveals complete absence of uterus, fallopian tubes and ovaries

Negative (male) nuclear chromatin, XY (male) chromosomal pattern

XY

Urinary gonadotropins normal

17-KS normal or slightly elevated

Estrogen (normal levels for female)

Section of testis typical of cryptorchidism (adenoma in upper left corner)

Possible Complications: There is a 25%–30% risk of malignant gonadal tumor formation if the testes are not removed (rare before age 25).

Expected Outcome: These patients are phenotypically, behaviorally, and psychologically female and continue to lead normal lives with the exception of infertility and amenorrhea.

MISCELLANEOUS

Pregnancy Considerations: These patients are infertile.

ICD-9-CM Codes: 257.8.

REFERENCES

American College of Obstetricians and Gynecologists. *Amenorrhea.* Washington, DC: ACOG; 1989. Technical Bulletin 128.

Griffin JE. Androgen resistance–the clinical and molecular spectrum. *N Engl J Med* 1992;326:611.

Morris JM. The syndrome of testicular feminization in male pseudohermaphrodites. *Am J Obstet Gynecol* 1953;65:1192.

Morris JM, Mahesh VB. Further observations on the syndrome "testicular feminization." *Am J Obstet Gynecol* 1963;87:731.

Speroff L, Glass RH, Kase NG, eds. *Clinical Gynecologic Endocrinology and Infertility.* 5th ed. Baltimore, Md: Williams & Wilkins; 1994:339, 420.

ANOVULATION

INTRODUCTION

Description: Absence of ovulation in woman of reproductive age.

Prevalence: Up to 30% of infertile couples.

Predominant Age: Reproductive.

Genetics: No genetic pattern, some chromosomal abnormalities are associated with premature ovarian failure (deletions on the X chromosome).

ETIOLOGY AND PATHOGENESIS

Causes: Physiologic—menopause (normal or premature), pregnancy; hormonal—elevated prolactin, hypothyroidism; functional—exercise (excessive), malnutrition, obesity, weight loss; drug-induced—alkylating chemotherapy, hormonal contraception, marijuana, tranquilizers; neoplasia—craniopharyngioma, hypothalamic hamartoma, pituitary adenoma (prolactin-secreting), small cell carcinoma of lung; psychogenic—anorexia nervosa, anxiety, pseudocyesis, stress; other—adrenal androgenization, central nervous system trauma, chronic medical illness, hemochromatosis, histiocytosis X, internal carotid artery aneurysms, irradiation, juvenile diabetes mellitus, polycystic ovary syndrome, Sheehan's syndrome (postpartum ischemic necrosis), syphilitic gummas, tuberculosis, uremia.

Risk Factors: Factors noted above.

CLINICAL CHARACTERISTICS

Signs and Symptoms:

Amenorrhea (primary or secondary)

Absence of premenstrual molimina (prodromal symptoms)

DIAGNOSTIC APPROACH

Differential Diagnosis:

Pregnancy must always be considered

Menopause

Congenital abnormality of the outflow tract causing amenorrhea

Cervical stenosis resulting in amenorrhea

Associated Conditions: Infertility, dysfunctional uterine bleeding, endometrial hyperplasia, and endometrial cancer.

Workup and Evaluation

Laboratory: Follicle-stimulating hormone (FSH), prolactin, thyroid function studies (eg, sensitive thyroid-stimulating hormone [TSH]), others as indicated clinically.

Imaging: No imaging indicated.

Special Tests: Basal body temperature charting may be used to detect ovulation, but other laboratory tests are more specific for establishing the cause.

Diagnostic Procedures: Endometrial biopsy performed during the presumed luteal phase.

Pathologic Findings

Endometrial—proliferative changes only, hyperplasia possible with prolonged anovulation.

MANAGEMENT AND THERAPY

Nonpharmacologic

General Measures: Evaluation.

Specific Measures: If pregnancy is desired, induction of ovulation. If pregnancy is not desired, periodic progestin therapy.

Diet: No specific dietary changes indicated.

Activity: No restriction.

Patient Education: Reassurance, American College of Obstetricians and Gynecologists Patient Education Pamphlet AP002 (*Infertility: Causes and Treatments*), AP095 (*Abnormal Uterine Bleeding*), AP049 (*Menstruation*), AP047 (*The Menopause Years*).

Drug(s) of Choice

Ovulation induction—clomiphene citrate 50 mg PO qd on days 5–10 of the menstrual cycle, may be increased to 100 mg PO qd on days 5–10 of the menstrual cycle if ovulation does not occur

Progestin withdrawal—medroxyprogesterone acetate 5–10 mg for 1–14 days each month

Contraindications: Undiagnosed amenorrhea or bleeding.

Precautions: Progestins should not be used until pregnancy has been ruled out.

Alternative Drugs

Norethindrone acetate 5–10 mg for 10–14 days each month.

FOLLOW-UP

Patient Monitoring: Normal health maintenance.

Prevention/Avoidance: None.

Possible Complications: Infertility, dysfunctional uterine bleeding, endometrial hyperplasia.

Expected Outcome: For many patients, normal ovulation and fertility may be restored.

MISCELLANEOUS

Pregnancy Considerations: No effect on pregnancy once pregnancy is achieved.

ICD-9-CM Codes: 628.0.

Assessment of Ovulation

Ovulatory phase
Hormonal and physical findings indicate ovulation occurred

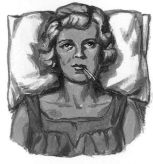

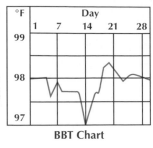

BBT Chart

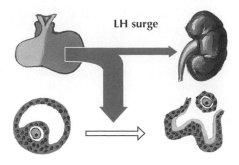

LH surge

Basal body temperature (BBT). Detects signs of ovulation

Preovulatory follicle   Ruptured follicle

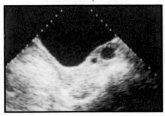

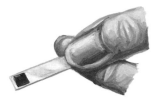

Serial follicular ultrasonography. Monitors follicular rupture

Ovulation detection kit detects urinary metabolites of luteinizing hormone (LH)

Luteal phase
Hormonal and physical findings indicate functioning corpus luteum

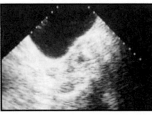

Progesterone

Corpus luteum

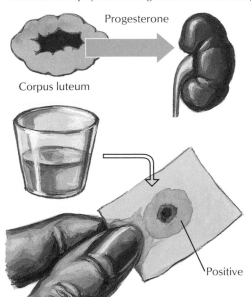

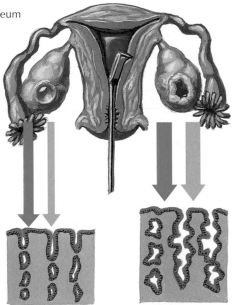

Positive

Spot urine test. Detects urinary metabolites of progesterone (measure of corpus luteum function)

Proliferative phase   Secretory phase

Endometrial biopsy and dating. Provides evidence of functioning corpus luteum and end organ response

JOHN A. CRAIG—AD
© ICON

REFERENCES

Alpert MM, Garner PR. Premature ovarian failure: its relationship to autoimmune disease. *Obstet Gynecol* 1985;66:27.

American College of Obstetricians and Gynecologists. *Infertility.* Washington, DC: ACOG; 1989. ACOG Technical Bulletin 125.

Liu JH. Hypothalamic amenorrhea: Clinical perspectives, pathophysiology, and management. *Am J Obstet Gynecol* 1990;163:1732.

Pettersson F, Fries H, Nillius SJ. Epidemiology of secondary amenorrhea. I. Incidence and prevalence rates. *Am J Obstet Gynecol* 1973;117:80.

Reindollar RH, Novak M, Tho SPT, McDonough PG. Adult-onset amenorrhea: a study of 262 patients. *Am J Obstet Gynecol* 1986;155:531.

Smith RP. *Gynecology in Primary Care.* Baltimore, Md: Williams & Wilkins; 1997:25, 339.

ASSISTED REPRODUCTION

THE CHALLENGE

To use advanced reproductive technology to assist couples who experience difficulty conceiving through normal means.

Scope of the Problem: Ten percent to fifteen percent of infertile couples require or benefit from assisted reproductive technologies.

Objectives of Management: To achieve a successful pregnancy (carried to term) with a minimum of intervention. The treatment of an infertile couple is based on identifying the impediment to fertility and overcoming or bypassing it to achieve pregnancy. A number of techniques are available to accomplish this end. Most are less exotic than their acronyms suggest (see table). Among infertile couples seeking treatment, 85%–90% can be treated with conventional medical and surgical procedures and do not require assisted reproductive technologies such as in vitro fertilization.

TACTICS

Relevant Pathophysiology: The success of treatment depends to a great extent on the identified cause of infertility because some problems are more easily overcome than others. It must be recognized that success is also a function of the age of the woman. It is also true that the rate of spontaneous pregnancy loss increases rapidly after age 35, adversely impacting success.

Strategies: Often a good starting point in the treatment of infertility is a frank and open discussion about sexuality and the physiology of conception. When couples have intercourse four or more times per week, more than 80% achieve pregnancy in the first 6 months of trying. By contrast, only about 15% of couples conceive when intercourse happens less than once a week. Intercourse should be maintained on an every-other-day cycle for the period from 3–4 days before the presumed ovulation until 2–3 days after that time. When ovulation disorders are encountered, ovulation induction or control may be used to enhance the likelihood of pregnancy. Tubal factor infertility may be addressed by either surgical repair of the damage or by bypassing the tubes completely through in vitro fertilization and embryo transfer (IVF/ET). Success rates for surgical repair, including the reversal of previous sterilization procedure, are highly variable. Technologies such as intracellular sperm injection may allow fertility with as few as one sperm per oocyte.

Patient Education: Reassurance, American College of Obstetricians and Gynecologists Patient Education Pamphlet AP002 (*Infertility: Causes and Treatments*).

ABBREVIATIONS FOR TECHNIQUES

Abbreviation	Technique
AID	Artificial insemination, donor (using donor sperm, occasionally referred to as *TDI* or *therapeutic donor insemination*)
AIH	Artificial insemination, homologous (using the partner's sperm)
BT	Basal body temperature
GIFT	Gamete intrafallopian transfer (gametes placed in the fallopian tube for fertilization)
HSG	Hysterosalpingogram or uterine cavity radiograph
ICSI	Intracytoplasmic sperm injection
IUI	Intrauterine insemination (placement of either donor or husband sperm directly into the uterine cavity)
IVF/ET	In vitro fertilization with embryo transfer
PCT	Postcoital test or Huhner-Sims test
SPA	Sperm penetration assay (also known as a hamster egg test or zona-free egg penetration test)
AFT	Zygote intrafallopian transfer (fertilization takes place in vitro and the zygote is transferred to the fallopian tube to be transported into the uterine cavity)

IMPLEMENTATION

Special Considerations: Infertility patients are extremely motivated, following to the letter any suggestion made by the health care team. For this reason, care must be taken that during the evaluation and treatment of infertility the couple's relationship is not destroyed in the process. In the end, there is no guarantee that efforts will result in a conception, so the health care team must not damage what is present in the quest of something that may not be. Couples should be reminded that "If you miss having intercourse at the 'right time' in a given month, remember that ovulations are like commuter trains—there is probably another one on its way." If the couple is in the mood for "making love," in any of its myriad forms, they should not worry about what the temperature chart is doing. To do otherwise is the fodder of cinematic comedy and divorce lawyers. Because in-

fertility threatens neither life nor health, many insurance providers do not cover the cost of its evaluation or treatment. A frank and open discussion about the time and expense involved in an infertility evaluation allows the couple to make informed choices and avoids unnecessary financial or emotional hardship in the future.

REFERENCES

American College of Obstetricians and Gynecologists. *Infertility.* Washington, DC: ACOG; 1989. ACOG Technical Bulletin 125.

American College of Obstetricians and Gynecologists. *New Reproductive Technologies.* Washington, DC: ACOG; 1990. ACOG Technical Bulletin 140.

Office of Technology Assessment. *Infertility: Medical and Social Choices.* Washington, DC: Congress of the United States; 1988:25.

Smith RP. *Gynecology in Primary Care.* Baltimore, Md: Williams & Wilkins; 1997:339.

Gonadotropins and HCG by injection

Superovulating ovary with mature follicles

In vivo fertilization

JOHN A.CRAIG —AD

HCG triggers superovulation, providing numerous ova for potential fertilization

Sperm fraction concentrate

Transcervical insemination bypasses interactive factor

Timed intrauterine insemination with sperm fraction concentrate within 24 hours after ovulation increases potential for fertilization

In Vitro Fertilization

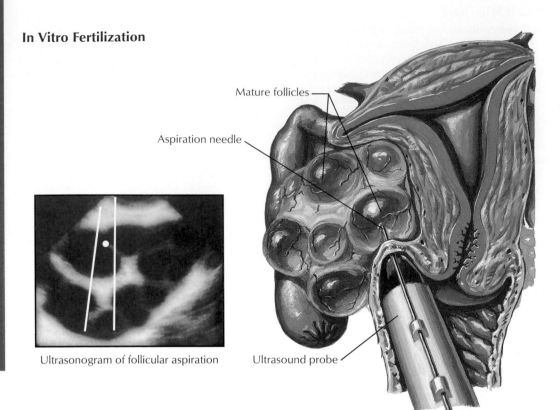

Mature follicles

Aspiration needle

Ultrasonogram of follicular aspiration

Ultrasound probe

In superovulating ovary, ova harvested from mature follicles transvaginally with ultrasound-guided needle

JOHN A. CRAIG—AD
© ICON

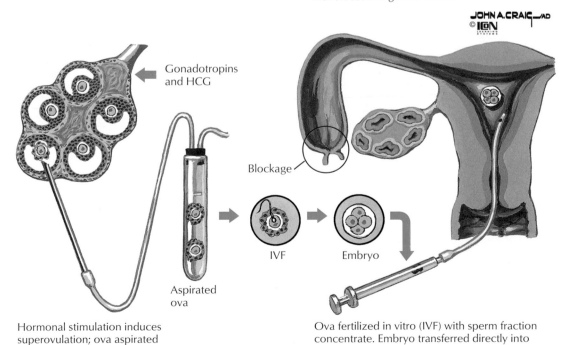

Gonadotropins and HCG

Blockage

IVF

Embryo

Aspirated ova

Hormonal stimulation induces superovulation; ova aspirated from mature follicles

Ova fertilized in vitro (IVF) with sperm fraction concentrate. Embryo transferred directly into uterus, bypassing tubal occlusion

Gamete Intrafallopian Transfer (GIFT) and Zygote Intrafallopian Transfer (ZIFT)

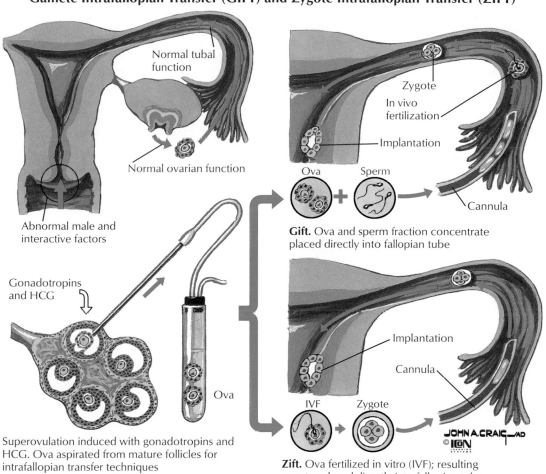

Normal tubal function

Normal ovarian function

Abnormal male and interactive factors

Gonadotropins and HCG

Ova

Superovulation induced with gonadotropins and HCG. Ova aspirated from mature follicles for intrafallopian transfer techniques

Zygote

In vivo fertilization

Implantation

Ova   Sperm

Cannula

Gift. Ova and sperm fraction concentrate placed directly into fallopian tube

Implantation

Cannula

IVF   Zygote

Zift. Ova fertilized in vitro (IVF); resulting zygotes placed directly into fallopian tube

JOHN A. CRAIG—AD
©ICON

DOWN SYNDROME

INTRODUCTION

Description: A syndrome of physical and mental symptoms that have their origin in the presence of extragenetic material from chromosome 21. This may be due to errors of duplication or the translocation of genetic material that results in effective duplication. These patients exhibit a spectrum of changes that range from mild to profound.

Prevalence: Based on maternal age.

Predominant Age: Most patients with Down syndrome are identified at birth; life-span is generally shortened.

Genetics: Ninety percent caused by nondisjunction resulting in an extra chromosome 21, 5% caused by translocation, 5% caused by mosaicism.

ETIOLOGY AND PATHOGENESIS

Causes: Nondisjunction of chromosome 21, resulting in two copies from one parent and one from the other, with a net of three. Balanced translocation of chromosome 21q material onto another chromosome (most often 12, 13, or 15) in 90% of patients. During cell division, this is inherited independently from the normal chromosome 21s, resulting in extra genetic material. Roughly one half of these duplications are new occurrences; one half have a parental carrier. Mosaicism of two cell lines: one normal and one with trisomy 21. This is generally associated with milder clinical manifestations.

Risk Factors: Maternal age, known carrier state (translocation), prior chromosomal abnormality. Screening based on age identifies only 25% of all cases (the remainder are born to low risk mothers).

CLINICAL CHARACTERISTICS

Signs and Symptoms:
  Brachycephaly (100%)
  Hypotonia at birth (80%)
  Posterior third fontanel
  Small or low set ears
  Prominent epicanthal folds, mongoloid eyes (90%)
  Enlarged tongue (75%)
  Depressed nasal bridge
  Cardiac murmur (50%)
  Mental retardation (IQ = 40–45)
  Abnormal dermatoglyphics (single palmar crease, absent plantar whorl)

DIAGNOSTIC APPROACH

Differential Diagnosis: Familial structural mimics (mongoloid faces)

Associated Conditions: Renal and cardiac anomalies, mental retardation, bowel obstruction, Hirschsprung's disease, and thyroid disease.

Workup and Evaluation

Laboratory: Maternal serum α-fetoprotein (MSAFP) screening between 15 and 22 weeks of gestation (16–18 optimal) may be abnormally low, suggesting the presence of an infant with Down syndrome.

Imaging: Imaging of the urinary tract should be considered to look for anomalies.

Special Tests: Karyotyping should be performed to look for translocation—useful for genetic counseling of parents. Chorionic villus sampling or amniocentesis may be performed for diagnosis.

Diagnostic Procedures: History, physical examination, chromosomal analysis (antenatal or after birth). (The presence of a whorl on the ball of the foot generally indicates a normal child, not a trisomy.)

Pathologic Findings

Physical changes as noted. Alzheimer's plaques common after age 20.

MANAGEMENT AND THERAPY

Nonpharmacologic

General Measures: Genetic and cardiac evaluation and counseling. Assessment of abilities and assistance with activities of daily living as appropriate.

Specific Measures: Based on the needs of the individual. Parental support and counseling are vital.

Diet: No specific dietary changes indicated.

Activity: No restriction, except if cardiac abnormalities are present.

Patient Education: American College of Obstetricians and Gynecologists Patient Education Pamphlet AP094 (*Genetic Disorders*), AP060 (*Later Childbearing*), AP107 (*Amniocentesis and Chorionic Villus Sampling*).

Drug(s) of Choice

None.

FOLLOW-UP

Patient Monitoring: Normal health maintenance, monitor for renal or cardiac complications.

Down (Trisomy 21) Syndrome

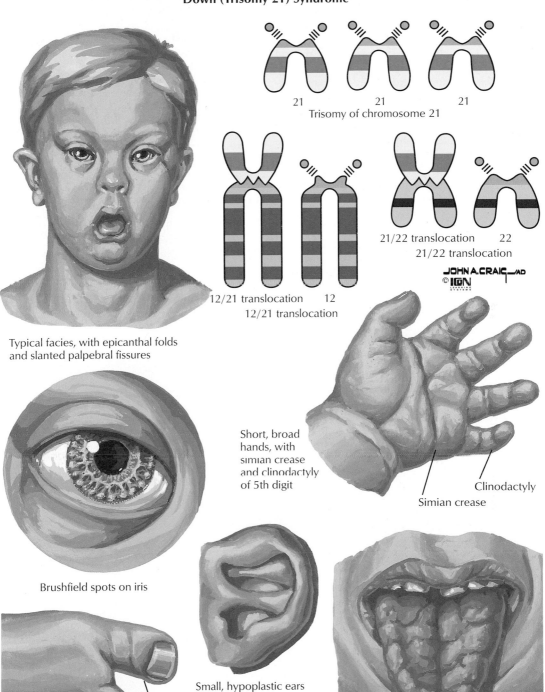

21   21   21

Trisomy of chromosome 21

12/21 translocation   12

12/21 translocation

21/22 translocation   22

21/22 translocation

JOHN A. CRAIG—AD
©ICN

Typical facies, with epicanthal folds
and slanted palpebral fissures

Short, broad
hands, with
simian crease
and clinodactyly
of 5th digit

Clinodactyly

Simian crease

Brushfield spots on iris

Wide gap between
1st and 2nd toes

Small, hypoplastic ears

Fissured tongue in adults

Prevention/Avoidance: Recurrence rate is 1% for true trisomy, 16%–20% for translocation, 100% for trisomy involving chromosome 12.

Possible Complications: Congenital heart disease (50%), bowel obstruction (10%), Hirschsprung's disease (3%), thyroid disease (5%–8%), and Alzheimer's disease.

Expected Outcome: One third of patients have normal development during the first year of life; growth, language, and mental development slows thereafter. Life expectancy is reduced by cardiac and other associated anomalies. Life potential varies from ability to live and work within sheltered environment to profound restriction. Premature aging is common with life expectancy of 50–60 years.

MISCELLANEOUS

Pregnancy Considerations: Chorion villus sampling (9–10 weeks) or amniocentesis (13–15 weeks) should be offered for patients at risk by age or other factors. MSAFP (low) or triple screening (MSAFP, β-human chorionic gonadotropin, estriol) should be performed at 14–16 weeks.

Pregnancy is possible for patients with Down syndrome; recurrence rate is 50%.

ICD-9-CM **Codes:** 758.0.

REFERENCES

American College of Obstetricians and Gynecologists. *Maternal Serum Screening.* Washington, DC: ACOG; 1996. ACOG Technical Bulletin 228.

American College of Obstetricians and Gynecologists. *Antenatal Diagnosis of Genetic Disorders.* Washington, DC: ACOG; 1987. ACOG Technical Bulletin 228.

Ardinger RH Jr. Genetic counseling in congenital heart disease. *Pediatr Ann* 1997;26:99.

Benacerraf BR. The second-trimester fetus with Down syndrome: detection using sonographic features. *Ultrasound Obstet Gynecol* 1996;7:147.

Gray JC, Dunstan FD, Nix AB. Detection rates and false positive rates for Down syndrome screening: how precisely can they be estimated? *Early Hum Dev* 1996;47(suppl):S59.

Saller DN Jr, Canick JA. Maternal serum screening for fetal Down syndrome: clinical aspects. *Clin Obstet Gynecol* 1996;39:783.

Takashima S. Down syndrome. *Curr Opin Neurol* 1997;10:148.

GONADAL DYSGENESIS

INTRODUCTION

Description: A developmental abnormality of patients who do not carry the stigmata of Turner's syndrome but still suffer absent menarche because of chromosomal abnormalities. These patients are generally tall (>150 cm), are more normal in appearance, and are a chromosomally heterogeneous group: 46,XX, 46,XY, or mosaic X/XY karyotypes.

Prevalence: Appears in 1 of 2500 female births.

Predominant Age: Present at birth, may not be detected until puberty is delayed.

Genetics: Sporadic, loss of part or all of one X chromosome (amenorrhea more common with long arm loss; short stature with short arm loss).

ETIOLOGY AND PATHOGENESIS

Causes: Pure gonadal dysgenesis 45,XO (Turner's syndrome); 46,XY gonadal dysgenesis (Swyer syndrome); 46,XX q5 X chromosome long-arm deletion, mixed or mosaic.

Risk Factors: Translocations involving the X chromosome (rare).

CLINICAL CHARACTERISTICS

Signs and Symptoms (Based on the Amount of Chromatin Lost):

  Primary amenorrhea and infertility (the most common cause of failure to begin menstruation is gonadal dysgenesis; In approximately 60% of women with primary amenorrhea, an abnormality of gonadal differentiation or function has occurred during the fetal or neonatal period)

  Absent or grossly abnormal gonad development

DIAGNOSTIC APPROACH

Differential Diagnosis:

  Polycystic ovary disease

  Hypothyroidism

  Growth hormone deficiency or glucocorticoid excess

  Androgen insensitivity syndrome (male pseudohermaphroditism, testicular feminization)

  Intersex abnormality

  Enzymatic defects (such as 17α-hydroxylase deficiency)

  Structural genital tract abnormalities (uterine and/or vaginal agenesis or an imperforate hymen)

  Ovarian insensitivity syndrome (Savage's syndrome)

  Follicular depletion (autoimmune disease, infection [mumps], infiltrative disease processes [tuberculosis, galactosemia])

Associated Conditions: Amenorrhea, infertility, incomplete or abnormal external genitalia, and premature menopause.

Workup and Evaluation

Laboratory: FSH and LH levels are high (nonspecific). (FSH is usually elevated in gonadal dysgenesis.) Assessment of thyroid function, prolactin, or growth hormone if indicated by the differential diagnosis being considered.

Imaging: Pelvic ultrasound studies to evaluate the presence and condition of upper genital tract organs.

Special Tests: Karyotype.

Diagnostic Procedures: History, physical examination, karyotyping.

Pathologic Findings

Abnormal karyotype. Germ cell involution occurs soon after they migrate into the undifferentiated gonad. This results in fibrous streak gonads that are hormonally inactive.

MANAGEMENT AND THERAPY

Nonpharmacologic

General Measures: Evaluation, screening for associated defects, counseling about menstrual and fertility issues.

Specific Measures: Hormone replacement therapy. When there is a mosaicism involving a Y chromosome, surgical extirpation of the gonads must be performed because of a 25%–30% risk of malignant gonadal tumors. Timing of gonadal removal in patients with a Y chromosome is controversial; removal as soon as the diagnosis is made versus delaying removal until pubertal changes are complete.

Diet: No specific dietary changes indicated.

Activity: No restriction.

Patient Education: Extensive counseling about sexual maturation and fertility.

Drug(s) of Choice

Adolescents are much more sensitive to the effects of estrogen than are postmenopausal women, allowing doses in the range of 0.3 mg of conjugated estrogen, 0.5 mg of estradiol, or their equivalent, daily. After 6–12 months of therapy at this level, the dose should be doubled and a progestin (eg, medroxyprogesterone acetate, 10 mg for the first 12 days of the month) added, or the patient's treatment should be switched to combination oral

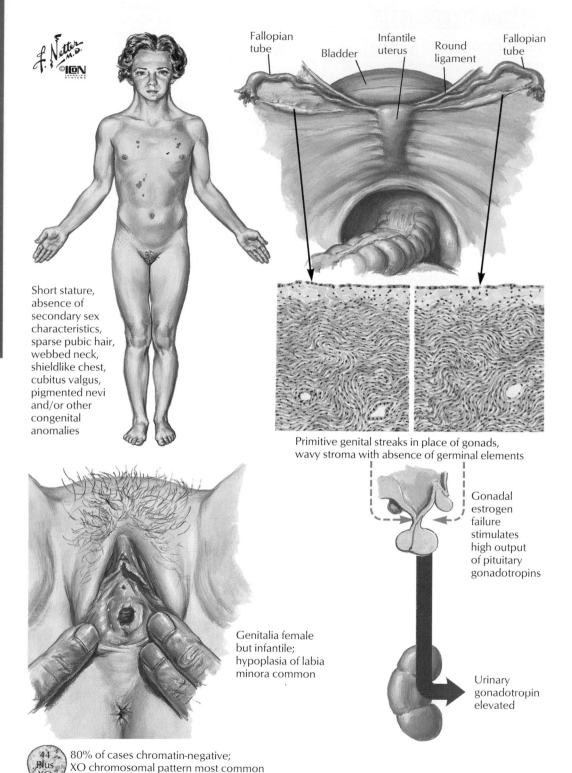

Fallopian tube

Bladder

Infantile uterus

Round ligament

Fallopian tube

Short stature, absence of secondary sex characteristics, sparse pubic hair, webbed neck, shieldlike chest, cubitus valgus, pigmented nevi and/or other congenital anomalies

Primitive genital streaks in place of gonads, wavy stroma with absence of germinal elements

Gonadal estrogen failure stimulates high output of pituitary gonadotropins

Urinary gonadotropin elevated

Genitalia female but infantile; hypoplasia of labia minora common

44 Plus XO

80% of cases chromatin-negative; XO chromosomal pattern most common

contraceptives. This generally results in regular menstruation, and normal pubertal development proceeds on its own when the patient reaches a bone age of 13.

Contraindications: Undiagnosed amenorrhea.

FOLLOW-UP

Patient Monitoring: Normal health maintenance.

Prevention/Avoidance: Prenatal chromosomal analysis for those known to carry translocations (detection only, not prevention although the couple may choose not to continue the pregnancy based on the findings).

Possible Complications: Gonadal malignancy or virilization in those with Y chromatin present. Others based on cause.

Expected Outcome: Reasonably normal lives with the exception of fertility.

MISCELLANEOUS

Pregnancy Considerations: These patients may be infertile. In pure gonadal dysgenesis and XX/XY mosaicism, a uterus is present. Consequently, some patients may achieve pregnancy. Pregnancy is associated with a 50% chance of aneuploidy.

ICD-9-CM Codes: 752.0.

REFERENCES

American Academy of Pediatrics Committee on Genetics. Health supervision for children with Turner syndrome. *Pediatrics* 1995;96:1166.

American College of Obstetricians and Gynecologists. *Amenorrhea.* Washington, DC: ACOG; 1989. Technical Bulletin 128.

Hall JG, Gilchrist DM. Turner's syndrome and its variants. *Pediatr Clin North Am* 1990;37:1421.

McDonough PG, Byrd JR. Gonadal dysgenesis. *Clin Obstet Gynecol* 1977;20:565.

Simpson JL, Meyers CM. Gonadal dysgenesis associated with 46,XX or 46,XY chromosomal patterns. In: Sciarra JJ, ed. *Gynecology and Obstetrics.* Vol 5. Philadelphia, Pa: Lippincott-Raven, 1994;86:1.

Simpson JL, Shulman LP. Gonadal dysgenesis associated with abnormal chromosomal complements. In: Sciarra JJ, ed. *Gynecology and Obstetrics.* Vol 5. Philadelphia, Pa: Lippincott-Raven, 1997;86:1.

HIRSUTISM

INTRODUCTION

Description: Hirsutism refers to increased or excessive hair growth only. It may be idiopathic (hypertrichosis) or caused by androgen-stimulated excessive growth. Hypertrichosis involves increased hair on the extremities and tends to be ethnic, racial, or familial in origin. This is not considered hirsutism.

Prevalence: Five percent to twenty-five percent of women, variable within ethnic groups, 60% of women with Cushing's disease.

Predominant Age: After puberty.

Genetics: Influenced by the number of hair follicles present, a function of race and ethnicity.

ETIOLOGY AND PATHOGENESIS

Causes: Familial, idiopathic, increased hair follicle androgens (5α-reductase). Increased androgen production—ovarian (polycystic ovary disease, hilus cell hyperplasia/tumor, arrhenoblastoma, adrenal rest), adrenal (congenital adrenal hyperplasia [10%–15% of hirsute women], Cushing's disease, virilizing carcinoma or adenoma). Drugs (minoxidil, androgens [including Danocrine], phenytoin, diazoxide). Other (hypothyroidism, hyperprolactinemia).

Risk Factors: Androgen use, danazol sodium, minoxidil, phenytoin, and diazoxide.

CLINICAL CHARACTERISTICS

Signs and Symptoms:

Increased or excessive hair growth, primarily along the angle of the jaw, upper lip, and chin. (For most patients, hirsutism dates from puberty.)

Menstrual irregularity or amenorrhea (60%)

Acne (40%)

DIAGNOSTIC APPROACH

Differential Diagnosis:

Virilization (especially when hirsutism is in a male pattern)

Familial hypertrichosis

Cushing's disease (truncal obesity, facial rounding, cervicodorsal fat deposition [buffalo hump], and red or purple striae are often not fully developed)

Polycystic ovary disease

Iatrogenic hirsutism (patients may use steroids for a number of reasons, legal and otherwise, and may not recognize the possibility of virilizing side effects; the use of danazol sodium, eg, for endometriosis ther-

apy, may be associated with increased hair growth as well)

Acromegaly

Hypothyroidism

Hyperprolactinemia

Anorexia nervosa

Associated Conditions: Obesity, menstrual irregularity, amenorrhea, infertility, acne, oily skin, increased libido, alopecia, acanthosis nigricans.

Workup and Evaluation

Laboratory: Evaluation for possible virilizing process (prolactin, dehydroepiandrosterone sulfate [DHEA-s], FSH, thyroid screening). (Patients suspected of having adrenal sources of hyperandrogenicity may be screened by measuring 24-hour urinary-free cortisol, by performing adrenocorticotropic hormone [ACTH] stimulation tests, or an overnight dexamethasone suppression test.) Circulating testosterone is generally normal or only mildly elevated (<1.5 ng/mL). Eighty percent of patients with idiopathic hirsutism have elevated levels of 3α-diol-G (metabolite of 5α-reductase).

Imaging: No imaging indicated, except as indicated by physical or laboratory findings.

Special Tests: Clitoral index may be useful if virilization is suspected. (The clitoral index is defined as the vertical dimension times the horizontal dimension, in millimeters. The normal range is from 9–35 mm, with borderline values in the range of 36–99 mm. Values above 100 mm indicate severe hyperandrogenicity and should prompt aggressive evaluation and referral.) Hirsutism may be quantified using the Ferriman-Gallwey scoring system.

Diagnostic Procedures: History and physical examination, Ferriman-Gallwey score >8.

Pathologic Findings

Based on underlying pathophysiologic conditions.

MANAGEMENT AND THERAPY

Nonpharmacologic

General Measures: Evaluation, shaving, depilatories, or electrolysis. Topical treatment of acne (if present). Weight reduction if obesity is present.

Specific Measures: Suppressive therapies reduce the growth of new hair, but once a hair follicle is *induced,* or turned on, it continues to grow. For this reason, shaving, depilatories, or electrolysis may be required. These are satisfactory only if combined with other therapies to reduce new growth.

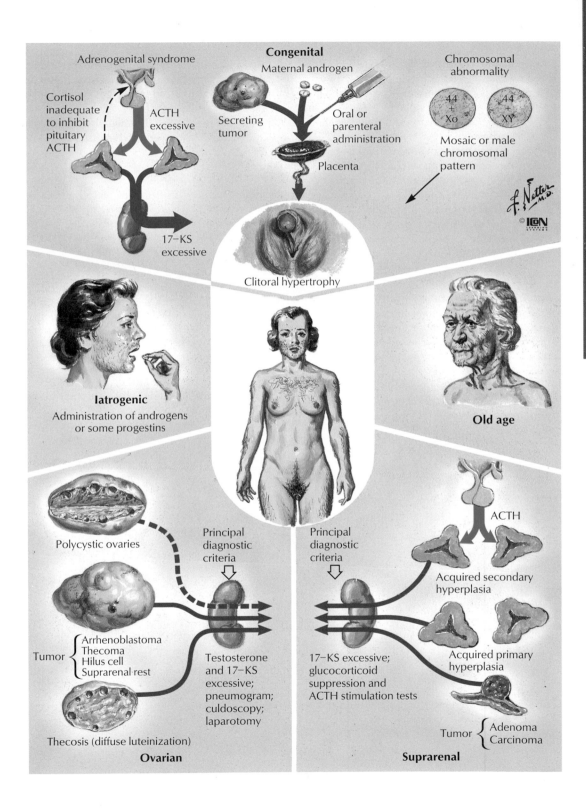

Adrenogenital syndrome

Cortisol inadequate to inhibit pituitary ACTH

ACTH excessive

17–KS excessive

Congenital

Maternal androgen

Secreting tumor

Oral or parenteral administration

Placenta

Chromosomal abnormality

44 + Xo

44 + XY

Mosaic or male chromosomal pattern

Clitoral hypertrophy

Iatrogenic

Administration of androgens or some progestins

Old age

Polycystic ovaries

Tumor { Arrhenoblastoma, Thecoma, Hilus cell, Suprarenal rest }

Thecosis (diffuse luteinization)

Ovarian

Principal diagnostic criteria

Testosterone and 17–KS excessive; pneumogram; culdoscopy; laparotomy

Principal diagnostic criteria

17–KS excessive; glucocorticoid suppression and ACTH stimulation tests

ACTH

Acquired secondary hyperplasia

Acquired primary hyperplasia

Tumor { Adenoma, Carcinoma }

Suprarenal

Diet: No specific dietary changes indicated.
Activity: No restriction.

Drug(s) of Choice

5α-Reductase inhibitors (finasteride 5 mg PO daily)

Polycystic ovary syndrome—combination oral contraceptives: spironolactone (100–200 mg PO daily), medroxyprogesterone acetate (Depo-Provera 150–300 mg IM q3 mo)

Hyperandrogenicity of adrenal origin—cortisol administration. If DHEA-s is elevated, dexamethasone (0.25–0.5 mg PO qhs) may be added.

Contraindications: Pregnancy. (Spironolactone and finasteride are category X drugs; patients using them and able to become pregnant must use reliable contraception.)

FOLLOW-UP

Patient Monitoring: Normal health maintenance once a diagnosis is established. Contraception and weight maintenance should also be addressed. There is an increased risk of diabetes for patients with polycystic ovaries.

Prevention/Avoidance: None.

Possible Complications: Permanent induction of hair changes. Chronic anovulation is associated with increased risk of endometrial hyperplasia and cancer.

Expected Outcome: Approximately 70% response after 1 year of therapy may be expected.

MISCELLANEOUS

Pregnancy Considerations: No effect on pregnancy, although some metabolic causes of hirsutism may result in reduced fertility or virilization of a fetus.

ICD-9-CM Codes: 704.1. Clitomegally, 642.2, (excludes that found in endocrine disorders 255.2, 256.1)

REFERENCES

American College of Obstetricians and Gynecologists. *Evaluation and Treatment of Hirsute Women.* Washington, DC: ACOG; 1995. ACOG Technical Bulletin 203.

Carr BR, Breslau NA, Givens C, Byrd W, Barnett-Hamm C, Marshburn PB. Oral contraceptive pills, gonadotropin-releasing hormone agonists, or use in combinations for treatment of hirsutism: a clinical research center study. *J Clin Endocrinol Metab* 1995;80:1169.

Ferriman D, Gallwey JD. Clinical assessment of body hair growth in women. *J Clin Endocrinol Metab* 1961; 21:1440.

Fruzzetti F, De Lorenzo D, Parrini D, Ricci C. Effects of finasteride, a 5α-reductase inhibitor, on circulating androgens and gonadotropin secretion in hirsute women. *J Clin Endocrinol Metab* 1994;79:831.

Kuttenn F, Couillin P, Girard F, et al. Late-onset adrenal hyperplasia in hirsutism. *N Engl J Med* 1985;313:224.

Rittmaster RS, Loriaux DL. Hirsutism. *Ann Intern Med* 1987;106:95.

HYPERPROLACTINEMIA

INTRODUCTION

Description: Pathologic elevation of serum prolactin levels. The finding of elevated levels of prolactin is nonspecific as to cause, requiring careful clinical evaluation.

Prevalence: Uncommon; reports vary from 1% to 30% depending on the population studied.

Predominant Age: Reproductive.

Genetics: No genetic pattern.

ETIOLOGY AND PATHOGENESIS

Causes: Pituitary adenoma (most common), pharmacologic (most often those that affect dopamine or serotonin), herpes zoster, chest wall/breast stimulation or irritation, physiologic during pregnancy, or after childbirth and/or nursing.

Risk Factors: Exposure to known pharmacologic agents, specific disease processes (see table).

CLINICAL CHARACTERISTICS

Signs and Symptoms:
Asymptomatic
Bilateral, spontaneous milky discharge from both breasts (75%)
Amenorrhea (30%)
Large adenoma, clinical appearance of impingement on the optic nerve or adjacent structures

DIAGNOSTIC APPROACH

Differential Diagnosis:
Pregnancy
Breast cancer
Chronic nipple stimulation
Hypothyroidism
Sarcoidosis
Lupus
Cirrhosis or hepatic disease
Radiculopathy (herpetic)

Associated Conditions: One third of patients with elevated prolactin levels experience amenorrhea or infertility. Prolonged amenorrhea is associated with an increased risk of osteoporosis.

Workup and Evaluation

Laboratory: Serum prolactin level. Pregnancy should always be considered if menses are absent.

Imaging: Computed tomography (CT) or magnetic resonance imaging (MRI) to evaluate the pituitary and surrounding bony structures; MRI now preferred.

Special Tests: Assessment of visual fields may be indicated.

Diagnostic Procedures: History, physical examination, and laboratory determination of prolactin levels.

Pathologic Findings

None.

MANAGEMENT AND THERAPY

Nonpharmacologic

General Measures: When prolactin levels are low and a coned-down view of the sella turcica is normal, observation alone may be sufficient. If observation is chosen, periodic reevaluation is required to check for the emergence of slow-growing tumors.

Specific Measures: Treatment with bromocriptine is recommended for patients who desire pregnancy or for those with distressing degrees of galactorrhea or to suppress intermediate sized pituitary tumors. Rapidly growing tumors, tumors that are large at the time of discovery, or those that do not respond to bromocriptine therapy may have to be treated surgically.

Diet: No specific dietary changes indicated.

Activity: No restriction.

Patient Education: American College of Obstetricians and Gynecologists Patient Education Pamphlet AP102 (*Infertility*).

Drug(s) of Choice

Bromocriptine (Parlodel) 2.5 mg daily increased gradually to tid.

Contraindications: Uncontrolled hypertension, pregnancy.

Precautions: With medical therapy—may experience nausea, orthostasis, drowsiness, or syncope: rarely may produce hypertension or seizures.

Interactions: Medical therapy may interact with phenothiazines or butyrophenones.

Alternative Drugs

Intravaginal bromocriptine.
Dopamine agonists (cabergoline) may become available.

FOLLOW-UP

Patient Monitoring: Normal health maintenance. If a pituitary adenoma is present, periodic assessment of visual fields should be considered.

Prevention/Avoidance: None.

Possible Complications: Visual field loss, symptoms may return after medication is discontinued.

SOURCES OF ELEVATED PROLACTIN LEVELS

Pharmacologic (Examples)	Pathophysiologic Causes
Anesthetics	Central nervous system
Central nervous system— dopamine-depleting agents	Cavernous sinus thrombosis
α-Methyldopa	Infection
Monoamine oxidase inhibitors	Neurofibromas
Reserpine	Temporal arteritis
Dopamine receptor blocking agents	Tumors and cysts (all types)
Domperidone	Hypothalamic
Haloperidol	Craniopharyngioma
Metoclopramide	Glioma
Phenothiazines	Granulomas
Pimozide	Histiocytosis disease
Sulpiride	Sarcoid
Dopamine reuptake blockers	Tuberculosis
Nomifensine	Irradiation damage
Histamine H_2-receptor antagonists	Pituitary stalk transection
Cimetidine	Surgical
Hormones	Traumatic
Estrogens	Pseudocyesis (functional)
Oral contraceptives	Pituitary lesions
Thyrotropin-releasing hormone	Acromegaly
Opiates	Mixed growth hormone or adrenocorticotropic hormone-prolactin secreting adenoma
Stimulators of serotoninergic inhibitors	Prolactinoma
Amphetamines	Somatic sources
Hallucinogens	Breast augmentation or reduction
	Bronchogenic carcinoma
	Chest wall trauma
	Chronic nipple stimulation
	Cushing syndrome
	Herpes zoster
	Hypernephroma
	Hypothyroidism
	Pregnancy
	Renal failure
	Upper abdominal surgery

Hyperprolactinemia

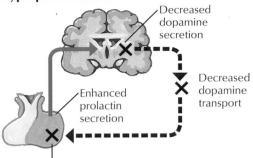

Decreased dopamine secretion

Decreased dopamine transport

Enhanced prolactin secretion

Decreased inhibition by dopamine

Conditions in which normal dopamine short-loop inhibition is blocked or prolactin secretion is enhanced cause clinically evident hyperprolactinemia

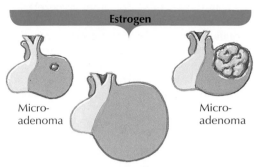

Estrogen

Micro-adenoma

Micro-adenoma

Hyperplasia

Conditions that increase estrogen levels may cause pituitary hyperplasia and induce growth of adenomas, causing hyperprolactinemia

Conditions associated with hyperprolactinemia

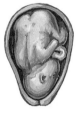

Pregnancy

Nursing

Chest wall stimulation

Drugs

Renal failure

Polycystic ovaries

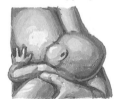

Infiltrating lesions of hypothalamus

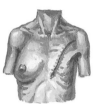

Pituitary stalk section

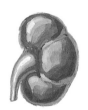

Pituitary tumor

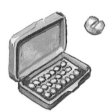

Hypothyroidism

JOHN A. CRAIG—AD
©ICON

Mechanisms in galactorrhea-amenorrhea syndromes

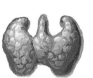

Dopamine

GnRH

LH

FSH

Failure of short-loop feedback inhibition

GnRH suppression

Hypogonadism amenorrhea anovulation

Galactorrhea

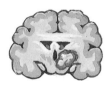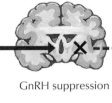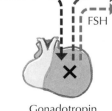

Gonadotropin suppression

Prolactin

Galactorrhea results from direct effect of prolactin on breast; amenorrhea and hypogonadism result from secondary prolactin effects (via dopamine) on GnRH and gonadotropin production and release

Chronic anovulation is associated with an increased risk of endometrial hyperplasia and cancer.

Expected Outcome: Generally good depending on cause. Prolactin levels should be measured every 6–12 months and visual fields reassessed yearly. The pituitary should be reevaluated every 2–5 years, based on initial diagnosis.

MISCELLANEOUS

Pregnancy Considerations: No effect on pregnancy. Pregnancy may cause adenomas to grow rapidly.

REFERENCES

American College of Obstetricians and Gynecologists. *Amenorrhea.* Washington, DC: ACOG; 1989. Technical Bulletin 128.

Detection, evaluation, and treatment of pituitary microadenomas in patients with galactorrhea and amenorrhea. *Am J Obstet Gynecol* 1977;128:356.

Schlechte J, Dolan K, Sherman B, Chapter F, Luciano A. The natural history of untreated hyperprolactinemia: a prospective analysis. *J Clin Endocrinol Metab* 1989; 68:412.

Smith RP. *Gynecology in Primary Care.* Baltimore, Md: Williams & Wilkins; 1997:405.

Speroff L, Glass RH, Kase NG. *Clinical Gynecologic Endocrinology and Infertility.* 5th Ed. Baltimore, Md: Williams & Wilkins; 1994:404, 555.

INFERTILITY

INTRODUCTION

Description: The inability to conceive or bear a child despite more than 1 year of trying. Under ordinary circumstances, 80%–90% of normal couples conceive during 1 year of attempting pregnancy. Infertility may be further subdivided into primary and secondary types based on the patient's past reproductive history: nulligravida infertility patients are in the primary infertility group; those who have become pregnant more than 1 year previously, regardless of the outcome of that pregnancy, are in the secondary infertility group. Slightly more than one half of infertility patients fall into the primary group.

Prevalence: Eight percent to eighteen percent of the American population; slightly higher for couples who have never conceived and slightly lower for couples who have conceived before.

Predominant Age: Reproductive. The prevalence of infertility increases with the age of the woman.

Genetics: No genetic pattern. Some chromosomal abnormalities are associated with reduced or absent fertility.

ETIOLOGY AND PATHOGENESIS

Causes: Approximately 35%–50% of infertility is due to a male factor, such as azoospermia. Female factors, such as tubal disease (20%–30%), ovulation disorders (10%–15%), and cervical factors (5%), contribute to the roughly 50%–60% of female causes. The remaining 10%–20% of couples have no identifiable cause for their infertility (idiopathic). Couples experiencing primary infertility are more likely to have idiopathic or chromosomal causes than are couples who have conceived previously.

Risk Factors: Factors that increase the risk of anovulation (obesity, athletic overtraining, exposure to drugs or toxins), pelvic adhesive disease (infection, surgery, endometriosis), impaired sperm production (mumps, varicocele), or sperm delivery (ejaculatory dysfunction).

CLINICAL CHARACTERISTICS

Signs and Symptoms:
Inability to conceive after 1 year of attempts

DIAGNOSTIC APPROACH

Differential Diagnosis:
Recurrent pregnancy loss
Primary infertility—Chromosomal abnormality (eg, 45,XO [Turner's syndrome], 46,XY gonadal dysgenesis [Swyer syndrome], 46,XX q5 X chromosome long-arm deletion)
Congenital abnormality of the genital tract (either partner)

Associated Conditions: Based on the pathologic condition causing the infertility.

Workup and Evaluation

Laboratory: Based on diagnoses being considered.

Imaging: Based on diagnoses being considered.

Special Tests: Half of all women found to have tubal factor infertility have no history of antecedent infections or surgery, supporting the need to evaluate tubal patency in patients regardless of their past history.

Diagnostic Procedures: Based on diagnoses being considered.

Pathologic Findings

None.

MANAGEMENT AND THERAPY

Nonpharmacologic

General Measures: Support—because infertility involves both members of the couple and intrudes on the most intimate aspects of their relationship, all with no promise of success, a great deal of support is vital.

Specific Measures: The treatment of an infertile couple is based on identifying the impediment to fertility and overcoming or bypassing it to achieve pregnancy.

Diet: No specific dietary changes indicated.

Activity: No restriction, unless athletic activities are thought to be adversely affecting fertility. While the evaluation of infertility proceeds, couples should be instructed to continue attempting pregnancy through intercourse timed to the most fertile days of the cycle.

Patient Education: Reassurance, American College of Obstetricians and Gynecologists Patient Education Pamphlet AP002 (*Infertility: Causes and Treatments*).

Drug(s) of Choice

(Based on diagnosis of cause)

Secondary infertility (ovulation induction)—clomiphene citrate 50 mg PO qd on days 5–10 of the menstrual cycle, may be increased to 100 mg PO qd on days 5–10 of the menstrual cycle if ovulation does not occur.

Contraindications: Undiagnosed infertility.

Precautions: The possibility of ovarian hyperstimulation must be considered and close follow-up maintained if ovulation induction is attempted.

Ovulatory Phase

Basal body temperature (BBT) detects signs of ovulation

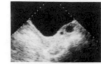

BBT chart

Preovulatory follicle

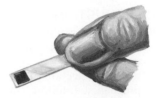

Ruptured follicle

Serial follicular ultrasound monitors follicular rupture

Ovulation detection kit detects urinary metabolites of luteinizing hormone (LH)

Luteal Phase

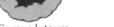

Corpus luteum

Progesterone

Endometrial biopsy and dating provides evidence of functioning corpus luteum and end organ response

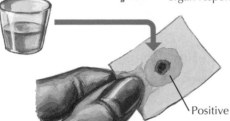

Positive

Spot urine test. Detects urinary metabolites of progesterone (measure of corpus luteum function)

Proliferative phase

Secretorys phase

Postcoital Analysis

Postcoital mucus specimen from endocervical canal placed on slide for testing

Motile sperm in orderly pattern

Ferning

Sluggish sperm in low numbers

Nonferning mucus

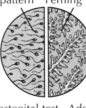
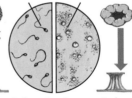

Optimal postcoital test. Adequate motile sperm and cervical mucus with high water content. Increased ferning and spinnbarkeit

Suboptimal postcoital test. Few sluggish sperm in thick, cellular mucus. Decreased ferning and spinnbarkeit

Semen Analysis

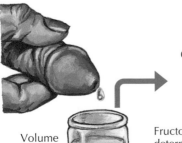

Volume

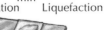

Fructose determination (if azospermic)

25–30 min

Coagulation

Liquefaction

morphology/motility

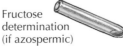

JOHN A. CRAIG—AD
© ICON
LEARNING SYSTEMS

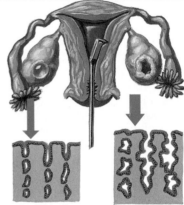
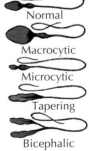

Normal

Macrocytic

Microcytic

Tapering

Bicephalic

Morphology

Alternative Drugs

Gonadotropin-releasing hormone (GnRH) agonists may be used to control the hormonal environment during ovulation induction. Human gonadotropins may be used to induce ovulation, but are associated with an increased risk of multiple ovulations and multiple gestations if pregnancy ensues.

FOLLOW-UP

Patient Monitoring: Normal health maintenance.

Prevention/Avoidance: None.

Expected Outcome: Less than 40% of couples with primary infertility conceive after 6 years of therapy compared with >50% of secondary infertility couples who conceive by 3 years.

MISCELLANEOUS

Pregnancy Considerations: No effect on pregnancy once pregnancy is achieved. Some causes of impaired fertility are associated with a greater risk of early pregnancy loss.

ICD-9-CM **Codes:** 628.9 (other more specific classifications based on cause).

REFERENCES

American College of Obstetricians and Gynecologists. *Infertility.* Washington, DC: ACOG; 1989. ACOG Technical Bulletin 125.

American College of Obstetricians and Gynecologists. *Male Infertility.* Washington, DC: ACOG; 1990. ACOG Technical Bulletin 142.

American College of Obstetricians and Gynecologists. *Managing the Anovulatory State: Medical Induction of Ovulation.* Washington, DC: ACOG; 1997. ACOG Technical Bulletin 142.

Office of Technology Assessment. *Infertility: Medical and social choices.* Washington, DC: Congress of the United States, 1988:25.

Mosher WD, Pratt WF. Fecundity and infertility in the United States, 1965–1988. *Advance Data* 1990;192:1.

Smith RP. *Gynecology in Primary Care.* Baltimore, Md: Williams & Wilkins; 1997:339.

MENOPAUSE

INTRODUCTION

Description: Endocrinopathy caused by the loss of normal ovarian steroidogenesis because of age, chemotherapy, radiation, or surgical therapy. (Menopause is now viewed as an endocrinopathy: the loss of an endocrine function with adverse health consequences.)

Prevalence: Of postmenopausal women who do not receive estrogen replacement, 100% risk health consequences.

Predominant Age: Median 51.5, 95% between 44 and 55 (or after surgical menopause).

Genetics: Loss of genetic material from the long arm of the X chromosome is associated with premature menopause.

ETIOLOGY AND PATHOGENESIS

Causes: Loss of estrogen production because of surgery, chemotherapy (alkylating agents), radiation, or natural cessation of ovarian function (menopause).

Risk Factors: Menopause may occur at a younger age in smokers, those with poor nutrition or chronic illness, or those who have a loss of genetic material from the long arm of the X chromosome.

CLINICAL CHARACTERISTICS

Signs and Symptoms:
- Absence of menstruation (with a normal uterus and outflow tract)
- Hot flashes, flushes, and night sweats
- Vaginal atrophy
- Dysuria, urgency, and urgency incontinence, urinary frequency, nocturia, and an increased incidence of stress urinary incontinence
- Decrease in libido
- Irregular bleeding common during the climacteric (perimenopausal) period

DIAGNOSTIC APPROACH

Differential Diagnosis:
- Pregnancy
- Hypothyroidism
- Polycystic ovary disease
- Prolactin-secreting tumor
- Hypothalamic dysfunction
- Hypothyroidism

Associated Conditions: Dyspareunia, vulvodynia, atrophic vulvitis, osteoporosis, increased risk of cardiovascular disease, hot flashes and flushes, sleep disturbances, stress urinary incontinence, and others.

Workup and Evaluation

Laboratory: Usually not necessary. When the diagnosis of ovarian failure must be confirmed, measurement of serum FSH is sufficient. Levels of greater than 100 mIU/mL are diagnostic, although lower levels (40–50 mIU/mL) may be sufficient to establish a diagnosis when symptoms are also present. Serum estradiol levels may be determined (generally less than 15 pg/mL) but are less reliable as a marker of ovarian failure. A pregnancy test is always indicated in sexually active perimenopausal women who are not using contraception.

Imaging: No imaging indicated. Standard imaging does not document bone loss of less than 30%.

Special Tests: A vaginal maturation index may be obtained, but is generally not required for diagnosis. Bone densitometry may be indicated for those at special risk. When noncyclic bleeding occurs in these patients, endometrial biopsy should be strongly considered. Women who have ovarian failure below age 30 should have a karyotype performed.

Pathologic Findings

Vaginal, vulvar, and endometrial atrophy. Thinned ovarian stroma with few, inactive oocytes. Accelerated calcium loss from bone.

MANAGEMENT AND THERAPY

Nonpharmacologic

General Measures: Health maintenance, annual mammogram, annual pelvic and rectal examinations, thyroid and cholesterol screening every 5 years or as indicated, tetanus booster shot every 10 years, *Pneumococcus* vaccine as indicated.

Specific Measures: Systemic estrogen (estrogen/progestin) therapy. (Less than 1% of women do not benefit from therapy. Only 17% of women use estrogen, 55% never try estrogen therapy, and 28% try but discontinue therapy.) Topical estrogen supplements.

Diet: Adequate dietary calcium (1000–1500 mg/d).

Activity: No restriction, weight-bearing activity to promote bone health, cardiovascular fitness training/maintenance.

Patient Education: Reassurance, American College of Obstetricians and Gynecologists Patient Education Pamphlet AP047 (*The Menopause Years*), AP066 (*Hormone Replacement Therapy*), AP048 (*Preventing Osteoporosis*), AP028 (*Vaginitis: Causes and Treatments*), AB008 (Menopause packet with 3 titles).

Pituitary and Ovarian Hormone Changes in Menopause

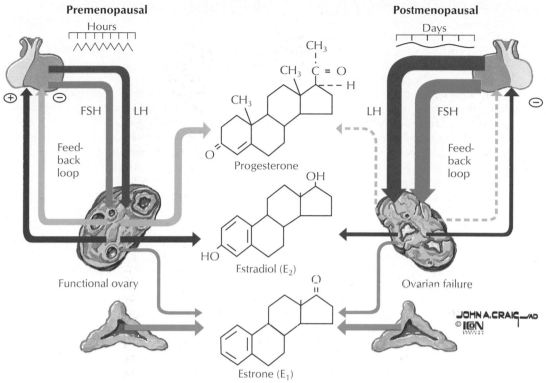

Premenopausal

Hours

FSH   LH

Feed-
back
loop

Functional ovary

Postmenopausal

Days

LH   FSH

Feed-
back
loop

Ovarian failure

CH_3
CH_3 C = O
CH_3 ‑‑‑ H
O
Progesterone

OH
HO
Estradiol (E_2)

O
Estrone (E_1)

JOHN A. CRAIG—AD
© ICON

Hormone levels increase and decrease cyclically during menstrual cycle. Modulation occurs by pulsatile releases of gonadotropins and positive and negative feedback loops

In postmenopausal period, gonadotropin levels increase and ovarian hormone levels decrease secondary to ovarian failure. Endogenous estrogen is primarily of adrenal origin, and E_1 to E_2 ratio is reversed

LH and FSH (mIU/ml)

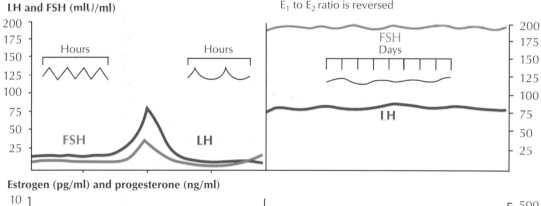

200
175
150
125
100
75
50
25

Hours   Hours

FSH   LH

FSH
Days

LH

200
175
150
125
100
75
50
25

Estrogen (pg/ml) and progesterone (ng/ml)

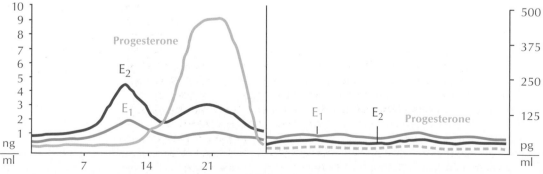

10
9
8
7
6
5
4
3
2
1
ng
ml

Progesterone

E_2
E_1

E_1 E_2 Progesterone

500

375

250

125

pg
ml

7   14   21

Drug(s) of Choice

(Most common drug doses shown)

Oral estrogens—conjugated equine estrogens (0.625–1.25 mg/d), diethylstilbestrol, esterified estrogens (0.625–1.25 mg/d), ethinyl estradiol (0.05 mg/d), micronized estradiol (0.5–1 mg/d), piperazine estrone sulfate, estropipate, quinestrol

Injectable estrogens—conjugated equine estrogens, estradiol benzoate, estradiol cypionate, estradiol valerate (oil), estrone (aqueous), ethinyl estradiol, polyestradiol phosphate

Topical estrogens—17β-estradiol (transdermal) (0.05–0.10 μg/d), conjugated equine estrogens (0.625 mg/g), estradiol (0.1 mg/g), estropipate (1.5 mg/g)

Contraindications: Systemic therapy:—active liver disease, carcinoma of the breast (current), chronic liver damage (impaired function), endometrial carcinoma (current), recent thrombosis (with or without emboli), unexplained vaginal bleeding. Relative contraindications/special considerations—endometriosis, familial hyperlipidemia, gallbladder disease, hypertension (uncontrolled), migraine headaches, seizure disorders, thrombophlebitis (unknown risk), uterine leiomyomas. Topical use—known sensitivity to vehicle.

Precautions: Continuous estrogen exposure without periodic or concomitant progestins increases the risk of endometrial carcinoma 6- to 8-fold. Continuous estrogen/progestin therapy frequently results in random vaginal bleeding, but biopsy or other investigation is still warranted. Patients receiving cyclic estrogen/progestin therapy should experience vaginal bleeding only after withdrawal of the progestin; biopsy or other investigation is warranted for other bleeding.

Interactions: Raloxifene should not be used with cholestyramine. Most therapies alter the effects of warfarin therapy.

Alternative Drugs

Raloxifene (Evista) 60 mg PO qd—no relief for hot flashes or vaginal dryness, but does reduce breast cancer risk

Progestin therapy (oral, vaginal, or injectable)—effective for hot flashes, may reduce bone loss, but has no effect on coronary artery disease or urogenital atrophy

Clonidine (oral or transdermal)

Bellergal-S (phenobarbital, ergotamine tartrate, belladonna)

Alendronate (Fosamax)—for osteoporosis.

Topical moisturizers for atrophic vaginitis

FOLLOW-UP

Patient Monitoring: Normal health maintenance. Continued (lifelong) compliance with medical therapy must be encouraged.

Prevention/Avoidance: Estrogen replacement therapy at menopause. The use of progestins is required if the patient retains her uterus to reduce the risk of iatrogenic endometrial hyperplasia or cancer. Therapy may be oral (such as medroxyprogesterone acetate [Provera] 5–10 mg PO qd for 12–14 days per month or 2.5 mg PO qd) or vaginal (progesterone bioadhesive gel [Crinone] 4%–8%, 45 mg [1.125 g] intravaginally every other day for six doses per month).

Possible Complications: Endometrial hyperplasia if the uterus is present and progestins not used, vaginal bleeding (predictable or otherwise).

Expected Outcome: Reversal of symptoms, reestablishment of normal physiology with treatment. Loss of symptoms with urogenital atrophy, osteoporosis and increased risk of coronary artery disease if untreated. Selective estrogen receptor modulators (also called *tissue specific estrogens*) may provide protection against cardiac, bone, and colon cancer and Alzheimer's disease with reduced rates of risk for both breast and endometrial cancer.

MISCELLANEOUS

Pregnancy Considerations: Menopause is associated with the loss of fertility.

ICD-9-CM Codes: 627.2 (Menopause or female climacteric states), 256.3 (Premature), 256.2 (Premature: post irradiation or surgical), 627.4 (Surgical).

REFERENCES

Albertazzi P, Pansini F, Bonaccorsi G, Zanotti L, Forini E, De Aloysio D. The effects of dietary soy supplementation on hot flushes. *Obstet Gynecol* 1998;91:6.

American College of Obstetricians and Gynecologists. *Hormone Replacement Therapy.* Washington, DC: ACOG; 1998. ACOG Technical Bulletin 247.

American College of Obstetricians and Gynecologists. *Health Maintenance for Perimenopausal Women.* Washington, DC: ACOG; 1995. ACOG Technical Bulletin 210.

Grodstein F, Stampfer MJ, Colditz GA. Postmenopausal hormone therapy and mortality. *N Engl J Med* 1997;336:1769.

Lobo RA. Benefits and risks of estrogen replacement therapy. *Am J Obstet Gynecol* 1995;173:982.

Sherwin BB. Hormones, mood and cognitive functioning in postmenopausal women. *Obstet Gynecol* 1996;87:20S.

Udoff L, Langenberg P, Adashi EY. Combined continuous hormone replacement therapy: a critical review. *Obstet Gynecol* 1995;86:306.

POLYCYSTIC OVARIAN DISEASE

INTRODUCTION

Description: A syndrome consisting of amenorrhea, hirsutism, insulin resistance, and obesity in association with enlarged, multicystic ovaries.

Prevalence: Up to 5% of women, 30% of secondary amenorrhea.

Predominant Age: Begins at menarche.

Genetics: No genetic pattern established, suggestion of increased family tendency.

ETIOLOGY AND PATHOGENESIS

Causes: The exact pathophysiology of polycystic ovarian disease is not well established, but increased amplitude of GnRH pulsation and abnormal secretion of FSH and LH during puberty are thought to result in androgen excess. Elevated levels of LH persist and may be used to help establish the diagnosis.

Risk Factors: Borderline adrenal hyperplasia, occult hypothyroidism, and childhood obesity.

CLINICAL CHARACTERISTICS

Signs and Symptoms:
Anovulation and amenorrhea (75%–80%)
Infertility (75%)
Excessive hair growth, primarily along the angle of the jaw, upper lip, and chin (70%)
Obesity (50%)
Acanthosis nigricans

DIAGNOSTIC APPROACH

Differential Diagnosis:
Virilization (especially when hirsutism is in a male pattern)
Familial hypertrichosis
Cushing's disease (truncal obesity, facial rounding, cervicodorsal fat deposition [buffalo hump], and red or purple striae are often not fully developed)

Associated Conditions: Increased risk of cardiovascular disease (adverse lipid profiles), diabetes (insulin resistance in 50% of patients), hypertension, and infertility.

Workup and Evaluation

Laboratory: Elevated levels of LH may be used to help establish the diagnosis. (A two to one ratio of LH to FSH is considered diagnostic.) Evaluation for possible virilizing process (prolactin, FSH, thyroid screening). (Patients suspected of having adrenal sources of hyperandrogenicity may be screened by measuring 24-hour urinary free cortisol, by performing ACTH stimulation tests, or an overnight dexamethasone suppression test.) Serum testosterone (total) is generally 70–120 ng/mL and androstenedione is 3–5 ng/mL. DHEA-s is elevated in roughly 50% of patients.

Imaging: Ultrasonography (abdominal or transvaginal) may identify ovarian enlargement or the presence of multiple small follicles. MRI or CT may be used to evaluate the adrenal glands.

Special Tests: None indicated.

Diagnostic Procedures: History, physical examination, imaging and laboratory evaluations. May be confirmed at laparoscopy, but seldom required for diagnosis.

Pathologic Findings

The ovaries are enlarged with a thickened white capsule. They contain multiple follicles in varying stages of development. Luteinization of theca cells may be present.

MANAGEMENT AND THERAPY

Nonpharmacologic

General Measures: Evaluation. Weight loss is often associated with resolution of symptoms and a return of menstrual function in patients with mild or early polycystic ovary disease.

Specific Measures: Medical therapy has replaced surgical treatment. Treatment depends on desire for pregnancy; if pregnancy is desired then ovulation induction may be required.

Diet: No specific dietary changes indicated, weight loss or control desirable.

Activity: No restriction.

Patient Education: American College of Obstetricians and Gynecologists Patient Education Pamphlet AP121 (*Polycystic Ovary Syndrome*).

Drug(s) of Choice

Combination oral contraceptives (less than 50 μg formulation and a progestin other than norgestrel)
If DHEA-s is elevated, dexamethasone (0.25–0.5 mg PO qhs) may be added to oral contraceptives
Spironolactone (100–200 mg PO daily)

Contraindications: Pregnancy. (Spironolactone is a category X drug; patients using it and able to become pregnant must use reliable contraception.)

Alternative Drugs

GnRH analogs and clomiphene citrate may be used.

FOLLOW-UP

Patient Monitoring: Normal health maintenance once diagnosis and management have been implemented. There is an increased risk of diabetes in patients with polycystic ovaries. Weight control and contraception should also be addressed.

Prevention/Avoidance: Role of normalized weight debated.

Possible Complications: Chronic anovulation is associated with osteoporosis and endometrial hyperplasia or carcinoma.

Expected Outcome: Generally good response to medical therapy.

MISCELLANEOUS

Pregnancy Considerations: No effect on pregnancy, although fertility is often reduced.

ICD-9-CM Codes: 256.4.

REFERENCES

DeVane GW, Czekala NM, Judd HL, Yen SS. Circulating gonadotropins, estrogens, and androgens in polycystic ovarian disease. *Am J Obstet Gynecol* 1975;121:496.

Franks S. Polycystic ovarian disease. *N Engl J Med* 1995;333:853.

Goldzieher JW. Polycystic ovarian syndrome. *Fertil Steril* 1981;35:371.

Goldzieher JW, Axelrod LR. Clinical and biochemical features of polycystic ovarian disease. *Fertil Steril* 1963;14:631.

Hall JE. Polycystic ovarian disease as a neuroendocrine disorder of the female reproductive axis. *Endocrinol Metab Clin North Am* 1993;22:75.

Luciano AA, Chapler FK, Sherman BM. Hyperprolactinemia in polycystic ovary syndrome. *Fertil Steril* 1984;41:719.

Plymate SR, Fariss BL, Basset ML, Matej L. Obesity and it s role in polycystic ovary syndrome. *J Clin Endocrinol Metab* 1981;52:1246.

Tagitz GE, Kopher RA, Nagel TC, Okagaki T. The clitoral index: a bioassay of androgenic stimulation. *Obstet Gynecol* 1979;54:562.

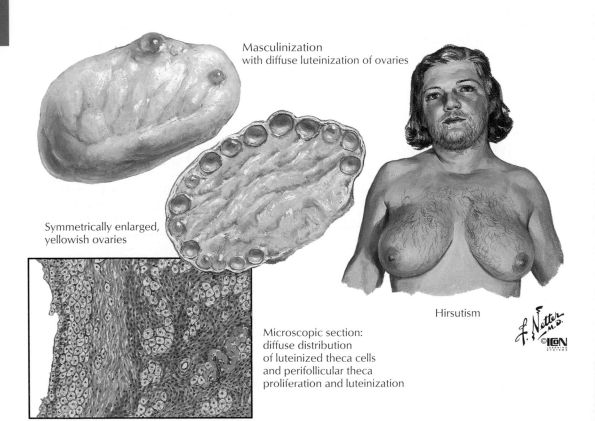

Masculinization with diffuse luteinization of ovaries

Symmetrically enlarged, yellowish ovaries

Microscopic section: diffuse distribution of luteinized theca cells and perifollicular theca proliferation and luteinization

Hirsutism

PUBERTY: ABNORMAL

THE CHALLENGE

To evaluate patients who do not experience the normal events of puberty when expected and to provide reassurance when appropriate or timely diagnosis and intervention when more sinister processes are at work.

Scope of the Problem: For all patients with precocious puberty (pubertal changes before age 8 or cyclic menstruation before age 10), the possibility of a serious process, either central or peripheral, must be evaluated. Precocious puberty is customarily divided into two classifications: true or GnRH-dependent, and precocious pseudopuberty that is independent of GnRH control. For most girls older than 4, no specific cause is usually discovered for the early development. By contrast, the most common cause of precocious change in girls younger than 4 is a central nervous system lesion, most often hamartomas of the hypothalamus. Even when the sequence of events appears normal, a serious process (such as a slowly progressing brain tumor) must be aggressively sought initially and watched for with long-term continuing follow-up. Delayed puberty is a relatively uncommon problem in girls. When it occurs, the possibility of a genetic or hypothalamic-pituitary abnormality must be considered, along with a moderately large number of other possibilities. Based on the average age and normal variation of puberty, any girl who has not exhibited breast budding by age 13 requires preliminary investigation. Similarly, girls who do not menstruate by age 15 or 16, regardless of other sexual development, should be evaluated. Patients should also be evaluated any time there is a disruption in the normal sequence of puberty or there is patient or parental concern. Patients with significant abnormalities of either height or weight should be evaluated for chromosomal abnormalities or endocrinopathies.

Objectives of Management: To establish the cause of delayed events of puberty with appropriate speed and care, without adding to the trauma of adolescence.

TACTICS

Relevant Pathophysiology: True precocious puberty, also known as complete, isosexual, or central precocity, is related to early activation of the hypothalamic-pituitary-gonadal axis. In three fourths of patients, there is no indication of how or why the normal processes of puberty are accelerated. In the remaining one fourth, a central nervous system abnormality is the cause. A number of central nervous system pathologic conditions may result in activation of GnRH secretion and the early onset of pubertal changes. Precocious pseudopuberty is also referred to as incomplete or peripheral and may be isosexual or heterosexual. In these patients, there may be secretion of sex steroids or human chorionic gonadotropin from sources other than the pituitary. More than 10% of girls with precocious puberty have an ovarian tumor. These tumors are palpable in 80% of patients or may be readily detected by ultrasonography or tomographic studies. Bleeding is heavy and irregular in character, befitting escape from the normal control mechanisms. One of the most common chromosomal causes of absent (delayed) menstruation is the premature ovarian failure found in patients with Turner's syndrome (45,X). The absence of one X chromosome results in accelerated ovarian follicular atresia, to the extent that by the age of puberty, no functionally competent follicles remain. The appearance of these patients is noteworthy for short stature, webbed neck (pterygium colli), a shield-like chest with widely spaced nipples, and an increased carrying angle of the arms (cubitus valgus). Buccal smears do not demonstrate Barr bodies and chromosomal analysis confirms the diagnosis. Because these women will not undergo any secondary sexual maturation, referral to a specialist for counseling and management of replacement hormonal manipulations is advisable. Deletions of only a part of the long arm of the X chromosome have been shown to be associated with premature ovarian failure, with the earliest failures associated with the greatest deletions.

Strategies: The evaluation of patients with precocious puberty is focused on detecting possible life-threatening disease and defining the velocity of the process. When the diagnosis of true precocious puberty is established, generally by exclusion, treatment with GnRH agonists usually halts the progression of change. This therapy is expensive and is effective only if the observed changes are under central control. Suppression of GnRH may also be carried out using medroxyprogesterone acetate (Depo-Provera), in doses of 100–200 mg given intramuscularly every 2–4 weeks. This therapy is less likely to control bone growth abnormalities than is GnRH agonist treatment. The eval-

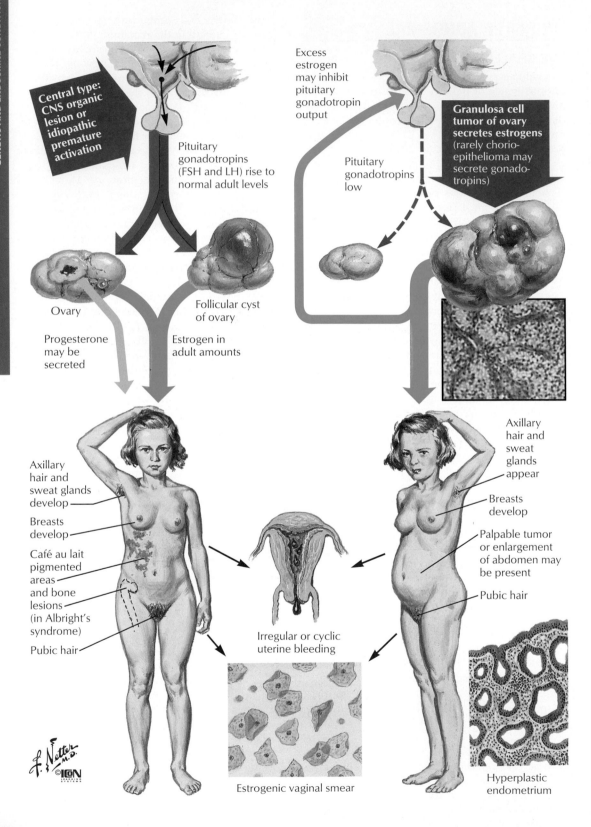

Central type: CNS organic lesion or idiopathic premature activation

Pituitary gonadotropins (FSH and LH) rise to normal adult levels

Excess estrogen may inhibit pituitary gonadotropin output

Pituitary gonadotropins low

Granulosa cell tumor of ovary secretes estrogens (rarely chorio-epithelioma may secrete gonado-tropins)

Ovary

Follicular cyst of ovary

Progesterone may be secreted

Estrogen in adult amounts

Axillary hair and sweat glands develop

Breasts develop

Café au lait pigmented areas and bone lesions (in Albright's syndrome)

Pubic hair

Axillary hair and sweat glands appear

Breasts develop

Palpable tumor or enlargement of abdomen may be present

Pubic hair

Irregular or cyclic uterine bleeding

Estrogenic vaginal smear

Hyperplastic endometrium

uation of patients with delayed pubertal development must begin with a general history, including general health, weight and height records, and family history including the pubertal experience of others in the family. Physical examination should identify the type and degree of sexual development present. The presence of breast changes generally indicates the production of estrogen, and the development of pubic or axillary hair indicates the production of androgens. Laboratory evaluation should include serum FSH, LH, and prolactin measurements, skull radiographs, and thyroid function studies. Bone age, chromosomal or cytologic studies, and pelvic ultrasonography or other imagining studies may also be indicated. Because of the significance of the potential causes of disordered puberty, most of these patients should be evaluated by or in consultation with a specialist.

Patient Education: Reassurance, American College of Obstetricians and Gynecologists Patient Education Pamphlet AP041 (*Growing Up* [for ages 8–14]).

IMPLEMENTATION

Special Considerations: Although precocious puberty is most often heralded by the sequence of increased growth, thelarche, and adrenarche, these events may occur simultaneously, or menarche itself may be the first indication. Idiopathic or constitutional precocious puberty is associated with a normal reproductive life and normal age of menopause. The greatest risk for abnormality comes from the early closure of the bony growth plates that often leaves these patients with short stature. (Half are shorter than 5 feet in height at maturity.) Therapy is worth considering for young children to achieve adult height and to avoid the social and emotional stresses that early maturation

can entail. If the cause of delayed puberty is found to be hypogonadism, hormonal therapy initiates and sustains the development of normal secondary sex characteristics. Hormonal therapy also allows for normal height and bone mass deposition to be achieved. Adolescents require much less hormone therapy than do adults or postmenopausal women. Therapy usually begins with unopposed estrogen at a dose of 0.3 mg of conjugated estrogen, 0.5 mg of estradiol, or their equivalent daily. In 6–12 months, this dose is roughly doubled and medroxyprogesterone acetate is added (10 mg for the first 12 days of the month). This combination results in regular menstruation but is insufficient for contraception. Normal pubertal development generally proceeds when the patient reaches a bone age of 13.

REFERENCES

American College of Obstetricians and Gynecologists. *Pediatric Gynecologic Disorders.* Washington, DC: ACOG; 1995. ACOG Technical Bulletin 201.

American College of Obstetricians and Gynecologists. *The Adolescent Gynecologic Patient.* Washington, DC: ACOG; 1990. ACOG Technical Bulletin 145.

Lee PA. Normal ages of pubertal events among American males and females. *J Adolesc Health Care* 1980;1:26.

Reindollar RH, Byrd JR, McDonough PG. Delayed sexual development: a study of 252 patients. *Am J Obstet Gynecol* 1981;140:371.

Reindollar RH, McDonough PG. Pubertal aberrancy: etiology and clinical approach. *J Reprod Med* 1984; 29:391.

Stein DT. New developments in the diagnosis and treatment of sexual precocity. *Am J Med Sci* 1992;303:53.

Wheeler MD, Styne DM. The treatment of precocious puberty. *Endocrinol Metab Clin North Am* 1991;20:183.

Zacharias L, Rand WM, Wurtman RJ. A prospective study of sexual development and growth in American girls: the statistics of menarche. *Obstet Gynecol Surv* 1976;31:325.

GENETIC AND ENDOCRINE CONDITIONS

PUBERTY: NORMAL SEQUENCE

THE CHALLENGE

Adolescence with the onset of puberty is a time of great emotional and physical change. By understanding the normal sequence of events and being sensitive to the presence of abnormalities, the caregiver may be able to make the most of opportunities to improve health and well-being.

Scope of the Problem: The variety of decisions, concerns, and changes confronting an adolescent are formidable, not the least of which are health issues raised by rapid growth, sexual maturation, and emerging sexuality. Puberty involves physical, emotional, and sexual changes that mark the transition from childhood to adulthood. Despite the potential need for medical education and care, teenagers have the lowest rate of physician office visits of any group. Embarrassment, an inability to pay, a lack of familiarity with health care delivery options, and legal obstructions to access all contribute to this lack of care.

Objectives of Management: Understanding the normal sequence of events involved in sexual maturation is important for counseling young women who may be concerned about "being normal." It is also pivotal to the important task of identifying those in whom the progression is not normal so that timely evaluation and intervention may be achieved.

TACTICS

Relevant Pathophysiology: Hormonally, puberty involves a change from negative gonadal feedback to the establishment of circadian and ultradian gonadal rhythms and the positive feedback controls that result in monthly cycles and fertility. It appears that three elements must be present for puberty to progress normally: adequate body mass, adequate sleep, and exposure to light. These factors appear to facilitate or allow the complex hypothalamic, pituitary, and ovarian changes that must occur. As the hypothalamus matures there is a decrease in its sensitivity to estrogen, resulting in an increase in the production and release of GnRH. Consequently, FSH levels begin to rise at about the 8th to the 10th year of life, accompanied by a rise in estrogen levels. As the sensitivity of the hypothalamus to negative feedback further decreases, FSH and LH levels continue to rise. Eventually these hormones reach a suf-

ficient level that the follicles can respond, initiating cyclic ovulation and menstruation.

Strategies: The changes of puberty generally follow a predictable pattern. A growth spurt and the rounding of body curves generally herald puberty. Breast tissue begins to develop, there is darkening of the nipples, and fat is laid down in the shoulders, hips, buttocks, and in front of the pubic bone (the mons). Body hair begins to appear because of the influence of androgens made in small amounts by the ovary and adrenal glands. Height increases because of accelerated growth in the long bones of the body, capped off by the closure of the growth centers near the end of puberty. Generally this growth spurt begins approximately 2 years before the start of menstruation itself, with growth slowing about the same time menstruation begins.

Patient Education: American College of Obstetricians and Gynecologists Patient Education Pamphlet AP041 (*Growing Up* [for ages 8–14]).

IMPLEMENTATION

Special Considerations: The average age of first menstruation (menarche) is about 12.8, with a normal range of 8 to 16. Menarche generally occurs after the growth spurt and beginning of breast development, while changes in the pubic hair and labia are still under way. Although there is some variation in the normal progression of events, thelarche is the indication of pubertal change for most, followed by adrenarche, then peak growth velocity, and ending with the onset of menstruation. This sequence generally takes $4\frac{1}{2}$ years to run its course, with a range of $1\frac{1}{2}$ to 6 years.

REFERENCES

American College of Obstetricians and Gynecologists. *Pediatric Gynecologic Disorders.* Washington, DC: ACOG; 1995. ACOG Technical Bulletin 201.

American College of Obstetricians and Gynecologists. *The Adolescent Gynecologic Patient.* Washington, DC: ACOG; 1990. ACOG Technical Bulletin 145.

Lee PA. Normal ages of pubertal events among American males and females. *J Adolesc Health Care* 1980;1:26.

Reindollar RH, McDonough PG. Pubertal aberrancy: etiology and clinical approach. *J Reprod Med* 1984; 29:391.

Zacharias L, Rand WM, Wurtman RJ. A prospective study of sexual development and growth in American girls: the statistics of menarche. *Obstet Gynecol Sur* 1976;31:325.

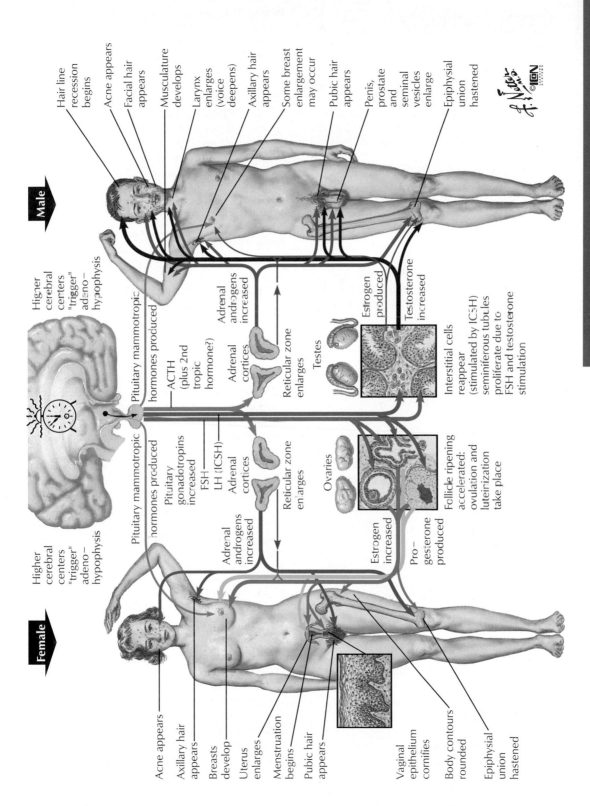

Male

Hair line recession begins

Acne appears

Facial hair appears

Musculature develops

Larynx enlarges (voice deepens)

Axillary hair appears

Some breast enlargement may occur

Pubic hair appears

Penis, prostate and seminal vesicles enlarge

Epiphysial union hastened

Higher cerebral centers "trigger" adeno-hypophysis

Pituitary mammotropic hormones produced

ACTH (plus 2nd tropic hormone?)

Adrenal cortices

Reticular zone enlarges

Adrenal androgens increased

Testes

Estrogen produced

Testosterone increased

Interstitial cells reappear (stimulated by ICSH) seminiferous tubules proliferate due to FSH and testosterone stimulation

Higher cerebral centers "trigger" adeno-hypophysis

Pituitary mammotropic hormones produced

Pituitary gonadotropins increased

FSH LH (ICSH)

Adrenal cortices

Reticular zone enlarges

Adrenal androgens increased

Ovaries

Estrogen increased

Progesterone produced

Follicle ripening accelerated; ovulation and luteirization take place

Female

Acne appears

Axillary hair appears

Breasts develop

Uterus enlarges

Menstruation begins

Pubic hair appears

Vaginal epithelium cornifies

Body contours rounded

Epiphysial union hastened

SEXUAL AMBIGUITY

INTRODUCTION

Description: Structural abnormalities present at birth may make the assignment of an appropriate sex of rearing (gender) difficult or impossible. The evaluation of these infants represents both a social and medical emergency because life-threatening conditions may be present.

Prevalence: Less than 1 of 2000 births.

Predominant Age: Present at birth.

Genetics: Some enzymatic defects may be inheritable. A history of a previously affected relative may be present for patients with androgen insensitivity or its variants.

ETIOLOGY AND PATHOGENESIS

Causes: Enzyme defects (5α-reductase, 11β- 17α-, or 21-hydroxylase deficiencies) (Most patients with ambiguous genitalia prove to be androgenized females with adrenal hyperplasia.), androgen insensitivity syndrome, intrauterine androgen exposure.

Risk Factors: In utero androgen exposure.

CLINICAL CHARACTERISTICS

Signs and Symptoms:

Incompletely formed or malformed external genitalia (varies from labial adhesion to clitoral hypertrophy and vaginal agenesis based on cause and genetic makeup of the individual)

Infants—rapid development of vomiting, diarrhea, dehydration, and shock

DIAGNOSTIC APPROACH

Differential Diagnosis:

Congenital adrenal hyperplasia (may be life-threatening—must be first consideration in any newborn with ambiguous genitalia or male babies with cryptorchidism; if gonads are not palpable, adrenal hyperplasia must be presumed until disproven)

Androgen exposure in utero (exogenous, luteoma of pregnancy)

Vaginal agenesis

Imperforate hymen

Other enzymatic defects

Associated Conditions: Premature puberty, infertility, sexual dysfunction, and gender dysphoria.

Workup and Evaluation

Laboratory: Electrolytes, hormonal and enzymatic function.

Imaging: Ultrasonography may be used to assess the internal genitalia, but is seldom necessary for initial diagnosis.

Special Tests: Karyotyping may be desirable, but a buccal smear to detect Barr bodies is often sufficient.

Diagnostic Procedures: Systematic examination of the genitalia (mons and groin, clitoris/phallus, urethral opening, labioscrotal folds, vaginal opening, posterior fourchette and perineum, anus and anal patency—the penis has a midline frenulum; the clitoris has two lateral folds that extend to the labia minora), karyotype, laboratory testing. A multidisciplinary team may be required to complete the evaluation.

Pathologic Findings

Based on cause.

MANAGEMENT AND THERAPY

Nonpharmacologic

General Measures: Rapid assessment. (The assignment of gender must be made as soon as possible after delivery but should be delayed until a gender can be established if at all possible. Many experts argue against the use of names that are gender ambiguous such as Leslie, Terry, or Jamie.)

Specific Measures: Therapy is medical and surgical—medical therapy to reverse the effects of enzyme defects; surgical therapy for cosmetics and sexual function. Surgery is often delayed until late infancy or adolescence (based on the type of reconstruction planned). If a Y-chromosome cell line is present, removal of the gonads is indicated.

Diet: No specific dietary changes indicated.

Activity: No restriction.

Drug(s) of Choice

None.

FOLLOW-UP

Patient Monitoring: Normal health maintenance, continuing support for enzymatic defects.

Prevention/Avoidance: Avoidance of agents with androgenic activity during pregnancy (drugs and food supplements).

Possible Complications: Failure to establish a clear, unambiguous gender (sex of rearing) can result in lifelong social and psychologic problems and may limit future surgical reconstruction and sexual options.

Expected Outcome: With early detection, successful growth and development appropriate to gen-

Ambiguous Genitalia
Clinical Considerations

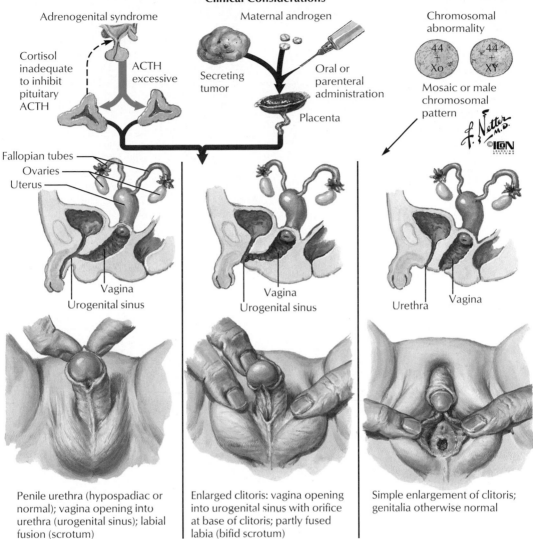

Adrenogenital syndrome

Cortisol inadequate to inhibit pituitary ACTH

ACTH excessive

Maternal androgen

Secreting tumor

Oral or parenteral administration

Placenta

Chromosomal abnormality

44 + Xo   44 + XY

Mosaic or male chromosomal pattern

Fallopian tubes
Ovaries
Uterus

Vagina
Urogenital sinus

Vagina
Urogenital sinus

Urethra   Vagina

Penile urethra (hypospadiac or normal); vagina opening into urethra (urogenital sinus); labial fusion (scrotum)

Enlarged clitoris: vagina opening into urogenital sinus with orifice at base of clitoris; partly fused labia (bifid scrotum)

Simple enlargement of clitoris; genitalia otherwise normal

Work-Up for Ambiguous Genitalia

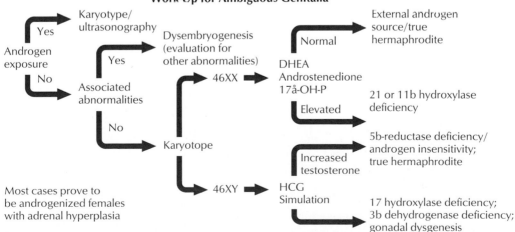

Androgen exposure

Yes → Karyotype/ultrasonography

No → Associated abnormalities

Yes → Dysembryogenesis (evaluation for other abnormalities)

No → Karyotope

46XX → DHEA Androstenedione 17å-OH-P

Normal → External androgen source/true hermaphrodite

Elevated → 21 or 11b hydroxylase deficiency

46XY → HCG Simulation

Increased testosterone → 5b-reductase deficiency/androgen insensitivity; true hermaphrodite

17 hydroxylase deficiency; 3b dehydrogenase deficiency; gonadal dysgenesis

Most cases prove to be androgenized females with adrenal hyperplasia

der may be anticipated. With reconstruction, even severe anatomic deformities can be corrected to provide cosmetic and sexually acceptable results.

MISCELLANEOUS

Pregnancy Considerations: Based on cause—androgenized females are fully fertile and have normal pregnancies; males with isolated hypospadias or cryptorchidism may be fertile; all others are sterile.

ICD-9-CM **Codes:** 752.7.

REFERENCES

Coran AG, Porley TZ. Surgical management of ambiguous genitalia in the infant and child. *J Pediatr Surg* 1991;26:812.

Donahoe PK, Powell DM, Lee MK. Clinical management of intersex abnormalities. *Curr Probl Surg* 1992;28:515.

Myers-Seifer CH, Charest NJ. Diagnosis and management of patients with ambiguous genitalia. *Semin Perinatol* 1992;16:332.

New MI. Female pseudo-hermaphroditism. *Semin Perinatol* 1992;16:289.

Speroff L, Glass RH, Kase NG. *Clinical Gynecologic Endocrinology and Infertility.* 5th Ed. Baltimore, Md: Williams & Wilkins; 1994:350.

White PC, New MI, DuPont B. Congenital adrenal hyperplasia. *N Engl J Med* 1987;316:1519.

Wilson JD, George FW, Griffin JE. The hormonal control of sexual development. *Science* 1981;211:1278.

SHEEHAN'S SYNDROME

INTRODUCTION

Description: Loss of pituitary function resulting from damage or necrosis that occurs through anoxia, thrombosis, or hemorrhage. When associated with pregnancy, it is called *Sheehan's syndrome;* when unrelated to pregnancy it is called *Simmonds' disease.*

Prevalence: Rare, less than 1 of 10,000 deliveries.

Predominant Age: Reproductive.

Genetics: No genetic pattern.

ETIOLOGY AND PATHOGENESIS

Causes: Anoxia, thrombosis, or hemorrhage that results in damage or necrosis of the pituitary gland. (The exact mechanism of pituitary damage is unknown.)

Risk Factors: Postpartum hemorrhage with hypotension.

CLINICAL CHARACTERISTICS

Signs and Symptoms:

Secondary amenorrhea

Secondary hypothyroidism

Adrenal insufficiency (the degree of pituitary damage and resultant loss is highly variable; as a result, the reduction of adrenal and thyroid hormone production seen is also variable, from slight to virtually complete loss)

Postpartum failure of lactation and loss of pubic and axillary hair (lactation following delivery virtually precludes pituitary necrosis)

Uterine superinvolution

DIAGNOSTIC APPROACH

Differential Diagnosis:

Lactational amenorrhea

Pregnancy

Exogenous hormone use

Metabolically active ovarian tumor

Other causes of secondary amenorrhea

Associated Conditions: Hypothyroidism, adrenal insufficiency, and postpartum hemorrhage.

Workup and Evaluation

Laboratory: FSH, LH, TSH, and ACTH levels are diagnostic.

Imaging: CT of the pituitary is suggestive but not diagnostic.

Special Tests: None indicated.

Diagnostic Procedures: History and laboratory evaluation.

Pathologic Findings

Necrosis of the pituitary gland.

MANAGEMENT AND THERAPY

Nonpharmacologic

General Measures: Evaluation (rapid, potentially life-threatening through loss of adrenal and thyroid hormones).

Specific Measures: Hormone replacement (thyroid, adrenal, and ovarian steroids).

Diet: No specific dietary changes indicated.

Activity: No restriction.

Patient Education: Patients must be carefully instructed in the need for continuing adrenal and thyroid hormone replacement therapy.

Drug(s) of Choice

Hormone replacement (thyroid, adrenal, and ovarian steroids).

FOLLOW-UP

Patient Monitoring: Careful follow-up of thyroid and adrenal function is required.

Prevention/Avoidance: Maintenance of adequate perfusion and oxygenation when postpartum hemorrhage occurs.

Possible Complications: Failure to diagnose the loss of pituitary function can result in life-threatening adrenal insufficiency and hypothyroidism.

Expected Outcome: With timely diagnosis and hormone replacement, normal life and function may be expected.

MISCELLANEOUS

Pregnancy Considerations: Without ovulation induction and assisted reproduction, pregnancy is unlikely.

ICD-9-CM Codes: 253.2.

REFERENCES

Ammini AC, Mathur SK. Sheehan syndrome: an analysis of possible aetiological factors. *Aust N Z J Obstet Gynecol* 1994;34:534.

Barkiri R, Bendib SE, Maoui R, Bendib A, Benmiloud M. The sella turcica in Sheehan's syndrome: computerized tomographic study in 54 patients. *J Endocrinol Invest* 1991;14:193.

Cunningham FG, MacDonald PC, Gant NF, et al, eds. *Williams Obstetrics.* 20th ed. Stamford, Conn: Appleton & Lange; 1997:763.

Grimes HG, Brooks MH. Pregnancy in Sheehan's syndrome. Report of a case and review. *Obstet Gynecol Surv* 1980;35:481.

Whitehead R. The hypothalamus in post-partum hypopituitarism. *J Pathol Bacteriol* 1963;86:55.

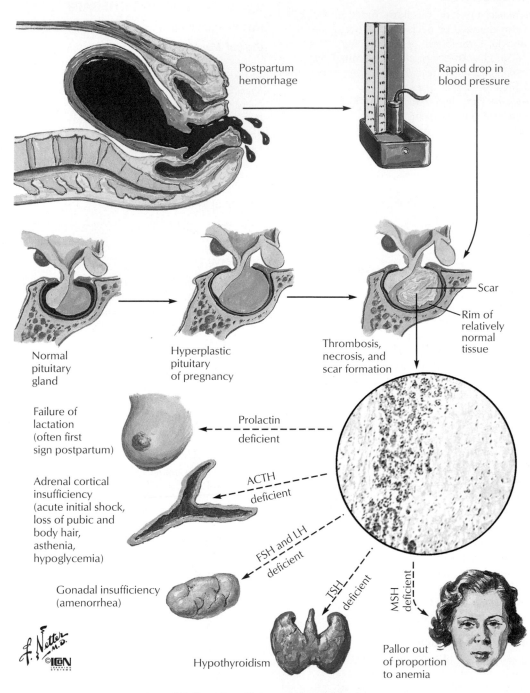

Postpartum hemorrhage

Rapid drop in blood pressure

Scar

Rim of relatively normal tissue

Normal pituitary gland

Hyperplastic pituitary of pregnancy

Thrombosis, necrosis, and scar formation

Failure of lactation (often first sign postpartum)

Prolactin deficient

Adrenal cortical insufficiency (acute initial shock, loss of pubic and body hair, asthenia, hypoglycemia)

ACTH deficient

FSH and LH deficient

Gonadal insufficiency (amenorrhea)

TSH deficient

MSH deficient

Hypothyroidism

Pallor out of proportion to anemia

Pituitary insufficiency of variable degree usually <u>without</u> diabetes insipidus

TURNER'S SYNDROME

INTRODUCTION

Description: Caused by the absence of one X chromosome, Turner's syndrome is a collection of stigmata that include edema of the hands and feet, webbing of the neck, short stature, left-sided heart or aortic anomalies, and gonadal dysgenesis resulting in primary amenorrhea and infertility. These patients have normal mental abilities but may have difficulty with mathematics, visual-motor coordination, and spatial-temporal processing.

Prevalence: One of 2700 female births.

Predominant Age: Present at birth, may not be detected until puberty is delayed.

Genetics: Sporadic, loss of one X chromosome (45,XO, 60% of cases, others partial losses: amenorrhea with long arm loss; short stature with short arm loss). Ninety-eight percent of conceptuses with only one X chromosome abort in early pregnancy.

ETIOLOGY AND PATHOGENESIS

Causes: Monosomy for the X chromosome.

Risk Factors: Translocations involving the X chromosome (rare).

CLINICAL CHARACTERISTICS

Signs and Symptoms:
- Short stature (<150 cm) (98%)
- Gonadal dysgenesis, amenorrhea (95%)
- Short neck, high palate, low hairline, and wide-spaced, hypoplastic nipples (80%)
- Broad (shield) chest, nail hypoplasia (75%)
- Lymphedema, cubitus valgus, prominent anomalous ears, multiple nevi, hearing impairment (70%)
- Webbing of the neck, short fourth metacarpal (65%)
- Renal and cardiac anomalies

DIAGNOSTIC APPROACH

Differential Diagnosis:
- Pure gonadal dysgenesis
- Polycystic ovary disease
- Noonan's syndrome
- Hypothyroidism
- Familial short stature
- Growth hormone deficiency or glucocorticoid excess
- Hereditary congenital lymphedema
- Pseudohypoparathyroid

Associated Conditions: Renal and cardiac anomalies, amenorrhea, infertility, short stature, hearing difficulties, Hashimoto's thyroiditis, hypothyroidism (10%), alopecia, vitiligo, and autoimmune disorders. Gonadoblastomas or virilization may occur if the individual is mosaic for 45 X/46 XY.

Workup and Evaluation

Laboratory: FSH and LH levels are high but do not need to be tested to establish the diagnosis (nonspecific).

Imaging: Renal and cardiac ultrasound studies to evaluate the possibility of anomalies.

Special Tests: Karyotype (40% of those thought to have Turner's syndrome have a mosaic karyotype or have an abnormal X or Y chromosome), electrocardiogram, blood pressure in each arm or arm and leg (to screen for coarctation of the aorta).

Diagnostic Procedures: Karyotyping, physical examination.

Pathologic Findings

A 45,X karyotype, gonadal dysgenesis (with rudimentary streak gonads), horseshoe kidney or double collecting system (60%), bicuspid aortic valve, coarctation of the aorta, aortic valvular stenosis, and bone dysplasia.

MANAGEMENT AND THERAPY

Nonpharmacologic

General Measures: Evaluation, screening for associated defects, counseling about stature and fertility issues.

Specific Measures: Hormone replacement therapy, growth hormone therapy if diagnosis is established before age 10. Removal of the gonadal tissue in individuals with X/XY mosaic.

Diet: No specific dietary changes indicated. (There is a tendency for obesity.)

Activity: No restriction (based on cardiac and renal status).

Patient Education: Extensive counseling about stature, sexual maturation, and fertility.

Drug(s) of Choice

Adolescents are much more sensitive to the effects of estrogen than are postmenopausal women, allowing doses in the range of 0.3 mg of conjugated estrogen, 0.5 mg of estradiol, or their equivalent daily. After 6–12 months of therapy at this level, the dose should be doubled and a progestin (eg, medroxyprogesterone acetate, 10 mg for the first 12 days of the month) should be added, or the patient's therapy should be switched to combination oral contraceptives. This generally results in regu-

GENETIC AND ENDOCRINE CONDITIONS

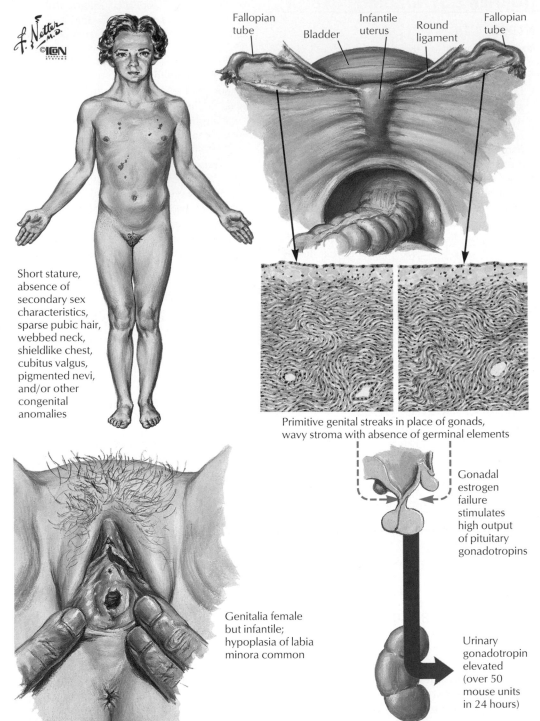

Short stature, absence of secondary sex characteristics, sparse pubic hair, webbed neck, shieldlike chest, cubitus valgus, pigmented nevi, and/or other congenital anomalies

Fallopian tube

Bladder

Infantile uterus

Round ligament

Fallopian tube

Primitive genital streaks in place of gonads, wavy stroma with absence of germinal elements

Gonadal estrogen failure stimulates high output of pituitary gonadotropins

Urinary gonadotropin elevated (over 50 mouse units in 24 hours)

Genitalia female but infantile; hypoplasia of labia minora common

 80% of cases chromatin-negative; XO chromosomal pattern most common

  20% of cases chromatin-positive; isochromosomes XX, translocation or deletion of X chromosomal fragment X^, mosaicism XO/XX/XY, or other

lar menstruation, and normal pubertal development proceeds on its own when the patient reaches a bone age of 13. Growth hormone (0.05 mg/kg SC qd) may be effective if given before age 10.

Contraindications: Undiagnosed amenorrhea.

FOLLOW-UP

Patient Monitoring: Screening for cardiac and renal anomalies, periodic hearing and thyroid testing (annual), monitor of growth. Screening of serum lipids and glucose should be performed annually as well as pelvic examinations to detect gonadal neoplasia.

Prevention/Avoidance: Prenatal chromosomal analysis for those known to carry translocations (detection only, not prevention although the couple may choose not to continue the pregnancy based on the findings).

Possible Complications: Renal or cardiac complications. New-onset breast growth or sexual hair growth should suggest the development of a gonadal tumor.

Expected Outcome: Reasonably normal life with the exception of infertility.

MISCELLANEOUS

Pregnancy Considerations: These patients are infertile. Individuals with a mosaic karyotype may be fertile but pregnancy is associated with a 50% chance of aneuploidy.

***ICD-9-CM* Codes:** 758.6.

REFERENCES

American Academy of Pediatrics Committee on Genetics. Health supervision for children with Turner syndrome. *Pediatrics* 1995;96:1166.

American College of Obstetricians and Gynecologists. *Amenorrhea.* Washington, DC: ACOG; 1989. Technical Bulletin 128.

Hall JG, Gilchrist DM. Turner's syndrome and its variants. *Pediatr Clin North Am* 1990;37:1421.

Lyons AL, Preece MA, Grant DB. Growth curve for girls with Turner syndrome. *Arch Dis Child* 1985;60:932.

Park E, Bailey JD, Cowell CA. Growth and maturation of patients with Turner's syndrome. *Pediatr Res* 1983;17:1.

Simpson JL, Shulman LP. Gonadal dysgenesis associated with abnormal chromosomal complements. In: Sciarra JJ, ed. *Gynecology and Obstetrics.* Vol 5. Philadelphia, Pa: Lippincott-Raven, 1997;86:1.

Singh RP, Carr DH. The anatomy and histology of XO human embryos and fetuses. *Anat Res* 1966;155:369.

UTERINE ANOMALIES: UTERINE AGENESIS

INTRODUCTION

Description: Failure of the müllerian system to fuse in the midline to form the uterus. Incomplete variations of this failure result in a didelphic, bicornuate, septate, or arcuate uterus.
Prevalence: One of 4000–5000 female births.
Predominant Age: Congenital.
Genetics: Isolated developmental defect except for androgen insensitivity syndrome.

ETIOLOGY AND PATHOGENESIS

Causes: Isolated developmental defect in most patients, production of antimüllerian hormone by Sertoli's cells in a fetal testes (in androgen resistance syndrome). 17α-Hydroxylase deficiency, 17, 20-desmolase deficiency, and agonadism may account for those rare individuals with no breast or uterine development and a male karyotype (vanishing testes syndrome).
Risk Factors: None known.

CLINICAL CHARACTERISTICS

Signs and Symptoms:
Primary amenorrhea (accounts for 15% of primary amenorrhea)
Shortened or absent vagina
Breast development may be absent in some syndromes

DIAGNOSTIC APPROACH

Differential Diagnosis:
Androgen resistance (testicular feminization)—may be ruled out by the presence of normal pubic hair
Vaginal agenesis
Imperforate hymen
Primary amenorrhea
Associated Conditions: Primary amenorrhea, infertility, urinary tract abnormalities (25%–40%), skeletal abnormalities (12%), congenital rectovaginal fistula, imperforate anus, and hypospadias.

Workup and Evaluation

Laboratory: Serum FSH (to differentiate hypogonadal hypogonadism and gonadal dysgenesis).
Imaging: No imaging indicated. Ultrasonography may be used to assist the diagnosis but is generally not indicated. Intravenous pyelography should be considered.
Special Tests: Measurement of height, weight, and arm span. (A karyotype or buccal smear may be performed, but is generally not necessary.)

Diagnostic Procedures: History, physical examination, imaging procedures.

Pathologic Findings

One or both fallopian tubes and some fibrous tissue may be present in the normal location of the uterus. Normal ovaries, with normal cyclic ovarian function, are usually present.

MANAGEMENT AND THERAPY

Nonpharmacologic

General Measures: Evaluation and education.
Specific Measures: Patients may require surgical removal of abnormal gonads (after puberty: age 18) because of an increased risk of malignancy. Fertility may be achieved through in vitro fertilization with implantation into a host uterus.
Diet: No specific dietary changes indicated.
Activity: No restriction.
Patient Education: Frank discussion about the syndrome and its effects (infertility and amenorrhea), American College of Obstetricians and Gynecologists Patient Education Pamphlet AP002 (*Infertility: Causes and Treatments*).

Drug(s) of Choice

None.

FOLLOW-UP

Patient Monitoring: Normal health maintenance.
Prevention/Avoidance: None.
Possible Complications: Renal, skeletal, and cardiac abnormalities are more common in these patients.
Expected Outcome: Normal life expectancy without reproductive capability. (Fertility may be achieved through in vitro fertilization with implantation into a host uterus.)

MISCELLANEOUS

Pregnancy Considerations: Normal pregnancy is not possible.
ICD-9-CM Codes: 752.3.

REFERENCES

Buttram VC. Müllerian anomalies and their management. *Fertil Steril* 1983;40:159.
Golan A, Langer R, Bukovsky I, Caspi E. Congenital anomalies of the müllerian system. *Fertil Steril* 1981;51:747.
Reinhold C, Hricak H, Forstner R, et al. Primary amenorrhea: evaluation with MR imaging. *Radiology* 1997;203:383.
Mayo-Smith WW, Lee MJ. MR imaging of the female pelvis. *Clin Radiol* 1995;50:667.
Williams EA. Uterovaginal agenesis. *Ann R Soc Med* 1970;63:40.

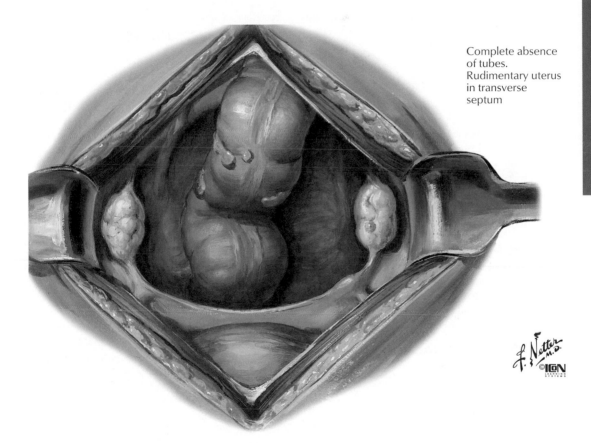

Complete absence
of tubes.
Rudimentary uterus
in transverse
septum

VAGINAL AGENESIS

INTRODUCTION

Description: Congenital absence of the vagina, most often associated with an absence of the uterus (Mayer-Rokitansky-Küster-Hauser syndrome).

Prevalence: Reported to vary from 1 of 4000 to 1 of 10,500 female births.

Predominant Age: Generally not diagnosed until puberty, often following a delay of 2–3 years or more.

Genetics: No genetic pattern (accident of development), although in some inbred communities there is a suggestion that an autosomal recessive gene is present.

ETIOLOGY AND PATHOGENESIS

Causes: Failure of the endoderm of the urogenital sinus and the epithelium of the vaginal vestibule to fuse and perforate during embryonic development. This process is normally completed by the 21st week of gestation. Patients with a congenital absence of the vagina but with a uterus present represent an extreme form of transverse vaginal septum.

Risk Factors: None known.

CLINICAL CHARACTERISTICS

Signs and Symptoms:
Vaginal obstruction (absence)
Primary amenorrhea
Cyclic abdominal pain
Hematometra (if uterus is present)

DIAGNOSTIC APPROACH

Differential Diagnosis:
Imperforate hymen
Hermaphroditism
Androgen insensitivity syndrome (testicular feminization)
Mayer-Rokitansky-Küster-Hauser syndrome (75% have vaginal agenesis, 25% have shortened vaginal pouch)
Transverse vaginal septum

Associated Conditions: Endometriosis, infertility, chronic pelvic pain, sexual dysfunction, hematometra (when uterus is present), urologic abnormalities (25%–40%), and skeletal abnormalities (10%–15%).

Workup and Evaluation

Laboratory: No evaluation indicated.

Imaging: Ultrasonography, MRI, or CT to determine the presence and status of the upper genital tract structures. Intravenous pyelography should be considered.

Special Tests: Karyotyping or buccal smear should be considered. Laparoscopy may be desirable in some patients to confirm the diagnosis, although this is generally not necessary.

Diagnostic Procedures: History and physical examination (including rectal examination).

Pathologic Findings

The ovaries are usually normal and the fallopian tubes are present.

MANAGEMENT AND THERAPY

Nonpharmacologic

General Measures: Evaluation and reassurance.

Specific Measures: Surgical creation of a vagina when intercourse is desired. May be created by a flap procedure (McIndoe procedure) or progressive perineal pressure techniques (Ingram dilators or bicycle seat). Patients with androgen insensitivity should have their gonads (testes) removed to prevent seminoma; patients with Mayer-Rokitansky-Küster-Hauser syndrome have normal ovaries and should not have them removed.

Diet: No specific dietary changes indicated.

Activity: No restriction.

Drug(s) of Choice

None.

FOLLOW-UP

Patient Monitoring: Normal health maintenance. Patients in whom a neovagina is created must be monitored for narrowing.

Prevention/Avoidance: None.

Possible Complications: Hematocolpos, endometriosis, sexual dysfunction. If a neovagina is created, it will scar and stenose if it is not used frequently or maintained with the use of a dilator.

Expected Outcome: Sexual function can generally be restored through the creation of a neovagina. The presence of a uterus is associated with cyclic pain and often must be removed. Except as an egg donor, fertility is unlikely to be restored.

MISCELLANEOUS

Pregnancy Considerations: Generally not a consideration. Patients may be able to achieve reproduction as egg donors.

ICD-9-CM Codes: 752.49.

REFERENCES

Baramki TA. The treatment of congenital anomalies in girls and women. *J Reprod Med* 1984;29:376.

Counsellor VS, Flor FS. Congenital absence of the vagina. *Surg Clin North Am* 1957;37:1107.

Greiss FC, Mauzy CH. Congenital anomalies in women: an evaluation of diagnosis, incidence, and obstetric performance. *Am J Obstet Gynecol* 1961;82:330.

Ingram JM. The bicycle seat stool in the treatment of vaginal agenesis and stenosis: a preliminary report. *Am J Obstet Gynecol* 1981;140:867.

Rock JA, Keenan DL. Surgical correction of uterovaginal anomalies In: Sciarra JJ, ed. *Gynecology and Obstetrics.* Vol 1. Philadelphia, Pa: JB Lippincott; 1992;70:1.

Stenchever MA. Congenital abnormalities of the female reproductive tract. In: Mishell DR, Stenchever MA, Droegemueller W, Herbst AL, eds. *Comprehensive Gynecology.* St Louis, Mo: Mosby; 1997:249.

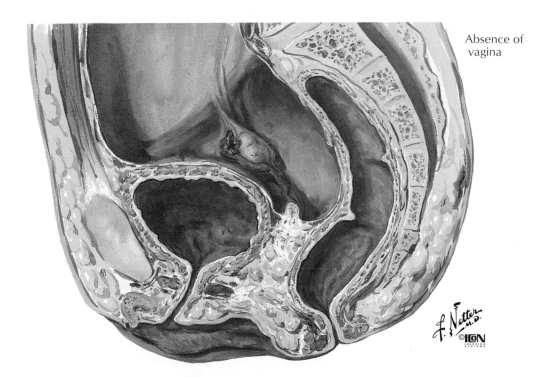

Absence of vagina

VIRILIZATION

INTRODUCTION

Description: Virilization refers to the loss of female sexual characteristics such as body contour and the acquisition of masculine qualities such as increased muscle mass, temporal balding, deepening of the voice, and clitoromegaly.

Prevalence: Uncommon.

Predominant Age: Reproductive.

Genetics: No genetic pattern.

ETIOLOGY AND PATHOGENESIS

Causes: Idiopathic ovarian (polycystic ovary disease, hilus cell hyperplasia/tumor, arrhenoblastoma, adrenal rest), adrenal (congenital adrenal hyperplasia [10%–15% of hirsute women], Cushing's disease, virilizing carcinoma or adenoma), drugs (minoxidil, androgens [including danazol {Danocrine}], phenytoin, diazoxide), pregnancy (androgen excess of pregnancy, luteoma, or hyperreactio luteinalis).

Risk Factors: None known.

CLINICAL CHARACTERISTICS

Signs and Symptoms:

    Amenorrhea (common but not universal)
    Temporal or frontal balding
    Deepening of the voice
    Clitoral enlargement
    Vaginal dryness
    Increased muscle mass
    Male pattern hair growth

DIAGNOSTIC APPROACH

Differential Diagnosis:

    Iatrogenic or exogenous steroid use
    Polycystic ovary disease
    Ovarian stromal hyperthecosis
    Ovarian tumors (Sertoli-Leydig tumors)
    Cushing's disease (truncal obesity, facial rounding, cervicodorsal fat deposition [buffalo hump], and red or purple striae are often not fully developed)
    Adrenal tumors
    Congenital adrenal hyperplasia (especially in infants and children)

Associated Conditions: Defeminization, amenorrhea, obesity, menstrual irregularity, amenorrhea, infertility, acne, oily skin, increased libido, and alopecia.

Workup and Evaluation

Laboratory: Prolactin, FSH, thyroid screening. Patients suspected of having adrenal sources of hyperandrogenicity may be screened by measuring 24-hour urinary free cortisol, by performing ACTH stimulation tests, or an overnight dexamethasone suppression test. DHEA-s and testosterone should be measured. The circulating testosterone level is generally ≥ 2 ng/mL.

Imaging: Despite the ability of transvaginal ultrasonography and computerized tomography to detect 90% of virilizing tumors, 5%–10% of tumors may not be detected, necessitating surgical exploration when these are suspected.

Special Tests: Clitoral index. (The clitoral index is defined as the vertical dimension times the horizontal dimension, in millimeters. The normal range is from 9 to 35 mm, with borderline values in the range of 36 to 99 mm. Values greater than 100 mm indicate severe hyperandrogenicity and should prompt aggressive evaluation and referral.)

Diagnostic Procedures: History, physical examination, and laboratory evaluation.

Pathologic Findings

Based on underlying pathophysiologic conditions.

MANAGEMENT AND THERAPY

Nonpharmacologic

General Measures: Evaluation and support, shaving, depilatories, or electrolysis. Topical treatment of acne (if present).

Specific Measures: Patients with polycystic ovary disease often do well with oral contraceptive suppression of ovarian function or with the use of spironolactone. Patients with hyperandrogenicity of adrenal origin respond well to cortisol administration, which results in a reduction of the production of androgenic precursors. Tumors require surgical removal.

Diet: No specific dietary changes indicated.

Activity: No restriction.

Drug(s) of Choice

Polycystic ovary syndrome—combination oral contraceptives, spironolactone (100–200 mg PO daily), medroxyprogesterone acetate (Depo-Provera 150–300 mg IM q3mo).

Hyperandrogenicity of adrenal origin—cortisol administration.

Contraindications: Pregnancy. (Spironolactone is teratogenic, patients using it and able to become pregnant must use reliable contraception.)

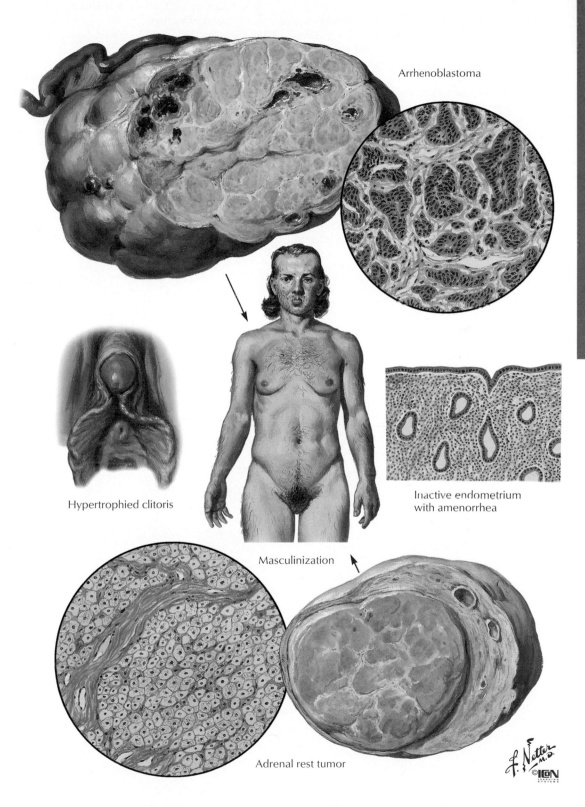

Arrhenoblastoma

Hypertrophied clitoris

Inactive endometrium with amenorrhea

Masculinization

Adrenal rest tumor

FOLLOW-UP

Patient Monitoring: Normal health maintenance once diagnosis and management have been implemented. There is an increased risk of diabetes in patients with polycystic ovaries.

Prevention/Avoidance: None.

Possible Complications: Permanent loss of feminine attributes and induction of hirsutism, lowering of voice, and others. Chronic anovulation is associated with increased risk of endometrial hyperplasia and cancer.

Expected Outcome: Good, with appropriate diagnosis and treatment.

MISCELLANEOUS

Pregnancy Considerations: No effect on pregnancy, although some metabolic causes of virilization of the mother may result in reduced fertility or virilization of a fetus.

ICD-9-CM **Codes:** 255.2 (others based on diagnosis).

REFERENCES

Bakri YN, Bakhashwain M, Hugosson C. Massive theca-lutein cysts, virilization, and hypothyroidism associated with normal pregnancy. *Acta Obstet Gynecol Scand* 1994;73:153.

Hall JE. Polycystic ovarian disease as a neuroendocrine disorder of the female reproductive axis. *Endocrinol Metab Clin North Am* 1993;22:75.

Ireland K, Woodruff JD. Masculinizing ovarian tumors. *Obstet Gynecol* Surv 1976;31:83.

Tagitz GE, Kopher RA, Nagel TC, Okagaki T. The clitoral index: a bioassay of androgenic stimulation. *Obstet Gynecol* 1979;54:562.

Women's Health/ Primary Care

ABUSE: PHYSICAL AND SEXUAL

INTRODUCTION

Description: A pattern of physical trauma that occurs within a continuing relationship. Although the definition of abuse requires only one episode of physical abuse, a pattern of escalating violence is more typical. (In at least one fourth of cases, there have been three or more episodes of violence in the 6 months preceding the report of abuse.) In the United States, women are at greater risk of injury or death at the hands of a domestic partner than from an unrelated attacker. Sexual abuse is a specific form of physical abuse that relates to trauma of a sexual nature or a pattern of coercive sexual activities. Sexual abuse includes, but is not limited to, disrobing, exposure, photography or posing, oral-genital contact, insertion of foreign bodies, and vaginal or rectal intercourse.

Prevalence: More than 1.5 million cases of domestic violence each year. It is estimated that between 5% and 25% of women treated for injuries in emergency rooms receive these injuries as a result of domestic violence. Twenty to forty percent of adults report abuse or sexual victimization before age 18, and 10%–25% of wives report one or more episodes of sexual abuse.

Predominant Age: Any, most common teens to 30s.

Genetics: Women are the primary victims of domestic violence, accounting for almost 95% of incidents.

ETIOLOGY AND PATHOGENESIS

Causes: Multiple factors. Alcohol or drugs are often involved, although not causative factors.

Risk Factors: Slightly higher rate among those of lower educational or socioeconomic status.

CLINICAL CHARACTERISTICS

Signs and Symptoms:
- Physical abuse—Highly variable signs and symptoms (In almost 85% of reported cases, the injuries sustained are sufficient to required medical treatment. Between 5% and 25% of women treated for injuries in emergency rooms receive these injuries as a result of domestic violence. The correct diagnosis is rendered in less than 5% of women. The most frequent locations for injuries are the head, neck, chest, abdomen, and breasts. Upper extremity injuries result from defensive efforts.)
- Sexual abuse—nonspecific

DIAGNOSTIC APPROACH

Differential Diagnosis:
- Depression (may mimic the vague complaints that should raise the suspicion of abuse)
- Coagulopathy (leading to bruising)

Associated Conditions: More than one half of men who abuse their wives abuse their children as well. Between one third and one half of all murders of women occur at the hands of a male partner.

Workup and Evaluation

Laboratory: No evaluation indicated.

Imaging: No imaging indicated unless fracture or other injury is suspected.

Special Tests: The five-question Abuse Assessment Screen increases the likelihood of detecting abuse. The longer it has been since an assault or when abuse is ongoing, the more likely it is for the presenting complaints to be unrelated to the underlying concerns generated by the attack. Somatic complaints and subtle behavioral changes may suggest the possibility of domestic violence or abuse.

Diagnostic Procedures: History and suspicion. Because one of the pivotal aspects of sexual assault is the loss of control, every effort should be made to allow the patient control over even the most trivial aspects of the physical examination.

Pathologic Findings

In the typical battering relationship three phases are usually present: a tension-building phase that gradually escalates; the battering incident, which may be triggered by almost any event; and a period of contrition during which the batterer apologizes and asks for forgiveness. This cycle tends to repeat and escalate with greater physical harm and risk and less remorse.

MANAGEMENT AND THERAPY

Nonpharmacologic

General Measures: Support, contact with social agencies, assistance with developing means for independence (eg, money, transportation, destination, childcare) should escape become necessary.

Specific Measures: Assessment and management of any injuries present. The patient should be given the telephone number of and directions to a shelter or safe house.

Diet: No specific dietary changes indicated.

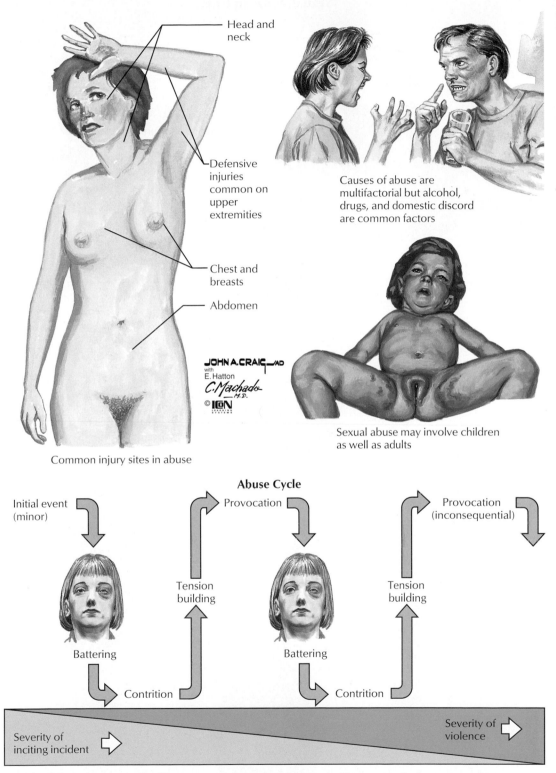

Head and neck

Defensive injuries common on upper extremities

Chest and breasts

Abdomen

Common injury sites in abuse

Causes of abuse are multifactorial but alcohol, drugs, and domestic discord are common factors

Sexual abuse may involve children as well as adults

Abuse Cycle

Initial event (minor)

Provocation

Provocation (inconsequential)

Tension building

Tension building

Battering

Battering

Contrition

Contrition

Severity of inciting incident

Severity of violence

Cycle of abuse is characterized by progressively smaller incidents inciting progressively greater violence interspersed with periods of remorse.

Sexual Abuse in Girls

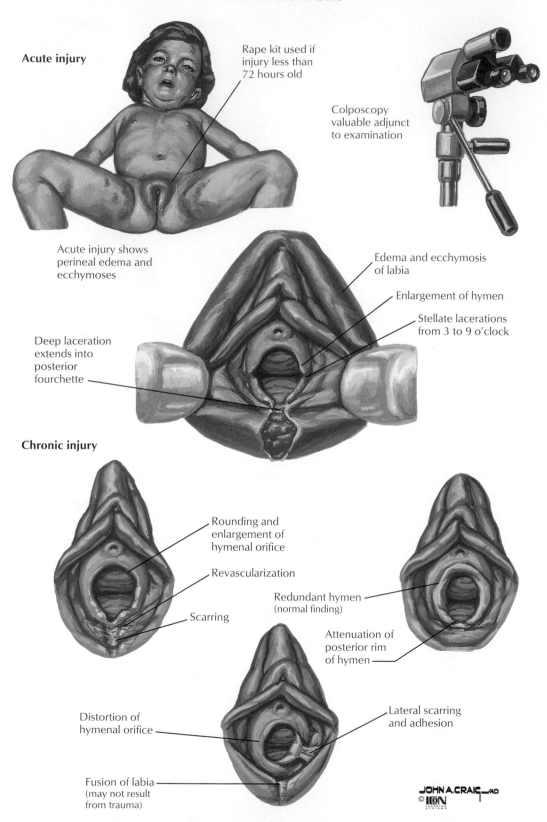

Acute injury

Rape kit used if injury less than 72 hours old

Colposcopy valuable adjunct to examination

Acute injury shows perineal edema and ecchymoses

Edema and ecchymosis of labia

Enlargement of hymen

Stellate lacerations from 3 to 9 o'clock

Deep laceration extends into posterior fourchette

Chronic injury

Rounding and enlargement of hymenal orifice

Revascularization

Scarring

Redundant hymen (normal finding)

Attenuation of posterior rim of hymen

Distortion of hymenal orifice

Lateral scarring and adhesion

Fusion of labia (may not result from trauma)

JOHN A. CRAIG—AD

© ICON

Activity: No restriction.

Patient Education: American College of Obstetricians and Gynecologists Patient Education Pamphlet AP083 (*The Abused Woman*).

Drug(s) of Choice

None indicated. Great care must be used with any antidepressants or other mood-altering drugs given in these situations.

FOLLOW-UP

Patient Monitoring: In many locations, suspected sexual assault must be reported to law enforcement authorities. In all locations, suspected abuse, sexual or otherwise, occurring to a minor must be reported.

Prevention/Avoidance: None. Patients must be told they are not at fault and that their efforts to change their spouse are unlikely to have an effect in reducing the number of future episodes.

Possible Complications: Escalating violence with an increasing risk of severe injury or death.

Expected Outcome: The pattern of physical or sexual abuse is ongoing. Acute management of trauma is only a part of the larger problem of interpersonal dysfunction. If the abuser receives counseling and treatment, the outcome can be good; without it there is great risk of continued or worsening abuse.

MISCELLANEOUS

Pregnancy Considerations: Ten percent to twenty percent of pregnant women report physical abuse during pregnancy. For these women, injuries to the breast and abdomen are more frequent.

ICD-9-CM **Codes:** 995.81, 995.85 (Multiple forms).

REFERENCES

AMA Council on Scientific Affairs. Violence against women: relevance for medical practitioners. *JAMA* 1992;267:3184.

American College of Obstetricians and Gynecologists. *The Battered Woman.* Washington, DC; ACOG; 1989. ACOG Technical Bulletin 124.

American College of Obstetricians and Gynecologists. *Sexual Assault.* Washington, DC: ACOG; 1992. ACOG Technical Bulletin 172.

American Medical Association. *Diagnostic and Treatment Guidelines on Domestic Violence.* Chicago: American Medical Association; 1992.

Chez RA. Woman battering. *Am J Obstet Gynecol* 1988; 158:1.

Hillard PJ. Physical abuse in pregnancy. *Obstet Gynecol* 1985;66:185.

Smith RP. *Gynecology in Primary Care.* Baltimore, Md: Williams & Wilkins; 1997:501.

ACNE

INTRODUCTION

Description: Inflammatory disorder of the sebaceous glands that results in comedones, papules, inflammatory pustules, and scarring. The significance of acne for a woman often exceeds that dictated by medical considerations. It is often a reason to either choose or discontinue the use of oral contraceptives. Acne, or the fear of it, is a major factor in poor compliance with oral contraceptives.

Prevalence: Most adolescents, 15% seek care.

Predominant Age: Early teens to 20s, may persist into 40s.

Genetics: No genetic pattern. Women generally have milder forms of acne than men, although the social consequences are often greater.

ETIOLOGY AND PATHOGENESIS

Causes: Increased turnover of keratin in sebaceous glands under the influence of androgens. This results in a keratin plug (comedone) that obstructs sebum drainage from the gland. Infection by *Propionibacterium acnes* results in inflammation and pustule formation.

Risk Factors: Increased androgen of adolescence, oily cosmetics or moisturizers, virilizing conditions, medications (oral contraceptives, iodides, bromides, lithium, phenytoins, corticosteroids), and poor local hygiene.

CLINICAL CHARACTERISTICS

Signs and Symptoms:
- Closed comedones (whiteheads)
- Open comedones (blackheads, black because of oxidation of sebum)
- Nodules and papules
- Pustules and cysts, with or without erythema and edema, may result in scarring
- Most lesions concentrated over the forehead, cheeks, nose, upper back, and chest

DIAGNOSTIC APPROACH

Differential Diagnosis:
- Chemical exposure (grease, oils, tars)
- Folliculitis
- Steroid acne
- Virilizing tumors

Concerns about acne may serve as a surrogate for other issues including sexual development, menstruation, and contraception.

Associated Conditions: Social or emotional withdrawal.

Workup and Evaluation

Laboratory: No evaluation indicated.

Imaging: No imaging indicated.

Special Tests: None indicated.

Diagnostic Procedures: History and physical examination.

Pathologic Findings

Increased oiliness of the skin, increased skin thickness with hypertrophic sebaceous glands, perifolliculitis, and scarring.

MANAGEMENT AND THERAPY

Nonpharmacologic

General Measures: General hygiene, nail clipping (to reduce secondary trauma and infections), twice-a-day cleansing with a mild soap, oil-free sunscreens.

Specific Measures: Comedone extraction (with extractor), topical medical therapy.

Diet: No specific dietary changes indicated. (None have been shown to be effective.)

Activity: No restriction.

Patient Education: General hygiene measures, need for long-term treatment, American College of Obstetricians and Gynecologists Patient Education Pamphlet AP014 (*Growing Up* [for ages 8–14]).

Drug(s) of Choice

Benzoyl peroxide 5% applied to skin qhs.
Tretinoin (retinoic acid) 0.025% cream applied to skin qhs (applying ½ hour after washing reduces side effects).
Topical antibiotics—erythromycin, clindamycin (2%) in water base.
Systemic antibiotics—tetracycline 250 mg PO qid for 7–10 days then tapering to lowest effective dose, erythromycin 250 mg PO qid for 7–10 days then tapering to lowest effective dose.
Oral contraceptives.

Contraindications: Known or suspected allergy, hepatic dysfunction for oral agents, pregnancy (tetracycline and isotretinoin).

Precautions: Tetracycline may cause photosensitivity.

Interactions: Tetracycline should not be given with antacids, dairy products, or iron. Erythromycin should not be given with terfenadine (Seldane) and astemizole because it may cause cardiac abnormalities including arrhythmias and death. Broad-spectrum antibiotics may (theoretically) interfere with oral contraceptive efficacy.

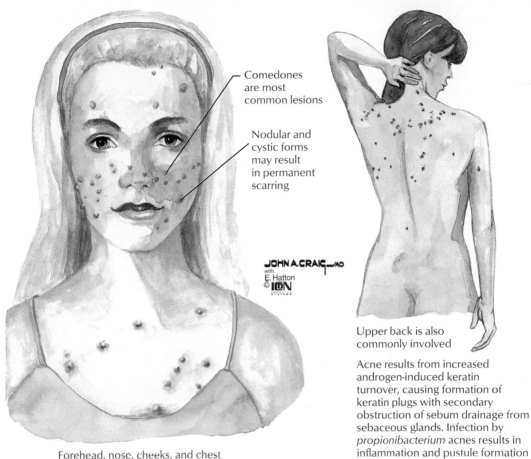

Comedones are most common lesions

Nodular and cystic forms may result in permanent scarring

JOHN A.CRAIG—AD
with E. Hatton ©

Forehead, nose, cheeks, and chest are commonly involved by acne

Upper back is also commonly involved

Acne results from increased androgen-induced keratin turnover, causing formation of keratin plugs with secondary obstruction of sebum drainage from sebaceous glands. Infection by *propionibacterium* acnes results in inflammation and pustule formation

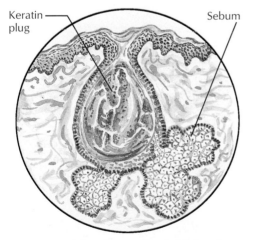

Keratin plug

Sebum

Section of closed comedone (whitehead) showing keratin plug and accumulated sebum in sebaceous glands

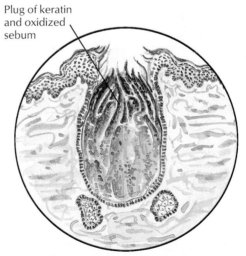

Plug of keratin and oxidized sebum

Section of open comedone (blackhead) showing plug of keratin and oxidized sebum

WOMEN'S HEALTH/PRIMARY CARE

Alternative Drugs

Tretinoin (retinoic acid) 0.025% gel applied chest or back qhs.

Isotretinoin (Accutane) 0.5–1.0 mg/kg/d in two doses for 12–16 weeks with a second course possible after an 8-week interval (associated with significant side effects including dry skin, dryness of the mucous membranes, and cheilitis).

FOLLOW-UP

Patient Monitoring: Periodic follow-up (monthly) until control is obtained. For patients receiving isotretinoin, liver function, lipid concentrations, and the possibility of pregnancy should be monitored.

Prevention/Avoidance: None.

Possible Complications: Scarring, hypo- or hyperpigmentation, keloidal scarring on the sternum or shoulders.

Expected Outcome: Gradual improvement over time and with therapy.

MISCELLANEOUS

Pregnancy Considerations: Pregnancy may cause a flair-up or remission of acne. Isotretinoin and erythromycin should not be used during pregnancy.

ICD-9-CM **Codes:** 706.1.

REFERENCES

Leyden JJ. Retinoids in acne. *J Am Acad Dermatol* 1988; 19:164.

McClintoch JH, Arpey CJ, Whitaker DC. Dermatologic disease common to women. In: Ling FW, Laube DW, Nolan TE, Smith RP, Stovell TG, eds. *Primary Care in Gynecology.* Baltimore, Md: Williams & Wilkins; 1996:369.

Shalita AR, Leyden JE Jr, Pochi PE, et al. Acne vulgaris. *J Am Acad Dermatol* 1987;16:410.

ALZHEIMER'S DISEASE

INTRODUCTION

Description: Degenerative organic mental syndrome characterized by progressive intellectual deterioration and dementia.

Prevalence: Four million cases annually, 40% of patients older than 85.

Predominant Age: Older than 65.

Genetics: Two- to three-fold more common in women, increased familial risk (50% of patients). Markers have been found on chromosomes 1 and 14 for early onset and 12 and 19 for late onset.

ETIOLOGY AND PATHOGENESIS

Causes: Unknown. Proposed—slow virus, aluminum exposure, accelerated aging, autoimmune process, genetic alteration in amyloid production or metabolism.

Risk Factors: Aging, head trauma, Down syndrome, and family history.

CLINICAL CHARACTERISTICS

Signs and Symptoms:
- Loss of mental function (calculation, abstraction, memory, aphasia)
- Social withdrawal (anhedonia, apathy, personality change, anxiety, depression)
- Delusions and confabulation
- Dementia
- Sleep disturbances and restlessness

DIAGNOSTIC APPROACH

Differential Diagnosis:
- Dementia (vascular, infarct, Parkinson's disease)
- Multiple sclerosis
- Brain tumor (primary or metastatic)
- Alcohol or drug use/abuse
- Drug reaction
- Depression
- Hepatic or renal failure leading to toxicity
- Neurosyphilis
- Hypothyroidism

Associated Conditions: Down syndrome, depression, and insomnia.

Workup and Evaluation

Laboratory: Screening to rule out other causes as indicated.

Imaging: Computed tomography (CT) or magnetic resonance imaging (MRI) may show characteristic changes, but are not required to make the diagnosis.

Special Tests: Spinal tap as indicated by the diagnoses being considered. Special paper and pencil tests are available to help with the assessment of cognitive function.

Diagnostic Procedures: History and clinical characteristics.

Pathologic Findings

β-Amyloid deposits in neuritic plaques and on arteriolar walls characterize the disease. Pyramidal cell loss, decreased cholinergic innervation, and neuritic senile plaques are also seen.

MANAGEMENT AND THERAPY

Nonpharmacologic

General Measures: Support, exercise to reduce restlessness and improve sleep, continued cognitive challenge, family support.

Specific Measures: Estrogen replacement is associated with a 50% reduction in risk and a delay in onset of symptoms in some studies, although more recent studies do not confirm these findings. For those with Alzheimer's changes, estrogen replacement seems to improve function.

Diet: No specific dietary changes indicated.

Activity: No restriction except those imposed by ability.

Patient Education: Reassurance, extensive educational materials are available from support groups, Internet sites, and the Alzheimer's Association (Chicago).

Drug(s) of Choice

None. Studies on agents to enhance memory (donepezil [Aricept] 5–10 mg daily) are ongoing; they provide some improvement for 30%–50% of patients with severe disease. Drugs may be used to improve specific manifestations such as insomnia or depression.

Contraindications: Avoid anticholinergic drugs, such as tricyclic antidepressants and antihistamines.

Precautions: Tacrine (Cognex) may cause liver toxicity. Benzodiazepines may produce paradoxical excitation. Triazolam (Halcion) can produce memory loss, confusion, or psychotic reactions. Care must be taken in the use of all drugs in these patients; they tend to tolerate them poorly and confusion may lead to dosing errors.

FOLLOW-UP

Patient Monitoring: Watch for problems with nutrition, further mental deterioration, and drug

Testing for Defects of Higher Cortical Function

A. Appearance and interpersonal behavior

Pleasant, neatly dressed, good spirits

Depressed, sloppily dressed, careless

Belligerent

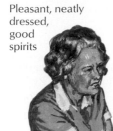
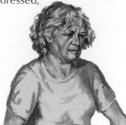
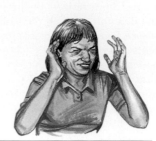

B. Language

Doctor: "Write me a brief paragraph about your work"

Good

I have been an executive secretary to the vice president of the Zilch corporation for many years. My working conditions are satisfactory and I look forward to each day's business activity. I tend to many details for and supervise other ...

Defective

I don't mush much do it yestiday way loszy day five alock when no to go to a job when

C. Memory

Doctor: "Here are three objects: a pipe, a pen and a picture of Abraham Lincoln. I want you to remember them and in 5 minutes, I will ask you what they were"

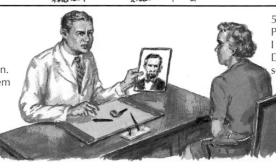

5 minutes later. Patient: "I'm sorry, I can't remember. Did you show me something?"

D. Constructional praxis and visual-spatial function

Doctor: "Draw me a simple picture of a house"

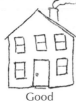

Good   Abnormal

"Draw a clock face for me"

Good   Abnormal

E. Reverse counting

Doctor: "Count backward from five to one for me"
Patient: "5...3...4..., sorry, I can't do it"

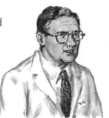
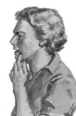

Doctor: "Spell the word "worlds" backward for me"
Patient: "W..L..R..D..S"

use. Provide continuing and aggressive family support. Periodically evaluate the need for nursing home placement or other assistance.

Prevention/Avoidance: None.

Possible Complications: Progressive deterioration with metabolic changes, dehydration, drug overdose, falls, depression, and suicide.

Expected Outcome: Poor—progressive deterioration with 8- to 10-year average survival.

MISCELLANEOUS

ICD-9-CM Codes: 331.0 290.0 (Senile dementia, uncomplicated), 290.10 (Presenile dementia, uncomplicated).

REFERENCES

Agency for Health and Research. *Recognition and initial assessment of Alzheimer's disease and related dementias: Clinical Practice Guidelines 19.* Rockville, Md: US Dept of Health and Human Services; 1996. AHCPR publication 97-0702.

Geldmacher DS, Whitehouse PJ. Evaluation of dementia. *N Engl J Med* 1996;335:330.

Progress Report on Alzheimer's Disease 1996. Washington, DC: National Institute on Aging, US Dept of Health and Human Services; 1996. NIH publication 96-4137.

Pendlebury W, Solomon PR. Alzheimer's disease. *Ciba Clin Symp* 1996;48:1.

ANEMIA

INTRODUCTION

Description: A reduction below normal in the oxygen-carrying capacity of the blood as reflected by the hemoglobin or hematocrit values. Women are at higher risk because of menstrual blood loss.

Prevalence: More than 20% of women, 50%–60% of pregnant women.

Predominant Age: Reproductive most common for women.

Genetics: Hemoglobinopathies such as sickle cell disease, thalassemia, and others are associated with anemia.

ETIOLOGY AND PATHOGENESIS

Causes: Abnormalities of production (eg, iron deficiency, chronic disease, chemotherapy, radiation). Abnormalities of destruction or loss (eg, hemorrhage, hemolysis, sickle cell disease).

Risk Factors: Excessive blood loss (menorrhagia), poor diet, pica, malabsorption, chronic disease, endocrinopathy (thyroid). Smokers have slightly higher hemoglobin values (0.5–1.0 g/dL).

CLINICAL CHARACTERISTICS

Signs and Symptoms:
- Asymptomatic
- Fatigue, palpitations, dyspnea, exhaustion (late signs)
- Ice craving, spooning or ridging of fingernails (iron deficiency anemia)
- Sore mouth or dysphagia (B_{12} or iron deficiency anemia)
- Joint and bone pain (sickle cell anemia)

DIAGNOSTIC APPROACH

Differential Diagnosis: See illustration.

Associated Conditions: Stomatitis, ridging and spooning of fingernail, hypersegmented polymorphonuclear neutrophils (megaloblastic anemia).

Workup and Evaluation

Laboratory: Mean corpuscular volume, reticulocyte count, blood smear, iron studies, hemoglobin electrophoresis; others based on individual patient—serum iron, total iron binding capacity, serum ferritin.

Imaging: No imaging indicated.

Special Tests: Bone marrow analysis (not necessary for the majority of patients).

Diagnostic Procedures: Laboratory evaluation.

Pathologic Findings

Based on underlying cause.

MANAGEMENT AND THERAPY

Nonpharmacologic

General Measures: Evaluation, diet counseling, control of menstrual abnormalities.

Specific Measures: Based on cause.

Diet: Adequate iron (7–12 mg/d) and folate (1–5 mg/d).

Activity: No restriction.

Patient Education: Diet counseling, American College of Obstetricians and Gynecologists Patient Education Pamphlet AP001 (*Nutrition During Pregnancy*).

Drug(s) of Choice

Iron supplements (ferrous sulfate 300–350 mg PO tid) for 6–12 months or longer (Parenteral iron may be given to patients with severe anemia or to those who do not comply with oral therapy.)

For pernicious anemia—vitamin B_{12} 100 μg IM monthly. (Treatment of megaloblastic anemia due to B_{12} deficiency with folate will reverse anemia but progressive and irreversible neurologic damage may result. B_{12} levels should always be checked if this is suspected.)

Precautions: Anaphylaxis may occur with parenteral iron.

Interactions: Ascorbic acid increases absorption of iron.

FOLLOW-UP

Patient Monitoring: Normal health maintenance, periodic evaluation of blood count.

Prevention/Avoidance: Good diet, control of excessive menstrual blood loss.

Possible Complications: Progressive and irreversible neurologic damage may result with untreated vitamin B_{12} deficiency.

Expected Outcome: Generally good response to iron therapy (iron deficiency type).

MISCELLANEOUS

Pregnancy Considerations: Anemia more common in pregnancy.

ICD-9-CM Codes: 285.9 (others based on cause).

REFERENCES

Millman RS, Ault KA. *Hematology in Clinical Practice. A Guide to Diagnosis and Management.* New York, NY: McGraw-Hill; 1995.

Signs and symptoms

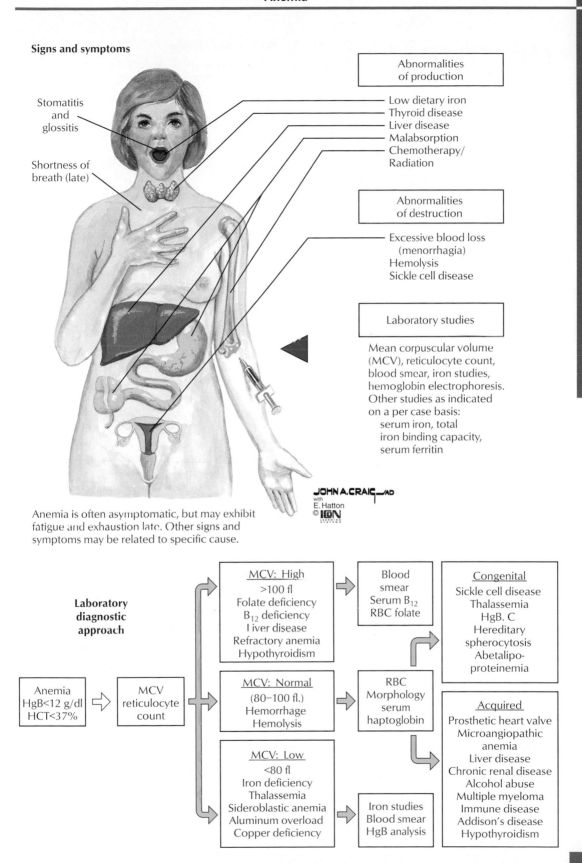

Stomatitis and glossitis

Shortness of breath (late)

Abnormalities of production

Low dietary iron
Thyroid disease
Liver disease
Malabsorption
Chemotherapy/ Radiation

Abnormalities of destruction

Excessive blood loss (menorrhagia)
Hemolysis
Sickle cell disease

Laboratory studies

Mean corpuscular volume (MCV), reticulocyte count, blood smear, iron studies, hemoglobin electrophoresis. Other studies as indicated on a per case basis: serum iron, total iron binding capacity, serum ferritin

JOHN A.CRAIG—AD
with
E. Hatton
© ICON
LEARNING SYSTEMS

Anemia is often asymptomatic, but may exhibit fatigue and exhaustion late. Other signs and symptoms may be related to specific cause.

Laboratory diagnostic approach

Anemia
HgB<12 g/dl
HCT<37%

MCV reticulocyte count

MCV: High
>100 fl
Folate deficiency
B_{12} deficiency
Liver disease
Refractory anemia
Hypothyroidism

Blood smear
Serum B_{12}
RBC folate

Congenital
Sickle cell disease
Thalassemia
HgB. C
Hereditary spherocytosis
Abetalipo-proteinemia

MCV: Normal
(80–100 fl.)
Hemorrhage
Hemolysis

RBC Morphology serum haptoglobin

Acquired
Prosthetic heart valve
Microangiopathic anemia
Liver disease
Chronic renal disease
Alcohol abuse
Multiple myeloma
Immune disease
Addison's disease
Hypothyroidism

MCV: Low
<80 fl
Iron deficiency
Thalassemia
Sideroblastic anemia
Aluminum overload
Copper deficiency

Iron studies
Blood smear
HgB analysis

ANORECTAL FISTULA

INTRODUCTION

Description: A communication between the anal or rectal canal and the perineum.
Prevalence: Common.
Predominant Age: Any.
Genetics: No genetic pattern.

ETIOLOGY AND PATHOGENESIS

Causes: Anorectal fistulae may arise spontaneously or result from the drainage of a perirectal abscess. Patients with anal fistulae should be evaluated for the possibility of inflammatory bowel disease.
Risk Factors: Although Crohn's disease and tuberculosis are recognized risk factors, in most patients a predisposing cause is not apparent. Other risk factors include tears, puncture wounds, and internal hemorrhoids.

CLINICAL CHARACTERISTICS

Signs and Symptoms:
- Intermittent perineal drainage or discharge
- Perianal lump or mass
- Pain (external sphincter) with defecation
- Anal bleeding
- Most fistulae have involvement of the posterior midline and origin in the anorectal crypts

DIAGNOSTIC APPROACH

Differential Diagnosis:
- Inflammatory bowel disease (Crohn's disease)
- Pilonidal sinus
- Perianal or other abscess
- Rectal carcinoma

Associated Conditions: Crohn's disease.

Workup and Evaluation

Laboratory: No evaluation indicated.
Imaging: If inflammatory bowel disease is suspected, lower gastrointestinal series.
Special Tests: None indicated.
Diagnostic Procedures: History, physical examination, probe of fistulous tract. Anoscopy, proctoscopy, or sigmoidoscopy may be helpful.

Pathologic Findings

Inflammation and granulation change from chronic infection. Tract may be single or multiple. Internal opening is generally within an anal crypt.

MANAGEMENT AND THERAPY

Nonpharmacologic

General Measures: Evaluation, stool softening, and sitz baths.
Specific Measures: The only effective treatment is surgical, often carried out under general or spinal anesthesia in an ambulatory surgery unit. Fistulectomy or fistulotomy should not be performed in the presence of diarrhea or active inflammatory bowel disease.
Diet: High-fiber diet advisable.
Activity: No restriction.
Patient Education: Perianal care, sitz baths

Drug(s) of Choice

Although the only effective treatment is surgery, the use of stool softeners is often beneficial.

FOLLOW-UP

Patient Monitoring: Close follow-up during postoperative period, routine health care thereafter.
Prevention/Avoidance: None.
Possible Complications: Constipation, rectovaginal fistula, recurrence.
Expected Outcome: Healing is generally good after surgical excision, although recurrence resulting from underlying disease is common.

MISCELLANEOUS

Pregnancy Considerations: No effect on pregnancy, although may affect the choice of an episiotomy site.
ICD-9-CM Codes: 565.1.

REFERENCES

American College of Obstetricians and Gynecologists. *Genitourinary Fistulas.* Washington, DC: ACOG; 1985. ACOG Technical Bulletin 83.

Bassford T. Treatment of common anorectal disorders [review]. *Am Fam Physician* 1992;45:1787.

Hancock BD. ABC of colorectal diseases. Anal fissures and fistulas [review]. *BMJ* 1992;304:904.

Smith RP, Ling FW. *Procedures in Women's Health Care.* Baltimore, Md: Williams & Wilkins; 1997:153, 163, 175, 201.

Appearance and Management or Anorectal Crohn's Disease

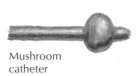

Mushroom catheter

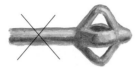

Malecot catheter (allows ingrowth of fibrous tissue, making removal difficult)

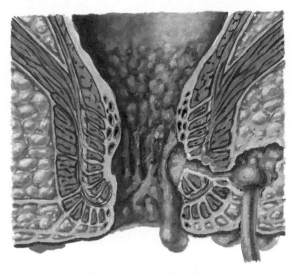

Abscess drained by placing small mushroom catheter as close to anus as possible to avoid subsequent long fistula tract

JOHN A. CRAIG—AD
© ICN

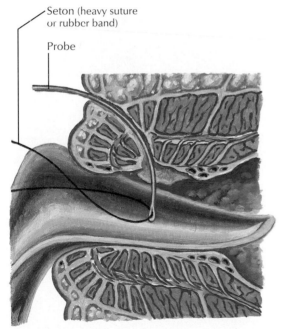

Seton (heavy suture or rubber band)

Probe

Sepsis of fistula tract controlled by placing seton (avoids fistulotomy wounds, which heal poorly)

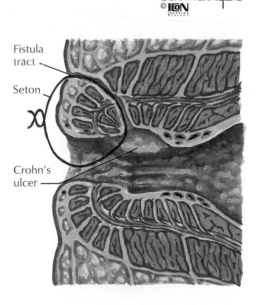

Fistula tract

Seton

Crohn's ulcer

Seton left in place between internal and external openings to prevent abscess formation and further destruction of sphincter mechanism

Anorectal Fistula

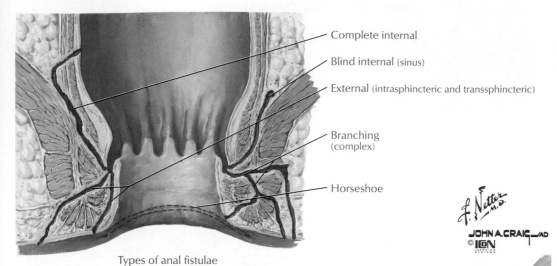

Complete internal

Blind internal (sinus)

External (intrasphincteric and transsphincteric)

Branching (complex)

Horseshoe

Types of anal fistulae

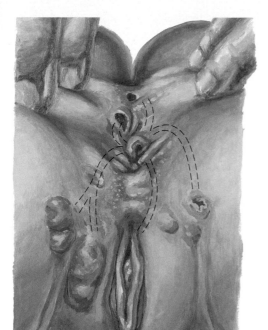

Unusually located (often multiple) anal fistulas, abscesses, ulcers and edematous hemorrhoidal skin tags

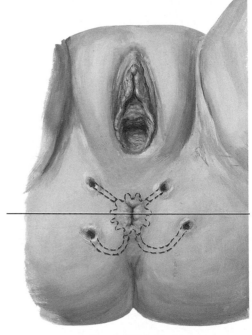

Goodsall-Salmon Law

ANXIETY

INTRODUCTION

Description: Anxiety is a common acute or chronic emotion, associated with physical symptoms, which is two to three times more common in women. Subtypes include situational anxiety, adjustment disorders, panic disorders, phobias, and post-traumatic stress disorder. Obsessive compulsive disorders are often classified in this group as well.

Prevalence: Eighteen percent of women, 40 million Americans.

Predominant Age: 20–45.

Genetics: Increased risk of panic disorders within monozygotic twins. Panic disorder, social phobia, and obsessive compulsive disorders have a genetic base.

ETIOLOGY AND PATHOGENESIS

Causes: Psychosocial stressors, abnormality of the neurotransmitter system (serotonin, norepinephrine, γ-aminobutyric acid).

Risk Factors: Social, family or financial stress, medical illness, family history, and a lack of social support network.

CLINICAL CHARACTERISTICS

Signs and Symptoms (Vary with Subtype):
- Unrealistic or excessive worry
- Sense of impending doom
- Nervousness or instability
- Palpitations or tachycardia
- Hyperventilation or sense of suffocation
- Systemic systems (nausea, abdominal pain, paresthesias, diaphoresis, chest tightness, dizziness, muscle tension, headaches, and backaches)

DIAGNOSTIC APPROACH

Differential Diagnosis:
- Cardiovascular (ischemic heart disease, valvular disease, cardiomyopathies, arrhythmias, mitral valve prolapse)
- Respiratory (asthma, emphysema, pulmonary embolism)
- Central nervous system (transient ischemia, psychomotor epilepsy, essential tremor)
- Metabolic (hyperthyroidism, adrenal insufficiency, pheochromocytoma, Cushing's syndrome, hypoglycemia, hypokalemia, hyperparathyroidism, myasthenia gravis)
- Nutritional (thiamine, pyridoxine, or folate deficiency)
- Medication/drugs (caffeinism, alcohol, cocaine, sympathomimetics, amphetamine)

Associated Conditions: Mitral valve prolapse, irritable bowel syndrome (IBS), depression, agoraphobia, substance abuse, and somatoform disorders.

Workup and Evaluation

Laboratory: No specific evaluation indicated. Tests should be based on the diagnoses being considered (eg, thyroid function studies).

Imaging: No imaging indicated.

Special Tests: None indicated.

Diagnostic Procedures: History and psychologic testing.

Pathologic Findings

None.

MANAGEMENT AND THERAPY

Nonpharmacologic

General Measures: Evaluation and assessment of cause and subtype, screening for substance abuse, counseling, establishing ties to support systems, beginning exercise program, and maintaining frequent follow-up.

Specific Measures: Psychotherapy, medications.

Diet: No specific dietary changes indicated.

Activity: No restriction.

Patient Education: American College of Obstetricians and Gynecologists Patient Education Pamphlet AP068 (*Alcohol and Women*), AP083 (*The Abused Woman*).

Drug(s) of Choice

Acute anxiety or adjustment disorders—short-term benzodiazepines (alprazolam, 0.25 mg two to three times daily, increase in 0.25 mg increments if needed).

Generalized anxiety—azaperones (buspirone [BuSpar] 5 mg PO bid–tid, increased every 2–3 days to a maximum of 60 mg/d).

Panic disorders and phobias—selective serotonin reuptake inhibitors (SSRIs) (fluoxetine [Prozac] 4 mg PO, increased by 4 mg q5d to maximum of 40 mg, sertraline [Zoloft] 25 mg PO, increased by 25 mg q5d, paroxetine [Paxil]) 10 mg PO increased by 10 mg q5d).

Obsessive compulsive disorders—SSRIs or clomipramine (Anafranil) 25 mg PO bid, increased to 250 mg/d).

Contraindications: Benzodiazepines are contraindicated in the first trimester of pregnancy, in patients with acute alcohol intoxication,

Clinical Features

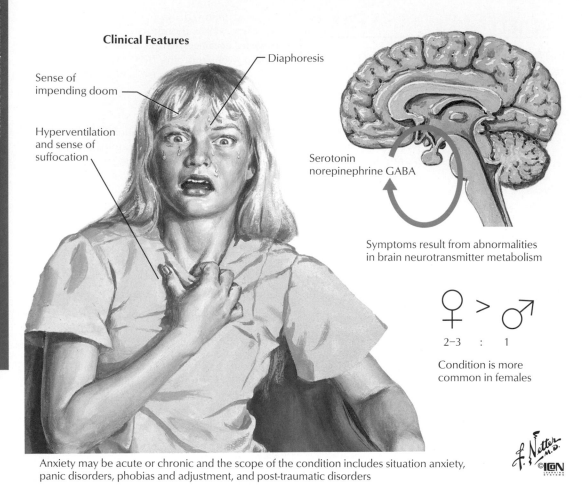

Sense of impending doom

Diaphoresis

Hyperventilation and sense of suffocation

Serotonin norepinephrine GABA

Symptoms result from abnormalities in brain neurotransmitter metabolism

2–3 : 1

Condition is more common in females

Anxiety may be acute or chronic and the scope of the condition includes situation anxiety, panic disorders, phobias and adjustment, and post-traumatic disorders

Systemic Somatic Symptoms

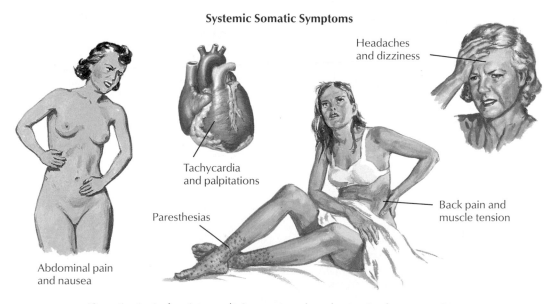

Headaches and dizziness

Tachycardia and palpitations

Paresthesias

Back pain and muscle tension

Abdominal pain and nausea

"Somatization" of anxiety results in symptoms in various systemic organ systems

and in patients with sleep apnea or open angle glaucoma.

Precautions: Agents with short half-lives (eg, alprazolam) have a high potential for dependency and withdrawal symptoms; acute withdrawal may precipitate panic attacks or seizures. Hepatic and renal function should be monitored in patients using benzodiazepines or buspirone. Breast-feeding should be discouraged in women on chronic or high dose benzodiazepines.

Interactions: Buspirone should not be used with monamine oxidase inhibitors.

Alternative Drugs

Panic disorders and phobias—imipramine (Tofranil) 10–25 mg PO qhs, increased by 10–25 mg/d every 2 weeks to a maximum of 300 mg/d in adults, 100 mg/d in adolescents and elderly patients).

FOLLOW-UP

Patient Monitoring: Frequent follow-up, identification and treatment of associated depression, periodic assessment of renal and hepatic function (based on medical therapy chosen).

Prevention/Avoidance: Stress management, relaxation training.

Possible Complications: Social withdrawal or isolation, drug dependence or side effects.

Expected Outcome: Generally good outcome. (Obsessive compulsive disorders and post-traumatic stress disorders are more difficult to treat.)

MISCELLANEOUS

Pregnancy Considerations: Medical therapy must be adjusted based on risk and need.

ICD-9-CM Codes: 300.00 (others based on cause).

REFERENCES

Katon W. Panic disorders: somatization, medical utilization and treatment. *Am J Med* 1992;92(suppl 1A):1s.

Linzer M, Kindy P, Williams JM, et al. Anxiety and depression: role of the gynecologists in diagnosis and therapy. In: Ling FW, Laube DW, Nolan TE, Smith RP, Stoval TG, eds. *Primary Care in Gynecology.* Baltimore, Md: Williams & Wilkins; 1997:325.

Parry BL. Reproductive factors affecting the course of affective illness in women. *Psychiatr Clin North Am* 1989;12:207.

Roy-Byme PP. Integrated treatment of panic disorder. *Am J Med* 1992;suppl 1A:495–545.

Spitzer R, Williams JBW, Kroenke K, et al. The PRIME-MD study: description, validation and clinical utility of a new procedure for diagnosing mental disorders in primary care. *JAMA* 1994;272:1749.

ASTHMA

INTRODUCTION

Description: Intermittent or chronic obstructive tracheobronchial condition characterized by wheezing or cough. Adult onset asthma is more common in women and poses potential problems during pregnancy.

Prevalence: Ten percent of the population.

Predominant Age: Adult 16–40 (50% of patients are younger than 10).

Genetics: Familial association with reactive airway disease, ectopic dermatitis, and allergic rhinitis.

ETIOLOGY AND PATHOGENESIS

Causes: Allergic factors (airborne pollens, molds, house dust, animal dander, feather pillows), smoke or pollutants, viral upper respiratory infections, aspirin or nonsteroidal antiinflammatory agents, exercise, gastrointestinal reflux.

Risk Factors: Family history, viral pneumonitis in infancy.

CLINICAL CHARACTERISTICS

Signs and Symptoms:
- Wheezing and coughing (one or both)
- Prolonged exhalation
- Decreased breath sounds, hyperresonant chest
- Periodic (especially nocturnal) attacks
- Cyanosis and tachycardia
- Pulsus paradoxus, accessory muscle use for breathing, flattened diaphragms on chest radiographs or physical examination

DIAGNOSTIC APPROACH

Differential Diagnosis:
- Recurrent pneumonia
- Chronic bronchitis
- Viral or fungal infection
- Aspiration (foreign body)
- Cystic fibrosis
- Tuberculosis
- Mitral valve prolapse
- Congestive heart failure
- Chronic obstructive pulmonary disease

Associated Conditions: Reflux esophagitis, sinusitis.

Workup and Evaluation

Laboratory: Complete blood count, arterial blood gases (severe cases).

Imaging: No imaging indicated. (Chest radiograph shows hyperinflation, atelectasis, or air leak, but is nonspecific.)

Special Tests: Sweat chloride test (childhood), nasal eosinophils, pulmonary function testing (peak expiratory flow rate), allergy testing (selected patients).

Diagnostic Procedures: History, physical examination, pulmonary function testing (forced expiratory volume in 1 second, FEV1). An excellent office screening test is to ask the patient to blow out a lit match held at arm's length. Patients with reduced FEV1 are unable to accomplish this task.

Pathologic Findings

Narrowing of large and small airways because of bronchial smooth muscle spasm, edema, and inflammation of the bronchial mucosa with increased mucus production characterize acute attacks. Chronic inflammatory changes are seen histologically. Biochemical factors related to inflammation mediators include chemical, eosinophil, and neutrophil chemotactic factors, bradykinins, and others.

MANAGEMENT AND THERAPY

Nonpharmacologic

General Measures: Evaluation, eliminate irritants, education, caffeine for mild symptoms.

Specific Measures: Mild—intermittent β-agonists via inhaler or cromolyn sodium qid plus low-dose inhaled steroids (beclomethasone dipropionate 400 μg/d) may add slow-release xanthines. Severe—cromolyn sodium plus high-dose inhaled steroids plus theophylline (therapeutic level 10–20 μg/mL), inhaled β-agonist to reverse airflow obstruction. During asthma attacks patients should avoid fluid loading, intermittent positive pressure breathing, or airway mist or humidification; these worsen symptoms.

Diet: No specific dietary changes indicated. Avoid known allergens (if any).

Activity: No restriction or restriction based on pulmonary function except for those with exercise-induced asthma (eg, cold weather, excessive activity).

Patient Education: Understanding of disease and use of inhalers, education about triggering factors and allergens.

Drug(s) of Choice

Cromoglycate and nedocromil, steroids (beclomethasone, prednisone), β-agonists (albuterol, bitolterol, salmeterol, terbutaline), methylxanthines (theophylline), anticholinergics (atropine, ipratropium bromide), leukotriene antagonists.

Postulated Mechanisms of Airway Hyperreactivity Causing Asthma

A. Immunologic response

Antigen

B. β-adrenergic blockade caused by

Infection
Metabolites
Adenylcyclase deficiency
Drugs

C. Cholinergic dominance

Central influences ?

D. β-adrenergic amine deficiency

E. Intrinsic smooth muscle defect

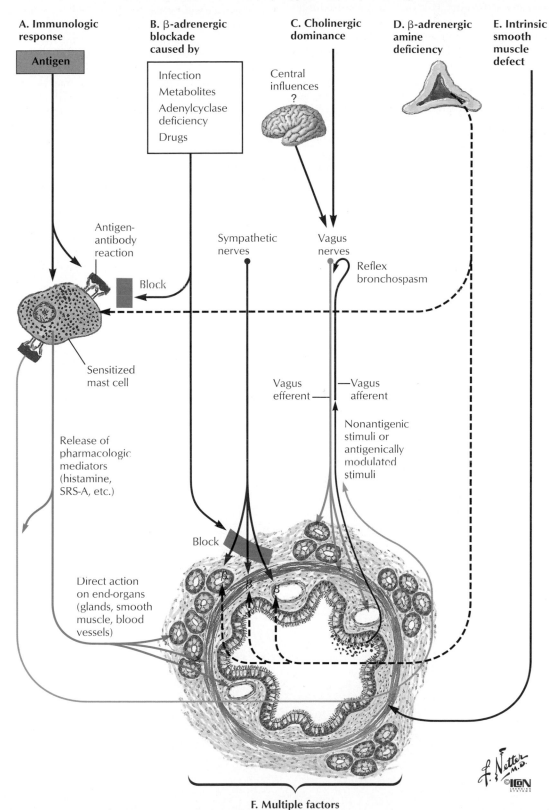

Antigen-antibody reaction

Block

Sympathetic nerves

Vagus nerves

Reflex bronchospasm

Sensitized mast cell

Vagus efferent

Vagus afferent

Release of pharmacologic mediators (histamine, SRS-A, etc.)

Nonantigenic stimuli or antigenically modulated stimuli

Block

β β β

Direct action on end-organs (glands, smooth muscle, blood vessels)

F. Multiple factors

Contraindications: Sedatives, mucolytics.

Precautions: β-Agonists should only be used intermittently.

Interactions: Erythromycin and ciprofloxacin slow theophylline clearance and can increase levels by 15%–20%.

Alternative Drugs

Histamine H_1-antagonists, methotrexate.

FOLLOW-UP

Patient Monitoring: Normal health maintenance.

Prevention/Avoidance: Avoid known allergens, aspirin, nonsteroidal antiinflammatory and β-adrenergic blocking drugs. Have a prearranged action plan for acute attacks. Obtain annual influenza immunization. Avoid food additives known to precipitate attacks (sulfites and tartrazine).

Possible Complications: Respiratory failure, atelectasis, and pneumothorax, death. (Mortality increases with more than three emergency visits or more than two hospital admissions per year, nocturnal symptoms, history of intensive care unit admission or mechanical ventilation, steroid dependence, and history of syncope with attacks.)

Expected Outcome: Excellent with careful management.

MISCELLANEOUS

Pregnancy Considerations: Roughly 50% of patients have no change in symptoms, 25% improve, and 25% worsen. Asthma is found in 1% of pregnant patients, 15% of whom have one or more significant attacks during the gestation: the effects are highly variable, but may include chronic hypoxia, intrauterine growth restriction, and rarely fetal death.

ICD-9-CM Codes: 493.9 (others based on type and cause).

REFERENCES

Bank DE, Rug SE. New approaches to upper airway disease [review]. *Emerge Med Clin North Am* 1995;13:473.

Barsky HE. Asthma and pregnancy: a challenge for everyone concerned. *Postgrad Med* 1991;89:125.

Clark SL. Management of asthma during pregnancy. National Asthma Education Program Working Group in Asthma and Pregnancy. National Institutes of Health, National Heart, Lung and Blood Institute. *Obstet Gynecol* 1993;82:1036.

Greenberger PA. Asthma in pregnancy. *Clin Chest Med* 1992;13:597.

Nolan TE. Upper respiratory and pulmonary problems [review]. *Clin Obstet Gynecol*. 1995;38:147.

Moore GJ. Asthma in pregnancy. *Br J Obstet Gynecol* 1994;101:658.

Schatz M. Asthma during pregnancy: interrelationships and management *Ann Allergy* 1992;68:23.

CHOLELITHIASIS

INTRODUCTION

Description: The formation of stones in the gall-bladder or biliary collecting system. Most stones are the result of precipitation of super-saturated cholesterol. Women are three times more likely than men to form gallstones.

Prevalence: Ten percent of the population, 1 million cases per year.

Predominant Age: Seventy percent of patients older than 40.

Genetics: Ratio of women to men 3:1, some races at greater risk (eg, Pima Indians).

ETIOLOGY AND PATHOGENESIS

Causes: The metabolic alteration leading to choles-terol stones is thought to be a disruption in the balance between hydroxymethylglutaryl coen-zyme A (HMG-CoA) reductase and cholesterol 7α-hydroxylase. HMG-CoA controls cholesterol synthesis, while cholesterol 7α-hydroxylase controls the rate of bile acid formation. Patients who form cholesterol stones have elevated lev-els of HMG-CoA and depressed levels of cho-lesterol 7α-hydroxylase. This change in ratio in-creases the risk of precipitation of cholesterol as stones.

Risk Factors: Age, female gender, parity (75% of af-fected patients have had one or more pregnan-cies), obesity (15–20 pounds overweight 2-fold increase in risk, 50–75 pounds excess weight 6-fold increase in risk), estrogen use (oral), cir-rhosis, diabetes, and Crohn's disease. A family history of cholelithiasis in siblings or children results in a 2-fold increase in risk.

CLINICAL CHARACTERISTICS

Signs and Symptoms:
- Asymptomatic (60%–70%) (50% become symptomatic, 20% develop complications)
- Fatty food intolerance
- Variable right upper quadrant pain with ra-diation to the back or scapula
- Nausea or vomiting (often mistaken for "indigestion")
- Fever usually associated with cholangitis

DIAGNOSTIC APPROACH

Differential Diagnosis:
- Gastroenteritis
- Esophageal reflux
- Malabsorption
- IBS
- Peptic ulcer disease
- Coronary artery disease
- Pneumonia
- Appendicitis

Associated Conditions: Cirrhosis, pancreatitis, and ileus.

Workup and Evaluation

Laboratory: Supportive, but often not diagnostic—complete blood count, serum bilirubin, amy-lase, alkaline phosphatase, and aminotrans-ferase measurements.

Imaging: Ultrasonography of the gallbladder (96% accuracy for diagnosing sludge or a stone in the gallbladder).

Special Tests: None indicated.

Diagnostic Procedures: History, physical examina-tion, ultrasonography, and laboratory investi-gation.

Pathologic Findings

Supersaturated bile, inflammation when accom-panied by infection or obstruction.

MANAGEMENT AND THERAPY

Nonpharmacologic

General Measures: Watchful waiting and dietary modifications.

Specific Measures: Oral therapy, surgical extirpa-tion, lithotripsy.

Diet: Reduced fatty food and cholesterol intake.

Activity: No restriction.

Patient Education: American College of Obstetri-cians and Gynecologists Patient Education Pamphlet AP064 (*Weight Control: Eating Right and Keeping Fit*).

Drug(s) of Choice

Ursodeoxycholic acid (Actigall) 8–10 mg/kg/d as two to three doses.

Contraindications: Known allergy, acute cholecysti-tis, abnormal liver function, calcified stones (not cholesterol based).

Precautions: The rate of stone dissolution (approxi-mately 1 mm/mo) limits applicability for stones greater than 1.5–2 cm in size.

Interactions: None.

FOLLOW-UP

Patient Monitoring: Normal health maintenance

Prevention/Avoidance: Low-fat and low-cholesterol diet may delay symptoms. Oral prophylaxis during rapid weight loss has been advocated for those otherwise at risk.

Possible Complications: Acute cholecystitis, pancre-atitis, ascending cholangitis, peritonitis, inter-

Pathogenesis of Gallstones

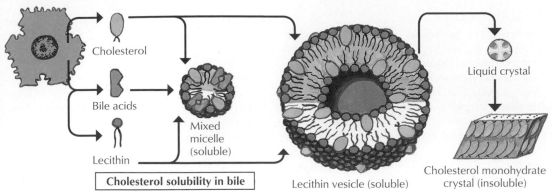

Cholesterol solubility in bile

Lecithin vesicle (soluble)

Cholesterol monohydrate crystal (insoluble)

Solubility of cholesterol in bile depends on incorporation of cholesterol in bile acid–lecithin micelles and lecithin vesicles. When bile becomes saturated with cholesterol, vesicles fuse to form liposomes, or liquid crystals, from which crystals of cholesterol monohydrate nucleate

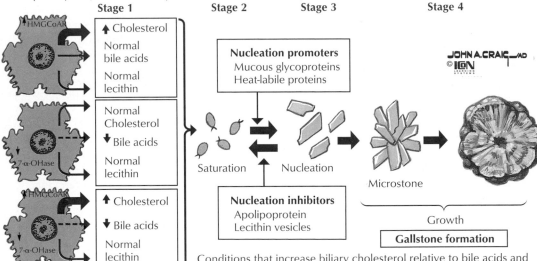

Stage 1 Stage 2 Stage 3 Stage 4

Conditions that increase biliary cholesterol relative to bile acids and lecithin favor saturation of bile and formation of gallstones

Gallstone formation

Predisposing factors

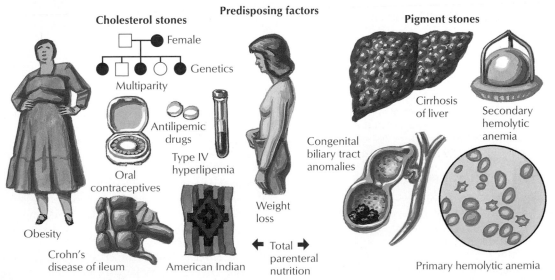

Cholesterol stones

Female

Genetics

Multiparity

Antilipemic drugs

Type IV hyperlipemia

Oral contraceptives

Obesity

Crohn's disease of ileum

American Indian

Weight loss

Total parenteral nutrition

Pigment stones

Cirrhosis of liver

Secondary hemolytic anemia

Congenital biliary tract anomalies

Primary hemolytic anemia

nal fistulization. Stones reform in approximately 50% of patients treated with oral therapy, although the majority (85%) remain asymptomatic. Those who have recurrent symptoms respond to additional courses of oral therapy.

Expected Outcome: Generally good with either oral or surgical therapy. Oral therapy results in resolution of symptoms in 2–3 months.

MISCELLANEOUS

Pregnancy Considerations: Three percent to four percent of pregnant patients experience gallstone symptoms. Women with increased parity and multifetal pregnancies are at greatest risk.

ICD-9-CM Codes: 574.2 (others based on obstruction or inflammation).

REFERENCES

Everson GT, McKinley C, Kern F Jr. Mechanisms of gallstone formation in women. *J Clin Invest* 1991;87:237.

Fromm H. Gallstone dissolution therapy: current status and future prospects. *Gastroenterology* 1986;91:1560.

Ikard RW. Gallstones, cholecystitis and diabetes. *Surg Gynecol Obstet*. 1990;171:528.

Maclure KM, Hayes KC, Colditz GA, Stampfer MJ, Willett WC. Dietary predictors of symptom-associated gallstones in middle-aged women. *Am J Clin Nutr* 1990;52:916.

McSherry CK, Ferstenberg H, Calhoun WF, Lahman E, Virshup M. The natural history of diagnosed gallstone disease in symptomatic and asymptomatic patients. *Ann Surg* 1985;202:59.

Smith RP, Nolan TE: Gallbladder disease and women: etiology, diagnosis and therapy. *Female Patient* 1992;17:99.

CONSTIPATION

INTRODUCTION

Description: The infrequent passage of hard stools, often associated with mechanical or other means to stimulate bowel movements. Often also related to changes in the size, consistency, and ease of bowel movement in the subjective definition of constipation.

Prevalence: Very common as a sporadic problem, 8%–10% of women.

Predominant Age: Any, more common in youth and old age.

Genetics: No genetic pattern.

ETIOLOGY AND PATHOGENESIS

Causes: Inadequate dietary fiber and fluid intake, altered gastrointestinal motility (drugs, illness, injury, laxative abuse), metabolic (hypothyroidism, diabetes), mechanical (obstruction, impaction).

Risk Factors: Poor diet and fluid intake, inactivity, medications (narcotics, iron therapy), and sedentary lifestyle.

CLINICAL CHARACTERISTICS

Signs and Symptoms:
- Bowel movements less than three times per week
- Hard stools
- Straining to have a bowel movement
- Inability to have bowel movements without medical or mechanical interventions (enemas, manual evacuation)

DIAGNOSTIC APPROACH

Differential Diagnosis:
- Hypothyroidism
- Rectocele
- Laxative abuse
- Dehydration
- Inappropriate expectation

Associated Conditions: Diverticulitis, abdominal pain.

Workup and Evaluation

Laboratory: No evaluation indicated.

Imaging: Radiography (abdominal plain film [kidneys, ureter, bladder], barium enema, defecography) may help to identify the source of the problem, but it is not required for diagnosis.

Special Tests: Rectal examination, flexible sigmoidoscopy, or colonoscopy should be considered for older patients.

Diagnostic Procedures: History and physical examination.

Pathologic Findings

None.

MANAGEMENT AND THERAPY

Nonpharmacologic

General Measures: Fluids, dietary fiber, fiber supplements, and physical activity.

Specific Measures: Mechanical assistance (enemas), mechanical disimpaction.

Diet: Increased dietary fiber and adequate fluids, fiber supplements as needed.

Activity: No restriction, activity encouraged.

Patient Education: Reassurance, diet counseling, American College of Obstetricians and Gynecologists Patient Education Pamphlet AP001 (*Nutrition During Pregnancy*), AA005 (*Healthy Mother's Food Wheel*), AP064 (*Weight Control: Eating Right and Keeping Fit*).

Drug(s) of Choice

Fiber supplements, stool softeners (docusate sodium 100 mg PO bid), laxatives (use with caution).

Contraindications: Bowel obstruction, peritonitis.

Precautions: Laxative abuse and dependence are common. Patients should be warned about their appropriate use.

FOLLOW-UP

Patient Monitoring: Normal health maintenance.

Prevention/Avoidance: Adequate fiber and fluid, physical activity.

Possible Complications: Impaction, fluid or electrolyte imbalance with laxative abuse, possible increase in the risk of colon cancer (proposed, but unproven).

Expected Outcome: Good with adequate diet, fluid, and activity.

MISCELLANEOUS

Pregnancy Considerations: No effect on pregnancy, although pregnancy (and associated iron supplementation) may make constipation worse.

ICD-9-CM Codes: 564.0, 306.4 (Psychogenic).

REFERENCES

Leonard-Jones JE. Clinical management of constipation. *Pharmacology* 1993;47(suppl 1):216.

Rapkin AJ, Mayer EA. Gastroenterologic causes of chronic pelvic pain. *Obstet Gynecol Clin North Am* 1993;20:663.

Snape WJ Jr. Disorders of gastrointestinal motility. In: Wyngaarden JB, Smith LH Jr, Bennett JC, eds. *Cecil Textbook of Medicine.* 19th ed. Philadelphia, Pa: WB Saunders; 1992:671.

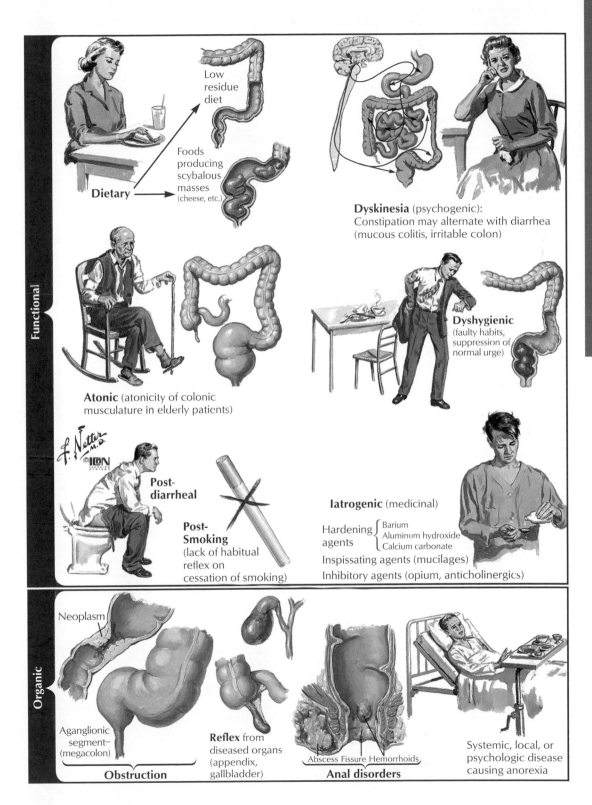

Functional

Dietary → Low residue diet

Foods producing scybalous masses (cheese, etc.)

Dyskinesia (psychogenic): Constipation may alternate with diarrhea (mucous colitis, irritable colon)

Atonic (atonicity of colonic musculature in elderly patients)

Dyshygienic (faulty habits, suppression of normal urge)

Post-diarrheal

Post-Smoking (lack of habitual reflex on cessation of smoking)

Iatrogenic (medicinal)

Hardening agents { Barium, Aluminum hydroxide, Calcium carbonate }

Inspissating agents (mucilages)

Inhibitory agents (opium, anticholinergics)

Organic

Neoplasm

Aganglionic segment— (megacolon)

Obstruction

Reflex from diseased organs (appendix, gallbladder)

Abscess Fissure Hemorrhoids

Anal disorders

Systemic, local, or psychologic disease causing anorexia

CROHN'S DISEASE

INTRODUCTION

Description: An idiopathic inflammatory bowel disease characterized by transmural involvement resulting in severe gastrointestinal symptoms and significant morbidity.

Prevalence: Two to ten of 10,000.

Predominant Age: 15–30.

Genetics: First-degree relative for 15% of patients, more common in whites and Jews.

ETIOLOGY AND PATHOGENESIS

Causes: The inflammatory process in Crohn's disease is transmural and involves both the large and small bowel in 50% of patients.

Risk Factors: Cigarette smoking (postulated but unproven).

CLINICAL CHARACTERISTICS

Signs and Symptoms:

- Abdominal pain (80%–85%, often lasting for days or weeks) (the pain described is frequently located in the mid abdomen or right lower quadrant, although generalized pain is often present)
- Diarrhea (voluminous, watery, with occasional blood [20%])
- Fever
- Dyspareunia
- Vulvar or perineal fissures or fistulae or occasionally vulvar granulomas
- Arthritis, sclerosing cholangitis (5%–10%)

DIAGNOSTIC APPROACH

Differential Diagnosis:

- IBS
- Ulcerative colitis
- Enteric pathogens
- Lymphoma
- Pelvic inflammatory disease (PID) (acute episodes)
- Endometriosis

Associated Conditions: Arthritis, dyspareunia, vulvar or perineal fissures or fistulae, vulvar granulomas, erythema nodosum, and sclerosing cholangitis.

Workup and Evaluation

Laboratory: Complete blood count, sedimentation rate.

Imaging: Barium enema, upper gastrointestinal radiograph with small bowel followthrough.

Special Tests: Sigmoidoscopy, colonoscopy, or rectal biopsy.

Diagnostic Procedures: History, sigmoidoscopy, or colonoscopy, radiologic studies, or rectal biopsy.

Pathologic Findings

Transmural inflammation with ulceration and distortion. Areas of normal bowel (skip areas). Granulomas may be found in 15% of patients.

MANAGEMENT AND THERAPY

Nonpharmacologic

General Measures: Maintenance of weight and nutrition, perineal care.

Specific Measures: Surgical therapy (resection) often required.

Diet: No specific dietary changes indicated, increased dietary fiber sometimes recommended.

Activity: No restriction.

Drug(s) of Choice

Mesalamine (5-aminosalicylic acid), methotrexate, or azathioprine (Imuran) for maintenance and suppression.

Prednisone (20–40 mg PO daily, tapered after 4–6 weeks) or sulfasalazine or mesalamine at increased doses for acute exacerbations.

Precautions: Folic acid supplements should be used with mesalamine.

FOLLOW-UP

Patient Monitoring: Weight and symptoms, periodic blood count and sedimentation rate. Endoscopy to monitor disease (as needed).

Prevention/Avoidance: None.

Possible Complications: Bowel thickening, stenosis, and internal fistula formation are common. Short bowel syndromes and malabsorption are common after repeated surgery.

Expected Outcome: Need for eventual or repeated surgery very likely.

MISCELLANEOUS

Pregnancy Considerations: No effect on pregnancy.

ICD-9-CM Codes: 555.9.

REFERENCES

Hannauer SB. Inflammatory bowel disease. *N Engl J Med* 1996;334:841.

Hannauer SB. Inflammatory bowel disease. In: Wyngaarden JB, Smith LH Jr, Bennett JC, eds. *Cecil Textbook of Medicine.* 19th ed. Philadelphia, Pa: WB Saunders; 1992:699.

Rapkin AJ, Mayer EA. Gastroenterologic causes of chronic pelvic pain. *Obstet Gynecol Clin North Am* 1993;20:663.

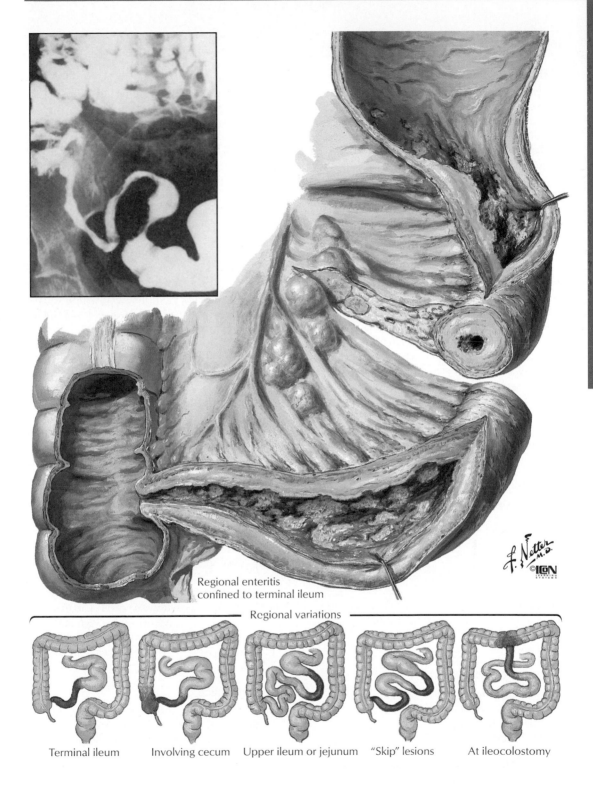

Regional enteritis
confined to terminal ileum

Regional variations

Terminal ileum · Involving cecum · Upper ileum or jejunum · "Skip" lesions · At ileocolostomy

DEPRESSION (UNIPOLAR)

INTRODUCTION

Description: A biochemically mediated state in which anger, frustration, loss of pleasure, and withdrawal predominate. This must be separated from normal stress reactions and grief.

Prevalence: Twenty million American adults per year, 1 in 6–8 lifetime risk, 6%–14% of primary care visits, 2:1 female to male ratio. Depression is the fourth most common reason to seek medical care.

Predominant Age: Rare before puberty, commonly begins in 20s–30s, average 40.

Genetics: Possible defect on chromosome 11 or X.

ETIOLOGY AND PATHOGENESIS

Causes: Proposed—alteration in norepinephrine or serotonin through impaired synthesis of neurotransmitters, increased breakdown or metabolism of neurotransmitters, increased uptake of neurotransmitters.

Risk Factors: Strong family history (depression, suicide, alcoholism, substance abuse). Women are at greatest risk during adolescence (up to 60% meet criteria), the premenstrual period, pregnancy, the postpartum period, and perimenopause, after pregnancy loss (3 times risk) and with infertility (2 times risk).

CLINICAL CHARACTERISTICS

Signs and Symptoms (Five or More over a 2-Week Period):
- Depressed mood
- Anhedonia
- Weight loss
- Sleep changes
- Psychomotor changes
- Fatigue
- Feeling of worthlessness or guilt
- Inability to concentrate
- Thoughts of death

DIAGNOSTIC APPROACH

Differential Diagnosis:
- Endocrine disorders (diabetes, pituitary, adrenal, thyroid)
- Malignancies
- Infections
- Neurologic disorders (organic brain disease)
- Autoimmune disease
- Cardiovascular, hepatic, or renal disease
- Vitamin or mineral deficiency or excess
- Medication side effect (cardiovascular drugs, hormones, anticancer agents, antiinflammatory or antiinfective agents, amphetamines [withdrawal], L-dopa, cimetidine, ranitidine)

Associated Conditions: Chronic pain, sexual dysfunction, weight changes (up or down), bipolar disorders (manic depression), schizophrenia, and substance abuse.

Workup and Evaluation

Laboratory: No evaluation indicated (clinical diagnosis only).

Imaging: No imaging indicated unless organic brain syndrome is being considered.

Special Tests: Zung's Self-Rating Depression Scale, Beck's Depression Inventory, Criteria for Epidemiologic Studies-Depression Scale, Children's Depression Inventory, or similar tests.

Diagnostic Procedures: Complete evaluation to rule out organic cause. Depression scales are helpful but are not required.

Pathologic Findings

None.

MANAGEMENT AND THERAPY

Nonpharmacologic

General Measures: Evaluation, support, and evaluation of support systems available to the patient.

Specific Measures: Psychotherapy (patients with mild depression without psychosis), medical therapy (choose agent to optimize benefit and decrease risk and avoid drug interactions), electroshock therapy in patients with refractory conditions (controversial).

Diet: No specific dietary changes indicated.

Activity: No restriction.

Patient Education: Reassurance, careful instruction on medication use, American College of Obstetricians and Gynecologists Patient Education Pamphlet AP057 (*Premenstrual Syndrome*), AP106 (*Depression*).

Drug(s) of Choice

Tricyclic agents—amitriptyline (50–300 mg/d), doxepin (75–300 mg/d), imipramine (50–300 mg/d), nortriptyline (50–200 mg/d).

Monoamine oxidase (MAO) inhibitors.

Selective serotonin reuptake inhibitors (SSRIs)—fluoxetine (10–80 mg/d), fluvoxamine (100–300 mg/d), paroxetine (10–50 mg/d), sertraline (50–200 mg/d).

Serotonin-norepinephrine reuptake inhibitors—venlafaxine (75–375 mg/d).

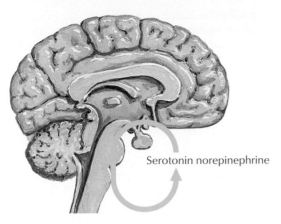

Serotonin norepinephrine

Depression is a biochemically mediated state most likely based on abnormalities in metabolism of serotonin and norepinephrine

♀ > ♂
2 : 1

Female gender predominates

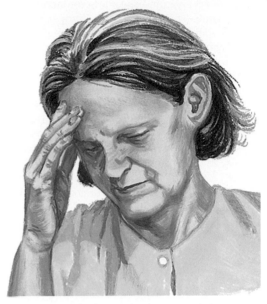

Clinical syndrome characterized by withdrawal, anger, frustration, and loss of pleasure

Associated Symptoms and Comorbidities

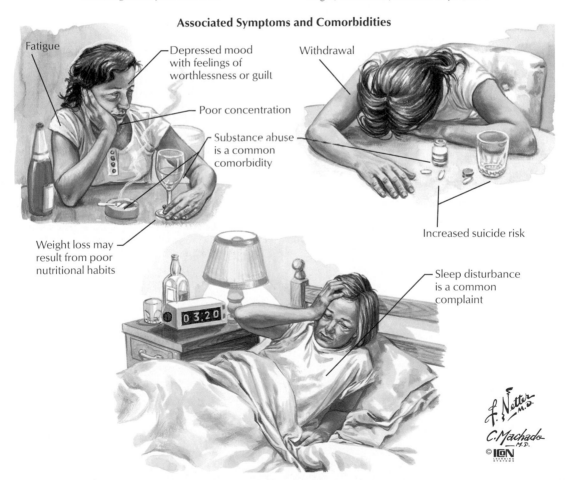

Fatigue

Depressed mood with feelings of worthlessness or guilt

Poor concentration

Substance abuse is a common comorbidity

Weight loss may result from poor nutritional habits

Withdrawal

Increased suicide risk

Sleep disturbance is a common complaint

Noradrenergic and specific serotonergic agents—mirtazapine (15–45 mg/d).

Miscellaneous agents—nefazodone (200–600 mg/d), trazodone (150–400 mg/d), bupropion (300–400 mg/d).

Contraindications: See individual agents. Most agents are pregnancy category B. Many are contraindicated in patients with seizure disorders or cardiac arrhythmias(tricyclic agents).

Precautions: MAO inhibitors are associated with both treatment and adverse reactions that appear as emergencies. Overdoses may be lethal. SSRI agents are associated with nausea (20%–35%) and sexual dysfunction (10%–30%). Some agents can alter the dose or effectiveness of other drugs such as antihypertensive agents, digoxin, and antiseizure medications. Fluoxetine, sertraline, and paroxetine are best given in the morning.

Interactions: MAO inhibitors and SSRIs or SNRIs may have lethal interactions and must not be used together. (Allow at least 2 weeks to elapse between therapies.) Avoid use of nonprescription drugs with pseudoephedrine, phenylephrine, or phenylpropanolamine.

Alternative Drugs

Additional tricyclic agents include clomipramine (100–250 mg/d), desipramine (50–300 mg/d), protriptyline (14–60 mg/d), and trimipramine (75–300 mg/d).

FOLLOW-UP

Patient Monitoring: Normal health maintenance. Monitor for recurrence, substance abuse, or suicide. Patients must be monitored every 1–2 weeks after they start medication and reassessed at 6 weeks. Follow-up up of treatment should continue every 3 months while therapy is maintained (6 months to 2 years).

Prevention/Avoidance: None.

Possible Complications: Increased risk of general medical disorders and worsened prognosis, disability, impaired function (family, work, social, sexual), chronic pain, mortality ($\geq$30,000 suicides per year in United States; adolescent girls at greatest risk).

Expected Outcome: Medical therapy is associated with 85%–90% success rates.

MISCELLANEOUS

Pregnancy Considerations: Up to 70% of patients have depressive symptoms and 10%–15% meet the diagnostic criteria during pregnancy. Symptoms often mimic those of pregnancy itself. Depression may result in poor nutrition, increased substance abuse, and poor fetal outcome. Drug therapy should be avoided or used sparingly in pregnancy.

ICD-9-CM Codes: 311 (Depressive disorder, not elsewhere classified), 296.2 (Major depressive disorder, single episode), 296.3 (Recurrent), 625.4 (Premenstrual syndrome).

REFERENCES

Association of Professors of Gynecology and Obstetrics. *Depressive Disorders in Women: Diagnosis, Treatment, and Monitoring.* Washington, DC: APGO; 1997.

American College of Obstetricians and Gynecologists. *Depression in Women.* Washington, DC: ACOG; 1993. ACOG Technical Bulletin 182.

Beck A. *Depression Inventory.* Philadelphia, Pa: Center for Cognitive Therapy; 1991.

McGrath E, Ketia GP, Strickland BR, Russo NF. *Women and Depression: Risk Factors and Treatment Issues.* Washington, DC: American Psychological Association; 1990.

Notman MT. Depression in women. Psychoanalytic concepts. *Psychiatr Clin North Am* 1989;12:221.

Nurnberg HG. An overview of somatic treatments of psychotic depression during pregnancy and postpartum. *Gen Hosp Psychiatry* 1989;11:328.

DIVERTICULAR DISEASE

INTRODUCTION

Description: Herniation of colon mucosa through the muscular wall. These herniations are most common in the sigmoid and distal colon, increase in prevalence with age, and can lead to significant morbidity when rupture or abscess formation occurs. Diverticulosis is the presence of these herniations, whereas diverticulitis is the symptomatic state.

Prevalence: Twenty percent of patients, increasing with age to 40%–50% by 60–80.

Predominant Age: Rare below 40, most common in patients older than 50.

Genetics: No genetic pattern.

ETIOLOGY AND PATHOGENESIS

Causes: Speculative, not clearly established. Proposed—defect in colon motility with increased intraluminal pressure, exacerbated by a low-fiber diet or an intrinsic defect in the colon wall.

Risk Factors: Low-fiber diet, age older than 40, and previous diverticulitis.

CLINICAL CHARACTERISTICS

Signs and Symptoms:
- Asymptomatic (75%–90%) (diverticulosis)
- Left lower quadrant abdominal pain (worse after eating, better after bowel movement or flatus)
- Diarrhea or constipation
- Fever or chills
- Anorexia, nausea, vomiting
- Abdominal distension
- Peritonitis (rebound tenderness, guarding, rigidity, depressed bowel sounds)
- Rectal tenderness or mass on rectal examination

DIAGNOSTIC APPROACH

Differential Diagnosis:
- IBS
- Lactose intolerance
- Inflammatory bowel disease (ulcerative colitis, Crohn's disease)
- Carcinoma of the colon
- Infectious colitis
- Appendicitis
- Ectopic pregnancy (in reproductive age women)
- Tubo-ovarian abscess

Associated Conditions: IBS.

Workup and Evaluation

Laboratory: Complete blood count, sedimentation rate, urinalysis with culture.

Imaging: Barium enema generally demonstrates diverticulosis. Supine and upright abdominal radiograph may demonstrate free air in the peritoneal cavity if rupture has occurred.

Special Tests: Colonoscopy or flexible sigmoidoscopy.

Diagnostic Procedures: History and physical examination, imaging or endoscopy.

Pathologic Findings

Herniation of colon mucosa through the muscularis, usually at the site of a perforating artery lying between two layers of serosa in the mesentery. Increased thickness of the muscular wall and narrowing of the gut lumen. With inflammation, necrosis and perforation occur.

MANAGEMENT AND THERAPY

Nonpharmacologic

General Measures: For diverticulosis—increased dietary fiber, stool softeners. Fiber supplements may be considered. For diverticulitis—evaluation, possible hospitalization (2%–5% of patients).

Specific Measures: Patients with diverticulitis may become acutely ill with sepsis, toxicity, and peritonitis. These patients require hospitalization, fluid support, and aggressive antibiotic treatment. Surgical resection may be considered in patients with multiple attacks, fistulae, or abscesses that do not respond to medical therapy.

Diet: Increased dietary fiber is desirable both as prevention and to decrease the risk of complications in established disease. Acutely ill patients should receive nothing by mouth.

Activity: No restriction. Activity is encouraged to foster normal bowel function.

Patient Education: Reassurance, counseling regarding diet and the need for periodic flexible sigmoidoscopy or colonoscopy screening.

Drug(s) of Choice

Antispasmodics and adjuncts—hyoscyamine (Levsin) 0.125 mg PO one to two q4h ≤ 12/24 hours), buspirone (BuSpar) 15–30 mg PO qd.

Antibiotics (ambulatory)—metronidazole (Flagyl) 250–500 mg PO q8h plus amoxicillin 500 mg PO q8h or ciprofloxacin (Cipro) 500 mg PO bid.

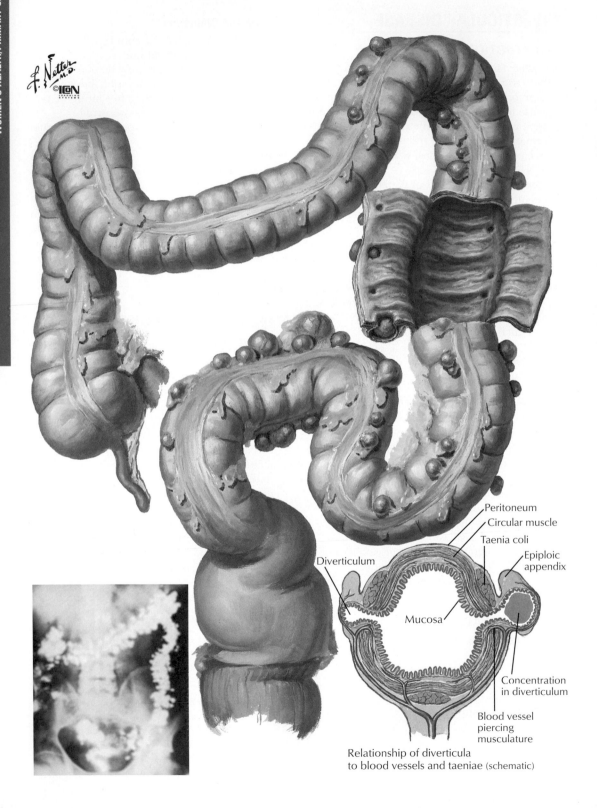

Peritoneum
Circular muscle
Taenia coli
Epiploic appendix
Diverticulum
Mucosa
Concentration in diverticulum
Blood vessel piercing musculature

Relationship of diverticula
to blood vessels and taeniae (schematic)

Symptomatic control of diarrhea or constipation as needed.

Contraindications: See individual agents. Contraindications to flexible sigmoidoscopy: absolute—active diverticulitis, acute abdomen, blood dyscrasia, or coagulopathy, cardiopulmonary disease (acute or severe), inadequate bowel preparation, subacute bacterial endocarditis or prosthetic heart valve without adequate antibiotic prophylaxis, suspected bowel perforation; relative—active infection, peritonitis, pregnancy, recent abdominal surgery.

Precautions: If narcotic pain relievers are needed, meperidine (Demerol) is preferred; others should be avoided because they cause changes in bowel motility. Aminoglycosides may be associated with renal toxicity.

Interactions: See individual agents.

Alternative Drugs

Tobramycin may be used in combination with metronidazole.

FOLLOW-UP

Patient Monitoring: Normal health maintenance. Monitor for development of symptoms; perform routine flexible sigmoidoscopy and fecal occult blood screening.

Prevention/Avoidance: High-fiber diet and good bowel habits.

Possible Complications: Diverticulitis develops in 5% of patients with diverticulosis each year; lifetime risk is 50%. Enterocutaneous, enterovaginal, and perirectal fistulae may occur.

Acutely, hemorrhage, perforation, abscess formation, peritonitis (with toxicity and collapse), and bowel obstruction may all occur.

Expected Outcome: With early detection and dietary change, the prognosis is good. With aggressive management of the first episode of diverticulitis, two thirds of patients do not have a recurrence. Up to 20% of those with rectal bleeding caused by diverticular disease have a recurrence of bleeding.

MISCELLANEOUS

Pregnancy Considerations: No direct effect on pregnancy, uncommon in reproductive age women.

ICD-9-CM Codes: 562.10 (Diverticulosis of colon), 562.11 (Diverticulitis of colon).

REFERENCES

Naliboff JA, Longmire-Cook SJ. Diverticulitis mimicking a tuboovarian abscess. Report of a case in a young woman. *J Reprod Med* 1996;41:921.

Tancer ML, Veridiano NP. Genital fistulas caused by diverticular disease of the sigmoid colon. *Am J Obstet Gynecol* 1996;174:1547.

Wedell J, Banzhaf G, Chaoui R, Fischer R. Reichmann J. Surgical management of complicated colonic diverticulitis. *Br J Surg* 1997;84:380.

Wong SK, Ho YH, Leong AP, Seow-Choen F. Clinical behavior of complicated right-sided and left-sided diverticulosis. *Dis Colon Rectum* 1997;40:344.

Zarling EJ, Bernsen MB. The effect of gender on the rates of hospitalization for gastrointestinal illnesses. *Am J Gastroenterol* 1997;92:621.

Zielke A, Hasse C, Nies C, et al. Prospective evaluation of ultrasonography in acute colonic diverticulitis. *Br J Surg* 1997;84:385.

DYSMENORRHEA: PRIMARY AND SECONDARY

INTRODUCTION

Description: Primary dysmenorrhea is painful menstruation without a clinically identifiable cause. Secondary dysmenorrhea is recurrent menstrual pain resulting from a clinically identifiable cause or abnormality.

Prevalence: Ten percent to fifteen percent of all women are unable to function because of pain, 90% have discomfort with at least one cycle.

Predominant Age: Late teens to early 30s (primary), prevalence follows the occurrence of underlying conditions for secondary dysmenorrhea. Dysmenorrhea that begins after the age of 25 is most often secondary.

Genetics: No genetic pattern.

ETIOLOGY AND PATHOGENESIS

Causes: Primary—increased production of prostaglandin $F_2\alpha$ ($PGF_2\alpha$) resulting in increased uterine contractions (dysrhythmic) and markedly elevated intrauterine pressures (up to 400 mm Hg), possible increased sensitivity to $PGF_2\alpha$ as well. Secondary—uterine (adenomyosis, cervical stenosis and cervical lesions), congenital abnormalities (outflow obstructions, uterine anomalies), infection (chronic endometritis), intrauterine contraceptive devices, myomas (generally intracavitary or intramural), polyps; extrauterine (endometriosis, inflammation, and scarring [adhesions]); nongynecologic causes (musculoskeletal, gastrointestinal, urinary); "pelvic congestive syndrome" (debated); psychogenic (rare); tumors (myomas, benign or malignant tumors of ovary, bowel, or bladder).

Risk Factors: None known.

CLINICAL CHARACTERISTICS

Signs and Symptoms:
- **Primary**—Crampy, midline, lower abdominal pain (often demonstrated by a fist opening and closing)
- Nausea, vomiting, and diarrhea common
- Syncope
- Headache
- **Secondary**—Midline lower abdominal or low back pain accompanying menstruation
- Pelvic heaviness or pressure
- Symptoms specifically associated with the underlying condition

DIAGNOSTIC APPROACH

Differential Diagnosis:
- Endometriosis
- IBS
- Inflammatory bowel disease
- Somatization (rare)

Abrupt onset of painful menstruation should suggest the possibility of a complication of pregnancy (abortion or ectopic pregnancy).

Associated Conditions: Menorrhagia is commonly associated.

Workup and Evaluation

Laboratory: Infrequently required, based on suspected or confirmed cause.

Imaging: For selected patients with secondary dysmenorrhea, ultrasonography of the pelvic organs may be indicated.

Special Tests: None indicated. Sigmoidoscopy may be helpful in selected patients with secondary dysmenorrhea.

Diagnostic Procedures: The absence of abnormality on pelvic examination, combined with historical characteristics, is diagnostic of primary dysmenorrhea. A pelvic examination that reveals a possible cause defines secondary dysmenorrhea.

Pathologic Findings

Based on the causative condition.

MANAGEMENT AND THERAPY

Nonpharmacologic

General Measures: Rest, analgesics (nonsteroidal antiinflammatory agents or pain relievers), heat (heating pad, hot water bottle, self-heating pads [ThermaCare]).

Specific Measures: Primary—medical management most effective, heat (heating pad, hot water bottle, or self-heating pads [ThermaCare]), transcutaneous electrical nerve stimulation (TENS) effective for selected patients, biofeedback suggested, but success poor or variable. Secondary—measures directed toward the underlying pathologic condition, modification of periods (oral contraceptives, menstrual suppression [depot medroxyprogesterone acetate, gonadotropic-releasing hormone (GnRH) agonists]), TENS effective for selected patients, surgery for specific pathologic conditions.

Diet: No specific dietary changes indicated.

Activity: No restriction; based on patient comfort.

Patient Education: Reassurance, American College of Obstetricians and Gynecologists Patient Ed-

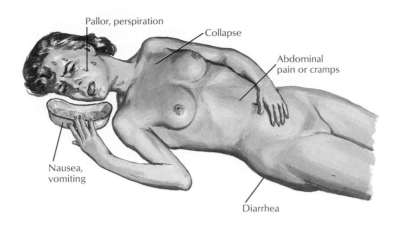

Pallor, perspiration

Collapse

Abdominal
pain or cramps

Nausea,
vomiting

Diarrhea

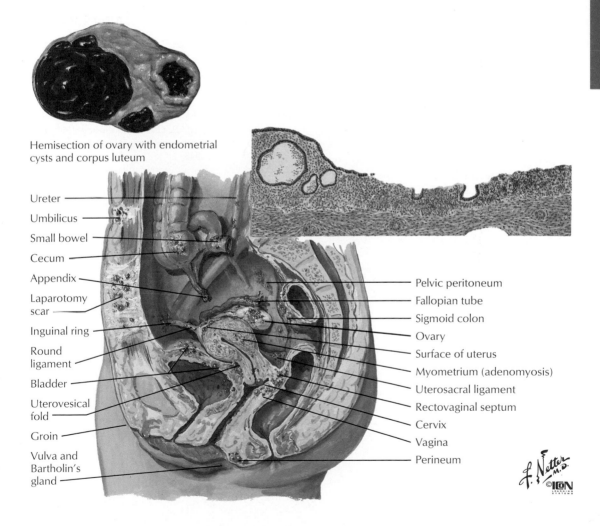

Hemisection of ovary with endometrial
cysts and corpus luteum

Ureter

Umbilicus

Small bowel

Cecum

Appendix

Laparotomy
scar

Inguinal ring

Round
ligament

Bladder

Uterovesical
fold

Groin

Vulva and
Bartholin's
gland

Pelvic peritoneum

Fallopian tube

Sigmoid colon

Ovary

Surface of uterus

Myometrium (adenomyosis)

Uterosacral ligament

Rectovaginal septum

Cervix

Vagina

Perineum

ucation Pamphlet AP046 (*Dysmenorrhea*), others related to underlying causes: AP013 (*Important Facts about Endometriosis*), AP074 (*Uterine Fibroids*), AP077 (*Pelvic Inflammatory Disease*) AP099 (*Pelvic Pain*).

Drug(s) of Choice

Primary—nonsteroidal antiinflammatory drugs (NSAIDs): ibuprofen 800 mg, two at onset of flow and one every 4–6 hours prn pain; naproxen sodium 275 mg, two at onset of flow and one every 6–8 hours prn pain; meclofenamate 100 mg, one at onset of flow and one every 4–6 hours prn pain, mefenamic acid 250 mg, two at onset of flow and one every 4–6 hours prn pain.

Secondary—based on pathophysiologic condition. NSAIDs or analgesics may be used.

Contraindications: Aspirin-sensitive asthma, ulcers, inflammatory bowel disease.

Precautions: Some patients experience increased stomach upset with NSAIDs; this may be reduced by taking them with food.

Interactions: Other over-the-counter pain relievers containing NSAID compounds.

Alternative Drugs

Other rapidly acting NSAIDs may be used. Combination oral contraceptives generally provide milder periods (and contraception if necessary). Centrally acting analgesics may be added with care to avoid interaction with NSAIDs. Suppression of menstruation (depot medroxyproges-terone acetate, GnRH agonists) may be indicated for patients with severe pain.

FOLLOW-UP

Patient Monitoring: Normal health maintenance.
Prevention/Avoidance: None.
Possible Complications: Most commonly side effects of medication. Anemia (if menorrhagia is present), others based on underlying cause.
Expected Outcome: Primary dysmenorrhea—significant relief of symptoms with medical therapy. If medical therapy does not produce pronounced improvement, the diagnosis should be reevaluated. The prevalence of primary dysmenorrhea declines with time. Secondary dysmenorrhea—based on cause and mode of therapy, resolution of symptoms is generally possible with NSAIDs, analgesics, or period modification.

MISCELLANEOUS

Pregnancy Considerations: No effect on pregnancy.
ICD-9-CM Codes: 625.3, 302.76 (Psychogenic) (others based on underlying cause).

REFERENCES

Akin MD, Weingand KW, Hengehold DA, Goodale MB, Hinkle RT, Smith RP. Use of continuous low-level topical heat in the treatment of dysmenorrhea. *Obstet Gynecol* 2001;97:343.

American College of Obstetricians and Gynecologists. *Dysmenorrhea.* March 1983, Washington, DC: ACOG; 1983. Technical Bulletin 68.

Dawood MY. Dysmenorrhea. *Clin Obstet Gynecol* 1990; 33:168.

DYSPAREUNIA: DEEP THRUST

INTRODUCTION

Description: Abdominal, pelvic, or vaginal pain that arises during sexual thrusting, especially with deep penetration.

Prevalence: Roughly 15% of women each year (severe—less than 2% of women).

Predominant Age: Reproductive age and beyond.

Genetics: No genetic pattern.

ETIOLOGY AND PATHOGENESIS

Causes: Gynecologic—extrauterine (adhesions, chronic pelvic infection, cysts, endometriosis, pelvic relaxation [cystocele, urethrocele, rectocele, enterocele], prolapsed adnexa or adnexa adherent to vaginal apex, retained ovary syndrome, shortening of the vagina after surgery or radiation); uterine (adenomyosis, fibroids, malposition [retroversion]). Urologic—chronic urinary tract infection, detrusor dyssynergia, interstitial cystitis, urethral syndrome. Gastrointestinal—chronic constipation, diverticular disease, inflammatory bowel disease, Crohn's disease, ulcerative colitis, IBS. Musculoskeletal—fibromyositis, hernias (abdominal, femoral), herniated disk. Other—inadequate arousal (failure of vaginal apex expansion), pelvic tumors (benign or malignant). Care must be taken to avoid labeling any dyspareunia as purely physical or purely emotional in origin. Most often a mixture of factors cause or contribute to the problem.

Risk Factors: Positions or practices that result in particularly deep or forceful penetration, such as male superior or rear entry positions.

CLINICAL CHARACTERISTICS

Signs and Symptoms:
- Ache-like pain, burning, a sense of fullness, or like something being bumped during deep sexual thrusting. Occasionally the pain is sharp and abrupt in character. Pain often depends on the type of sexual activity involved or the positions used.

DIAGNOSTIC APPROACH

Differential Diagnosis:
- Vulvitis
- Vestibulitis
- Vaginitis
- Bartholin's gland infection, abscess, cyst
- Atrophic change
- Anxiety, depression, phobia
- Sexual or other abuse

- Pelvic mass (uterine leiomyomata, ovarian cyst)
- Shortening of the vagina after surgery or radiation

Associated Conditions: Vaginismus, orgasmic dysfunction.

Workup and Evaluation

Laboratory: No evaluation indicated.

Imaging: No imaging indicated, pelvic (abdominal or transvaginal) ultrasonography for specific indications.

Special Tests: None indicated.

Diagnostic Procedures: History (general and sexual) and careful pelvic examination. (If discomfort is produced, it is important to be sure that the sensation matches that experienced during intercourse.)

Pathologic Findings

None.

MANAGEMENT AND THERAPY

Nonpharmacologic

General Measures: Evaluation, reassurance, relaxation measures.

Specific Measures: Because dyspareunia is ultimately a symptom, the specific therapy for any form of sexual pain is focused on the underlying cause. Vaginal lubricants (water-soluble or long-acting agents such as Astro-Glide, Replens, Lubrin, K-Y Jelly, and others), local anesthetics (for vulvar lesions), or pelvic relaxation exercises may be appropriate while more specific therapy is underway.

Diet: No specific dietary changes indicated.

Activity: No restriction.

Patient Education: Reassurance, relaxation training, alternate sexual positions and forms of expression, American College of Obstetricians and Gynecologists Patient Education Pamphlet AP020 (*Pain During Intercourse*), AP042 (*You and Your Sexuality*).

Drug(s) of Choice

The judicious use of anxiolytics or antidepressant medications for selected patients may be appropriate, but for short periods of time only.

ALTERNATIVE THERAPIES

Modifying sexual techniques used by the couple may reduce pain with intercourse. Delaying penetration until maximal arousal has been achieved improves vaginal lubrication, ensures vaginal apex expansion, and provides an element of con-

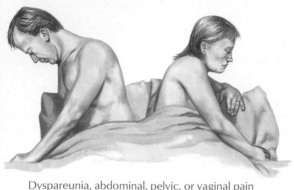

Etiologic Considerations in Dyspareunia

Dyspareunia, abdominal, pelvic, or vaginal pain during sexual thrusting affects approximately 15% of women each year

Vaginismus may be cause of dyspareunia

Failure of arousal and decreased vaginal lubrication may underlie dyspareunia

JOHN A.CRAIG—MD
C.Machado—M.D.
D. Mascaro
© ICON LEARNING SYSTEMS

Other Sources of Pain in Dyspareunia

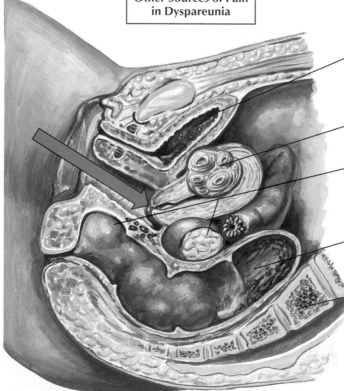

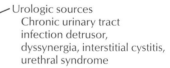

Urologic sources
  Chronic urinary tract infection detrusor, dyssynergia, interstitial cystitis, urethral syndrome

Uterine sources
  Adenomyosis, fibroids, malposition

Extra uterine
  Pelvic relaxation, adhesions, chronic pelvic infection, endometriosis, vaginal shortening, tumors

Gastrointestinal
  Chronic constipation, inflammatory bowel disease, irritable bowel syndrome

Musculoskeletal
  Herniated disc, femoral and abdominal hernia

Deep thrusting may elicit pain from adnexal structures, as well as gynecologic

trol for the female partner. Sexual positions that allow the women to control the direction and depth of penetration (such as woman astride) may also be of help.

FOLLOW-UP

Patient Monitoring: Normal health maintenance. Watch for signs of abuse, anxiety, or depression.
Prevention/Avoidance: None.
Possible Complications: Marital discord, orgasmic or libidinal dysfunction.
Expected Outcome: With diagnosis and treatment of the underlying cause, response should be good.

MISCELLANEOUS

Pregnancy Considerations: No effect on pregnancy.
ICD-9-CM Codes: 625.0.

REFERENCES

Fink P. Dyspareunia: current concepts. *Med Aspects Hum Sex* 1972;6:28.
Fordney DS. Dyspareunia and vaginismus. *Clin Obstet Gynecol* 1978;21:205.
Fullerton W. Dyspareunia. *BMJ* 1971;2:31.
Lamont JA. Female dyspareunia. *Am J Obstet Gynecol* 1980;136:282.
Steege JF. Dyspareunia and vaginismus. *Clin Obstet Gynecol* 1984;27:750.
Steege JF, Ling FW. Dyspareunia. A special type of chronic pelvic pain. *Obstet Gynecol Clin North Am* 1993;20:779.

DYSURIA

INTRODUCTION

Description: Painful passage of urine.

Prevalence: Common in women, 10%–20% per year.

Predominant Age: Any.

Genetics: No genetic pattern.

ETIOLOGY AND PATHOGENESIS

Causes: Infection and inflammation in the urethra and suburethral tissues. Most urinary tract infections in women ascend from contamination of the vulva and meatus, acquired via instrumentation, trauma, or sexual intercourse. (A history of intercourse within the proceeding 24–48 hours is present in up to 75% of patients with acute urinary tract infection.) Coliform organisms, especially *Escherichia coli*, are the most common organisms responsible for asymptomatic bacteriuria, cystitis, and pyelonephritis. Ninety percent of first infections and 80% of recurrent infections are caused by *E. coli*, with between 10% and 20% resulting from *Staphylococcus saprophyticus*. Infection with other pathogens such as *Klebsiella* species (5%) and *Proteus* species (2%) account for most of the remaining infections. Infection with *Neisseria gonorrhoeae, Chlamydia trachomatis, Mycoplasma*, and *Ureaplasma* should all be considered when urethritis is suspected. Chemical irritation, allergic reactions, or vulvitis may all produce symptoms of dysuria.

Risk Factors: Sexual activity, instrumentation, more virulent pathogens, altered host defenses, infrequent or incomplete voiding, foreign body or stone, obstruction, or biochemical changes in the urine (diabetes, hemoglobinopathies, pregnancy) estrogen deficiency, diaphragm use, spermicides.

CLINICAL CHARACTERISTICS

Signs and Symptoms:
- Painful urination
- Frequency, urgency, nocturia (commonly associated, indicate irritation of the bladder wall)
- Pelvic pressure (if cystitis is present)
- Pyuria (more than 5 white blood cells per high power field in a centrifuged specimen, most prominent in first one third of voided specimen)

DIAGNOSTIC APPROACH

Differential Diagnosis:
- Cystitis
- Traumatic trigonitis
- Urethral syndrome
- Interstitial cystitis
- Bladder tumors or stones
- Vulvitis and vaginitis (may give rise to external dysuria as in herpetic vulvitis)
- Urethral diverticulum
- Infection in the Skene's glands
- Detrusor instability

Associated Conditions: Dyspareunia, cystitis.

Workup and Evaluation

Laboratory: Nonpregnant women with a first episode of classic symptoms suggestive of urinary tract infection do not need laboratory confirmation of the diagnosis, but may be treated empirically. For others urinalysis and culture should be performed. For uncentrifuged urine samples, the presence of more than 1 white blood cell per high power field is 90% accurate for detecting infection. Gram's stain of urine samples or sediments may help establish the diagnosis or suggest a possible pathogen.

Imaging: No imaging indicated.

Special Tests: A sterile swab inserted into the urethra may be used to obtain material for culture and Gram's stain to establish the diagnosis.

Diagnostic Procedures: History and physical examination, urinalysis.

Pathologic Findings

Pyuria (hematuria may be present as well).

MANAGEMENT AND THERAPY

Nonpharmacologic

General Measures: Fluids, frequent voiding, and antipyretics. Urinary acidification (with ascorbic acid, ammonium chloride, or acidic fruit juices), and urinary analgesics (phenazopyridine [Pyridium]) may also be added based on the needs of the individual patient.

Specific Measures: Antibiotic therapy.

Diet: Increased fluids and reduction of caffeine.

Activity: No restriction.

Patient Education: Reassurance, American College of Obstetricians and Gynecologists Patient Education Pamphlet AP050 (*Urinary Tract Infections*).

Drug(s) of Choice (NONPREGNANT PATIENTS)

Single dose therapy: amoxicillin 3 g, ampicillin 3.5 g, a first-generation cephalosporin 2 g, nitrofurantoin 200 mg, sulfisoxazole 2 g, trimethoprim (TMP) 400 mg, TMP/sulfamethoxazole 300 (1600) mg.

Three- to seven-day therapy: amoxicillin 500 mg q8h, a first-generation

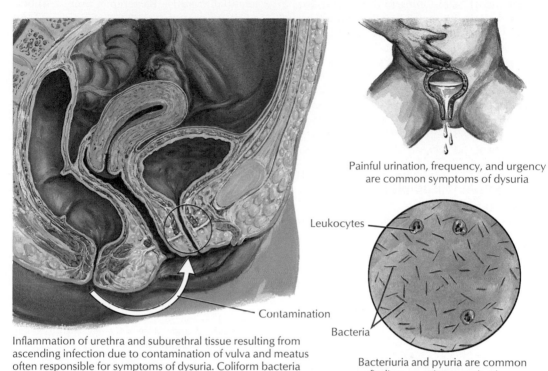

Painful urination, frequency, and urgency are common symptoms of dysuria

Leukocytes

Bacteria

Contamination

Inflammation of urethra and suburethral tissue resulting from ascending infection due to contamination of vulva and meatus often responsible for symptoms of dysuria. Coliform bacteria are most often the responsible organism

Bacteriuria and pyuria are common findings on urine examinations

Risk Factors | Evaluation

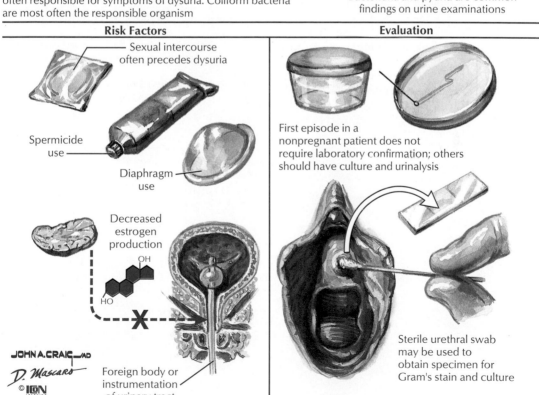

Sexual intercourse often precedes dysuria

Spermicide use

Diaphragm use

Decreased estrogen production

OH

HO

Foreign body or instrumentation of urinary tract

First episode in a nonpregnant patient does not require laboratory confirmation; others should have culture and urinalysis

Sterile urethral swab may be used to obtain specimen for Gram's stain and culture

JOHN A. CRAIG—MD

D. Mascaro

© ICON
LEARNING
SYSTEMS

cephalosporin 500 mg q8h, ciprofloxacin 250 mg q12h, nitrofurantoin 100 mg q12h, norfloxacin 400 mg q12h, ofloxacin 200 mg q12h, sulfisoxazole 500 mg q6h, tetracycline 500 mg q6h, TMP/sulfamethoxazole 160/800 mg q12h, TMP 100 (200) mg q12h.

Contraindications: Known or suspected hypersensitivity.

Precautions: Urinary analgesics (phenazopyridine [Pyridium]) should be used for no longer than 48 hours and may stain some types of contact lenses.

Interactions: See individual medications.

Alternative Drugs (PREGNANT PATIENTS)

Seven-day therapy: amoxicillin 500 mg q8h, a first-generation cephalosporin 500 mg q6h, nitrofurantoin 100 mg q12h.

FOLLOW-UP

Patient Monitoring: No follow-up is necessary after single dose treatment, or multiday treatment for nonpregnant women who experience resolution of their symptoms. Cure for all other patients should be confirmed by urinalysis and culture. Recurrent lower tract infections require prompt evaluation. Possible causes include incorrect or incomplete (eg, noncompliant) therapy, mechanical factors (such as obstruction or stone), or compromised host defenses.

Prevention/Avoidance: Frequent voiding, adequate fluid intake, voiding after intercourse.

Possible Complications: Urethral syndrome and interstitial cystitis. Bacteremia, septic shock, adult respiratory distress syndrome, and other serious sequelae are associated with pyelonephritis.

Expected Outcome: For most patients, symptoms should resolve within 2–3 days after the initiation of therapy.

MISCELLANEOUS

Pregnancy Considerations: Asymptomatic bacteriuria is more common during pregnancy. Those at high risk (eg, diabetic patients) should be monitored carefully to avoid urethritis, cystitis, and ascending infection.

ICD-9-CM Codes: 788.1.

REFERENCES

American College of Obstetricians and Gynecologists. *Antimicrobial therapy for obstetric patients.* Washington, DC: ACOG; 1988. ACOG Technical Bulletin 117.

Bump RC. Urinary tract infection in women. Current role of single-dose therapy. *J Reprod Med* 1990;35:785.

Greenberg RN, Reilly PM, Luppen KL, et al. Randomized study of single-dose, three-day, and seven-day treatment of cystitis in women. *J Infect Dis* 1986; 153:277.

Pappas P. Laboratory in the diagnosis and management of urinary tract infections. *Med Clin North Am* 1991; 75:313.

Powers R. New directions in the diagnosis and therapy of urinary tract infections. *Am J Obstet Gynecol* 1991; 164:1387.

Smith RP. *Gynecology in Primary Care.* Baltimore, Md: Williams & Wilkins; 1997:577.

EATING DISORDERS: ANOREXIA NERVOSA AND BULIMIA

INTRODUCTION

Description: Anorexia nervosa is a syndrome characterized by an altered body image, significant weight loss, and amenorrhea that is not caused by physical disease. Bulimia is an eating disorder characterized by an altered body image, recurrent binge eating, with or without purging through self-induced vomiting, laxative abuse, or diuretics. Exercise excess is often a part of after-binge behavior. Both affect more women than men.

Prevalence: One percent to three percent of females. Subclinical eating disorders are common in university populations.

Predominant Age: Teens to early 20s.

Genetics: No genetic pattern.

ETIOLOGY AND PATHOGENESIS

Causes: Unknown (emotional).

Risk Factors: Anorexia nervosa—perfectionistic personality (high expectations, personal or external). Bulimia—impulsive character, low self-esteem, stress (eg, multiple responsibilities, tight schedules), early puberty. High risk for both: dancers, models, cheerleaders, athletes.

CLINICAL CHARACTERISTICS

Signs and Symptoms:

- Insidious onset (occasionally stress related)
- Significant weight loss (15% below expected weight)
- Denial of problem
- Preoccupation with weight or body image
- Anorexia nervosa—Impression of obesity rather than objective view of weight
- Reduced food intake or refusal (often associated with elaborate eating rituals)
- Excessive exercise (marathon running)
- Bulimia—High calorie binges followed by severe restriction
- Food collections or hoarding
- Medication abuse (laxatives, diuretics, ipecac, thyroid medication)
- Dental erosion and scarred knuckles (secondary to finger-induced vomiting)

DIAGNOSTIC APPROACH

Differential Diagnosis:

- Wasting disease (tumors)
- Depression
- Hypothalamic tumor
- Food phobia
- Gastrointestinal disease
- Other emotional disorders (conversion disorder, schizophrenia, body dysmorphic disorder)

Associated Conditions: Major depression (50%–75% of patients), obsessive-compulsive disorders (10%–13% of patients), bipolar disorders, sexual disinterest, depression, growth arrest, hypotension and bradycardia, hypothermia, peripheral edema. Prolonged amenorrhea is associated with an increased risk of osteoporosis, which may not be reversible. Bulimia—social phobia and anxiety disorders, substance abuse, shoplifting common.

Workup and Evaluation

Laboratory: No evaluation specific for anorexia. For patients with bulimia there may be laboratory changes consistent with repeated vomiting (hypokalemia, hypomagnesemia, or hypochloremia).

Imaging: No imaging indicated.

Special Tests: Assessment of body fat.

Diagnostic Procedures: History and physical examination, Eating Attitudes Test.

Pathologic Findings

Anorexia nervosa—Dry, cracked skin, sparse scalp hair, fine lanugo hair on extremities, face and trunk, arrested maturation, pathologic fractures, cognitive defects. Bulimia—eroded dental enamel, esophagitis, Mallory-Weiss tears, parotid enlargement, gastric dilatation.

MANAGEMENT AND THERAPY

Nonpharmacologic

General Measures: Psychologic evaluation and support, supervised eating and exercise program, progressive increase in calories and activity as weight is regained (anorexia), limit access to bathroom for 2 hours after eating (bulimia).

Specific Measures: Hospitalization may be required, including intensive psychologic assessment and therapy. Tube feedings and intravenous fluids may be required for patients with anorexia.

Diet: Supervised program of reeducation and behavior modification. For patients with anorexia, a gradual increase in caloric intake as part of a supervised program of reeducation and behavior modification.

Activity: Stepwise increase based on weight change, avoidance of goal-oriented activities.

Patient Education: Nutritional instruction, assistance with a food log, American College of Obstetri-

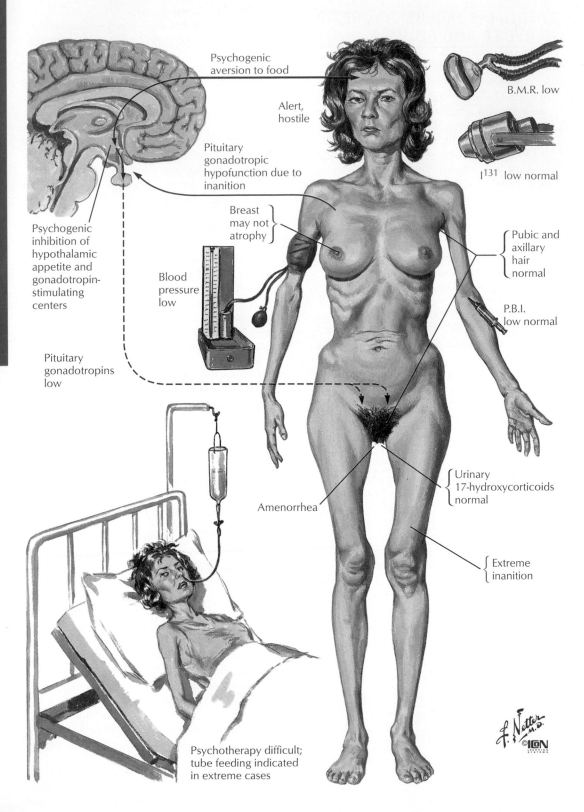

Psychogenic
aversion to food

Alert,
hostile

B.M.R. low

Pituitary
gonadotropic
hypofunction due to
inanition

I^{131} low normal

Psychogenic
inhibition of
hypothalamic
appetite and
gonadotropin-
stimulating
centers

Breast
may not
atrophy

Pubic and
axillary
hair
normal

Blood
pressure
low

P.B.I.
low normal

Pituitary
gonadotropins
low

Urinary
17-hydroxycorticoids
normal

Amenorrhea

Extreme
inanition

Psychotherapy difficult;
tube feeding indicated
in extreme cases

cians and Gynecologists Patient Education Pamphlet AP064 (*Weight Control: Eating Right and Keeping Fit*), AP045 (*Exercise and Fitness: A Guide for Women*).

Drug(s) of Choice

Fluoxetine (Prozac) 10–60 mg PO qd.

Oxazepam 15 mg or alprazolam 0.25 mg PO before meals to reduce anxiety about weight gain.

Contraindications: See specific agents.

Precautions: Starved patients tend to be more sensitive to medications or to have compromised renal, cardiac, or liver function.

Alternative Drugs

Imipramine (Tofranil) 10 mg gradually increased to 200 mg or desipramine (Norpramin) 25 mg increased gradually to 150 mg PO qd.

Lithium (Eskalith) 300 mg PO bid increased gradually until blood level of 0.6–1.2 mEq/L if bipolar disorder is present.

Cisapride (Propulsid) 10–20 mg before meals to increase gastric emptying.

Psyllium (Metamucil) 1 tablespoon qhs to prevent constipation.

FOLLOW-UP

Patient Monitoring: Periodic weight measurements (weekly until stable, then monthly). Monitor for depression or suicidal ideation.

Prevention/Avoidance: Encourage healthy attitudes about weight, eating, and exercise; enhance self-esteem; and reduce stress.

Possible Complications: Drug and alcohol use/abuse, suicide, cardiac arrhythmia or arrest (potassium depletion), cardiomyopathy, suicide, necrotizing colitis, osteoporosis and osteoporotic fractures. Depression is common.

Expected Outcome: Highly variable with relapses common, better outcome with inpatient care. Bulimia may spontaneously remit.

MISCELLANEOUS

Pregnancy Considerations: Amenorrhea and infertility common in anorexic women. For bulimic women, the binge–purge cycle may affect fetal nutrition and growth.

ICD-9-CM Codes: 307.1 (Anorexia), 783.6 (Bulimia).

REFERENCES

Abrams SA, Silber TJ, Esteban NV, et al. Mineral balance and bone turnover in adolescents with anorexia nervosa. *J Pediatr* 1993;123:326.

American College of Obstetricians and Gynecologists. *The Adolescent Gynecologic Patient.* Washington, DC. ACOG; 1990. ACOG Technical Bulletin 145.

Bachrach JK. Decreased bone density in adolescent girls with anorexia nervosa. *Pediatrics* 1990;86:440.

Beaumont PJ, Russell JD, Touyz SW. Treatment of anorexia nervosa. *Lancet* 1993;341:1635.

Centers for Disease Control and Prevention. Results from the National Adolescent Student Health Survey. *MMWR Morb Mortal Wkly Rep* 1989;38:147.

Crow SJ, Mitchell JE. Rational therapy in eating disorders. *Drugs* 1994;48:372.

Kurtzman FD, Yager J, Landvesk J, Wiesmeier E, Bodurka DC. Eating disorders among selected female student populations at UCLA. *J Am Diet Assoc* 1989;89:45.

Warren MP, Vande Wiele RL. Clinical and metabolic features of anorexia nervosa. *Am J Obstet Gynecol* 1973; 117:435.

GASTRITIS

INTRODUCTION

Description: An inflammatory condition affecting the stomach lining that results in acute or chronic indigestion, bloating, "gas," and heartburn.

Prevalence: Common.

Predominant Age: Any.

Genetics: No genetic pattern.

ETIOLOGY AND PATHOGENESIS

Causes: Generalized inflammation of the stomach lining, which, in some cases, may be infectious (*Helicobacter pylori*).

Risk Factors: Cigarette smoking, alcohol abuse, some medications (NSAIDs), bile reflux, radiation.

CLINICAL CHARACTERISTICS

Signs and Symptoms:
- Nausea, vomiting, dyspepsia, heartburn, and "gas" (symptoms are most common after large meals, consuming certain foods)
- Upper abdominal pain or tenderness
- Hiccups

DIAGNOSTIC APPROACH

Differential Diagnosis:
- Gastrointestinal Reflux
- Ulcer disease (gastric or duodenal)
- Esophageal cancer
- Linitis plastica

Associated Conditions: Bleeding, dysphagia, and gastric or duodenal ulcer.

Workup and Evaluation

Laboratory: No evaluation indicated.

Imaging: No imaging indicated.

Special Tests: Gastroscopy (with or without biopsy) establishes the diagnosis, but most often is not necessary.

Diagnostic Procedures: History and physical examination (suspicious), gastroscopy (diagnostic).

Pathologic Findings

Patchy erythema of the gastric mucosa (seldom full thickness) most common in the pyloric antrum.

MANAGEMENT AND THERAPY

Nonpharmacologic

General Measures: Dietary changes, elevation of the head of the bed, smoking cessation, alcohol in moderation only, antacids. (Antacids that coat [liquids] and those that tend to float on the surface of the stomach contents, such as Gaviscon, give better heartburn relief than other agents.)

Specific Measures: Eliminate medications that contribute to reduced esophageal pressure, such as diazepam and calcium channel blockers, or that may damage the esophagus (NSAIDs). Use acid-blocking therapy.

Diet: No specific dietary changes indicated.

Activity: No restriction.

Patient Education: Reassurance, diet counseling, behavior modification.

Drug(s) of Choice

Antacids.

Histamine H_2 antagonists (cimetidine 800 mg bid, ranitidine 400 mg qid, famotidine 20 mg bid, or nizatidine 150 mg bid).

Hydrogen potassium pump blocker (omeprazole 20–40 mg qd for 4–8 weeks, esomeprazole 20–40 mg qd for 4–8 weeks, or pantoprazole 40 mg qd for 8 weeks). Misoprostol (Cytotec, 100–200 μg PO qid) if mucosal injury is documented or suspected.

Contraindications: Know or suspected hypersensitivity. Misoprostol is contraindicated during pregnancy and lactation.

Precautions: If bismuth is prescribed, warn the patient about black stools. Because of a lack of long-term follow-up, hydrogen pump inhibitors may only be taken for 8–12 weeks.

Interactions: Multiple drug interactions are possible with agents such as cimetidine; check full prescribing information.

Alternative Drugs

In patients with *H pylori* infection, a combination of bismuth (Pepto-Bismol) and an antibiotic (metronidazole 250 mg q6h, tetracycline 500 q6h, or amoxicillin 500 mg q8h) has been recommended for 2 weeks. A 4-week treatment with clarithromycin (Bixin) and either omeprazole (Prilosec) or ranitidine bismuth citrate (Tritec) may also be used.

FOLLOW-UP

Patient Monitoring: Normal health maintenance. If significant gastric erosion is documented, repeat gastroscopy after 6 weeks is often recommended.

Prevention/Avoidance: Reduction of modifiable risk factors (eg, smoking).

Possible Complications: Chronic pain, ulcer formation, and perforation.

Expected Outcome: Generally good symptomatic relief, but long-term therapy is often required.

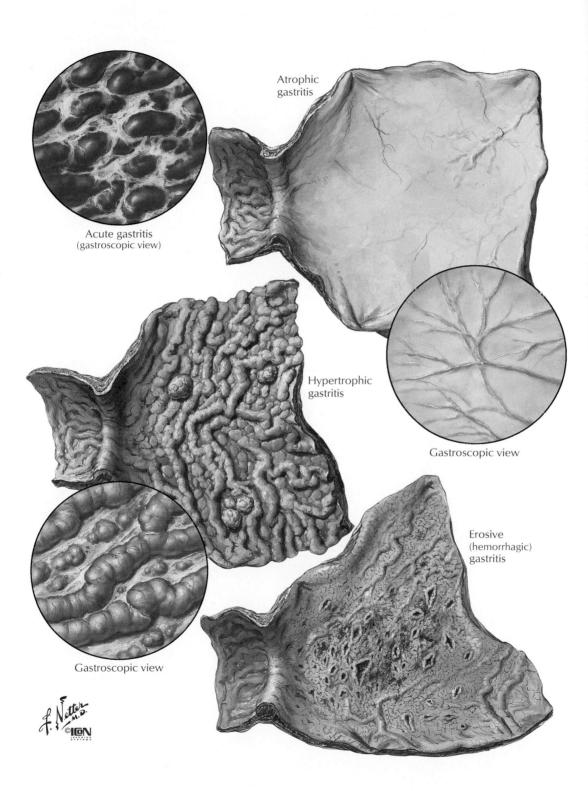

Acute gastritis
(gastroscopic view)

Atrophic
gastritis

Hypertrophic
gastritis

Gastroscopic view

Gastroscopic view

Erosive
(hemorrhagic)
gastritis

MISCELLANEOUS

Pregnancy Considerations: No direct effect on pregnancy, although severe gastritis may interfere with maternal nutrition.

***ICD-9-CM* Codes:** 535.5 (others based on cause).

REFERENCES

Graham DY, Malaty HM, Evans DG, Evans DJ, Jr, Klein PD, Adam E. Epidemiology of *Helicobacter pylori* in an asymptomatic population in the US. *Gastroenterology* 1991;100:1495.

Feldman M, Burton ME. Drug therapy: histamine2-receptor antagonists-standard therapy for acid-peptic disease. *N Engl J Med* 1990;323:1672, 1749.

Rapkin AJ, Mayer EA. Gastroenterologic causes of chronic pelvic pain. *Obstet Gynecol Clin North Am* 1993;20:663.

GASTROESOPHAGEAL REFLUX

INTRODUCTION

Description: The reflux of gastric acid to the sensitive esophagus causes heartburn, the cardinal manifestation of gastroesophageal reflux disease (GERD).

Prevalence: Common.

Predominant Age: Generally reproductive and beyond.

Genetics: No genetic pattern.

ETIOLOGY AND PATHOGENESIS

Causes: The most common cause is decreased tone of the lower esophageal sphincter. This is complicated in pregnant patients by the reduced gastric emptying and reduced esophageal sphincter tone that occurs during pregnancy.

Risk Factors: Cigarette smoking, alcohol abuse, some medications or foods, pregnancy, scleroderma, sliding hiatal hernia.

CLINICAL CHARACTERISTICS

Signs and Symptoms:
- Upper abdominal pain, nausea, vomiting, dyspepsia, heartburn, chest pain, and "gas" (70%–85%, symptoms most common after large meals, consuming certain foods, and upon assuming the recumbent position)
- Dysphagia (15%–20%, suggests stricture)
- Bronchospasm/asthma (15%–20%)

DIAGNOSTIC APPROACH

Differential Diagnosis:
- Ulcer disease (gastric or duodenal)
- Chemical or infectious esophagitis
- Crohn's disease of the esophagus
- Angina pectoris
- Achalasia
- Esophageal cancer

Associated Conditions: Dysphagia. Nocturnal aspiration may occur and be mistaken for asthma.

Workup and Evaluation

Laboratory: No evaluation indicated.

Imaging: Barium swallow may demonstrate hiatal hernia or esophageal narrowing. For patients who are pregnant, this should be reserved for after completion of the pregnancy.

Special Tests: Upper gastrointestinal endoscopy eliminates other potential causes of GERD that include esophageal motility disorders, erosive esophagitis, and peptic ulcer disease (gastric or duodenal).

Diagnostic Procedures: History (>80% accurate), physical examination, endoscopy, barium swallow.

Pathologic Findings

Acute inflammatory changes and hyperplasia of the basal layers of epithelium (85%). Squamous metaplasia of the lower esophagus may occur with chronic exposure to reflux acid (Barrett's syndrome), which may undergo dysplasia or malignant change.

MANAGEMENT AND THERAPY

Nonpharmacologic

General Measures: Dietary changes, elevation of the head of the bed, smoking cessation, alcohol in moderation only, weight loss, antacids. (Antacids that coat [liquids], and those that tend to float on the surface of the stomach contents, such as Gaviscon, give better heartburn relief than other agents.).

Specific Measures: Eliminate medications that contribute to reduced esophageal pressure, such as diazepam and calcium channel blockers, or that may damage the esophagus (NSAIDs). Use acid-blocking therapy.

Diet: Avoid spicy or acidic meals, chocolate, onions, garlic, peppermint, and large meals before bedtime.

Activity: No restriction.

Patient Education: Reassurance, diet counseling, behavior modification.

Drug(s) of Choice

Antacids.

Histamine H_2-antagonists (cimetidine 800 mg bid, ranitidine 400 mg qid, famotidine 20 mg bid, or nizatidine 150 mg bid).

Hydrogen potassium pump blocker (omeprazole 20–40 mg qd for 4–8 weeks, esomeprazole 20–40 mg qd for 4–8 weeks, or pantoprazole 40mg qd for 8 weeks).

Cisapride (10–20 mg qid, ac, and qhs.

Misoprostol (Cytotec, 100–200 μg PO qid) if mucosal injury is documented or suspected.

Contraindications: Know or suspected hypersensitivity. Misoprostol is contraindicated during pregnancy and lactation.

Precautions: Because of a lack of long-term follow-up, hydrogen pump inhibitors may only be taken for 8–12 weeks.

Interactions: Multiple drug interactions are possible with agents such as cimetidine; check full prescribing information.

Alternative Drugs

Bethanechol, antiemetics, phenobarbital if necessary.

FOLLOW-UP

Patient Monitoring: Normal health maintenance

Prevention/Avoidance: Reduction of modifiable risk factors (eg, smoking, weight loss, diet).

Possible Complications: Esophageal stricture, bleeding. Prolonged exposure of acid to the esophagus may lead to stricture formation and dysphagia. Epithelial changes induced in the lower esophagus are also associated with an increased risk of esophageal cancer.

Expected Outcome: Generally good symptomatic relief, but long-term therapy is often required.

MISCELLANEOUS

Pregnancy Considerations: No effect on pregnancy, although may worsen during pregnancy because of reduced esophageal tone and increased intraabdominal pressure caused by the expanding uterus.

ICD-9-CM Codes: 530.11.

REFERENCES

DeVault KR, Castell DO. Guidelines for the diagnosis and treatment of gastroesophageal reflux disease. *Arch Intern Med* 1995;155:2165.

Feldman M, Burton ME. Drug therapy: histamine2-receptor antagonists-standard therapy for acid-peptic disease. *N Engl J Med* 1990;323:1672, 1749.

Fennerty MB, Sampliner RE, Garewall HS. Barrett's oesophagus—cancer risk, biology and therapeutic management. *Aliment Pharmacol Ther* 1993;7:339.

Kahrilas PJ. Gastroesophageal reflux disease. *JAMA* 1996;276:983.

Rapkin AJ, Mayer EA. Gastroenterologic causes of chronic pelvic pain. *Obstet Gynecol Clin North Am* 1993;20:663.

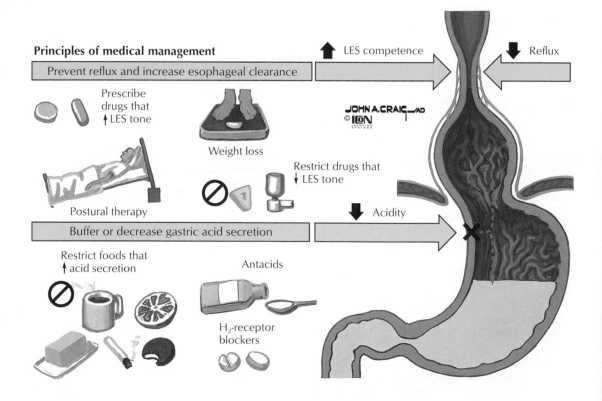

Principles of medical management

Prevent reflux and increase esophageal clearance

LES competence   Reflux

Prescribe drugs that ↑LES tone

Weight loss

Restrict drugs that ↓LES tone

Postural therapy

Acidity

Buffer or decrease gastric acid secretion

Restrict foods that ↑acid secretion

Antacids

H₂-receptor blockers

JOHN A. CRAIG—AD
© ICON

HAIR LOSS

INTRODUCTION

Description: Patients often experience hair loss in the early stages of pregnancy in the immediate postpartum period, or in the postmenopausal years. For some this may be of sufficient volume to cause concern or cosmetic problems.

Prevalence: Of postmenopausal women, 37% have some hair loss. Loss of hair 1–2 months after delivery (telogen effluvium) is common.

Predominant Age: Older than 50.

Genetics: Androgenic alopecia follows autosomal dominance with incomplete penetrance.

ETIOLOGY AND PATHOGENESIS

Causes: Accelerated hair loss may come about any time there is an abrupt change in hormonal patterns and is the result of a higher number of hair follicles entering into the resting, or telogen, phase of hair growth. Hair follicles have cycles of growth (anagen), followed by a resting phase (telogen) of 3–9 months, and then resumption of normal growth. Alterations in hormones may induce an increased number of follicles to enter telogen. If this is the situation, the lost hair will be regained in time. Stress and some medications (anticoagulants, retinoids, β-blockers, chemotherapeutic agents) may also cause similar hair loss. The relative androgen dominance found in postmenopausal women not receiving hormone replacement therapy might also cause male pattern hair loss (temporal balding, androgenic alopecia).

Risk Factors: Pregnancy, delivery, hormonal contraception, scalp disease, family history of baldness, nutritional deprivation, drug or toxin exposure.

CLINICAL CHARACTERISTICS

Signs and Symptoms:
- Hair loss
- Pruritus, scaling, and broken hairs (tinea)
- Tapered, easily removed hair near the edge of patches (alopecia areata)

DIAGNOSTIC APPROACH

Differential Diagnosis:
- Telogen effluvium (as seen after pregnancy)
- Anagen effluvium (loss that includes growing hairs and may progress to complete baldness)
- Cicatricial alopecia (resulting from scarring)
- Androgenic alopecia
- Traction alopecia (trauma)
- Tinea capitis
- Drug, poison, or chemotherapy exposure
- Local infection or dermatitis
- Endocrinopathy (polycystic ovaries, adrenal hyperplasia, pituitary hyperplasia)

Associated Conditions: Alopecia areata, Down syndrome, vitiligo, and diabetes; traction alopecia; behavior aberrations.

Workup and Evaluation

Laboratory: No evaluation indicated except as dictated by specific differential diagnoses being considered.

Imaging: No imaging indicated.

Special Tests: Inspection of hair shafts, skin scraping for fungi.

Diagnostic Procedures: History, physical examination, inspection of hair shafts.

Pathologic Findings

If the base of the hair shaft is smooth, it came from natural (telogen) loss, if the base has the follicular bulb still attached (a white swelling at the end), the loss may be due to dermatologic or other disease conditions and consultation is suggested.

MANAGEMENT AND THERAPY

Nonpharmacologic

General Measures: Evaluation, reassurance often is all that is required (telogen effluvium is self-limited).

Specific Measures: Based on cause, most are self-limited or reverse with correction of the underlying problem. For postmenopausal women, hormone replacement therapy often arrests or reverses hair loss.

Diet: No specific dietary changes indicated.

Activity: No restriction.

Patient Education: Reassurance and information about hair growth.

Drug(s) of Choice

For androgenic effluvium: topical minoxidil (Rogaine) 2% (approximately 40% response rate in 1 year).

For alopecia areata: high-potency topical steroids.

For tinea capitis: 6- to 8-week therapy with either griseofulvin (ultramicrosize) 250–375 mg PO qd or ketoconazole 200 mg PO qd and careful hand washing.

Contraindications: Griseofulvin is contraindicated in pregnant patients and in those with porphyria

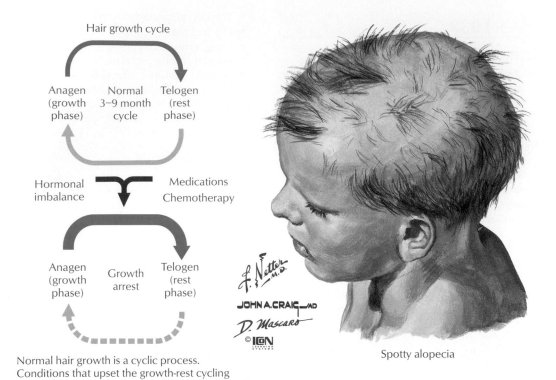

Hair growth cycle

Anagen (growth phase) — Normal 3–9 month cycle — Telogen (rest phase)

Hormonal imbalance — Medications Chemotherapy

Anagen (growth phase) — Growth arrest — Telogen (rest phase)

Normal hair growth is a cyclic process. Conditions that upset the growth-rest cycling may delay replacement of normal hair loss, resulting in alopecia. Such conditions are usually reversible

Spotty alopecia

Conditions associated with increased risk of hair loss

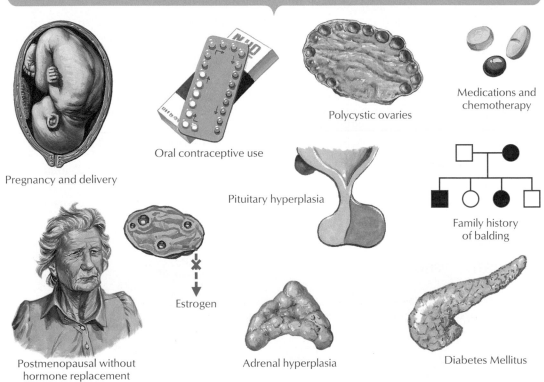

Pregnancy and delivery

Oral contraceptive use

Polycystic ovaries

Medications and chemotherapy

Pituitary hyperplasia

Family history of balding

Postmenopausal without hormone replacement

Estrogen

Adrenal hyperplasia

Diabetes Mellitus

and hepatocellular failure. Ketoconazole and itraconazole should not be used concomitantly with cisapride (Propulsid).

Precautions: Topical minoxidil can cause eye irritation. Griseofulvin use is associated with the possibility of photosensitivity, lupus-like syndromes, oral thrush, and granulocytopenia. Ketoconazole and itraconazole may be associated with hepatotoxicity.

Interactions: Minoxidil may potentiate the actions of other antihypertensive agents. Griseofulvin can interact with both barbiturates and warfarin. Ketoconazole and itraconazole may interact with warfarin, histamine H_2 blockers, digoxin, isoniazid, rifampin, and phenytoin.

Alternative Drugs

Finasteride (Propecia) has been used for male pattern baldness in men, but is ineffective for postmenopausal hair loss for women and is contraindicated during pregnancy.

FOLLOW-UP

Patient Monitoring: Normal health maintenance. With ketoconazole and itraconazole periodic assessment of liver function is prudent.

Prevention/Avoidance: None.

Possible Complications: Social withdrawal.

Expected Outcome: Most hair loss is not permanent; a gradual return may be expected in 3–6 months once any causes have been eliminated. Only cicatricial alopecia is associated with permanent damage to the hair follicles.

MISCELLANEOUS

Pregnancy Considerations: No effect on pregnancy although delivery is often the trigger for increased hair loss.

ICD-9-CM Codes: 704.02 (Telogen effluvium), 704.00 (Alopecia, unspecified), 704.01 (Alopecia areata), 704.09 (Other alopecias).

REFERENCES

Burfke KE. Hair loss. What causes it and what can be done about it. *Postgrad Med* 1989;85:52.5

Rook A, Dawber R. *Diseases of the Hair and Scalp.* 2nd ed. Boston, Mass: Blackwell Scientific Publications, 1992.

HEADACHE: TENSION, CLUSTER, AND MIGRAINE

INTRODUCTION

Description: The tension headache is the most common form of headache. Tension headaches are caused by abnormal neuronal sensitivity and pain facilitation and/or contracted muscles of the neck and scalp. Cluster headaches are a type of recurrent headache characterized as unilateral and "stabbing" that are associated with symptoms of histamine release such as nasal stuffiness. These occur in episodic waves of frequent headaches separated by days, weeks, or years of remission. Migraine headaches are recurrent severe headaches that last 4–72 hours and are accompanied by neurologic, gastrointestinal, and autonomic changes. These may or may not be preceded by a characteristic aura.

Prevalence: Ninety percent of women experience tension headaches. Cluster headaches occur in 4 of 100,000 women per year. Migraine headaches affect 15%–20% of women. Approximately 10% of tension headache suffers also have migraine headaches.

Predominant Age: Tensions headaches—any age, 60% begin after 20, rarely do they start after 50. Cluster headaches—20–30. Migraine headaches—25–55 (peak 30–49), first attack generally between adolescence and 20.

Genetics: Women are more often affected by tension headaches than men (88% versus 69%); 40% have a family history of headache. Cluster headaches are 4 times more common in women than in men; migraines are 3 times more common in women. Eighty percent of migraine suffers have a family history of headache.

ETIOLOGY AND PATHOGENESIS

Causes: Tension headache—abnormal neuronal sensitivity and pain facilitation; no correlation to muscle contraction. They generally build in intensity in relation to stress. Cluster headache—unknown; postulated: disorders of histamine release or sensitivity, serotonin metabolism or transmission, hypothalamic circadian rhythm, or cerebral artery autoregulation. Migraine headache—unknown; postulated: genetically linked vascular disruption secondary to neurochemical change, serotonin or norepinephrine metabolism, or tachykinin abnormality. These alterations may result in distension of and inflammation of cranial blood vessels. A strong relationship with female sex hormones is suspected.

Risk Factors: Tension headache—physical or emotional stress, poor posture, depression, obstructive sleep apnea, excess caffeine. Cluster headache—allergies, alcohol, tobacco, nitroglycerine, high altitudes, sleep cycle disruption, stress. Migraine headache—more common in upper-income patients (1.6 times), 60%–70% of women note a link with menstruation (14% of women have migraine headaches only during menses). Precipitating factors: some foods, stress or stress relief (let down), missed meals, excessive sleep.

CLINICAL CHARACTERISTICS

Signs and Symptoms:

- **Tension headache**—Dull, aching, and constant pain of mild to moderate intensity lasting from 30 minutes to 7 days, often located in the temples, around the head in a band, or up the back of the neck. Rare patients experience chronic tension-type headaches characterized by 15 days/month for 6 months or longer.
- Pressing or tightening quality (nonpulsating)
- Bilateral symmetry
- Not aggravated by physical activity
- No nausea or vomiting, photophobia, or phonophobia (may have one but not both)
- Teeth grinding common
- **Cluster headache**—Unilateral or orbital distribution (90% of headaches recur on the same side)
- Sharp, stabbing, or "ice pick" in character
- Symptoms of histamine release (nasal stuffiness and rhinorrhea, facial flushing, lacrimation, edema of eyelids)
- Symptoms are relieved when the patient is moving around
- Strong association with sleep
- Duration of less than 1 hour
- No aura or prodrome
- Annual recurrence common
- **Migraine headache**—May be preceded by aura (20%)
- May begin with dull ache
- Unilateral pain (30%–40%, may switch sides from attack to attack)
- Pulsating quality (60%), rapid onset
- Moderate to severe intensity
- Made worse by activity
- Frequently accompanied by nausea (90%), vomiting (60%), photophobia (80%), blurred vision, scalp tenderness and

neck stiffness, restlessness, irritability, nasal congestion, facial edema

- Menstrual migraine is characterized by onset between 1 day before and 4 days after menstruation. (Most common; first day.) This pattern is found in 15% of patients.

DIAGNOSTIC APPROACH

Differential Diagnosis:
- Depression
- Cervical spondylosis
- Temporomandibular joint syndrome
- Analgesic dependency
- Anemia
- Medication or toxin exposure
- Dental disease
- Chronic sinusitis (cluster, migraine)
- Temporal arteritis
- Trigeminal neuralgia
- Pheochromocytoma

Associated Conditions: Tension headache has been associated with an increased risk of epilepsy (4-fold). Cluster headaches are associated with seasonal allergy. Migraine headache are associated with increased risk of peptic ulcer and coronary heart disease. Epilepsy, depression, anxiety, Raynaud's phenomenon, mitral valve prolapse, stroke (debated), motion sickness, and panic disorders are more common in patients with migraine headaches.

Workup and Evaluation

Laboratory: No evaluation indicated.
Imaging: No imaging indicated. (CT, electroencephalogram, and other evaluations are not indicated unless there is the new onset of headaches after age 50.)
Special Tests: None indicated.
Diagnostic Procedures: History.

Pathologic Findings

None.

MANAGEMENT AND THERAPY

Nonpharmacologic

General Measures: Tension headache—over-the-counter analgesics, rest, fluids, massage of shoulders, neck, or temples. Cluster headache—over-the-counter analgesics, rest, fluids, avoidance of alcohol, bright lights, and noise. Migraine headache—rest, fluids, analgesics, avoidance of alcohol, bright lights, and noise. Compression over the temporal artery may help. Biofeedback has been suggested but results vary.

Specific Measures: Nonsteroidal antiinflammatory agents, stress reduction techniques, and biofeedback are indicated for tension headache. Prophylaxis is most effective for cluster headaches. Migraine headaches should be treated with medical therapy for acute attacks and prophylaxis against recurrent headaches.

Diet: No specific dietary changes indicated. (Caffeine restriction has been suggested.) Patients should avoid alcohol or food known to hasten attacks.

Activity: No restriction, avoidance of known precipitating activities. Improved general fitness and strengthening may reduce incidence. Bed rest for severe migraine attacks.

Patient Education: American College of Obstetricians and Gynecologists Patient Education Pamphlet AP124 (*Headache*).

Drug(s) of Choice

Tension headache—over-the-counter analgesics, nonsteroidal antiinflammatory agents, antidepressants (when appropriate).

Cluster headache—prophylaxis: ergotamine (1–2 mg PO 2 hours before likely attack, eg, sleep), verapamil (80 mg PO qid), lithium carbonate (Eskalith, 300 mg PO 2–4 times daily), methysergide (Sansert, 2 mg tid or qid); acute attacks: oxygen (100%, 7–10 L/min via mask for 10–15 minutes), sumatriptan (Imitrex, 6 mg SC or 100 mg PO, may repeat dose once in 24 hours when separated by at least 1 hour), dihydroergotamine mesylate (DHE 45, 1 mg IM or IV). Even though the symptoms of cluster headaches are consistent with histamine release, treatment with antihistamines is ineffective.

Migraine headache: nonsteroidal antiinflammatory agents (may provide relieve for some or may abort the headache if taken early in the attack), ergotamine preparations (ergotamine tartrate rectally at onset, may repeat in 1 hour or ergotamine tartrate 1 mg with caffeine 100 mg [Cafergot], 2 PO at onset, repeat q30 min up to six per day, DHE 1 mg IM or 2–3 mg intranasally at onset, 3 mg/24 h maximum), serotonin agonists (sumatriptan 6 mg SC or 100 mg PO or 5–20 mg intranasally at onset may repeat once in 24 hour with a minimum of 1 hour separation, naratriptan 1–2.5 mg PO, may repeat in 4 hours, 5 mg/24 h maximum, zolmitriptan 2.5 mg PO, may repeat in 2 hours, 10 mg/24 h maximum).

Muscle Contraction Headache

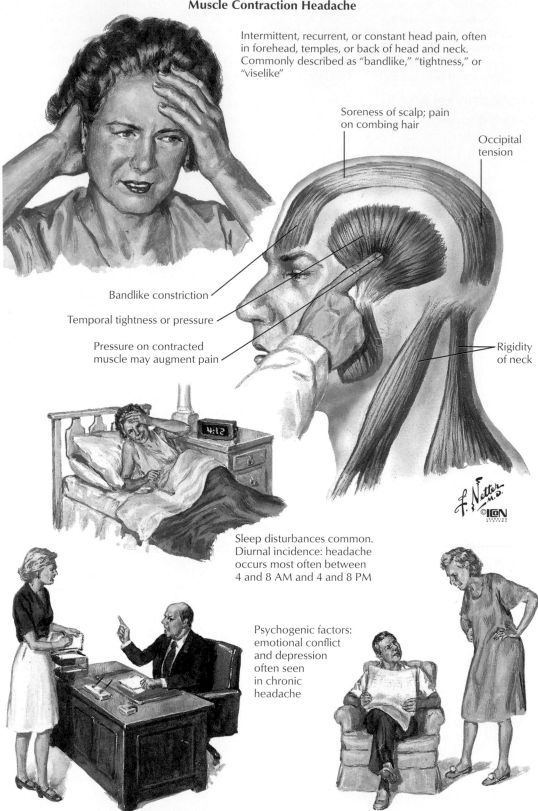

Intermittent, recurrent, or constant head pain, often in forehead, temples, or back of head and neck. Commonly described as "bandlike," "tightness," or "viselike"

Soreness of scalp; pain on combing hair

Occipital tension

Bandlike constriction

Temporal tightness or pressure

Pressure on contracted muscle may augment pain

Rigidity of neck

Sleep disturbances common. Diurnal incidence: headache occurs most often between 4 and 8 AM and 4 and 8 PM

Psychogenic factors: emotional conflict and depression often seen in chronic headache

Migraine Headache

Severe, throbbing headache; unilateral at first but may spread to opposite side

Local erythema may be present

Pallor, perspiration

Attack

Sonophobia

Photophobia

Speaks in low voice to avoid aggravating pain

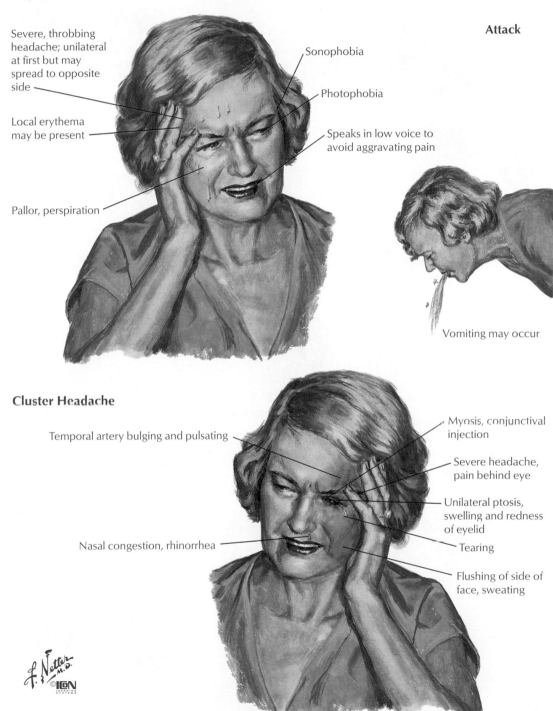

Vomiting may occur

Cluster Headache

Temporal artery bulging and pulsating

Nasal congestion, rhinorrhea

Myosis, conjunctival injection

Severe headache, pain behind eye

Unilateral ptosis, swelling and redness of eyelid

Tearing

Flushing of side of face, sweating

Triggers of Migraine

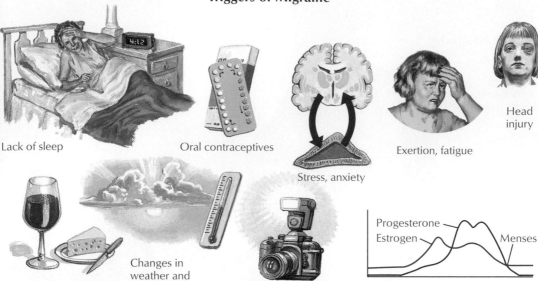

Lack of sleep

Oral contraceptives

Stress, anxiety

Exertion, fatigue

Head injury

Certain foods, alcohol

Changes in weather and temperature

Glare or dazzle

Menstruation

Progesterone — Estrogen — Menses

Common triggers

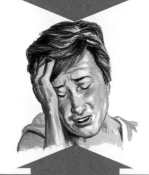

JOHN A. CRAIG—MD
C. Machado M.D.
© ICN

Common triggers

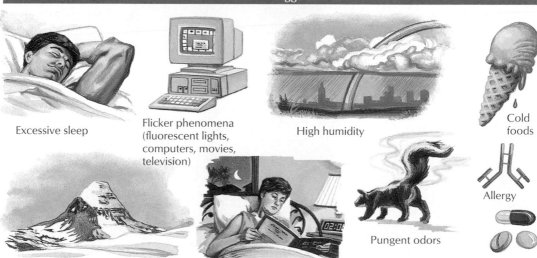

Excessive sleep

Flicker phenomena (fluorescent lights, computers, movies, television)

High humidity

Cold foods

High altitude

Reading or refractive errors

Pungent odors

Allergy

Drugs

Contraindications: Aspirin-sensitive asthma, known or suspected sensitivity. See individual medications for others.

Precautions: Overuse of analgesics may lead to habituation and "analgesic rebound headaches" perpetuating the cycle of headache and analgesic use. Avoid the use of narcotic analgesics, especially oral agents in patients with cluster headaches; may convert attack to chronic form. Significant side effects are possible with most migraine therapy—see individual agents. Use vasoactive agents with care in patients with cardiovascular disease.

Alternative Drugs

Cluster headache—indomethacin 25 mg PO qid, nifedipine 40–120 mg/d.

Migraine headache—antiemetics and phenothiazines may abort migraine headaches or help relieve associated symptoms. Metoclopramide may be used to reduce nausea. Narcotic analgesics may be used for patients who do not achieve relief with other measures or cannot take other agents.

FOLLOW-UP

Patient Monitoring: Normal health maintenance. Anticipate episodic recurrences for cluster and migraine headaches.

Prevention/Avoidance: Stress reduction, muscle strengthening and training, and biofeedback. For cluster headaches the prophylactic use of antihistamines should be considered during the times of year when the patient is most likely to have a recurrence. During the same period, alcoholic beverages and tobacco should be avoided because they may trigger an attack. These patients should also avoid sleep cycle disruption. Patients who suffer from migraine headache should have adequate rest and fluids and avoid known triggers. Prophylactic medical therapy may be warranted for patients with two or more attacks per month. Prophylaxis may be attempted using β-blockers, divalproex, calcium antagonists, antidepressants, or serotonin antagonists.

Possible Complications: Headaches that are of sudden onset, begin after age 50, are dramatically different from past experience, have an accelerating pattern or are brought on by exertion, sexual activity, coughing or sneezing, or are accompanied by focal neurologic signs are ominous and demand aggressive evaluation for possible intracranial or other pathologic cause. Patients with cluster or migraine headaches have an increased risk for peptic ulcers and gastrointestinal injury (from medications), caffeine dependence, coronary heart disease, and suicide.

Expected Outcome: Tension headaches generally resolve with rest and analgesics, although intermittent recurrence is common without lifestyle changes. Cluster headaches commonly have seasonal or annual recurrence patterns. Prolonged remission also is common. Migraines can generally be controlled, but recurrence is common. Severity and frequency tend to decline with age.

MISCELLANEOUS

Pregnancy Considerations: No effect on pregnancy. Pregnancy does not appear to affect the frequency of tension headaches. Cluster headaches are very rare in pregnancy. Migraine headaches may worsen in the first trimester of pregnancy and generally lessen in the second and third trimesters. Pregnancy may alter medical therapy because of adverse effects of medications on the pregnant patient or fetus.

ICD-9-CM Codes: 307.81 (Tension headache), 346.2 (Cluster headache), 346.9 (Migraine), 346.0 (Classical migraine).

REFERENCES

APGO Educational Series on Women's Health Issues. *Strategies for the Management of Headache.* Washington, DC: APGO; 1998.

Edelson RN. Menstrual migraine and other hormonal aspects of migraine. *Headache* 1985;25:376.

Granella F, Sances G, Zanferrari C, Costa A, Martignoni E, Manzoni GC. Migraine without aura and reproductive life events. A clinical epidemiologic study in 1300 women. *Headache* 1993;33:385.

Headache Classification Committee of the International Headache Society. Classification and diagnostic criteria for headache disorders, cranial neuralgia, and facial pain. *Cephalagia* 1988;8:1.

Kudrow L. The relationship of headache frequency to hormone use in migraine. *Headache* 1975;15:36.

Laube DW. Headache. In: Ling FW, Laube DW, Nolan TE, Smith RP, Stovall TG, eds. *Primary Care in Gynecology.* Baltimore, Md: Williams & Wilkins; 1996:87.

Silberstein SD. The role of sex hormones in headache. *Neurology* 1992;42:37.

HEMATURIA

INTRODUCTION

Description: The presence of blood, either microscopically or macroscopically, in the urine. Hematuria is a symptom only and requires further evaluation to establish a cause. Hematuria should be considered an indication of malignancy until proven otherwise.

Prevalence: Common in women.

Predominant Age: Any age, most common in reproductive years in association with urinary tract infections.

Genetics: No genetic pattern.

ETIOLOGY AND PATHOGENESIS

Causes: Disruption of the uroepithelium by infection, neoplasia (benign or malignant), or mechanical trauma (trauma, stone).

Risk Factors: Sexual activity, instrumentation, urinary tract infection, foreign body, or stone.

CLINICAL CHARACTERISTICS

Signs and Symptoms:

- Painless (or otherwise) passage of blood in the urine

DIAGNOSTIC APPROACH

Differential Diagnosis:

- Renal or bladder cancer
- Lower urinary tract infection (urethritis, cystitis)
- Pyelonephritis
- Urolithiasis
- Endometriosis involving the urinary tract
- Traumatic trigonitis
- Interstitial cystitis
- Coagulopathy (iatrogenic or natural)
- Contamination of the urine from another source (vaginal, rectal, anal, factitious)

Associated Conditions: Dysuria, urinary frequency, and urinary tract infections.

Workup and Evaluation

Laboratory: Urinalysis, urine culture, and sensitivity (based on other symptoms present).

Imaging: Intravenous or retrograde pyelography. Renal ultrasonography may reveal dilation of the collecting system.

Special Tests: Cystoscopy may be necessary for selected patients. Urine should be collected and passed through a fine screen or mesh if a stone is suspected.

Diagnostic Procedures: History and physical examination, urinalysis.

Pathologic Findings

Based on cause.

MANAGEMENT AND THERAPY

Nonpharmacologic

General Measures: Evaluation, hydration.

Specific Measures: Based on the underlying cause; infection should be treated with appropriate antibiotics; stones and tumors require more extensive diagnosis and eventual removal (or passage).

Diet: Adequate fluid intake.

Activity: No restriction except those imposed by the causative process.

Patient Education: Reassurance, American College of Obstetricians and Gynecologists Patient Education Pamphlet AP050 (*Urinary Tract Infections*).

Drug(s) of Choice

Based on cause.

FOLLOW-UP

Patient Monitoring: Normal health maintenance.

Prevention/Avoidance: None.

Possible Complications: Failure to diagnose a malignancy in a timely manner. With large-volume bleeding, clotting with urethral obstruction is theoretically possible.

Expected Outcome: For most patients, complete resolution of their symptoms occurs with appropriate treatment of the base problem.

MISCELLANEOUS

Pregnancy Considerations: No effect on pregnancy except that caused by the underlying condition.

ICD-9-CM Codes: 599.7.

REFERENCES

Ahmed Z, Lee J. Asymptomatic urinary abnormalities. Hematuria and proteinuria. *Med Clin North Am* 1977; 81:641.

Ahn JH, Morey AF, McAninch JW. Workup and management of traumatic hematuria. *Emerg Med Clin North Am* 1988;16:145.

Feld LG, Waz WR, Perez LM, Joseph DB. Hematuria. An integrated medical and surgical approach. *Pediatr Clin N Am* 1997;44:119.

Foresman WH, Messing EM. Bladder cancer: natural history, tumor markers, and early detection strategies. *Semin Surg Oncol* 1977;13:299.

Hematuria

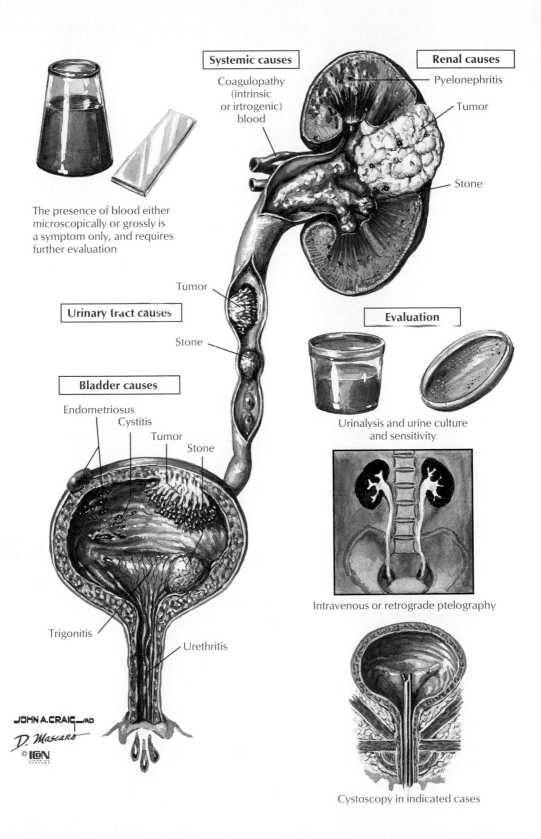

The presence of blood either microscopically or grossly is a symptom only, and requires further evaluation

Systemic causes

Coagulopathy (intrinsic or irtrogenic) blood

Renal causes

Pyelonephritis

Tumor

Stone

Urinary tract causes

Tumor

Stone

Bladder causes

Endometriosus

Cystitis

Tumor

Stone

Trigonitis

Urethritis

Evaluation

Urinalysis and urine culture and sensitivity

Intravenous or retrograde ptelography

Cystoscopy in indicated cases

JOHN A. CRAIG AD

D. Mascaro

© ICON
LEARNING SYSTEMS

Jayson M, Sanders H. Increased incidence of serendipitously discovered renal cell carcinoma. *Urology* 1998; 51:203.

Mahan JD, Turman MA, Mentser MI. Evaluation of hematuria, proteinuria, and hypertension in adolescents. *Pediatr Clin North Am* 1997;44:1573.

McCarthy JJ. Outpatient evaluation of hematuria: locating the source of bleeding. *Postgrad Med* 1997; 101:125.

HEMORRHOIDS

INTRODUCTION

Description: Symptomatic dilation of the hemorrhoidal venous plexus resulting in perianal swelling, itching, pain, hematochezia, and fecal soiling.

Prevalence: Fifty percent to eighty percent of all Americans.

Predominant Age: Adult, more common after pregnancy.

Genetics: No genetic pattern.

ETIOLOGY AND PATHOGENESIS

Causes: Dilated rectal venous plexus with varying degrees of inflammation.

Risk Factors: Pregnancy, obesity, chronic cough, constipation, heavy lifting, sedentary work or lifestyle, hepatic disease, colon malignancy, portal hypertension, loss of muscle tone resulting from age, surgery, episiotomy, anal intercourse, or neurologic disease (multiple sclerosis).

CLINICAL CHARACTERISTICS

Signs and Symptoms:
- Rectal bleeding
- Anal protrusion
- Anal itching and pain (especially with thrombosis or ulceration)
- Constipation and straining for bowel movement
- Rectal incontinence and soiling
- Hematochezia and stool mucous
- Anal fissure, infection or ulceration
- Hemorrhoidal thrombosis

DIAGNOSTIC APPROACH

Differential Diagnosis:
- Colon cancer
- Colon polyps
- Soiling caused by loss of anal tone (anal intercourse, multiple sclerosis, episiotomy)
- Pinworms
- Rectocele
- Fecal impaction
- Anal fissure or fistula

Associated Conditions: Liver disease, pregnancy, portal hypertension, and constipation.

Workup and Evaluation

Laboratory: No evaluation indicated.

Imaging: No imaging indicated.

Special Tests: None indicated.

Diagnostic Procedures: History and physical examination.

Pathologic Findings

Enlarged hemorrhoidal veins with stasis and inflammation are common.

MANAGEMENT AND THERAPY

Nonpharmacologic

General Measures: Stool softeners, bowel movement regulation, and topical medications.

Specific Measures: Surgical therapy is appropriate for those patients with debilitating symptoms or for whom medical therapy has failed (15%–20% of patients). Banding of internal hemorrhoids is better accepted by patients than traditional surgical therapy. Hemorrhoidal banding requires a minimum of equipment and is well suited to the office or outpatient surgical setting. Some aching is generally experienced for several days after hemorrhoid banding procedures. Sitz baths and topical analgesics such as witch hazel are generally sufficient.

Diet: Increased dietary fiber.

Activity: Avoid prolonged sitting, straining, or heavy lifting. Encourage physical fitness.

Patient Education: Reassurance, diet instruction.

Drug(s) of Choice

Dietary fiber supplements.

Stool softeners—docusate sodium (Colace, Dialose, Sof-Lax) 50–300 mg PO qd (larger doses are generally divided over the day).

Topical analgesic sprays or ointments—benzocaine (Americaine, Hurricaine) 20% spray or gel, dibucaine (Nupercainal) 1% ointment.

Antipruritics and antiinflammatory agents—hydrocortisone (Anusol-HC, Analpram-HC, Cortenema, Cortifoam, Epifoam, Proctofoam-HC), pramoxine 1% (Fleet rectal pads, Analpram-HC), witch hazel 50% (Tucks pads or gel).

Astringents—Preparation H.

Contraindications to Surgical Therapy: Acquired immunodeficiency syndrome (AIDS) or immunocompromise, anorectal fissures, bleeding diathesis or blood dyscrasia, inflammatory bowel disease, portal hypertension, rectal prolapse, undiagnosed anorectal tumor, undiagnosed rectal bleeding.

Precautions: See individual agents.

Interactions: Docusate sodium may potentiate the hepatotoxicity of other drugs; see individual agents.

FOLLOW-UP

Patient Monitoring: Normal health maintenance.

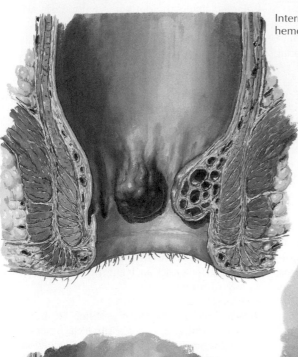

Internal hemorrhoids

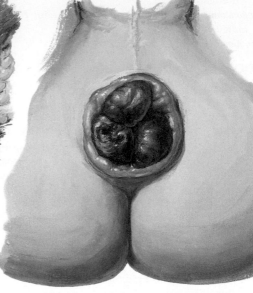

Prolapsed "rosette" of internal hemorrhoids

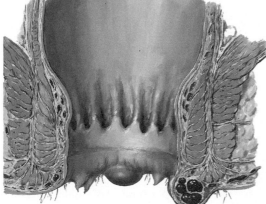

External hemorrhoids and skin tabs

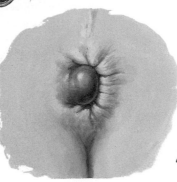

Thrombosed external hemorrhoid

Anal skin tabs

Prevention/Avoidance: Avoidance of constipation (bowel regularity), weight loss (if appropriate), physical fitness, avoidance of prolonged sitting, straining, or heavy lifting.

Possible Complications: Thrombosis, bleeding, secondary infection, ulceration, anemia, and rectal incontinence.

Expected Outcome: Resolution (spontaneous resolution or with medication), recurrence common.

MISCELLANEOUS

Pregnancy Considerations: No effect on pregnancy. Hemorrhoids are extremely common as pregnancy progresses. Dietary prophylaxis and symptomatic therapy early reduces the severity of symptoms. At least partial resolution after delivery is expected.

ICD-9-CM **Codes:** 455.6, 455.3 (External), 455.0 (Internal), 455.7 (Thrombosed).

REFERENCES

Bassford T. Treatment of common anorectal disorders [review]. *Am Fam Physician* 1992;45:1787.

Bleday R, Pena JP, Rothenberger DA, Goldberg SM, Buls JG. Symptomatic hemorrhoids: current incidence and complications of operative therapy. *Dis Colon Rectum* 1992;35:477.

Devine R, Ory S. Treatment of hemorrhoids in pregnancy. *J Fam Pract* 1992;17:65.

Guthrie JF. The current management of hemorrhoid. *Pract Gastroenterol* 1987;11:56.

Mazier WP. Hemorrhoids, fissures, and pruritus ani [review]. *Surg Clin North Am* 1994;74:1277.

Medich DS, Fazio VW. Hemorrhoids, anal fissure, and carcinoma of the colon, rectum, and anus during pregnancy. *Surg Clin North Am* 1995;75:77.

Schussman LC, Lutz LJ. Outpatient management of hemorrhoids. *Primary Care* 1986;13:527.

HYPERTHYROIDISM

INTRODUCTION

Description: Excess production of thyroid hormone. Hyperthyroidism is 3 times more common in women and may result in menstrual irregularity, fertility disturbances, or complicate pregnancy. It may occur because of Graves' autoimmune disease (most common) or toxic single or multinodular goiters. Rarely, trophoblastic tumors or dermoid cysts may be the cause.

Prevalence: One of 1000 women.

Predominant Age: 20–40 years.

Genetics: Graves' disease may follow a familial pattern.

ETIOLOGY AND PATHOGENESIS

Causes: Graves' disease—an autoimmune disease in which thyroid-stimulating immunoglobulins bind to thyroid-stimulating hormone (TSH) receptors mimicking the action of TSH and causing excess secretion of triiodothyronine (T_3) and thyroxine (T_4). Goiter and exophthalmos are common. Toxic single or multinodular goiter—one or more autonomous benign nodules that slowly grow. Exophthalmos and myxedema are generally absent.

Risk Factors: Family history, other autoimmune disorders, and iodine deprivation followed by replacement.

CLINICAL CHARACTERISTICS

Signs and Symptoms:
- Nervousness (85%)
- Palpitations, tachycardia (>100 beats/min) and dyspnea (75%)
- Heat intolerance (70%)
- Fatigue and weakness (60%)
- Weight loss (50%), increased appetite (40%)
- Palpable goiter (90%)
- Tremor (65%)
- Exophthalmos (35%)

DIAGNOSTIC APPROACH

Differential Diagnosis:
- Physiologic changes of pregnancy
- Anxiety
- Malignancy
- Diabetes
- Pregnancy
- Menopause
- Pheochromocytoma
- Substance abuse (caffeine, diet preparations, cocaine)
- Struma ovarii

Associated Conditions: Other autoimmune diseases (Graves' disease).

Workup and Evaluation

Laboratory: Sensitive TSH (below normal), T_3 radioimmunoassay (RIA) (>200 ng/mL), T_4 RIA (>160 nmol/L), free thyroxine index (>12).

Imaging: Radioiodine thyroid scan (diffuse uptake in Graves' disease; focal uptake in nodular goiter).

Special Tests: None indicated.

Diagnostic Procedures: History, physical examination, and laboratory studies.

Pathologic Findings

Graves' disease—diffuse hyperplasia; toxic nodules—discrete nodule formation.

MANAGEMENT AND THERAPY

Nonpharmacologic

General Measures: Evaluation, education about the need for continuing therapy, β-blockers for symptoms of tachycardia or tremor.

Specific Measures: Antithyroid medication, therapeutic radioiodine, surgical reduction of thyroid or excision of nodules.

Diet: No specific dietary changes indicated. Maintain adequate calories to avoid weight loss.

Activity: No restriction, as tolerated.

Patient Education: Education regarding need for compliance with medication and follow-up.

Drug(s) of Choice

For thyrotoxic crisis—propylthiouracil (PTU) 15–20 mg PO q4h during the first day in addition to other therapies. Initial treatment: PTU 30–300 mg PO tid (no more than 300 mg/d during pregnancy), maintain at 25–300 PO bid, methimazole (Tapazole, MMI) 15–60 mg PO qd, maintain at 5–30 mg PO qd; radioiodine therapy: sodium iodine (^{131}I); adjunctive therapy: propranolol (Inderal) 40–240 mg PO qd.

Contraindications: Radioiodine therapy is contraindicated in pregnancy (may cause fetal hypothyroidism or malformation). Propranolol is contraindicated in the presence of congestive heart failure, asthma, chronic bronchitis, and hypoglycemia and during pregnancy.

Precautions: Both PTU and MMI may cause agranulocytosis, dermatitis, or hepatotoxicity.

Interactions: PTU may potentiate the actions of anticoagulants.

Alternative Drugs

Ipodate sodium (Oragrafin) 0.5 g PO qid.

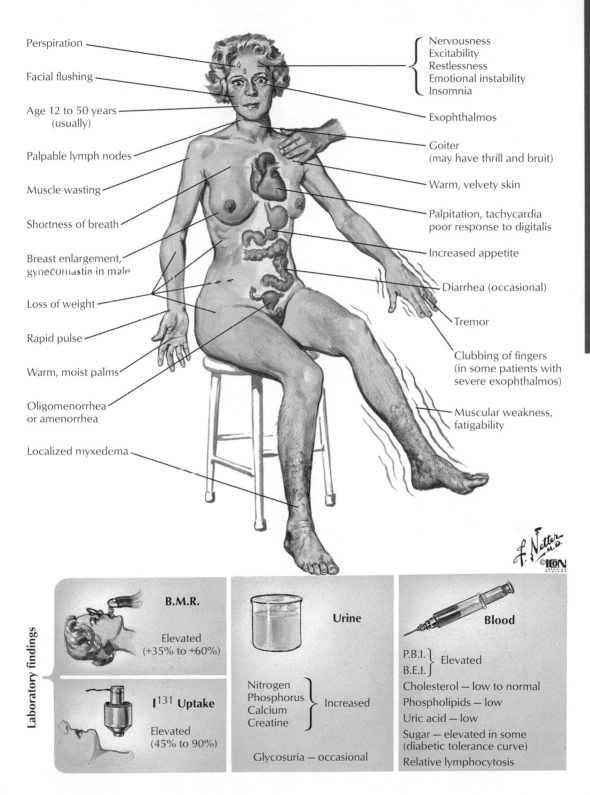

Perspiration

Facial flushing

Age 12 to 50 years (usually)

Palpable lymph nodes

Muscle wasting

Shortness of breath

Breast enlargement, gynecomastia in male

Loss of weight

Rapid pulse

Warm, moist palms

Oligomenorrhea or amenorrhea

Localized myxedema

Nervousness
Excitability
Restlessness
Emotional instability
Insomnia

Exophthalmos

Goiter (may have thrill and bruit)

Warm, velvety skin

Palpitation, tachycardia poor response to digitalis

Increased appetite

Diarrhea (occasional)

Tremor

Clubbing of fingers (in some patients with severe exophthalmos)

Muscular weakness, fatigability

Laboratory findings

B.M.R.
Elevated (+35% to +60%)

I¹³¹ Uptake
Elevated (45% to 90%)

Urine

Nitrogen
Phosphorus
Calcium
Creatine } Increased

Glycosuria — occasional

Blood

P.B.I.
B.E.I. } Elevated

Cholesterol — low to normal

Phospholipids — low

Uric acid — low

Sugar — elevated in some (diabetic tolerance curve)

Relative lymphocytosis

FOLLOW-UP

Patient Monitoring: Normal health maintenance, follow thyroid function test twice yearly. After radioiodine therapy, thyroid function should be checked at 6 and 12 weeks, 6 months, and then yearly.

Prevention/Avoidance: None.

Possible Complications: Hypothyroidism after medical therapy, vision change or loss caused by ophthalmopathy, pretibial myxedema or cardiac failure, muscle wasting and proximal muscle weakness. Surgical therapy—hypoparathyroidism, recurrent laryngeal nerve damage, hypothyroidism.

Expected Outcome: With early diagnosis and adequate treatment a good outcome is expected.

MISCELLANEOUS

Pregnancy Considerations: Difficult to diagnose in pregnancy. Increased risk of spontaneous abortion. Thyrotoxicosis often improves during pregnancy only to relapse postpartum—must be alert for this possibility. Any goiter is abnormal. Doses of PTU and MMI must be reduced. Radioiodine therapy is contraindicated.

***ICD-9-CM* Codes:** Based on cause.

REFERENCES

American College of Obstetricians and Gynecologists. *Thyroid Disease in Pregnancy.* Washington, DC: ACOG; 1993. ACOG Technical Bulletin 181.

Amino N, Mori H, Iwatani Y, et al. High prevalence of transient post-partum thyrotoxicosis and hypothyroidism. *N Engl J Med* 1982;306:849.

Amino N, Tanizawa O, Mori H, et al. Aggravation of thyrotoxicosis in early pregnancy and after delivery in Graves' disease. *J Clin Endocrinol Metab* 1982; 55:108.

Burrow GN. The management of thyrotoxicosis in pregnancy. *N Engl J Med* 1985;313:562.

Davis LE, Lucas MJ, Hankins GDV, Roark ML, Cunningham FG. Thyrotoxicosis complicating pregnancy. *Am J Obstet Gynecol* 1989;160:63.

Jansson R, Dahlberg PA, Winsa B, Meirik O, Säfwenberg J, Karlsson A. The postpartum period constitutes an important risk for the development of clinical Graves' disease in young women. *Acta Endocrinol (Copenh)* 1987;116:321.

HYPOTHYROIDISM

INTRODUCTION

Description: Reduced or inadequate circulating levels of thyroid hormone. Women are 5 to 10 times more likely to suffer from hypothyroidism than are men. Menstrual disturbances may be the first indication of this abnormality. Some women develop a transient (3–4 months) hypothyroid state (painless subacute thyroiditis) after delivery.

Prevalence: Five to ten of 1000 general population, 6%–10% of women older than 65.

Predominant Age: Older than 40.

Genetics: No genetic pattern for idiopathic type, may be associated with type II autoimmune polyglandular syndrome (HLA-DR3, -DR4).

ETIOLOGY AND PATHOGENESIS

Causes: Idiopathic or autoimmune (most common when goiter is present)—after ablative medical or surgical therapy. Postpartum thyroiditis (silent)—abnormalities of TSH or thyrotropin-releasing hormone (TRH) production or release.

Risk Factors: Age, other autoimmune disease, ablative therapy.

CLINICAL CHARACTERISTICS

Signs and Symptoms:
- Weakness, lethargy, fatigue
- Cold intolerance, hypothermia
- Menstrual disturbances (dysfunctional bleeding, amenorrhea, menorrhagia)
- Decreased memory, hearing loss
- Constipation
- Dry, coarse skin
- Periorbital puffiness, swelling of hands and feet
- Bradycardia, narrowed pulse pressure
- Anemia
- Cardiomegaly, pericardial effusion

DIAGNOSTIC APPROACH

Differential Diagnosis:
- Depression
- Congestive heart failure
- Dementia
- Amyloidosis
- Nephrotic syndrome
- Chronic nephritis

Associated Conditions: Anemia, bipolar disorder, depression, diabetes mellitus, hypercholesterolemia, hyponatremia, idiopathic adrenocorticoid deficiency, mitral valve prolapse, myasthenia gravis, vitiligo.

Workup and Evaluation

Laboratory: Sensitive TSH (>20 μU/mL), triiodothyronine (T_3) resin uptake (increased), thyroxine (T_4) radioimmunoassay (decreased), free thyroxine index (low).

Imaging: No imaging indicated.

Special Tests: None indicated.

Diagnostic Procedures: History, physical examination, and laboratory studies.

Pathologic Findings

The thyroid may be small and atrophic, normal, or enlarged.

MANAGEMENT AND THERAPY

Nonpharmacologic

General Measures: Evaluation, education about need for continuing therapy.

Specific Measures: Thyroid replacement mediation.

Diet: High-bulk diet to avoid constipation.

Activity: No restriction.

Patient Education: Education regarding need for compliance with medication and follow-up.

Drug(s) of Choice

Levothyroxine (Synthroid, Levothroid) 50–100 μg PO qd, increase by 25 μg/d every 4–6 weeks until TSH is in normal range.

Contraindications: Adrenocorticoid insufficiency (uncorrected), thyrotoxic heart disease.

Precautions: The initial dose should be reduced in elderly patients.

Interactions: The dose of insulin, oral hypoglycemics, and anticoagulants may need to be adjusted after thyroid therapy is initiated. Other possible interactions may be seen with oral contraceptives and estrogen and cholestyramine. Ferrous sulfate may decrease the absorption of thyroid replacement medications.

FOLLOW-UP

Patient Monitoring: Thyroid status should be checked every 6 weeks until stable, then every 6 months. Because of the prevalence of hypothyroidism in older women, a baseline assessment should be obtained at age 45 and periodic screening (biannually) is recommended in patients older than 60.

Prevention/Avoidance: None.

Possible Complications: Life threatening—coma (myxedema coma) and hypothermia. Others—treatment-induced congestive heart failure, increased susceptibility to infection, megacolon, organic psychosis with paranoia, infertility

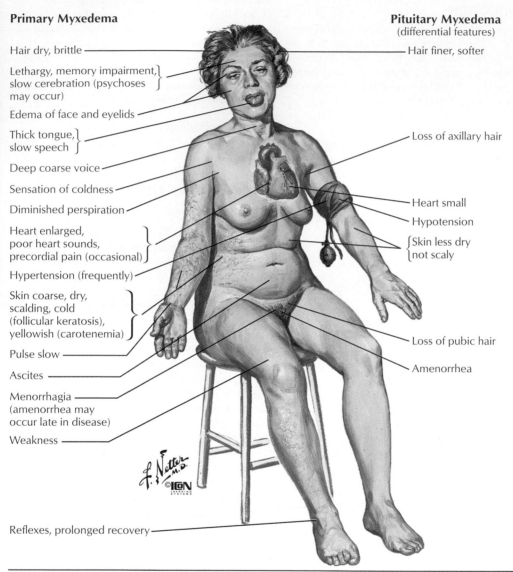

Primary Myxedema

Hair dry, brittle

Lethargy, memory impairment, slow cerebration (psychoses may occur)

Edema of face and eyelids

Thick tongue, slow speech

Deep coarse voice

Sensation of coldness

Diminished perspiration

Heart enlarged, poor heart sounds, precordial pain (occasional)

Hypertension (frequently)

Skin coarse, dry, scalding, cold (follicular keratosis), yellowish (carotenemia)

Pulse slow

Ascites

Menorrhagia (amenorrhea may occur late in disease)

Weakness

Reflexes, prolonged recovery

Pituitary Myxedema
(differential features)

Hair finer, softer

Loss of axillary hair

Heart small

Hypotension

Skin less dry not scaly

Loss of pubic hair

Amenorrhea

P.B.I. and B.E.I.; low — no rise after TSH	Low, but rise after TSH
I^{131}; 24-hour uptake low — no rise after TSH	Low, but rise after TSH
Cholesterol; elevated (usually)	Normal (usually)
Uric acid; elevated in males and postmenopausal females	Same
Urinary gonadotropins; positive	Absent
17-Ketosteroids; low	Lower
B.M.R.; usually low, but very variable	Same

and amenorrhea, or osteoporosis resulting from overtreatment.

Expected Outcome: With treatment, return to normal function. Relapse will occur if therapy is discontinued.

MISCELLANEOUS

Pregnancy Considerations: Medication may need to be adjusted. TSH levels should be checked monthly during the first trimester. TSH levels should be checked at 6 weeks' postpartum. Women who develop postpartum thyroiditis have a 30% chance of hypothyroidism in the future. Any goiter during pregnancy is abnormal.

***ICD-9-CM* Codes:** Based on cause.

REFERENCES

American College of Obstetricians and Gynecologists. *Thyroid Disease in Pregnancy.* Washington, DC: ACOG; 1993. ACOG Technical Bulletin 181.

Amino N, Mori H, Iwatani Y, et al. High prevalence of transient post-partum thyrotoxicosis and hypothyroidism. *N Engl J Med* 1982;306:849.

Barzel US. Hypothyroidism: Diagnosis and management. *Clin Geriatr Med* 1995;11:239.

Davis LE, Leveno KJ, Cunningham FG. Hypothyroidism complicating pregnancy. *Obstet Gynecol* 1988;72:108.

Felicetta JV. Thyroid changes with aging: Significance and management. *Geriatrics* 1987;42:86.

Mandel SJ, Larsen PR, Seely EW, Brent GA. Increased need for thyroxine during pregnancy in women with primary hypothyroidism. *N Engl J Med* 1990;323:91.

Ridgway EC. Modern concepts of primary thyroid gland failure. *Clin Chem* 1996;42:179.

INFERTILITY: GENERAL CONSIDERATIONS

THE CHALLENGE

To assist couples who experience difficulty conceiving through normal means.

Scope of the Problem: The inability to conceive and bear children affects 8%–18% of the American population. Under ordinary circumstances, 80%–90% of normal couples conceive during 1 year of attempting pregnancy. Infertility is generally defined as failure to conceive after 1 year of regular, unprotected intercourse. Infertility may be further subdivided into primary and secondary types based on the patient's past reproductive history; nulligravida infertility patients are in the primary infertility group; those who have achieved a pregnancy more than 1 year previously, regardless of the outcome of that pregnancy, are grouped in the secondary infertility group. Slightly more than one half of infertility patients fall into the primary group.

Objectives of Management: To establish the relevant cause or causes and develop strategies that result in conception and delivery. With improved understanding of the physiology of conception and a wide range of technologies that may be brought to bear to assist with procreation, 85% of "infertile" couples may be helped.

TACTICS

Relevant Pathophysiology: The male partner brings to the union sperm-laden semen, which is deposited in the vagina during intercourse. The average ejaculate has a volume of between 1 and 15 mL and contains more than 20 million spermatozoa. The survival of sperm in the female genital tract is thought to be at least 96 hours, and may be as long as 8 days. However, it is probable that sperm are capable of fertilizing an egg for only the first 24 to 48 hours after ejaculation. The woman's gametic contribution, the oocyte, is released from the ovary during the mid-cycle process of ovulation, 14 days before the onset of menstruation, regardless of the total cycle length. Progesterone is produced by the luteinized follicle, producing a characteristic rise of between 0.5° and 1° F in basal body temperature. The oocyte may be fertilized during the first 24 hours after ovulation only. Generally, fertilization takes place in the distal portion of the fallopian tube. Pregnancy does not result unless the zygote passes into the uterine cavity at the correct time (3–5 days after fertilization), encounters a re-

ceptive endometrium, and can successfully implant and grow.

Strategies: To achieve pregnancy, three critical elements must be in place: (1) a sperm must be available, (2) an egg must be available, and (3) the sperm and egg must meet at a time and place conducive to fertilization. It is the investigation of these three elements that constitutes the evaluation of the infertile couple.

Patient Education: Reassurance, American College of Obstetricians and Gynecologists Patient Education Booklet AP002 (*Infertility: Causes and Treatments*).

IMPLEMENTATION

Special Considerations: While the evaluation of infertility proceeds, couples should be instructed to continue attempting pregnancy through intercourse timed to the most fertile days of the cycle. Between one third and one half of all infertility problems may be diagnosed in the first phase of evaluation. The medical definition of infertility differs from that of fecundity, which refers to the physical ability of a woman to have children. Women with impaired fecundity include those who find it physically difficult or medically inadvisable to conceive and those who fail to conceive after 36 months of regular, unprotected intercourse. In short, fecundity deals with childbearing ability and fertility deals with childbearing performance. When dealing with the question of infertility, establishing the diagnosis is not the problem; the problem is identifying the underlying pathophysiologic causes. Unlike most areas of medicine, the provider must deal with two patients at the same time because it is the couple that is infertile, not the man or woman. When the relative frequency of causes is considered, it is apparent that male and female factors are present in roughly equal proportion, with a small remainder that are idiopathic. This is important to keep in mind during counseling. The distribution of causes is also helpful in designing a logical and efficient strategy for the evaluation of the infertile couple.

REFERENCES

American College of Obstetricians and Gynecologists. *Infertility.* Washington, DC: ACOG; 1989. ACOG Technical Bulletin 125.

American College of Obstetricians and Gynecologists. *New Reproductive Technologies.* Washington, DC: ACOG; 1990. ACOG Technical Bulletin 140.

American College of Obstetricians and Gynecologists. *Managing the Anovulatory State: Medical Induction of Ovulation.* Washington, DC: ACOG; 1997. ACOG Technical Bulletin 142.

Infertility

Ovulatory Phase

Basal body temperature (BBT) detects signs of ovulation

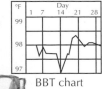

BBT chart

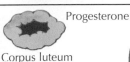

Preovulatory follicle

Ruptured follicle

Serial follicular ultrasound monitors follicular rupture

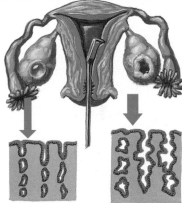

Ovulation detection kit detects urinary metabolites of luteinizing hormone (LH)

Luteal Phase

Corpus luteum

Progesterone

Endometrial biopsy and dating provides evidence of functioning corpus luteum and end organ response

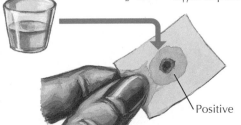

Positive

Spot urine test. Detects urinary metabolites of progesterone (measure of corpus luteum function)

Proliferative phase

Secretorys phase

Postcoital Analysis

Postcoital mucus specimen from endocervical canal placed on slide for testing

Motile sperm in orderly pattern   Ferning

Sluggish sperm in low numbers   Nonferning mucus

Optimal postcoital test. Adequate motile sperm and cervical mucus with high water content. Increased ferning and spinnbarkeit

Suboptimal postcoital test. Few sluggish sperm in thick, cellular mucus. Decreased ferning and spinnbarkeit

Semen Analysis

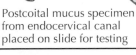
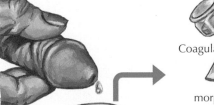

Volume

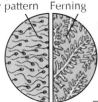

25–30 min

Coagulation   Liquefaction

morphology/motility

Fructose determination (if azospermic)

JOHN A.CRAIG—AD
© ICON
LEARNING SYSTEMS

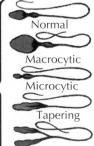

Normal

Macrocytic

Microcytic

Tapering

Bicephalic
Morphology

Office of Technology Assessment. *Infertility: Medical and Social Choices.* Washington, DC: Congress of the United States; 1988:25.

Mosher WD, Pratt WF. Fecundity and infertility in the United States, 1965–1988. *Advance Data* 1990; 192:1.

IRRITABLE BOWEL SYNDROME

INTRODUCTION

Description: A syndrome of intermittent abdominal pain, constipation, and diarrhea related to hypermotility of the gut.

Prevalence: First described in 1818 and accounts for 50% of all visits to gastroenterologists; 2.4–3.5 million physician visits per year and an estimated 2.2 million prescriptions. Despite the prevalence of irritable bowel syndrome (IBS), only approximately 25% of those with IBS seek care, and only 1% of those with IBS are referred to specialists or become chronic health care users.

Predominant Age: Young to middle age.

Genetics: No genetic pattern, 2:1 female/male ratio.

ETIOLOGY AND PATHOGENESIS

Causes: Colonic wall motility is altered in these patients with evidence suggesting altered colonic wall sensitivity. Patients with IBS have altered motor reactivity to various stimuli, including meals, psychologic stress, and balloon distention of the rectosigmoid, resulting in altered transit time, which in turn results in pain, constipation, and diarrhea. Studies of patients with and without IBS have shown that there are significantly higher levels of 5-hydroxytryptamine (5-HT) in those patients with IBS, supporting a possible causal role.

Risk Factors: None known.

CLINICAL CHARACTERISTICS

Signs and Symptoms:
- Intermittent abdominal pain (often worse before menses)
- Bloating and nausea
- Alternating constipation and diarrhea

Symptoms are generally worse 1–1½ hours after meals, with 50% of patients experiencing pain that lasts for hours or days, and may last for weeks in up to 20% of patients. Pain is generally worse with high-fat meals, stress, depression, or menstruation and is better after bowel movements. There are three common clinical variants: (1) "spastic colitis" characterized by chronic abdominal pain and constipation; (2) intermittent diarrhea, which is usually painless; and (3) a combination of both with alternating diarrhea and constipation (see box).

DIAGNOSTIC APPROACH

Differential Diagnosis:
- Bacterial or parasitic infections
- Somatization
- Laxative abuse
- Iatrogenic diarrhea (dietary—eg, tea, coffee, food poisoning)
- Ulcerative colitis or Crohn's disease
- Lactose intolerance
- Diverticular disease

Associated Conditions: High prevalence of psychopathologic conditions among IBS suffers; a greater likelihood of somatization disorders, stress, anxiety disorders, depression, hysteria, and hypochondriases.

Workup and Evaluation

Laboratory: No evaluation indicated.

Imaging: No imaging indicated.

Special Tests: Flexible sigmoidoscopy or colonoscopy may be considered for selected patients.

Diagnostic Procedures: History and exclusion of other pathologic conditions.

Pathologic Findings

None.

MANAGEMENT AND THERAPY

Nonpharmacologic

General Measures: Because many of these patients have hysterical, depressive, and bipolar personality disorders, psychologic support is important. In some studies, placebo response rates are as high as 80%.

ROME II DIAGNOSTIC CRITERIA FOR IRRITABLE BOWEL SYNDROME

At least 12 weeks, which need not be consecutive, in the preceding 12 months, of abdominal discomfort or pain that has two of three features:
• Relieved with defecation
• Onset associated with a change in frequency of stool
• Onset associated with a change in form (appearance) of stool

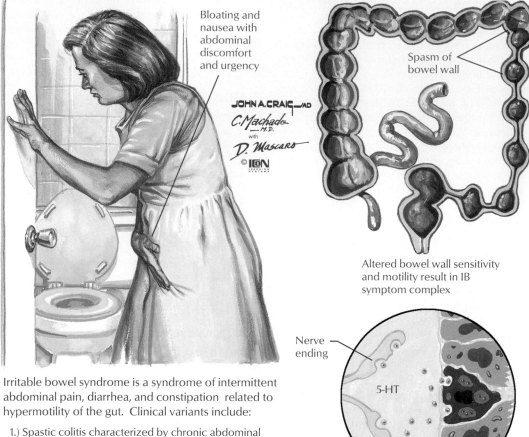

Bloating and nausea with abdominal discomfort and urgency

Spasm of bowel wall

Altered bowel wall sensitivity and motility result in IB symptom complex

Nerve ending

5-HT

Actions of gut wall 5-hydroxytryptamine (5-HT) may underlie anomalies of motility

Irritable bowel syndrome is a syndrome of intermittent abdominal pain, diarrhea, and constipation related to hypermotility of the gut. Clinical variants include:

1.) Spastic colitis characterized by chronic abdominal pain and constipation
2.) Intermittent diarrhea that is usually painless
3.) Combination of both with alternating diarrhea and constipation

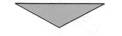

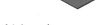

Rome II diagnostic criteria for irritable bowel syndrome	Symptoms suggestive of diagnoses beyond functional bowel disease
12 week history out of past 12 months of abdominal pain and discomfort incorporating 2 of 3 features: 1.) Relieved by defecation 2.) Onset associated with change in stool frequency 3.) Onset associated with change in stool form (appearance)	1.) Anemia 2.) Fever 3.) Persistent diarrhea 4.) Rectal bleeding 5.) Severe constipation 6.) Weight loss 7.) Nocturnal GI symptoms 8.) Family history of GI cancer, inflammatory bowel disease, or celiac disease 9.) New onset of symptoms after age 50

Specific Measures: Mild sedation with phenobarbital and tranquilizers may afford some relief, although long-term success is generally poor.

Diet: Bulk agents and increased dietary fiber, reduction in alcohol, fat, caffeine, and sorbitol.

Activity: No restriction.

Patient Education: Diet (increased fiber) and stress management. Biofeedback and relaxation techniques may be of some help.

Drug(s) of Choice

Bulk-forming agents including Guar gum. Emerging 5-HT$_3$ receptor-blocking agents.

Contraindications: Bowel obstruction or fecal impaction, known or suspected allergy to agent or any component.

Precautions: Empiric therapy may be started during the process of evaluation, but should not be continued indefinitely without the establishment of a diagnosis. Bulk-forming agents must be taken with adequate fluid intake to prevent obstruction and provide optimal effects.

FOLLOW-UP

Patient Monitoring: Normal health maintenance.

Prevention/Avoidance: High-fiber diet, stress reduction.

Possible Complications: Continued dependency on others, adverse effects of work, school, or home functions. Relapses are common.

Expected Outcome: Transient response is often good with most therapies. Long-term relapse is common.

MISCELLANEOUS

Pregnancy Considerations: No effect on pregnancy.

ICD-9-CM Codes: 564.1.

REFERENCES

American Gastroenterological Association Patient Care Committee. American Gastroenterological Association medical position statement: irritable bowel syndrome. *Gastroenterology* 1997;112: 2118.

American Gastroenterological Association. Irritable bowel syndrome: a technical review for practice guideline development. *Gastroenterology* 1997;112:2120.

Bearcroft CP, Perrett D, Farthing MJG. Postprandial plasma 5-hydroxytryptamine in diarrhea predominant irritable bowel syndrome: a pilot study. *Gut* 1998;42:42.

Drossman DA, Thompson WG. The irritable bowel syndrome: review and a graduated multicomponent treatment approach. *Ann Intern Med* 1992;116:1009.

Gershon MD. Review article: roles played by 5-hydroxytryptamine in the physiology of the bowel. *Aliment Pharmacol Ther* 1999;13(suppl 2):15.

Hannauer SB. Inflammatory bowel disease. In: Wyngaarden JB, Smith LH Jr, Bennett JC, eds. *Cecil Textbook of Medicine.* 19th ed. Philadelphia, Pa: WB Saunders; 1992:699.

Humphrey PPA, Bountra C, Clayton N, Kozlowski K. Review article: the therapeutic potential of 5-HT3 receptor antagonists in the treatment of irritable bowel syndrome. *Aliment Pharmacol Ther* 1999;13(suppl 2):31.

Mitchell CM, Drossman DA. The irritable bowel syndrome: understanding and treating a biopsychosocial illness disorder. *Ann Behav Med* 1987;9:13.

Paterson WG, Thompson WG, Vanner SJ, et al. Recommendations for the management of irritable bowel syndrome in family practice. *Can Med Assoc J* 1999; 161:154.

Rapkin AJ, Mayer EA. Gastroenterologic causes of chronic pelvic pain. *Obstet Gynecol Clin North Am* 1993;20:663.

Snape WJ Jr. Disorders of gastrointestinal motility. In: Wyngaarden JB, Smith LH Jr, Bennett JC, eds. *Cecil Textbook of Medicine.* 19th ed. Philadelphia, Pa: WB Saunders; 1992:671.

LOW BACK PAIN

INTRODUCTION

Description: Pain located in the lower portion of the back (generally between the level of the iliac spines and the lower ribs) with radiation to the abdomen, pelvis, legs, or trunk. In women, gynecologic processes are often implicated (correctly or incorrectly) in this complaint. Low back pain is especially common during pregnancy.
Prevalence: Common (80% suffer some form of low back pain during their lifetime).
Predominant Age: 25–45.
Genetics: No genetic pattern.

ETIOLOGY AND PATHOGENESIS

Causes: Normal aging aggravated by trauma, injury, or pregnancy.
Risk Factors: Obesity, poor posture, improper lifting, age, sedentary lifestyle, osteoporosis, psychosocial factors (secondary gain), and trauma.

CLINICAL CHARACTERISTICS

Signs and Symptoms:
- Pain and discomfort between the level of the iliac spines and the lower ribs, generally sudden in onset after an injury or gradually over the subsequent 24 hours
- Radiation of pain to buttocks or posterior thighs (stopping at the knees), referred pain, not radicular: back pain greater than leg pain
- Pain aggravated by back motion, lifting, coughing, straining, bending, or twisting, relieved by rest
- Normal sensory, motor and reflex findings, decreased range of motion

DIAGNOSTIC APPROACH

Differential Diagnosis:
- Gynecologic disease (pregnancy, endometriosis, PID)
- Gastrointestinal disease (duodenal ulcer, pancreatitis, IBS, diverticulitis)
- Urinary tract disease (pyelonephritis, nephrolithiasis)
- Disc herniation or degenerative disease
- Osteoporotic fracture
- Fibromyalgia
- Spinal stenosis
- Spondylolisthesis
- Ankylosing spondylitis
- Arthritis (hip or back)
- Neoplasia (primary or metastatic)
- Fictitious complaint (somatization, secondary gain)

Associated Conditions: Chronic pain states (pelvic pain, headaches), radiculopathy, obesity, and psychosocial disease. Secondary gain often complicates both the diagnosis and treatment of low back pain. Warning signs of significant secondary gain include pending litigation or compensation, depression, hostility, and prolonged use of potent analgesics.

Workup and Evaluation

Laboratory: No evaluation indicated unless suggested by nonmechanical symptoms or atypical patterns of pain.
Imaging: Generally not required. When indicated (persistent pain, atypical symptoms)—anteroposterior, lateral, and spot films of L_5–S_1 area. Bone scan if tumor, trauma, or infection is suspected.
Special Tests: CT, MRI, or myelography only for specific cause.
Diagnostic Procedures: History and physical examination (with special attention to the back and hips).

Pathologic Findings

Based on cause.

MANAGEMENT AND THERAPY

Nonpharmacologic

General Measures: Bed rest, short-term analgesics or antiinflammatory agents, massage, or manipulation.
Specific Measures: Muscle relaxants, Williams' flexion exercises, physical therapy.
Diet: No specific dietary changes indicated. Weight reduction if appropriate.
Activity: Restricted activity for 3–6 weeks, then a gradual return to normal activity as tolerated. Patients should begin Williams' flexion exercises as prevention for future injuries.
Patient Education: Posture and activity counseling, home back exercises, American College of Obstetricians and Gynecologists Patient Education Pamphlet AP115 (*Easing Back Pain During Pregnancy*).

Drug(s) of Choice

NSAIDs, muscle relaxants—cyclobenzaprine (Flexeril) 10 mg PO tid, diazepam (Valium) 5–10 mg PO bid.
Contraindications: See individual agents. Aspirin-sensitive asthma for most agents.
Precautions: See individual agents. Ulcer or renal disease for most agents.
Interactions: See individual agents.

Effects of Lumbar Hyperlordosis on Spinal Nerve Roots

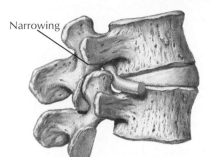

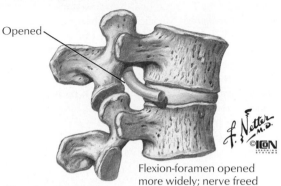

Narrowing

Opened

Hyperlordosis-intervertebral foramen greatly narrowed

Flexion-foramen opened more widely; nerve freed

Treatment of Lumbar Strain

Acute	Chronic and prophylactic
Absolute bed rest	Reduction of weight
Warm tub baths, heat pad, hydrocollator	Correction of posture
Sedation	Firm mattress, bed board
Firm mattress, bed board	Daily low back exercises
Diathermy, massage	Regular sports activity compatible
Local anesthetic infiltration to trigger zones	with age and physique
Occasionally corset, brace, or strapping	

Exercises for chronic lumbar strain (starting positions in outline)

1. Lie on back, arms on chest, knees bent. Press small of back firmly down to floor, tightening muscles of abdomen and buttocks, thus tilting pubis forward, exhale simultaneously. Hold for count of 10, relax and repeat

2. Lie on back, arms at sides, knees bent. Draw knees up and pull them firmly to chest with clasped hands several times. Relax and repeat. Also, repeat exercise using one leg at a time

3. Lie on back, knees bent, arms folded on chest or at sides. Sit up using abdominal muscles and reach forward. Return slowly to starting position

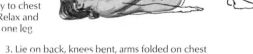

4. Begin in a runner's starting position (one leg extended, the other forward as shown, hands on floor) Press downward and forward several times, flexing front knee and bringing abdomen to thigh. Repeat with legs reversed

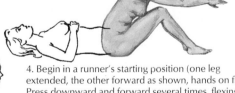

6. Sit on chair, hands folded in lap. Bend forward, bringing chin between knees. Return slowly to starting position while tensing abdominal muscles. Relax and repeat

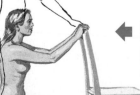

5. Stand with hands on back of chair. Squat, straightening hollow of back. Return to starting position and repeat

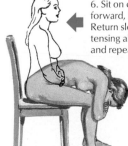

Exercises are best done on hard, padded surface like carpeted floor. Start slowly. Do each only once or twice a day, then progressively to 10 or more times within limits of comfort. Pain, but not mild discomfort, is indication to stop

FOLLOW-UP

Patient Monitoring: Normal health maintenance.

Prevention/Avoidance: Muscle-strengthening exercises, care in lifting, maintenance of reasonable weight. Avoid tasks that aggravate (heavy lifting, bending, twisting, sudden movements). Weight reduction, if appropriate.

Possible Complications: Chronic low back pain, pain medication dependence, and dependency state resulting from secondary gain.

Expected Outcome: Gradual improvement with analgesics, muscle relaxants, massage, and exercise (1–6 weeks).

MISCELLANEOUS

Pregnancy Considerations: No effect on pregnancy, although pregnancy (and the postural changes brought about by it) may worsen existing low back pain. Some relief is gained when the fetus descends into the pelvis in the last days of the gestation, but the sudden return to upright and the constant bending to care for a newborn make this improvement short-lived.

ICD-9-CM Codes: Based on cause.

REFERENCES

American Academy of Orthopedic Surgeons: *Clinical Policy; Low Back Musculoligamentous Injury (Sprain/Strain)*. Rosemont, Ill: AAOS; 1991. AAOS Bulletin 3638.

American College of Obstetricians and Gynecologists. *Chronic Pelvic Pain*. Washington, DC: ACOG; 1996. ACOG Technical Bulletin 223.

Chadwick PR. Examination, assessment and treatment of the lumbar spine. *Physiotherapy* 1984;70:2.

Cipriano JJ. *Photographic Manual of Regional Orthopaedic and Neurological Tests*. Baltimore, Md: Williams & Wilkins; 1991:48.

International Association for the Study of Pain. Classification of chronic pain, descriptions of chronic pain syndromes and definitions of pain terms. *Pain* 1986;3(suppl):S1.

Ling FW, ed. Contemporary management of chronic pelvic pain. *Obstet Gynecol Clin North Am* 1993;20:627.

Smith RP, Ling FW. Back examination. In: *Procedures in Women's Health Care*. Baltimore, Md: Williams & Wilkins; 1997:367.

MELANOMA

INTRODUCTION

Description: Malignant degeneration of cells from the melanocytic (pigment) system. Although generally a skin lesion, melanomas may arise in any pigmented tissue (such as the eye). The vulva accounts for 5% to 10% of all malignant melanomas in women despite containing only 1% of the skin surface.

Prevalence: Found in 4.5 of 100,000, 1995—38,000 cases, 6,700 deaths.

Predominant Age: 20–40 years (50% of patients).

Genetics: Familial dysplastic nevus syndrome (if history includes a family member with melanoma, lifetime risk is 100%).

ETIOLOGY AND PATHOGENESIS

Causes: Unknown, may be related to ultraviolet (A + B) light exposure.

Risk Factors: Previous dysplastic nevi, multiple pigmented lesions, fair complexion, freckling, blue eyes and blond hair, adolescent blistering sunburn (2-fold increase in risk), family history of melanoma.

CLINICAL CHARACTERISTICS

Signs and Symptoms:
- Asymptomatic
- Pigmented lesion with irregular border and variegation in color
- Bleeding, scaling, size, or texture change in any pigmented lesion (ABCDE mnemonic—asymmetry, border irregularity, color variegation, diameter >6 mm on back or lower leg [whites] or hand, feet, and nails [blacks], elevation above the skin surface)

DIAGNOSTIC APPROACH

Differential Diagnosis:
- Junctional nevus
- Dysplastic nevus
- Malignant melanoma (the risk of malignancy is greatest in nevi that are more than 5 mm in diameter, have irregular borders, asymmetry, or variegated coloration)
- Pigmented basal or squamous cell carcinoma
- Seborrheic keratoses

Associated Conditions: Junctional nevus, dysplastic nevus.

Workup and Evaluation

Laboratory: No evaluation indicated.

Imaging: No imaging indicated, used only to evaluate metastases (brain, bone, lymph nodes).

Special Tests: Excisional biopsy for all vulvar nevi or suspicious nevi anywhere on the body. All lesions should be submitted for histologic examination, never removed destructively.

Diagnostic Procedures: Physical examination and excisional biopsy.

Pathologic Findings

Superficial spreading melanoma (70% of cases), nodular (vertical growth, 15%), acral lentiginous (2%–8%), lentigo maligna (4%–10%).

MANAGEMENT AND THERAPY

Nonpharmacologic

General Measures: Evaluation, biopsy of suspicious lesions, instruction on prevention (sun screen use, excessive exposure avoidance).

Specific Measures: Surgical excision with 1 cm margin for lesions <2 mm thick, 3 cm for thicker lesions.

Diet: No specific dietary changes indicated.

Activity: Sun exposure reduction and protection.

Patient Education: Risks of sun exposure, use of sun screen products, characteristics of suspicious lesions.

Drug(s) of Choice

Adjuvant therapy with bacillus Calmette-Guérin and levamisole plus dacarbazine.

Contraindications: See individual agents.

Precautions: See individual agents.

Interactions: See individual agents.

FOLLOW-UP

Patient Monitoring: Frequent (every 3–6 months) total body inspection for abnormal or changing nevi. Annual chest radiograph (6% of recurrences diagnosed this way). Weekly self-examination.

Prevention/Avoidance: Avoidance of excessive sun exposure, especially blistering sunburn. Sun screen use.

Possible Complications: Disease progression or spread, cosmetic damage by excision.

Expected Outcome: Prognosis is based on staging—5-year survival if no local or distant spread 70%; <0.85 mm thick 95%–100%; lymphatic involvement 5%.

MISCELLANEOUS

Pregnancy Considerations: Although rarely seen, melanoma is exacerbated by pregnancy. Although any malignant metastasis to the fetus is rare, melanomas represent up to one third of all malignancies found. Melanoma is one of the few malignancies that spreads to the placenta, and metastatic melanoma is a threat to both the fetus and mother. If a woman has had a melanoma, it is recommended that she wait 2 or more years before planning a pregnancy.

ICD-9-CM Codes: Based on location and severity of disease.

REFERENCES

Blickstein I, Feldberg E, Dgani R, Ben-Hur H, Czernobilsky B. Dysplastic vulvar nevi. *Obstet Gynecol* 1991; 78:968.

Dunton CJ, Kautzky M, Hanau C. Malignant melanoma of the vulva: a review. *Obstet Gynecol Surv* 1995; 57:739.

Friedman RJ, Rigel DS, Kopf AW. Early detection of malignant melanoma: the role of physician examination and self-examination of the skin. *CA Cancer J Clin* 1985;35:130.

Koh HK. Cutaneous melanoma. *N Engl J Med* 1991; 325:171.

NIH Consensus Development Panel on Early Melanoma. Diagnosis and treatment of early melanoma. *JAMA* 1992;268:1314.

Silvers NC, Halperin AJ. Cutaneous and vulvar melanoma: an update. *Clin Obstet Gynecol* 1978;21:1117.

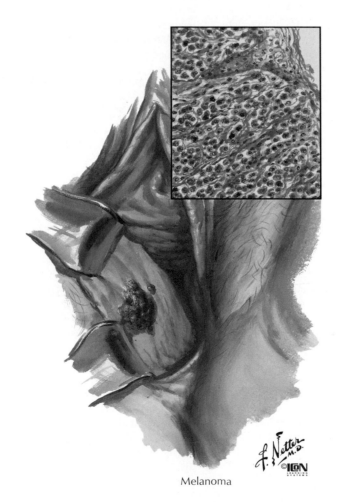

Melanoma

Melanoma

Clinical Considerations

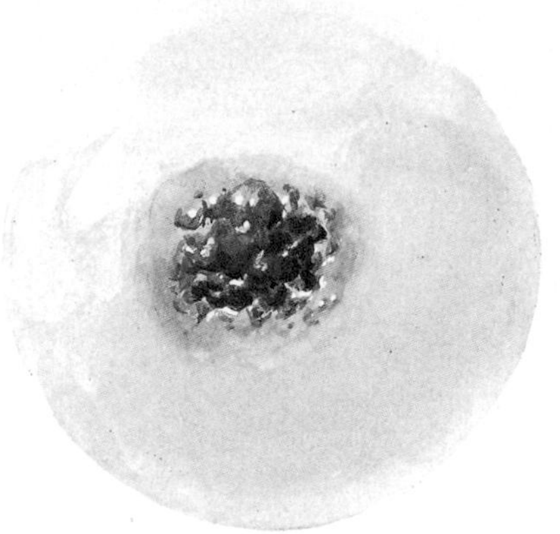

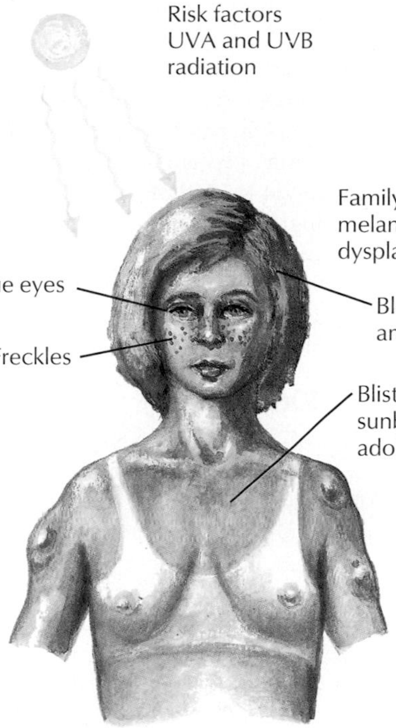

Risk factors
UVA and UVB
radiation

Family history of
melanoma or
dysplastic nevi

Blue eyes

Blonde hair
and fair skin

Freckles

Blistering
sunburn in
adolescence

Typical clinical appearance
of melanoma exhibiting
features of "ABCDE" mnemonic
A.) Asymmetry
B.) Border irregularity
C.) Color variegation
D.) Diameter >6 mm
E.) Elevation above skin surface

Excisions of Lesions

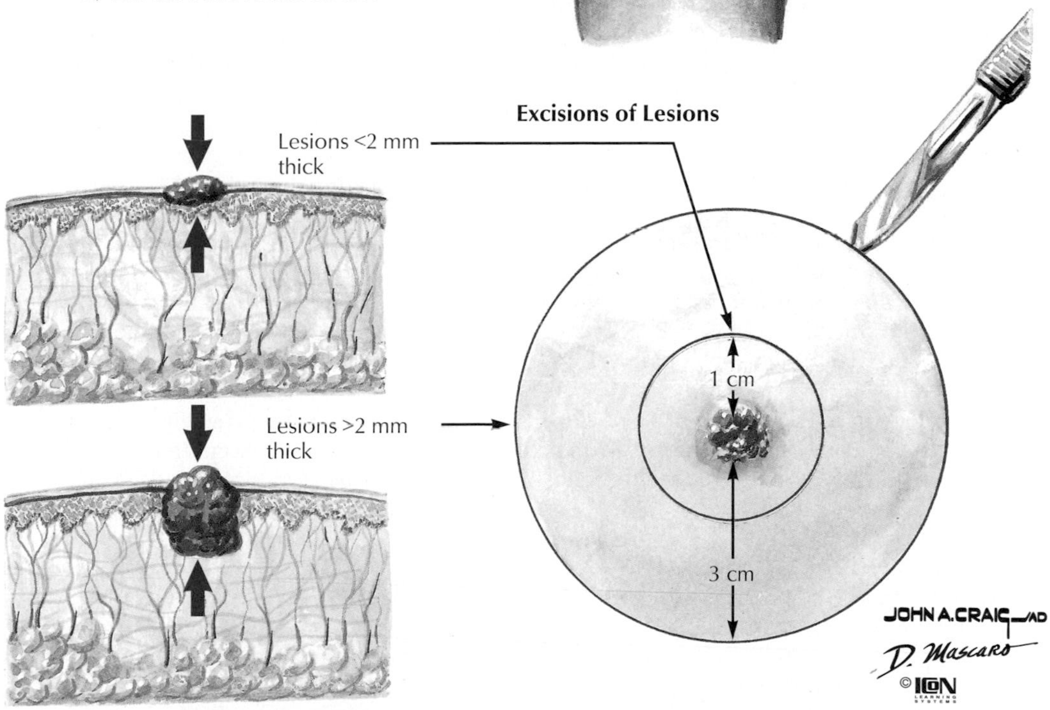

Lesions <2 mm
thick

Lesions >2 mm
thick

1 cm

3 cm

JOHN A. CRAIG——AD

D. Mascaro

© ICON
LEARNING
SYSTEMS

Wide excision of dysplastic nevi and suspected melanomas is based
on thickness of lesion—ICM border recommended for lesions less
than 2 mm thick, and 3 cm border for lesions greater than 2 mm thick

MYOFASCIAL SYNDROMES

INTRODUCTION

Description: A syndrome of muscular and fascial pain associated with localized tenderness and pain referred to sites that are often remote. Myofascial pain syndromes and fibromyalgia frequently demonstrate trigger-point involvement. These syndromes may present as chronic lower abdominal or pelvic pain that is easily confused with gynecologic causes.

Prevalence: Three percent of the population.

Predominant Age: Sedentary middle-aged women.

Genetics: No genetic pattern. More common in women.

ETIOLOGY AND PATHOGENESIS

Causes: Abnormal spasm of a small portion of a muscle resulting in an extremely taut, tender band of muscle (trigger point). Compression of this site elicits local tenderness and often reproduces the referred pain. Most trigger points are located at or near areas of moving or sliding muscle surfaces, although they are not limited to these locations.

Risk Factors: Stress, sleep deprivation, trauma, depression, and weather changes.

CLINICAL CHARACTERISTICS

Signs and Symptoms:
- Chronic pain referred to remote sites.
- "Trigger points" (hypersensitive areas overlying muscles that induce spasm and pain) that induce, or reproduce, the patient's symptoms (trigger points may be found throughout the body, but are most common in the abdominal wall, back, and pelvic floor when pelvic pain is the symptom)
- Pain worse in the morning, with stress or weather change, nonrestorative sleep and better with activity, stress reduction, rest

DIAGNOSTIC APPROACH

Differential Diagnosis:
- Somatization
- Sympathetic dystrophy
- Muscle strain or sprain
- Polymyalgia rheumatica
- Temporal arteritis
- IBS
- Low back strain or sprain

Associated Conditions: Chronic pain syndromes, IBS, depression, reduced physical endurance, and social withdrawal.

Workup and Evaluation

Laboratory: No evaluation indicated. Screening with an erythrocyte sedimentation rate (normal) may be helpful. Others based on diagnosis being considered.

Imaging: No imaging indicated.

Special Tests: None indicated.

Diagnostic Procedures: History and physical examination generally sufficient.

Pathologic Findings

A trigger point is often felt as an extremely taut band of muscle. (Normal muscle should not be tender to firm compression and does not contain taut bands.)

MANAGEMENT AND THERAPY

Nonpharmacologic

General Measures: Evaluation, analgesics, heat (hot packs, ultrasound therapy), and general conditioning exercises.

Specific Measures: TENS, trigger point injections. A 22-gauge needle is selected for trigger point injection because of the amount of movement within tissue often required to probe for and block a taut muscle bundle. Thinner needles may bend or break under these circumstances. The length of the needle should be sufficient to allow the entire trigger point to be reached without indenting the skin or having the hub at the skin surface. Superficial trigger points may also be treated with a "spray-and-stretch" technique. (The area overlying the trigger point is sprayed with a coolant or freezing spray [eg, ethyl chloride] for several seconds, and the muscle is forcibly stretched by passive extension.) Hypnosis may also be used.

Diet: No specific dietary changes indicated.

Activity: No restriction except that caused by pain.

Patient Education: American College of Obstetricians and Gynecologists Patient Education Pamphlet AP099 (*Pelvic Pain*).

Drug(s) of Choice

NSAIDs.

Sleep aids—flurazepam (Dalmane) 15 mg PO qhs, triazolam (Halcion) 0.125 mg PO qhs, amitriptyline (Elavil) 20–25 mg PO qhs.

Muscle relaxants—cyclobenzaprine (Flexeril) 10 mg PO tid.

Local anesthetic for injection (generally 1% lidocaine without epinephrine, limit injection to approximately 10 mL/site).

Myofascial Syndromes

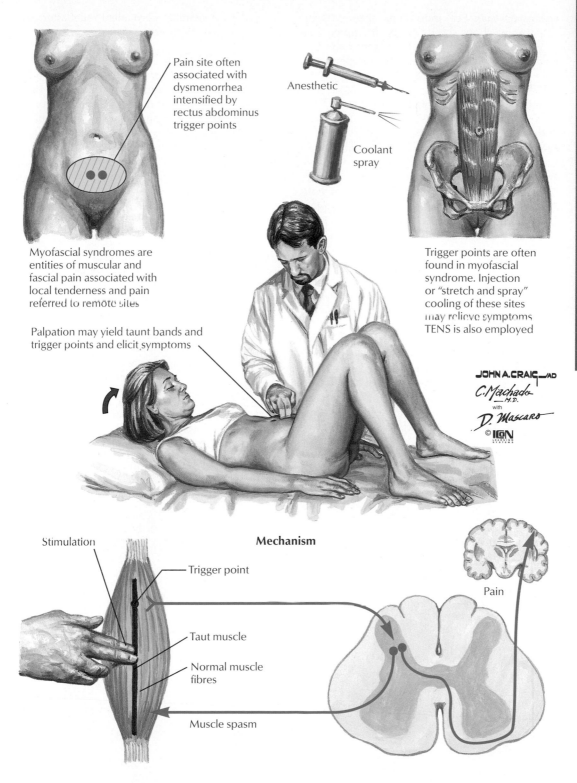

Pain site often associated with dysmenorrhea intensified by rectus abdominus trigger points

Anesthetic

Coolant spray

Myofascial syndromes are entities of muscular and fascial pain associated with local tenderness and pain referred to remote sites

Trigger points are often found in myofascial syndrome. Injection or "stretch and spray" cooling of these sites may relieve symptoms. TENS is also employed

Palpation may yield taunt bands and trigger points and elicit symptoms

JOHN A. CRAIG, MD
C. Machado M.D.
with
D. Mascaro
© ICN

Mechanism

Stimulation

Trigger point

Taut muscle

Normal muscle fibres

Muscle spasm

Pain

Symptoms cause abnormal spasm of small portion of muscle, resulting in extremely taut, tender band of muscle (trigger point). Compression of this site elicits local tenderness and often produces referred pain

Contraindications: See individual agents. Trigger point injections should not be attempted when infection is present near the planned site.

Precautions: Watch for side effects or dependence.

Alternative Drugs

Trazodone (Desyrel) 50 mg PO qhs.

FOLLOW-UP

Patient Monitoring: Normal health maintenance, monitor for medication side effects.

Prevention/Avoidance: Adequate restorative sleep, stress reduction, physical fitness, and activity.

Possible Complications: Depression, reduced physical endurance, social withdrawal, and chronic pain, work compromise, or absence. The most common complications of trigger point injection are local ecchymoses and anesthetic agent toxicity. The latter is best avoided by strictly limiting the total dose given. Infection is rare if the skin is first disinfected and areas of frank infection are avoided.

Expected Outcome: Improvement with medical therapy generally is seen in 2–4 weeks. With the identification of a specific trigger point and the use of trigger point injection, results should be good. (Response to trigger point injection routinely persists longer than the duration of action of the anesthetic agent used. This frequently extends to permanent relief after only one or two injections.)

MISCELLANEOUS

Pregnancy Considerations: No effect on pregnancy. Pregnancy may limit some therapies. Pregnancy is generally not a contraindication to trigger point injections.

***ICD-9-CM* Codes:** Based on type and location.

REFERENCES

Campbell SM. Regional myofascial pain syndromes. *Rheum Dis Clin North Am* 1989;15:31.

Garvey TA, Marks MR, Wiesel SW. A prospective, randomized, double-blind evaluation of trigger-point injection therapy for low-back pain. *Spine* 1989; 14:962.

Ling FW, Slocumb JC. Use of trigger point injections in chronic pelvic pain. *Obstet Gynecol Clin North Am* 1993;20:809.

McClaflin RR. Myofascial pain syndrome. Primary care strategies for early intervention. *Postgrad Med* 1994; 96:56.

Rothschild B. Diagnosing and treating fibrositis and fibromyalgia. *Geriatr Consultant* 1990;9:26.

Slocumb JC. Neurologic factors in chronic pelvic pain: trigger points and the abdominal pelvic pain syndrome. *Am J Obstet Gynecol* 1984;149:536.

Wolfe F, Smythe HA, Yunus MB, et al. The American College of Rheumatology criteria for the classification of fibromyalgia. *Arthritis Rheum* 1990;33:160.

OBESITY

INTRODUCTION

Description: Increased fat and lean body mass (>20% above ideal weight, body mass index [BMI] >28) associated with increase health risks. Obesity affects more women than men and is of special concern to adolescents and older women. Weight gained during pregnancy (in excess of that related to the pregnancy) is often not lost.

Prevalence: Varies with age: 30%–40% of women.

Predominant Age: Any.

Genetics: Of the variance in body mass, 20%–30% may be genetically determined. Rare genetic syndromes have been described.

ETIOLOGY AND PATHOGENESIS

Causes: Caloric consumption in excess of expenditure, insulinoma, hypothalamic disorders, Cushing's syndrome, corticosteroid drugs.

Risk Factors: Parental obesity, pregnancy, sedentary lifestyle, high-fat diet (higher calorie density), low socioeconomic status.

CLINICAL CHARACTERISTICS

Signs and Symptoms:
- Increased body mass and fat (Male pattern obesity [abdominal] is associated with the greatest health risk.)

DIAGNOSTIC APPROACH

Differential Diagnosis:
- Pathologic process other than excess dietary consumption

Associated Conditions: Increased morbidity and mortality (see complications).

Workup and Evaluation

Laboratory: No evaluation indicated. Consider thyroid testing in selected patients. Serum cholesterol, triglycerides, or glucose to assess risk factors for complications.

Imaging: No imaging indicated.

Special Tests: BMI = weight (kg)/height (m²), waist to hip circumference ration (normal female gynecoid pattern is greater than 0.85).

Diagnostic Procedures: Physical examination, BMI.

Pathologic Findings

Hypertrophy and/or hyperplasia of adipocytes. Cardiomegaly or hepatomegaly is common.

MANAGEMENT AND THERAPY

Nonpharmacologic

General Measures: Risk assessment, diet and exercise counseling. Assistance with diet planning or selection of a commercial program.

Specific Measures: Behavior modification and hypnosis have been applied with variable success. In rare patients (BMI >40) surgical intervention (stapling or bypass) may be indicated. Surgery is the most effective long-term therapy for morbid obesity.

Diet: Restriction to 500 kcal below maintenance generally provides the best sustainable loss (1 lb/wk). Very-low-calorie diets are associated with increased risk and occasional deaths.

Activity: A program of physical activity should accompany any calorie restriction diet. Activity by itself is generally ineffective.

Patient Education: Diet and exercise instruction, behavior modification, American College of Obstetricians and Gynecologists Patient Education Pamphlet AP045 (*Exercise and Health: A Guide for Women*), AP064 (*Weight Control: Eating Right and Keeping Fit*), AP101 (*Cholesterol and Your Health*).

Drug(s) of Choice

Drug therapy is not generally recommended. Orlistat [Xenical] 120 mg PO tid, taken during or up to 1 hour after meals; taken with meals containing fat).

Contraindications: See individual agents. Most are contraindicated in the presence of atherosclerosis or other heart disease, hypertension, hyperthyroidism, or glaucoma. Patients with chronic malabsorption syndromes or cholestasis should avoid orlistat.

Precautions: Relapse common, abuse potential is high for stimulants. Diarrhea, fatty stools, increased frequency of bowel movements, fecal incontinence, abdominal pain, and nausea may occur with orlistat therapy.

Interactions: Some agents may cause arrhythmias with general anesthetic agents. Orlistat can interact with cyclosporine, fat-soluble vitamin absorption, and warfarin.

Alternative Drugs

Phenylpropanolamine (over-the-counter preparations).

FOLLOW-UP

Patient Monitoring: Long-term follow-up, screening for complications of drug therapy or obesity itself.

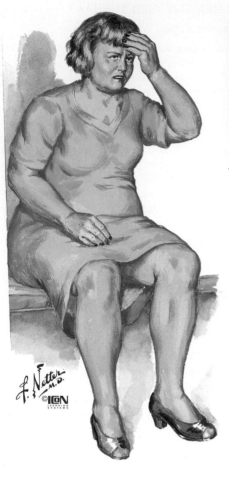

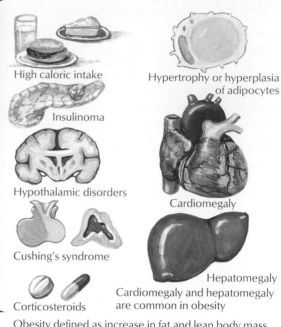

High caloric intake

Insulinoma

Hypothalamic disorders

Cushing's syndrome

Corticosteroids

Hypertrophy or hyperplasia of adipocytes

Cardiomegaly

Hepatomegaly

Cardiomegaly and hepatomegaly are common in obesity

Obesity defined as increase in fat and lean body mass greater than 20% above ideal body weight

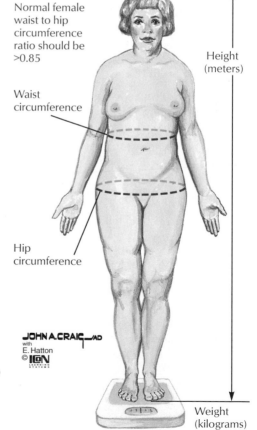

Normal female waist to hip circumference ratio should be >0.85

Waist circumference

Hip circumference

Height (meters)

Weight (kilograms)

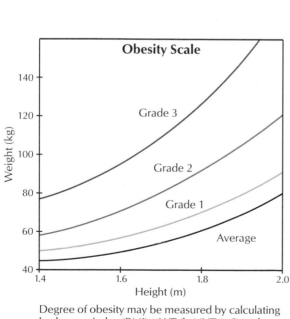

Obesity Scale

Grade 3

Grade 2

Grade 1

Average

Weight (kg): 40, 60, 80, 100, 120, 140

Height (m): 1.4, 1.6, 1.8, 2.0

Degree of obesity may be measured by calculating body mass index (BMI) = WT (kg)/HT (m²) and comparison with standardized charts.

$$\text{BMI} = \text{WT (kg)}/\text{HT (m}^2)$$

Prevention/Avoidance: Diet and exercise counseling (especially important for adolescents and children).

Possible Complications: Significant increase in risk for cardiovascular disease, diabetes mellitus, hypertension, hyperlipidemia, cholelithiasis, cholecystitis, osteoarthritis, gout, thromboembolism, and sleep apnea.

Expected Outcome: Long-term maintenance is difficult and relapses are common. Individual motivation is the best predictor of success.

MISCELLANEOUS

Pregnancy Considerations: Obesity complicates pregnancy, and pregnancy is often the time of onset of obesity for many women. Weight gain should be monitored and adjusted downward for obese patients. Orlistat is a category B medication.

ICD-9-CM Codes: 278.00, 278.01 (Morbid).

REFERENCES

Bray GA, ed. Obesity. *Endocrinol Metab Clin North Am* 1996;25.

Danford D, Fletcher JW. Methods for voluntary weight loss and control. National Institutes of Health Technology Assessment Conference. *Ann Intern Med* 1993;119 (7, pt 2):41.

Huang Z, Willett WC, Manson JE, et al. Body weight, weight change, and risk for hypertension in women. *Ann Intern Med* 1998;128:81.

Legato MJ. Gender-specific aspects of obesity. *Int J Fertil Womens Med* 1997;42:184.

Pasquali R, Casimirri F, Vicennati V. Weight control and its beneficial effect on fertility in women with obesity and polycystic ovary syndrome. *Hum Reprod* 1997;12(suppl 1):82.

Pettigrew R, Hamilton-Fairley D. Obesity and female reproductive function. *Br Med Bull* 1997;53:341.

Pujol P, Galtier-Dereure F, Bringer J. Obesity and breast cancer risk. *Hum Reprod* 1997;12(suppl 1):116.

Regulation of body weight. *Science* 1998;280:1363.

OSTEOPOROSIS

INTRODUCTION

Description: Loss of bone mass (calcium) that puts the patient at risk for fracture with minimal trauma or during activities of daily living. This process disproportionately affects older women and results in significant morbidity and mortality. Estimates of medical costs are as high as $10 billion each year in the United States.

Prevalence: Forty percent of women older than 75 (not receiving estrogen replacement) have spine, hip, or forearm fractures; 80% of hip fractures occur in this group.

Predominant Age: Postmenopausal.

Genetics: More common in some races (thought to be a function of peak bone mass).

ETIOLOGY AND PATHOGENESIS

Causes: Alcohol use/abuse, chronic illness, diabetes mellitus, estrogen loss, especially early menopause, excessive caffeine use, family history of osteoporosis, high parity, high protein intake, inactivity/sedentary lifestyle, inadequate vitamin D intake or sun exposure, low body weight, medical therapy (anticonvulsants, corticosteroids, excess thyroid hormone replacement, long-term heparin or tetracycline use, loop diuretics, chemotherapy), poor diet/inadequate calcium intake (<1000 mg/d), race white or oriental, radiation therapy, smoking.

Risk Factors: Menopause (without estrogen replacement), inactivity, presence of other causes as above. (Women suffer roughly a 10-fold increase in the normal rate of bone loss for a period of about 10 years beginning with the loss of ovarian function. This results in an average lifetime loss of approximately 35% of cortical bone mass and 50% of the more metabolically active trabecular bone. By comparison, men lose only about two thirds this amount.)

CLINICAL CHARACTERISTICS

Signs and Symptoms:
- Asymptomatic
- Spinal, hip, or forearm fractures (with or without pain, fractures should be suspected in idiopathic back pain in at-risk patients)
- Loss of height (up to 4–8 inches)
- Development of kyphoscoliosis ("dowager's hump")

DIAGNOSTIC APPROACH

Differential Diagnosis:
- Metastatic tumor (breast)
- Paget's disease (osteitis deformans)
- Multiple myeloma
- Unreported trauma (abuse, elder abuse)
- Cushing's disease

Associated Conditions: Dyspareunia, vulvodynia, atrophic vulvitis, increased risk of cardiovascular disease, hot flashes and flushes, sleep disturbances, urinary incontinence, and others associated with hypoestrogenic states.

Workup and Evaluation

Laboratory: No evaluation specifically indicated.

Imaging: Dual-photon absorptiometry or quantitative CT. Routine radiographic studies (eg, chest radiograph) do not detect changes until almost 30% of bone has been lost (approximately equal to fracture threshold, 1 gm/cm^2).

Special Tests: Urinary tests for bone metabolites are investigational only.

Diagnostic Procedures: Radiographic assessment of bone mass.

Pathologic Findings

Loss of bone calcium, thinning of trabeculae, microfractures, macrofractures (spine, hips, forearms).

MANAGEMENT AND THERAPY

Nonpharmacologic

General Measures: Smoking cessation, alcohol and caffeine intake in moderation, weight-bearing exercise, adequate dietary calcium or supplementation.

Specific Measures: Hormone replacement therapy, bisphosphonates, calcitonin (infrequently used, reserved for selected patients as a therapeutic agent, not as prevention).

Diet: Adequate dietary intake of calcium (1000–1500 mg/d) and vitamin D (400–800 IU daily). (Supplementation of vitamin D beyond this dose is generally not warranted.)

Activity: Weight-bearing exercise or exercise against resistance. Low-impact activities for those with established bone loss.

Patient Education: Reassurance, American College of Obstetricians and Gynecologists Patient Education Pamphlet AP048 (*Preventing Osteoporosis*), AP047 (*The Menopause Years*), AP045 (*Exercise and Fitness: A Guide for Women*), AP066 (*Hormone Replacement Therapy*).

Radiographic Findings in Axial Osteoporosis

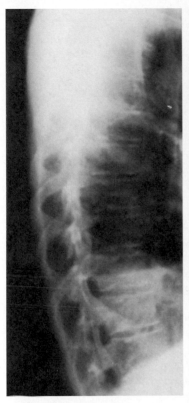

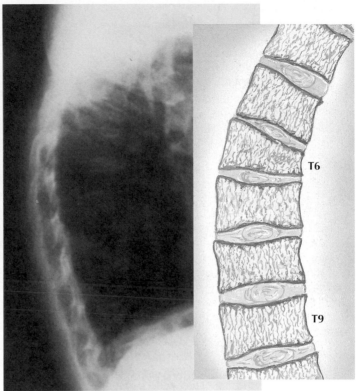

Mild osteopenia in post-
menopausal women. Vertebrae
appear "washed-out"; no
kyphosis or vertebral collapse

Anterior wedge compression at T6 in same patient 16½ years
later. Patient has lymphoma, with multiple biconcave ("codfish")
vertebral bodies and kyphosis. Focal lesion at T6 suggests
neoplasm

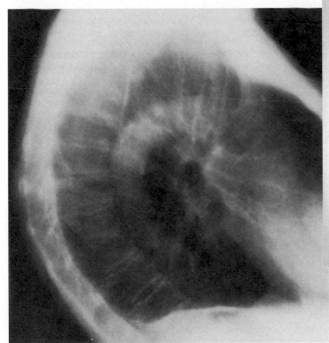

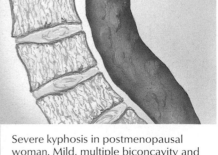

Severe kyphosis in postmenopausal
woman. Mild, multiple biconcavity and
wedging of vertebrae. Extensive
calcification of aorta

Drug(s) of Choice

Estrogen replacement therapy (with progesterone if indicated). See "Menopause" for
dosage options. (Estrogen's effect on bone
protection appears to depend on obtaining
a relatively normal [premenopausal] blood
level [40–60 pg/mL] and is not affected by
the route of therapy.)

Selective estrogen receptor modulators (also
known as tissue selective estrogens). Many
of these agents have bone activity and have
been shown to protect or increase bone
mass. For most there are no current data
showing a reduction in fracture rate, but
this is expected to be the case when studies
of longer-term use become available.

Bisphosphonates—alendronate sodium (Fosamax) 10 mg PO qd (must be taken upon
arising for the day, with a full glass of water, and nothing by mouth for 30 minutes).

Contraindications: See "Menopause." Alendronate is
contraindicated in patients with esophageal
stricture or difficulty swallowing and in nursing mothers.

Precautions: See "Menopause." Patients must remain upright after the ingestion of alendronate
to avoid esophageal irritation. Long-term use
may be associated with impaired mineraliza-
tion and therefore alendronate should be given
cyclically. Vitamin D should be used judi-
ciously, if at all, because doses that increase calcium absorption are close to doses that result
in bone resorption. If calcitonin is used, it must
be given with adequate calcium intake to avoid
secondary hyperparathyroidism.

Interactions: See "Menopause." Calcium supplements and antacids may interfere with the absorption of alendronate and must be taken
later in the day.

Alternative Drugs

Calcium supplements should be reserved for
those with inadequate intake or a food intolerance
that prevent achievement of sufficient dietary levels. Calcium carbonate provides the greatest percentage of elemental calcium, and calcium citrate
is highly absorbable, making both acceptable supplements. When used, these should be taken in di-

Progression of Scoliotic Curve in Adult

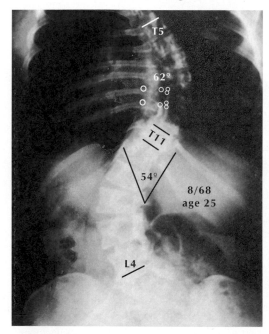

Right thoracic curve of 62° and left lumbar
curve of 54° in 25-year-old woman. Curve
and grade II spondylolisthesis of L5 detected
but not treated during adolescence. Curve
increased slowly during adulthood

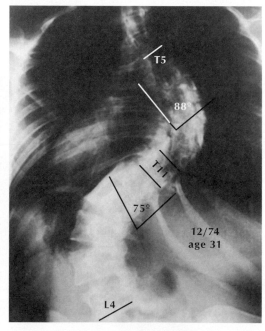

Increased curves in same woman at age 31
after two closely spaced pregnancies. Thoracic
curve progressed to 88° and lumbar curve to 75°
Spondylolisthesis increased to grade III

Reproduced from HA Keim. The Adolescent Spine. New York, Grune & Stratton, 1976.

vided doses over the course of the day. Excessive intake of calcium supplements has been associated with an increased risk of stone formation and should be discouraged.

FOLLOW-UP

Patient Monitoring: Normal health maintenance and continued (lifelong) compliance with medical therapy must be encouraged. Periodic measurement of height may detect asymptomatic spinal fractures.

Prevention/Avoidance: Estrogen replacement therapy at menopause, good diet (adequate calcium and vitamin D intake), and exercise.

Elimination or reduction of bone toxins (smoking and excess alcohol).

Possible Complications: After hip fracture, half of patients require assistance walking and 15%–30% are institutionalized, often for the rest of their lives. Roughly, 1 of 5 patients with a hip fracture die within 6 months of the fracture. Fracture of the hip is the twelfth leading cause of death for women.

Expected Outcome: The rate of bone loss may be slowed by medical interventions, but these are most successful if instituted early. Estrogen replacement is associated with a reduction by about 50% in the rate of hip and arm fractures

Progressive Spinal Deformity in Osteoporosis

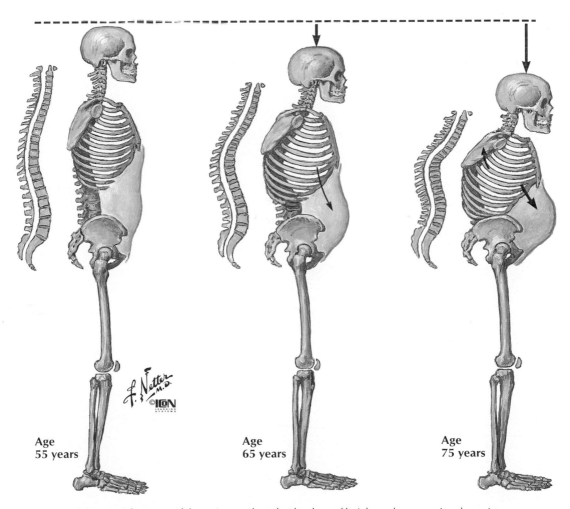

Compression fractures of thoracic vertebrae lead to loss of height and progressive thoracic kyphosis (dowager's hump). Lower ribs eventually rest on iliac crests, and downward pressure on viscera causes abdominal distention

in postmenopausal women. This value has been reported to rise to more than 90 when estrogen is used for more than 5 years. Vertebral fractures may be reduced by as much as 80% for these same women.

MISCELLANEOUS

Pregnancy Considerations: No effect on pregnancy (generally not a consideration). Alendronate is a pregnancy category C medication.

***ICD-9-CM* Codes:** 733.01 (Postmenopausal).

REFERENCES

American College of Obstetricians and Gynecologists. *Hormone Replacement Therapy.* Washington, DC: ACOG; 1998. ACOG Technical Bulletin 247.

American College of Obstetricians and Gynecologists. *Osteoporosis.* Washington, DC: ACOG; 1992. ACOG Technical Bulletin 167.

Hosking D, Chilvers CED, Christiansen C, et al. Prevention of bone loss with alendronate in postmenopausal women. *N Engl J Med* 1998;338:485.

Jones KP, ed. Estrogen replacement therapy. *Clin Obstet Gynecol* 1992;35:854.

Riggs BL. Osteoporosis. In: Wyngaarden JB, Smith LH JR, Bennett JC, eds. *Cecil Textbook of Medicine.* 19th ed. Philadelphia, Pa: WB Saunders, 1988:1426.

Riggs BL, Melton LJ III. Medical progress: involutional osteoporosis. *N Engl J Med* 1986;314:1676.

Smith RP. *Gynecology in Primary Care.* Baltimore, Md: Williams & Wilkins; 1997:281.

PESSARY THERAPY

THE CHALLENGE

To identify patients who may benefit from pessary therapy and to effectively select, fit, and monitor pessary use.

Scope of the Problem: As our population ages, the prevalence of pelvic relaxation disorders will increase. Pessary therapy offers an attractive, effective, nonsurgical therapy for many of these patients. Patients with symptomatic pelvic relaxation, uterine retroversion, cervical incompetence, or urinary incontinence may benefit from this form of therapy. It is estimated that 10%–15% of women suffer from anterior vaginal wall support failure, and this rises to 30%–40% after menopause.

Objectives of Management: To provide symptomatic relief for patients with pelvic relaxation, without causing iatrogenic harm.

TACTICS

Relevant Pathophysiology: Pessaries act either by using existing pelvic support mechanisms or by diffusing the forces acting on pelvic structures over a wide area so that support and reposition is achieved. Available in a variety of types and sizes, the most commonly used forms of pessaries for pelvic relaxation are the ring (or donut), the ball, and the cube. To varying degrees, the pessary occludes the vagina and holds the pelvic organs in a relatively normal position. The type of pessary chosen is based on the indications of the individual patient. Pessaries are available in both latex and polyurethane types. The latex type is often less expensive but tends to deteriorate over time; polyurethane pessaries are less likely to retain odor or cause irritation.

Strategies: Pessaries are fitted and placed in the vagina in much the same way as a contraceptive diaphragm. The pessary is lubricated with a water-soluble lubricant, folded or compressed, and inserted into the vagina. The pessary is next adjusted so that it is in the proper position based on the type: ring and lever pessaries should sit behind the cervix (when present) and rest in the retropubic notch; the Gellhorn pessary should be contained entirely within the vagina with the plate resting above the levator plane; the Gehrung pessary must bridge the cervix with the limbs resting on the levator muscles on each side; and the ball or cube pessaries should occupy and occlude the upper vagina. All pessaries must allow the easy passage of an examining finger between the pessary and the vaginal wall in all areas. Examination 5–7 days after initial fitting is required to confirm proper placement, hygiene, and the absence of pressure-related problems (vaginal trauma or necrosis). Earlier evaluation (in 24–48 hours) may be advisable for patients who are debilitated or require additional assistance.

Patient Education: Reassurance, American College of Obstetricians and Gynecologists Patient Education Pamphlet AP012 (*Pelvic Support Problems*), AP081 (*Urinary Incontinence*).

IMPLEMENTATION

Special Considerations: Pessaries offer an excellent alternative to surgical repair, but the use of a pessary requires the cooperation and involvement of the patient. Patients who are unable or unwilling to manage the periodic insertion and removal of the device are poor candidates for their use. Pessaries are not well tolerated and do not provide optimal support in patients who have low estrogen levels. For this reason, many suggest a minimum of 30 days of topical estrogen therapy (for those not already receiving estrogen replacement) before a trial of pessary therapy. Patients who are going to use a pessary should be instructed on both proper insertion and removal techniques. Ring pessaries should be removed by hooking a finger into the pessary's opening, gently compressing the device, and then withdrawing the pessary with gentle traction. Cube pessaries must also be compressed, but the suction created between the faces of the cube and the vaginal wall must be broken by gently separating the device from the vaginal sidewall. The locator string often attached to these pessaries should not be used for traction. Inflatable pessaries should be deflated before removal. Gellhorn and Gehrung pessaries are removed by a reversal of their insertion steps.

REFERENCES

American College of Obstetricians and Gynecologists. *Pelvic Organ Prolapse.* Washington, DC: ACOG; 1995. ACOG Technical Bulletin 214.

Deger RB, Menzin AW, Mikuta JJ. The vaginal pessary: past and present. *Postgrad Obstet Gynecol* 1993;13:1.

Greenhill JP. The nonsurgical management of vaginal relaxation. *Clin Obstet Gynecol* 1972;15:1083.

Miller DS. Contemporary use of the pessary. In; Sciarra JJ, ed. *Obstetrics and Gynecology.* Vol 1. Philadelphia, Pa: JB Lippincott; 1998;39:1.

Sulak PJ, Kuehl TJ, Shull BL. Vaginal pessaries and their use in pelvic relaxation. *J Reprod Med* 1993;38:919.

Smith RP, Ling FW. *Procedures in Women's Health Care.* Baltimore, Md: Williams & Wilkins; 1997:127.

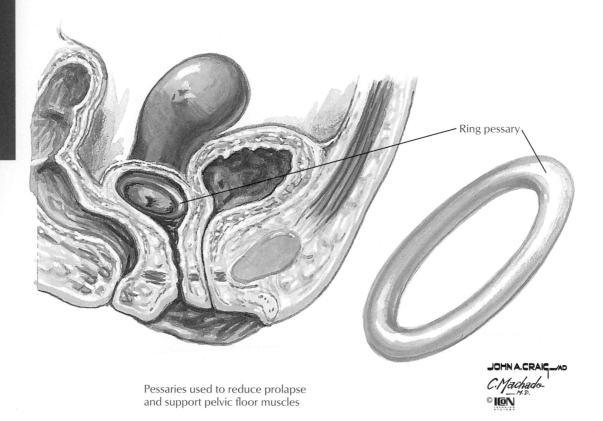

Ring pessary

Pessaries used to reduce prolapse
and support pelvic floor muscles

JOHN A. CRAIG__MD

C. Machado
__M.D.

©ICON
LEARNING
SYSTEMS

POSTCOITAL BLEEDING

INTRODUCTION

Description: Vaginal bleeding that follows intercourse.

Prevalence: Common.

Predominant Age: Reproductive age and beyond.

Genetics: No genetic pattern.

ETIOLOGY AND PATHOGENESIS

Causes: Uterine (pregnancy, endometrial polyps, endometrial hyperplasia, endometrial carcinoma, leiomyomata), cervical (polyps, cervicitis, cervical erosion, cervical dysplasia or neoplasia), vaginal (trauma, infection, atrophy), perineal (vulvar lesions, hemorrhoids).

Risk Factors: Hypoestrogen states (menopause without estrogen replacement, vigorous intercourse, and nonconsensual intercourse [rape]).

CLINICAL CHARACTERISTICS

Signs and Symptoms:
- Painless vaginal bleeding related to (after) intercourse

DIAGNOSTIC APPROACH

Differential Diagnosis:
- Pregnancy (normal or abnormal)
- Cervical polyps
- Endometrial polyps
- Uterine leiomyomata
- Cervicitis or cervical lesions (including cancer)
- Endometrial cancer
- Endometriosis
- Vaginitis (including atrophic vaginitis)
- Coagulopathy (acquired or iatrogenic)
- Nongynecologic sources of bleeding (eg, perineal or rectal)

Associated Conditions: Endometrial cancer, endometrial polyps or carcinoma, and uterine leiomyomata.

Workup and Evaluation

Laboratory: No evaluation indicated.

Imaging: No imaging indicated.

Special Tests: None indicated.

Diagnostic Procedures: History and physical examination often point to possible causes for further evaluation.

Pathologic Findings

Based on underlying pathologic condition.

MANAGEMENT AND THERAPY

Nonpharmacologic

General Measures: Evaluation.

Specific Measures: Focused on underlying cause.

Diet: No specific dietary changes indicated.

Activity: No restriction.

Patient Education: Reassurance, American College of Obstetricians and Gynecologists Patient Education Pamphlet AP095 (*Abnormal Uterine Bleeding*).

Drug(s) of Choice

Based on cause.

FOLLOW-UP

Patient Monitoring: Normal health maintenance.

Prevention/Avoidance: None.

Possible Complications: Sexual dysfunction (rare).

Expected Outcome: Return to normal sexual function with reassurance and correction of the causative process.

MISCELLANEOUS

Pregnancy Considerations: No effect on pregnancy. Slightly more common during pregnancy.

ICD-9-CM Codes: 626.7.

REFERENCES

American College of Obstetricians and Gynecologists. *Dysfunctional Uterine Bleeding.* Washington, DC: ACOG; 1989. ACOG Technical Bulletin 134.

Cowan BD, Morrison JC. Management of abnormal genital bleeding in girls and women. *N Engl J Med* 1991;324:1710.

Field CS. Dysfunctional uterine bleeding. *Primary Care* 1988;15:561.

Neese RE. Managing abnormal vaginal bleeding. *Postgrad Med* 1991;89:205.

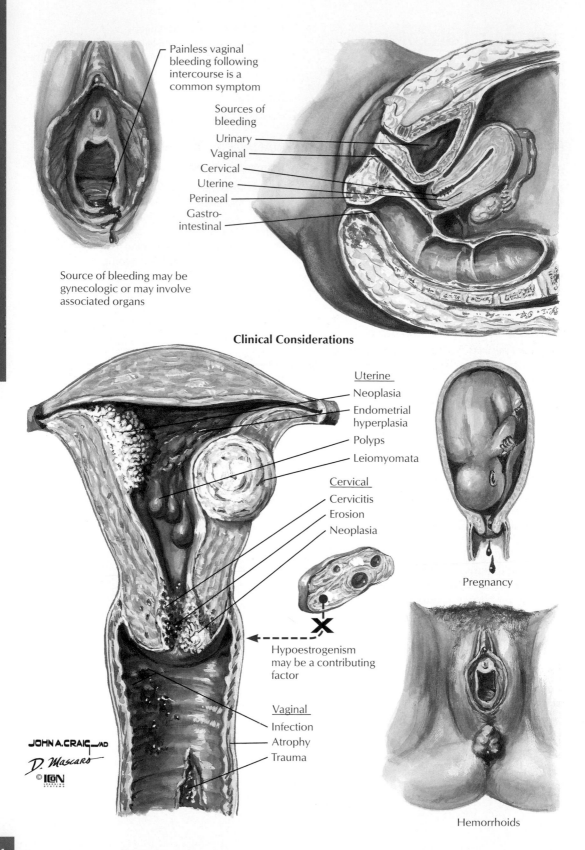

Painless vaginal bleeding following intercourse is a common symptom

Sources of bleeding

Urinary
Vaginal
Cervical
Uterine
Perineal
Gastro-intestinal

Source of bleeding may be gynecologic or may involve associated organs

Clinical Considerations

Uterine
Neoplasia
Endometrial hyperplasia
Polyps
Leiomyomata

Cervical
Cervicitis
Erosion
Neoplasia

Hypoestrogenism may be a contributing factor

Vaginal
Infection
Atrophy
Trauma

Pregnancy

Hemorrhoids

JOHN A.CRAIG—AD
D. Mascaro
©ICON LEARNING SYSTEMS

PREMENSTRUAL SYNDROME

INTRODUCTION

Description: A syndrome of physical and emotional symptoms characterized by its relationship to menses: symptoms are confined to a period of not more than 14 days before the onset of menstrual flow with complete resolution at, or soon after, the end of menstrual flow.

Prevalence: Reproductive (25%–85%; 2%–5% meet strict criteria).

Predominant Age: Reproductive; most commonly 30s and 40s.

Genetics: Family tendency, but no confirmed genetic pattern.

ETIOLOGY AND PATHOGENESIS

Causes: The physiologic foundations of premenstrual syndrome (PMS), premenstrual dysphoric disorder, and premenstrual magnification (PMM) have yet to be established. The most promising research into a cause of PMS has been in the areas of β-endorphins and serotonin.

Risk Factors: None known.

CLINICAL CHARACTERISTICS

Signs and Symptoms:
- Physical or emotional symptoms confined to a period or not more than 14 days before the onset of menstrual flow with complete resolution at, or soon after, the end of menstrual flow. More than 150 different signs and symptoms have been described under the rubric of PMS. (The character of the symptoms is not important, only the timing of their appearance. Symptoms that are present at all times but worsen before menses or those that appear at irregular intervals do not meet the criteria for PMS.)

DIAGNOSTIC APPROACH

Differential Diagnosis:
- Breast disorders
- Chronic fatigue states
- Drug and substance abuse
- Endocrinologic disorders
- Family, marital, and social stress
- Gastrointestinal conditions
- Gynecologic disorders
- Idiopathic edema
- Psychiatric and psychologic disorders

Associated Conditions: Bipolar disorders, sleep disorders, chronic pain states, and somatization.

Workup and Evaluation

Laboratory: Complete blood count, liver enzyme studies, endocrine studies (androgens, follicle-stimulating hormone [FSH]/luteinizing hormone [LH], glucose tolerance test, prolactin, thyroid function studies [highly sensitive TSH, thyronine, TRH stimulation])

Imaging: No imaging indicated.

Special Tests: Prospective menstrual calendar or other diary for a 3-month period to establish the diagnosis.

Diagnostic Procedures: History, physical examination, prospective menstrual calendar or diary. Research has shown that up to 80% of patients who present with self-diagnosed "PMS" fail to meet strict criteria for this diagnosis. Most are found to have other conditions ranging from mood disorders to irritable bowel disease or endometriosis. This observation makes it imperative that no therapy be instituted until the diagnosis can be firmly established.

Pathologic Findings

None.

MANAGEMENT AND THERAPY

Nonpharmacologic

General Measures: Lifestyle changes (aerobic exercise [20–45 minutes, three times weekly], smoking cessation, stress reduction), dietary changes and supplementation (adequate protein and complex carbohydrates, avoidance of alcohol, caffeine, and simple sugars, frequent small meals, fresh fruits and vegetables, reduction of dietary fat to <15%, salt restriction, increased dietary or supplemental fiber, calcium 1000 mg daily, magnesium 200 mg daily during luteal phase, vitamin B_6 50–200 mg daily, vitamin E 150–300 IU daily).

Specific Measures: Generally based on specific symptoms. A favorable response should be expected for 80% of patients with PMS and 50% of those with PMM.

Diet: See above.

Activity: Aerobic exercise (20–45 minutes, three times weekly).

Patient Education: Reassurance, American College of Obstetricians and Gynecologists Patient Education Pamphlet AP057 (*Premenstrual Syndrome*), AP106 (*Depression*).

Drug(s) of Choice

Hydrochlorothiazide 25–50 mg daily, luteal phase (for fluid retention).

Premenstrual Syndrome

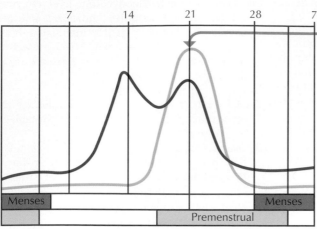

Cycle of premenstrual syndrome

Estrogen
Progesterone

Menses

Menses

Premenstrual

Syndrome characterized by pelvic pain, fluid retention, breast discomfort, and mood changes in days preceding menses

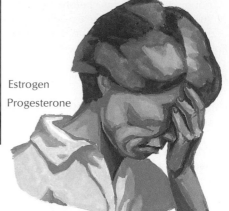

Depression, anxiety, and frequent mood changes predominate

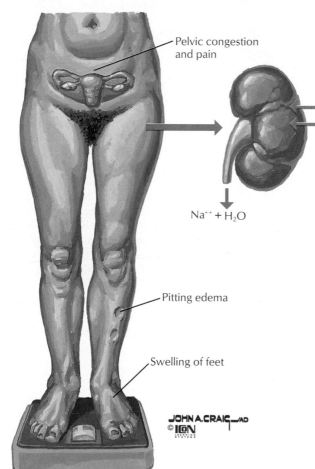

Pelvic congestion and pain

Pitting edema

Swelling of feet

$Na^{++} + H_2O$

JOHN A. CRAIG—AD
© ICON
LEARNING SYSTEMS

Generalized weight gain

Thiazides
Spironolactone

Diuretics effectively treat most signs and symptoms of fluid retention. Older patients may be less responsive to this treatment than younger women

Danazol

Danazol effectively reduces occurrence of breast cysts and relieves mastodynia

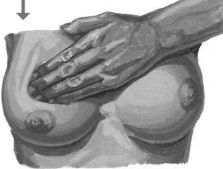

Breast pain and tenderness are common. Large cysts may develop in older patients

Alprazolam 0.25 mg three to four times daily or atenolol 25 mg two to three times daily (for agitation and anxiety).

Buspirone 5 mg three times daily or fluoxetine 20 mg daily (in the morning) (for mood swings).

Third-generation oral contraceptives (eg, desogestrel-containing).

Danazol sodium 200 mg daily, luteal phase or continuous GnRH agonists (depot leuprolide 3.75 mg IM monthly for a maximum of 6 months or nafarelin acetate nasal spray, 200 μg twice daily for a maximum of 6 months).

Contraindications: See individual agents.

Precautions: See individual agents.

FOLLOW-UP

Patient Monitoring: Normal health maintenance.

Prevention/Avoidance: General stress reduction appears to blunt the cyclic symptoms experienced.

Possible Complications: Social withdrawal or isolation, work or family disruption. The rate of suicide increases during the luteal phase.

Expected Outcome: Symptoms can generally be resolved through the process of diagnosis, providing insight and control to the patient, and pharmacologic intervention.

MISCELLANEOUS

Pregnancy Considerations: No effect on pregnancy. Patients with a history of PMS may have exaggerated response to the hormonal changes associated with pregnancy.

***ICD-9-CM* Codes:** 625.4.

REFERENCES

American College of Obstetricians and Gynecologists. *Premenstrual Syndrome.* Washington, DC: ACOG; 1995. ACOG Committee Opinion 155.

American Psychiatric Association. *Diagnostic and Statistical Manual of Mental Disorders.* 4th ed. Washington, DC: American Psychiatric Association; 1994.

Freeman E, Rickels K, Sondheimer S, Scharlop B. Diagnostic classifications from daily symptom ratings of women who seek treatment for premenstrual symptoms. *Am J Gynecol Health* 1987;1:17.

Garris PD, Sokol MS, Kelly K, Witman GF, Plouffe L Jr. Leuprolide acetate treatment of catamenial pneumothorax. *Fertil Steril* 1994;61:173.

Moline MI. Pharmacologic strategies for managing premenstrual syndrome. *Clin Pharm* 1993;12:181.

Plouffe L Jr, Trott EA. Premenstrual syndrome: new concepts and recent therapeutic breakthroughs. *Postgrad Obstet Gynecol* 1995;15:1.

Rubinow DR. The premenstrual syndrome: new views. *JAMA* 1992;268:1908.

PRURITUS ANI

INTRODUCTION

Description: Acute or chronic itching (generally intense) of the anal and perianal skin. Patients may also have complaints of vulvar itching or of a vaginal infection that has not responded to therapy.
Prevalence: Common.
Predominant Age: All ages.
Genetics: No genetic pattern.

ETIOLOGY AND PATHOGENESIS

Causes: Anal disease—fissures, fistulae, infection (bacterial, fungal, pin worms, scabies), neoplasia, hemorrhoids, leakage of stool. Dermatologic processes—psoriasis, eczema, fecal irritation, contact dermatitis, seborrheic dermatitis, vulvitis, chemical dermatitis (diarrheal irritation), dietary intolerance (coffee, cola, tomatoes, chocolate). Other—excessively zealous hygiene, psychologic problems.
Risk Factors: Hemorrhoids, obesity.

CLINICAL CHARACTERISTICS

Signs and Symptoms:
- Anal and perianal itching
- Perianal erythema
- Anal fissures
- Excoriation
- Bleeding after bowel movement

DIAGNOSTIC APPROACH

Differential Diagnosis:
- Vulvitis
- Vaginitis
- Pruritus vulvae
- Contact dermatitis
- Psoriasis
- Bacterial or fungal infection
- Parasites (pin worms, scabies)
- Diabetes mellitus
- Liver disease
- Anxiety
- Atopic dermatitis
- Menopausal perineal atrophy

Associated Conditions: Vaginitis, secondary infection, diabetes mellitus, psoriasis, and hemorrhoids.

Workup and Evaluation

Laboratory: No evaluation indicated. Selective testing based on differential diagnosis being considered (eg, fasting and postprandial glucose levels, skin scrapings for fungi, stool for ova and parasites).

Imaging: No imaging indicated.
Special Tests: None indicated. Anoscopy for anal diseases.
Diagnostic Procedures: History and physical examination.

Pathologic Findings

Excoriation common.

MANAGEMENT AND THERAPY
Nonpharmacologic

General Measures: Evaluation, perineal hygiene, cool sitz baths, moist soaks, or the application of soothing solutions such as Burow's solution. Patients should be advised to wear loose-fitting clothing and keep the area dry and well ventilated. Avoid soaps; water-moistened cotton balls or baby wipes provide a portable cleansing option. Nonmedicated talcum powder may be used to absorb moisture. If overnight itching and excoriation are a problem, patients should wear cotton gloves during sleep.
Specific Measures: Antihistamines, especially at night when itching is often intense and sedation may be desirable. Crotamiton (Eurax) may be applied topically, twice daily, to suppress itching. Occasionally, the use of a topical anesthetic, such as 2% lidocaine (Xylocaine) jelly, may be required. Other therapies based on causal agent.
Diet: No specific dietary changes needed. If food allergy or irritation is suspected, diet change is indicated (reduce caffeine, spices, citrus, vitamin C, milk products, alcohol).
Activity: No restriction.
Patient Education: Reassurance, counseling about perineal hygiene, risk reduction.

Drug(s) of Choice

Burow's solution (Domeboro, aluminum acetate 5% aqueous solution, three to four times daily for 30–60 minutes).
Crotamiton (Eurax) may be applied topically, twice daily.
Topical analgesic sprays or ointments—benzocaine (Americaine, Hurricane) 20% spray or gel, dibucaine (Nupercainal) 1% ointment.
Antipruritics and antiinflammatory agents—hydrocortisone (Anusol-HC, Analpram-HC, Cortenema, Cortifoam, Epifoam, Proctofoam-HC), pramoxine 1% (Fleet rectal pads, Analpram-HC), witch hazel 50% (Tucks pads or gel).
Astringents—Preparation H.

FOLLOW-UP

Patient Monitoring: Normal health maintenance.

Prevention/Avoidance: Perineal hygiene, hormone replacement therapy, and avoidance of local irritants and laxatives.

Possible Complications: Secondary infection caused by excoriation, lichenification.

Expected Outcome: With identification of underlying causation—good.

MISCELLANEOUS

Pregnancy Considerations: No effect on pregnancy

ICD-9-CM Codes: 698.0.

REFERENCES

Alexander S. Dermatological aspects of anorectal disease. *Clin Gastroenterol* 1975;4:651.

Beart RW. Common anorectal problems. In: Sciarra JJ, ed. *Gynecology and Obstetrics.* Vol 1. Philadelphia, Pa: JB Lippincott; 1992;97:1.

Schrock TR. Diseases of the rectum and anus. In: Wyngaarden JB, Smith LH Jr, Bennett JC, eds. *Cecil Textbook of Medicine.* 19th ed. Philadelphia, Pa: WB Saunders, 1992: 735.

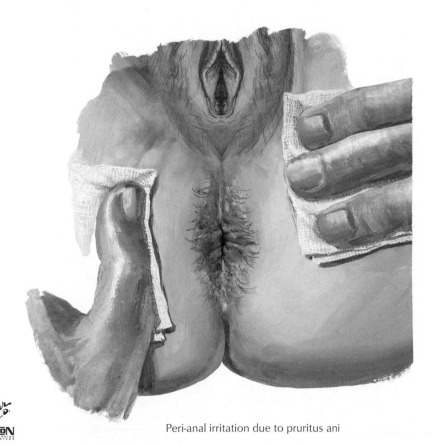

Peri-anal irritation due to pruritus ani

RAPE AND RAPE TRAUMA SYNDROME

INTRODUCTION

Description: Rape and sexual assault encompass manual, oral, and genital contact by one person without the consent of the other, in a way that is considered sexual in a consensual situation. It does not require penetration, ejaculation, force, or evidence of resistance, only the lack of consent. The legal definition varies slightly by location, but often includes elements of fear, fraud, coercion, or threat. In some areas, the mentally incompetent, those under the influence of drugs or alcohol, or the underage are deemed incapable of giving consent for any otherwise consensual sexual activity, resulting in "statutory rape." Rape trauma syndrome is a well-recognized set of behaviors that occur after a sexual assault. These responses are organized into three phases: The acute phase, lasting from hours to days; a middle, or readjustment, phase, lasting from days to weeks; and a final reorganization or resolution phase that involve lifelong changes.

Prevalence: Rape constitutes 5%–10% of violent crime, 60+ of 100,000 women. It is the most underreported crime in the United States. Rape trauma syndrome occurs in virtually every case.

Predominant Age: Any age.

ETIOLOGY AND PATHOGENESIS

Causes: One quarter to one half of all rapes occur at home (either the victim's or the attacker's), but only one third of these involve a male intruder. Most attackers are known to the victims. Of recurrent victims, about 25% have been raped by someone well known to them, such as an ex-lover, employer, coworker, neighbor, or relative, and two thirds are vulnerable because of mental impairment, substance abuse, or a psychiatric disorder. Weapons are used in 30%–50% of sexual assaults (handguns are most common). Approximately 50% of campus rapes occur during dates. Estimates of sexual violence occurring in the setting of a dating relationship indicate that 10%–25% of high school students and 20%–50% of college students have experienced some form of sexual violence. Rape trauma syndrome can follow rape or other forms of intense physical or emotional trauma.

Risk Factors: Studies indicate that alcohol use is involved in more than one half of all rapes of college students. Rape trauma syndrome is more common in those older than 40, those assaulted in their homes by a stranger, and those with a history of previous mental illness.

CLINICAL CHARACTERISTICS

Signs and Symptoms:
- **Rape**—History of nonconsensual sexual activity
- Physical signs of sexual activity (not limited to vaginal intercourse)
- Physical signs of trauma or coercion (including impairment resulting from drugs, alcohol, or mental abilities)
- **Rape trauma syndrome**—Acute (decompensation, inability to cope, volatile emotions, fear, guilt, anger, depression, and problems concentrating are common, flashbacks are frequent, ideation is often disturbed)
- Middle, or readjustment (resolution of many issues [may not be functional], flashbacks, nightmares, and phobias may develop)
- Reorganization (recognizes that event was an assault over which she could have no control)

DIAGNOSTIC APPROACH

Differential Diagnosis:
- Consensual intercourse
- Nonsexual trauma
- Rape trauma syndrome—Depression
- Mania
- Psychosis

Associated Conditions: Pregnancy, sexually transmissible infections, and depression.

Workup and Evaluation

Laboratory: As outlined in *Special Tests*, as well as serum pregnancy test, cervical cultures for sexually transmissible infections, a screening serologic test for syphilis and human immunodeficiency virus (HIV), hepatitis antigens, urinalysis (often with culture).

Imaging: No imaging indicated unless the possibility of internal injuries is suspected.

Special Tests: Special rape evaluation kits are available in many jurisdictions and should be used if available. Wood's light (ultraviolet light) causes semen stains to fluoresce.

Diagnostic Procedures: Examination under general anesthesia is also indicated any time the patient is unable to urinate or there is hematuria, lower abdominal tenderness, or signs of occult blood loss, such as hypovolemia.

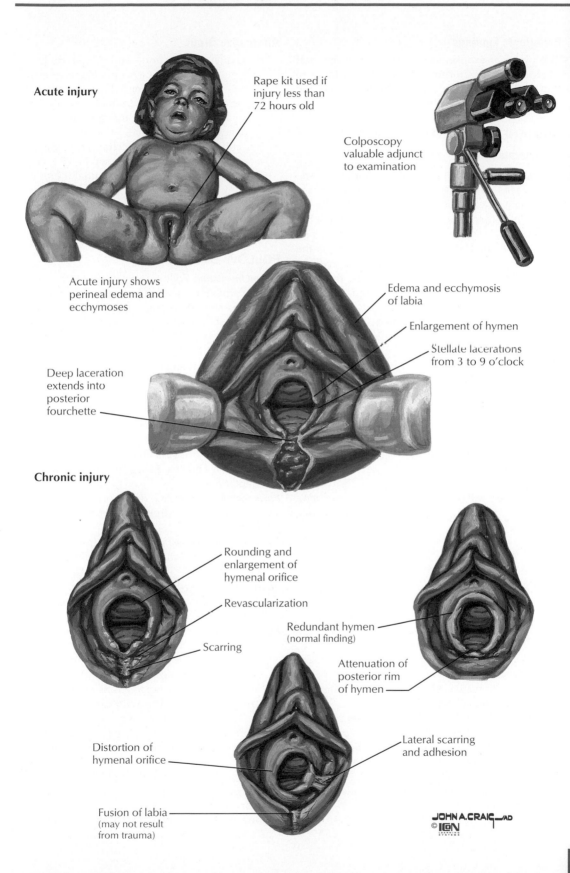

Acute injury

Rape kit used if injury less than 72 hours old

Colposcopy valuable adjunct to examination

Acute injury shows perineal edema and ecchymoses

Edema and ecchymosis of labia

Enlargement of hymen

Stellate lacerations from 3 to 9 o'clock

Deep laceration extends into posterior fourchette

Chronic injury

Rounding and enlargement of hymenal orifice

Revascularization

Scarring

Redundant hymen (normal finding)

Attenuation of posterior rim of hymen

Distortion of hymenal orifice

Lateral scarring and adhesion

Fusion of labia (may not result from trauma)

JOHN A. CRAIG—AD
© ICON

Pathologic Findings

The physical examination is normal in one half of rape victims. Common sites of lacerations are the vaginal wall, the lateral fornices, and the cul-de-sac.

MANAGEMENT AND THERAPY

Nonpharmacologic

General Measures: Support with compassion, care, and sensitivity. The primary goal is to provide reassurance and a return of control. Support and assistance should be provided in moving through the stages of resolution. Because one of the pivotal aspects of sexual assault is the loss of control, every effort should be made to allow the patient control over even the most trivial aspect of the physical examination.

Specific Measures: There are three basic responsibilities in the care of someone who may have been raped or abused: the detection and treatment of serious injuries, the preservation of evidence, and protection against sequelae. All women deserve intensive follow-up and counseling. Assistance in recognizing and adapting to the changes that make up the rape trauma syndrome.

Diet: No specific dietary changes indicated.

Activity: No restriction.

Patient Education: American College of Obstetricians and Gynecologists Patient Education Pamphlet AP114 (*Emergency Contraception*), AP009 (*How to Prevent Sexually Transmitted Diseases*).

Drug(s) of Choice

Pregnancy interdiction—diethylstilbestrol 25 mg PO bid for 5 days with prochlorperazine (Compazine) 10 mg PO q8h or ethinyl estradiol 0.05 mg plus norgestrel 0.5 mg (Ovral) two tablets PO bid for 2–5 days, ethinyl estradiol 50 μg plus levonorgestrel 0.25 mg (Preven) 2 PO q12h for two doses.

Sexually transmissible infection prophylaxis—ceftriaxone 250 mg IM or

Spectinomycin 2 g IM, both followed by tetracycline 500 mg PO qid for 7 days or

Doxycycline 100 mg PO bid for 7 days.

Prophylaxis—tetanus toxoid should be given if indicated.

Contraindications: Known or suspected allergy, preexisting pregnancy.

Precautions: Nausea is common with high-dose estrogen pregnancy interdiction.

Alternative Drugs

Pregnancy interdiction—ethinyl estradiol, 5 mg PO qd for 5 days or conjugated estrogen, 10 mg PO qid for 5 days. An intrauterine contraceptive device may be placed as an alternative to drug therapy for pregnancy interdiction.

Sexually transmissible infection prophylaxis—amoxicillin 3 g PO or ampicillin 3.5 g PO plus probenecid 1 g PO as initial therapy, then follow as above.

Erythromycin esterase 500 mg PO qid for 7 days may be substituted for tetracycline or doxycycline.

FOLLOW-UP

Patient Monitoring: Follow-up contacts by the health care provider, social service agencies, or support groups should be made early and often. Contacts at 1–2 weeks, a month, and periodically thereafter provide support and identify evolving problems. Physical reevaluation should be performed at 1 and 6 weeks to check for delayed symptoms or signs of pelvic infection, bleeding abnormalities, delayed menses, suicidal ideation, or other possible sequelae of the attack. Retesting for HIV and hepatitis B status should be done at 12–18 weeks. Health care providers should watch for a failure to move to resolution and the emergence of dysfunctional adaptations.

Prevention/Avoidance: Avoidance of high-risk situations, especially those involving alcohol or drugs.

Possible Complications: The risk of acquiring a sexually transmitted disease is uncertain but is estimated to be 3%–5% or less. The risk of becoming infected with HIV is unknown. Roughly one third of rape victims suffer long-term psychiatric problems.

Expected Outcome: If both physical and mental trauma are addressed in a proactive manner, results should be good. This must include risk avoidance to reduce the chance of recurrence. (Up to one fifth of rape victims have been victims previously.) Even with care and support, the last phase of the rape trauma syndrome is often accompanied by painful transitions, frequently involving significant changes in lifestyles, work, or friends. Insomnia, depression, somatic complaints, and poor self-esteem are common during this phase. For some, this phase can be extremely disruptive and prolonged. Roughly one third of rape victims suffer long-term psychiatric problems. The risk of this is greatest for those older than 40, those assaulted in their homes by a stranger, and those with a history of previous mental illness.

MISCELLANEOUS

Pregnancy Considerations: No effect on preexisting pregnancy. If pregnancy interdiction fails, the agents used are teratogenic and a therapeutic abortion is recommended.

***ICD-9-CM* Codes:** V71.5 (Alleged, observation or examination), 308 (Acute reaction to stress), 308.0 (Predominant disturbance of emotions), 308.3 (Other acute reactions to stress), 308.4 (Mixed disorders as reaction to stress).

REFERENCES

American College of Obstetricians and Gynecologists. *Adolescent Victims of Sexual Assault.* Washington, DC: ACOG; 1998. ACOG Technical Bulletin 252.

American College of Obstetricians and Gynecologists. *Sexual Assault.* Washington, DC: ACOG; 1992. ACOG Technical Bulletin 172.

Burgess WA, Holmstrom LL. Rape trauma syndrome. *Am J Psychiatry* 1974;131:981.

Burgess WA, Holmstrom LL. Adaptive strategies and recovery from rape. *Am J Psychiatry* 1979;136:1278.

Hampton HL. Care of the woman who has been raped. *N Engl J Med* 1995;332:234.

Hicks DJ. Rape: sexual assault. *Am J Obstet Gynecol* 1980; 137:931.

Smith RP. *Gynecology in Primary Care.* Baltimore, Md: Williams & Wilkins; 1997:501.

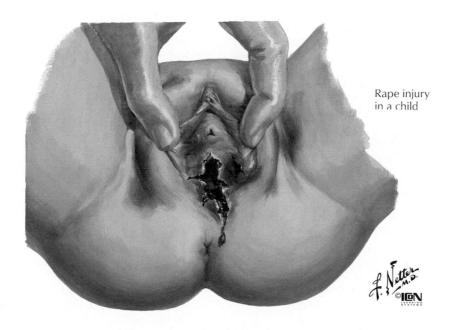

Rape injury in a child

SEXUALLY TRANSMITTED INFECTIONS: CHANCROID

INTRODUCTION

Description: Infection by *Haemophilus ducreyi* results in chancroid, one of a group of infrequently encountered sexually transmitted infections. Chancroid is more common than syphilis in some areas of Africa and Southeast Asia, but is uncommon in the United States.

Prevalence: In the United States, 1500 cases per year.

Predominant Age: Younger reproductive.

Genetics: No genetic pattern.

ETIOLOGY AND PATHOGENESIS

Causes: *H ducreyi* is not capable of infecting intact skin; thus the lesions of chancroid tend to be found in areas traumatized by sexual activity. Material from the vulvar ulcers is virulent and can infect other body sites.

Risk Factors: Sexual trauma and exposure to the infective agent, prostitution, and HIV infection.

CLINICAL CHARACTERISTICS

Signs and Symptoms:

- One to three painful "soft chancres" 3–10 days after exposure (these break down over about 2 weeks to form shallow, progressive ulcers with red, ragged, undermined edges, with little surrounding inflammation; autoinoculation is common, resulting in lesions at various stages of evolution)
- Unilateral adenopathy progressing to massive enlargement and inflammation ("buboes," 50%)

DIAGNOSTIC APPROACH

Differential Diagnosis:

- Herpes simplex
- Syphilis
- Granuloma inguinale
- Lymphogranuloma venereum

Associated Conditions: Other sexually transmitted infections, HIV.

Workup and Evaluation

Laboratory: Gram's stain and culture of material from open ulcers. Because of the growing association with HIV, serum testing for HIV infections is highly recommended.

Imaging: No imaging indicated.

Special Tests: None indicated.

Diagnostic Procedures: The diagnosis is established based on clinical findings, finding the gram-negative coccobacillus on smears from the primary lesion, or, rarely, on culture of aspirates of the bubo. Biopsy is also diagnostic, although not often performed.

Pathologic Findings

The *H ducreyi* bacillus is a gram-positive, nonmotile, facultative anaerobe that can be seen in chains on Gram's stain or in culture. Superficial and deep ulcers with granulomatous inflammation are found on biopsy.

MANAGEMENT AND THERAPY

Nonpharmacologic

General Measures: Evaluation, culture or Gram's stain, topical cleansing, and care.

Specific Measures: Antibiotic treatment for patient and her sexual partner(s). Fluctuant nodes may be drained by aspiration through adjacent normal tissue, but incision and drainage delay healing and should not be attempted.

Diet: No specific dietary changes indicated.

Activity: No sexual activity until lesions have healed.

Patient Education: American College of Obstetricians and Gynecologists Patient Education Pamphlet AP009 (*How to Prevent Sexually Transmitted Diseases*). Patients should be advised to have all sexual partners seen for diagnosis and treatment.

Drug(s) of Choice

Azithromycin 1 g PO single dose or ceftriaxone 250 mg IM single dose or ciprofloxacin 500 mg PO bid for 3 days or erythromycin 500 mg PO qid. Treatment must continue for no less than 10 days or until the lesions heal, which ever is longer.

Contraindications: Erythromycin estolate and ciprofloxacin are contraindicated in pregnancy and should not be used. Ciprofloxacin is contraindicated in patients younger than 18 years of age.

Precautions: See individual agents. The safety of azithromycin in pregnancy has not been established.

Interactions: See individual agents.

Alternative Drugs

Trimethoprim 160 mg plus sulfamethoxazole 800 mg PO bid. Treatment must continue for no less than 10 days or until the lesions heal, which ever is longer.

Amoxicillin 500 mg plus clavulanic acid 125 mg (Augmentin) PO q8h for 7 days.

FOLLOW-UP

Patient Monitoring: Follow-up evaluation for cure with culture or other tests should be carried out, as well as screening for other sexually transmitted diseases. (As with all sexually transmitted diseases, all sexual partners who have had sexual contact with the patient within the preceding 30 days should be screened and treated for probable infections.)

Prevention/Avoidance: Use of barrier contraception (condoms, diaphragm), limitation or elimination of risky behavior (sexual promiscuity).

Possible Complications: Buboes may rupture and drain, causing extensive soft tissue and skin damage. Chronic draining sinus tracts and abscesses may occur. Scarring is common.

Expected Outcome: If detected early, successful treatment with minimal sequelae may be expected. Buboes, if present, may take several weeks to resolve. Up to 10% of patients have a recurrence at the site of old ulcers.

MISCELLANEOUS

Pregnancy Considerations: No effect on pregnancy, although the possibility of vertical transmission of other associated conditions (such as HIV infection) should be considered.

ICD-9-CM Codes: 099.0.

REFERENCES

Abeck D, Freinkel AL, Korting HC, Szeimis RM, Ballard RC. Immunohistochemical investigations of genital ulcers caused by *Haemophilus ducreyi*. *Int J STD AIDS* 1997;8:585.

Centers for Disease Control and Prevention. 1998 guidelines for treatment of sexually transmitted diseases. *MMWR Morb Mortal Wkly Rep* 1998:47(RR-1):19.

Chen CY, Mertz KJ, Spinola SM, Morse SA. Comparison of enzyme immunoassays for antibodies to *Haemophilus ducreyi* in a community outbreak of chancroid in the United States. *J Infect Dis* 1997; 175:1390.

Dillon SM, Cummings M, Rajagopalan S, McCormack WC. Prospective analysis of genital ulcer disease in Brooklyn, New York. *Clin Infect Dis* 1997;24:945.

Eichmann A. Chancroid. *Curr Probl Dermatol* 1996;4:20.

Wilkinson EJ, Stone IK. *Atlas of Vulvar Disease*. Baltimore, Md: Williams & Wilkins; 1995:137.

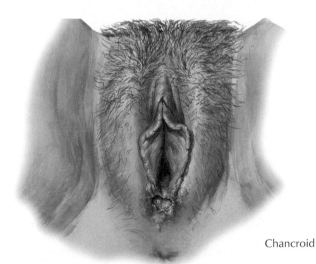

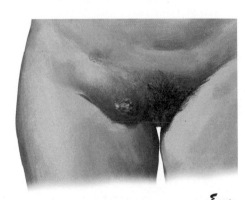

Chancroid

SEXUALLY TRANSMITTED INFECTIONS: *CHLAMYDIA TRACHOMATIS*

INTRODUCTION

Description: The second most common sexually transmitted disease (STD) and most common bacterial STD is infection caused by *Chlamydia trachomatis*. More common than *Neisseria gonorrhoeae* by as much as 10:1 in some studies, infections by *C trachomatis* can be the source of significant complications and infertility.

Prevalence: Twenty percent of pregnant patients, 30% of sexually active adolescent women. Up to 40% of all sexually active women have antibodies suggesting prior infection.

Predominant Age: 15–30 years (85%).

Genetics: No genetic pattern.

ETIOLOGY AND PATHOGENESIS

Causes: Infection by the obligate intracellular organism *C trachomatis*. *Chlamydia* has a long incubation period (average, 10 days) and may persist in the cervix as a carrier state for many years.

Risk Factors: The risk of contracting chlamydial infection is 5 times greater with three or more sexual partners and 4 times higher for patients using no contraception or nonbarrier methods of birth control. Other factors are age less than 25, new partner within the preceding 3 months, other sexually transmitted diseases, vaginal douching.

CLINICAL CHARACTERISTICS

Signs and Symptoms:
- Frequently asymptomatic
- Cervicitis, PID, or much less common, lymphogranuloma venereum
- Less common: nongonococcal urethritis and inclusion conjunctivitis
- Eversion of the cervix with mucopurulent cervicitis supports the diagnosis but not pathognomic

DIAGNOSTIC APPROACH

Differential Diagnosis:
- Gonorrhea
- PID
- Septic abortion
- Appendicitis
- Gastroenteritis

Associated Conditions: Infertility, ectopic pregnancy, mucopurulent cervicitis, PID, chronic pelvic pain, and endometritis.

Workup and Evaluation

Laboratory: Cultures on cycloheximide-treated McCoy cells are very specific and may be used to confirm the diagnosis, but these cultures are expensive, difficult to perform, and often not available. Two clinical screening tests are an enzyme-linked immunoassay (enzyme-linked immunosorbent assay) performed on cervical secretions and a monoclonal antibody test carried out on dried smears. When trying to obtain cervical cultures for *Chlamydia,* plastic- or metal-shafted rayon- or cotton-tipped swabs are preferred. Wood-shafted or calcium alginate swabs reduce the yield of material when transport media is used because of leeching of toxic products into the media.

Imaging: No imaging indicated. Ultrasonography may demonstrate free fluid in the cul-de-sac when pelvic inflammation is present.

Special Tests: None indicated.

Diagnostic Procedures: Physical examination, suspicion, and cervical culture.

Pathologic Findings

This infection tends to involve the mucosal layers and not the entire structure. As a result, extensive damage may occur without dramatic symptoms when the fallopian tubes become infected.

MANAGEMENT AND THERAPY

Nonpharmacologic

General Measures: Evaluation and diagnosis.

Specific Measures: Aggressive antibiotic therapy should be instituted in those suspected of infection. Approximately 45% of patients with chlamydial infection have coexisting gonorrhea; the therapy chosen should consider this.

Diet: No specific dietary changes indicated.

Activity: No restriction. (Sexual continence required until infection is resolved.)

Patient Education: American College of Obstetricians and Gynecologists Patient Education Pamphlet AP009 (*How to Prevent Sexually Transmitted Diseases*). Patients should be advised to have all sexual partners seen for diagnosis and treatment.

Drug(s) of Choice

Azithromycin (1 g PO, single dose) compares favorably with the standard 7-day course of doxycycline, while providing better compliance and fewer side effects.

Tetracycline (500 mg PO qid for 7 days) or doxycycline (100 mg PO bid for 7 days) may also be used.

Contraindications: Quinolones (Ofloxacin), tetracyclines (including doxycycline), and erythromycin estolate are contraindicated in pregnancy and should not be used.

Precautions: Pregnant patients with chlamydial infections should be treated with azithromycin, erythromycin base, or erythromycin ethylsuccinate.

Alternative Drugs

Erythromycin (erythromycin base 500 mg PO qid for 7 days, or erythromycin ethylsuccinate 800 mg PO qid for 7 days) may be substituted for tetracycline in tetracycline-sensitive or pregnant patients. For patients who cannot tolerate erythromycin, amoxicillin (500 mg PO tid for 7–10 days) may be substituted.

Ofloxacin (300 mg PO bid for 7 days).

FOLLOW-UP

Patient Monitoring: Follow-up evaluation for cure with culture or other tests should be carried out, as well as screening for other sexually transmitted diseases. (As with all sexually transmitted diseases, all sexual partners within the preceding 30 days should be screened and treated for probable infections.)

Prevention/Avoidance: Use of barrier contraception (condoms, diaphragm), limitation or elimination of risky behavior (sexual promiscuity).

Possible Complications: Infertility, chronic pelvic pain. If PID occurs, the risk of infertility roughly doubles with each subsequent episode resulting in a 40% rate of infertility after only three episodes. Women with documented salpingitis have a 4-fold increase in their rate of ectopic pregnancy and 5%–15% of women require surgery because of damage caused by PID.

Expected Outcome: If detected early, successful treatment with minimal sequelae may be expected. Significant permanent damage is common despite treatment because of the indolent course of most infections and thus the late institution of therapy.

MISCELLANEOUS

Pregnancy Considerations: No effect on pregnancy. Neonatal conjunctivitis and ophthalmia neonatorum may result if an infant does not receive

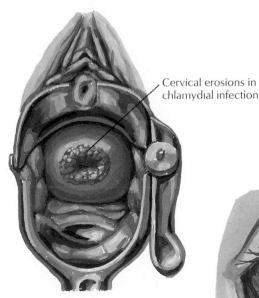

Cervical erosions in chlamydial infection

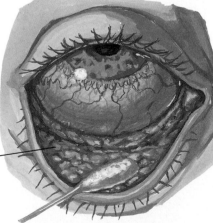

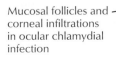

Mucosal follicles and corneal infiltrations in ocular chlamydial infection

JOHN A.CRAIG—AD
©ICON

adequate prophylaxis. Even with standard protection (1% AgNO3 or 0.5% erythromycin ointment) complete protection is not assured.
ICD-9-CM Codes: 099.5.

REFERENCES

American College of Obstetricians and Gynecologists. *Gonorrhea and Chlamydial Infections.* Washington, DC: ACOG; 1994. ACOG Technical Bulletin 190.

Centers for Disease Control and Prevention. 1998 guidelines for treatment of sexually transmitted diseases. *MMWR Morb Mortal Wkly Rep* 1998:47(RR-1):54.

Hammerschlag MR, Golden NH, Oh MK, et al. Single dose of azithromycin for the treatment of genital chlamydial infections in adolescents. *J Pediatr* 1993; 122:961.

Martin DH, Mroczkowski TF, Dalu ZA, et al. A controlled trial of a single dose of azithromycin for the treatment of chlamydial urethritis and cervicitis: the azithromycin for Chlamydial Infections Study Group. *N Engl J Med* 1992;327:921.

Pearlman MD, McNeeley SG. A review of the microbiology, immunology and clinical implications of *Chlamydia trachomatis* infections. *Obstet Gynecol* Surv 1992;47:448.

SEXUALLY TRANSMITTED INFECTIONS: CONDYLOMA ACUMINATA

INTRODUCTION

Description: Raised warty lesions caused by infection by the human papilloma virus.

Prevalence: Most common sexually transmitted disease, other than pregnancy: 500,000 cases per year.

Predominant Age: 16 to 25.

Genetics: No genetic pattern.

ETIOLOGY AND PATHOGENESIS

Causes: Caused by infection by human papilloma virus (HPV) (most frequently serotypes 6 and 11). This DNA virus is found in 2%–4% of all women and up to 60% of patients have evidence of the virus when polymerase chain reaction techniques are used. The virus is hardy and may resist even drying, making transmission and autoinoculation common. There is some evidence that fomite transmission could rarely occur. The virus is most commonly spread by skin-to-skin (generally sexual) contact and has an incubation period of 3 weeks to 8 months, with an average of 3 months. Roughly 65% of patients acquire the infection after intercourse with an infected partner.

Risk Factors: Multiple sexual partners, the presence of other vaginal infections such as candidiasis, trichomoniasis, or bacterial vaginosis.

CLINICAL CHARACTERISTICS

Signs and Symptoms:
- Asymptomatic (<2% have condyloma)
- Painless, raised, soft, fleshy, growths on the vulva, vagina, cervix, urethral meatus, perineum and anus (mild irritation or discharge may accompany secondary infections). Symmetrical lesions across the midline of the genital area common (condyloma may also be found on the tongue or within the oral cavity, the urethra, bladder, or rectum). (Roughly one third of women with vulvar lesions also have vaginal warts or intraepithelial neoplasia [VAIN], and approximately 40% have cervical involvement. Cervical condyloma are generally flatter and may be identified through colposcopic examination, Pap smear, or through the application of 3%–5% acetic acid to make apparent the raised, white, shiny plaques.)

- Abnormal cervical cytologic changes common

DIAGNOSTIC APPROACH

Differential Diagnosis:
- Condyloma lata (syphilis)
- Papilloma

Associated Conditions: Other sexually transmissible infections (*Trichomonas* infection or bacterial vaginosis), abnormal cervical cytologic changes, vulvar and vaginal neoplasia.

Workup and Evaluation

Laboratory: No evaluation indicated. (Tests for syphilis when indicated.)

Imaging: No imaging indicated.

Special Tests: Colposcopic examination, Pap smear, or the application of 3%–5% acetic acid to make apparent the raised, white, shiny plaques. Serotyping is not currently indicated.

Diagnostic Procedures: Physical examination, colposcopy, and biopsy.

Pathologic Findings

Sessile (keratotic) lesions.

MANAGEMENT AND THERAPY

Nonpharmacologic

General Measures: Local hygiene.

Specific Measures: The treatment of small, uncomplicated venereal warts is generally by cytolytic topical agents, such as podophyllin (*Podophyllum* resin), bichloracetic or trichloroacetic acid (TCA), or physical ablative methods such as laser, cryotherapy, or electrodesiccation. In rare selected patients, surgical excision or tangential shaving may be used.

Diet: No specific dietary changes indicated.

Activity: Sexual continence until partner(s) are examined and treated.

Patient Education: American College of Obstetricians and Gynecologists Patient Education Pamphlet AP009 (*How to Prevent Sexually Transmitted Diseases*). Patients should be advised to have all sexual partners seen for diagnosis and treatment.

Drug(s) of Choice

Podophyllin (20% in tincture of benzoin, 25% ointment), podophyllotoxin (0.5% solution, Condylox), bichloracetic or trichloroacetic acid (80%–100% solution), carefully applied to the warts, protecting the adjacent skin, and allowed to remain for between 30 minutes and 4 hours before being washed off the lesions. With most topical therapy, slough of the treated lesions happens in 2–4 days. Treatment may be repeated every 7–14 days as needed. Patients may self-apply podofilox (0.5% solution or gel, bid for 3 days) or Imiquimod (5% cream, Aldara, qhs three times per week for up to 16 weeks).

Contraindications: Podophyllin may not be used during pregnancy because of absorption, potentially resulting in neural or myelotoxicity.

Precautions: To limit toxicity with podophyllin, treatments should be limited to less than 0.5 mL total volume and less than 10 cm² in area. Imiquimod should be washed from the vulva in the morning (after 6–10 hours).

Alternative Drugs

Treatment with 5-fluorouracil 1% or 5% cream is often used as primary therapy or as an adjunct for cervical or vaginal lesions (applied daily until edema, erythema, or vesiculation occurs). Therapy with autologous vaccine, dinitrochlorobenzene, and interferon has been advocated but has yet to gain a significant place in clinical practice.

FOLLOW-UP

Patient Monitoring: The patient should be seen weekly, until no further lesions are found. Be-

cause these patients are at higher risk for cervical neoplasia, close follow up with Pap smears and/or colposcopy at 6- to 12-month intervals is recommended. Follow-up serologic testing for syphilis and HIV infection as indicated. The sexual partners of patients with HPV should also be screened for genital warts.

Prevention/Avoidance: Limitation or elimination of risky behavior (sexual promiscuity). The use of condoms has not been shown to reduce the spread of HPV, but should still be encouraged to reduce the spread of other sexually transmitted diseases.

Possible Complications: Those who are immunocompromised, such as transplant patients, patients with AIDS, or pregnant patients, may experience rapid and exuberant growth of condyloma. External factors that suppress the immune system (steroids, cigarette smoking, metabolic deficiencies, and infections with other viruses such as herpes) may have similar effects. Several subtypes (16, 18, 31, 33, 35, and others) are associated with the development of cervical neoplasia. Roughly 90% of patients with cervical squamous cell carcinoma have evidence of HPV DNA present in their cervical tissues. It is currently thought that a cocarcinogen, such as smoking, other viruses, or nutri-

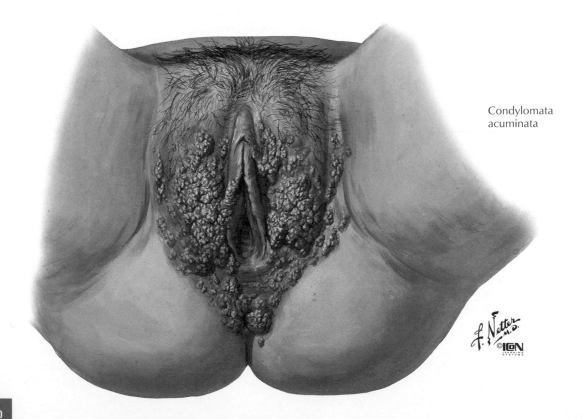

Condylomata acuminata

tional factors are required before malignant transformation may take place.

Expected Outcome: The success rate for resolution of overt warts is approximately 75%, with a recurrence rate of 65%–80%. If lesions persist or continually recur, cryosurgery, electrodesiccation, surgical excision, or laser vaporization may be required. If cryotherapy is chosen, three to six treatments are often required, but cure rates are higher than those for podophyllin and comparable with those for laser ablation (60%–80%). Even with laser ablation, recurrence rates are reported to vary from 25% to 100%. Scarring is rare.

MISCELLANEOUS

Pregnancy Considerations: Pregnant patients may experience rapid and exuberant growth of condyloma, and lesions are more resistant to therapy. Extensive vaginal or vulvar lesions may require delivery via cesarean section to avoid extensive lacerations and suturing problems.

***ICD-9-CM* Codes:** 078.11.

REFERENCES

American College of Obstetricians and Gynecologists. *Genital Human Papillomavirus Infections.* Washington, DC: ACOG; 1994. ACOG Technical Bulletin 193.

Bonnez W, Elswick RK Jr, Bailey-Farchione A, et al. Efficacy and safety of 0.5% podofilox solution in the treatment and suppression of anogenital warts. *Am J Med* 1994;96:420.

Centers for Disease Control and Prevention. 1998 guidelines for treatment of sexually transmitted diseases. *MMWR Morb Mortal Wkly Rep* 1998:47(RR-1):89.

Horowitz BJ. Interferon therapy for condylomatous vulvitis. *Obstet Gynecol* 1989;73:446.

Jha PK, Beral V, Peto J, et al. Antibodies to human papillomavirus and to other genital infectious agents and invasive cervical cancer risk. *Lancet* 1993;341:1116.

SEXUALLY TRANSMITTED INFECTIONS: GONORRHEA

INTRODUCTION

Description: Infection by this gram-negative intracellular diplococcus remains common, accounting for approximately 1 million cases of gonorrhea annually in the United States.

Prevalence: Roughly 3 of 1000 sexually active women and as many as 7% of pregnant patients.

Predominant Age: 15–30 (85%).

Genetics: No genetic pattern.

ETIOLOGY AND PATHOGENESIS

Causes: Infection by the gram-negative intracellular diplococcus, *Neisseria gonorrhoeae*.

Risk Factors: It is estimated that the rate of infection with one act of intercourse with an infected partner is 20% for men but 60%–80% for women. (For this reason, any patient exposed to gonorrhea within the preceding month should be cultured and treated presumptively.) This rate rises to 60%–80% for both sexes with four or more exposures. The groups with the highest risk are adolescents, drug users, and sex workers.

CLINICAL CHARACTERISTICS

Signs and Symptoms:
- Asymptomatic (50%)
- Malodorous, purulent discharge from the urethra, Skene's duct, cervix, vagina, or anus (even without rectal intercourse) 3–5 days after exposure (40%–60%)
- Simultaneous urethral infection (70%–90%)
- Infection of the pharynx (10%–20%)
- Gonococcal conjunctivitis (can rapidly lead to blindness)
- Polyarthritis
- Septic abortion or postabortal sepsis

DIAGNOSTIC APPROACH

Differential Diagnosis:
- Chlamydial infection
- PID
- Septic abortion
- Appendicitis
- Gastroenteritis

Associated Conditions: Infertility, ectopic pregnancy, mucopurulent cervicitis, PID, chronic pelvic pain, and endometritis.

Workup and Evaluation

Laboratory: Culture on Thayer-Martin agar plates kept in a CO_2-rich environment. Cervical cultures provide 80%–95% diagnostic sensitivity. Cultures should also be obtained from the urethra and anus, although these additional cultures do not significantly increase the sensitivity of testing. A Gram's stain of any cervical discharge for the presence of gram-negative intracellular diplococcus supports the presumptive diagnosis, but does not establish it (sensitivity 50%–70%, specificity 97%). A solid-phase enzyme immunoassay is available. Even when the diagnosis is established by other methods, all cases of gonorrhea should have cultures obtained to assess antibiotic susceptibility, although therapy should not be delayed pending the results.

Imaging: No imaging indicated. Ultrasonography may demonstrate free fluid in the cul-de-sac when pelvic inflammation is present.

Special Tests: None indicated.

Diagnostic Procedures: Physical examination, suspicion, and cervical culture.

Pathologic Findings

Gram-negative intracellular diplococcus associated with diffuse inflammatory reaction (transluminal in the fallopian tube).

MANAGEMENT AND THERAPY

Nonpharmacologic

General Measures: Evaluation and diagnosis.

Specific Measures: Aggressive antibiotic therapy should be instituted in patients suspected of having an infection.

Diet: No specific dietary changes indicated.

Activity: No restriction. (Sexual continence is required until the infection has resolved.)

Patient Education: American College of Obstetricians and Gynecologists Patient Education Pamphlet AP009 (*How to Prevent Sexually Transmitted Diseases*). Patients should be advised to have all sexual partners seen for diagnosis and treatment.

Drug(s) of Choice

Ceftriaxone 125 mg IM or cefixime 400 mg PO single dose or

Ciprofloxacin 500 mg PO single dose or

Ofloxacin 400 mg PO as single dose plus

Azithromycin 1 g PO single dose or doxycycline 100 mg PO bid for 7 days.

Contraindications: Quinolones (Ofloxacin), tetracyclines (including doxycycline), and erythromycin estolate are contraindicated in pregnancy and should not be used.

Precautions: See individual agents.

Interactions: See individual agents.

Gonorrhea in the Female

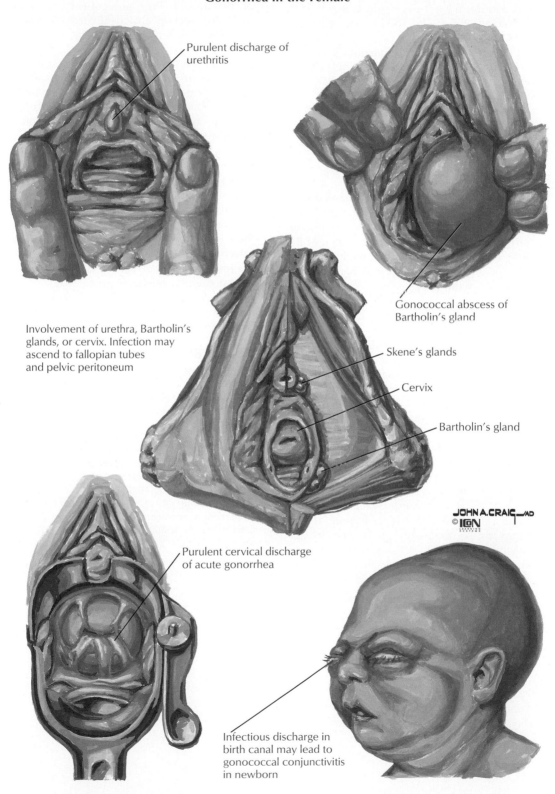

Purulent discharge of urethritis

Involvement of urethra, Bartholin's glands, or cervix. Infection may ascend to fallopian tubes and pelvic peritoneum

Gonococcal abscess of Bartholin's gland

Skene's glands

Cervix

Bartholin's gland

Purulent cervical discharge of acute gonorrhea

JOHN A.CRAIG—AD
© ICON
LEARNING SYSTEMS

Infectious discharge in birth canal may lead to gonococcal conjunctivitis in newborn

Alternative Drugs

Spectinomycin 2 g IM as single dose.

Ceftriaxone 125 mg IM and cefixime 400 mg PO as single dose.

Ceftizoxime 500 mg IM, cefotaxime 500 mg IM, or cefotetan 1 g IM, all as single dose.

Cefoxitin 2 g IM plus probenecid 1 g PO.

Cefuroxime axetil 1 g PO or cefpodoxime proxetil 200 mg PO, both as single dose.

Enoxacin 400 mg PO, lomefloxacin 400 mg PO, or norfloxacin 800 mg PO, all as single dose.

FOLLOW-UP

Patient Monitoring: When patients are treated with the currently recommended ceftriaxone-doxycycline, therapy failure is rare and a follow-up culture is not necessary. Reexamination of the patient in 1–2 months for the possibility of reinfection may be warranted in high-risk patients. (As with all sexually transmitted diseases, all sexual partners within the preceding 30 days should be screened and treated for probable infections.)

Prevention/Avoidance: Use of barrier contraception (condoms, diaphragm), limitation or elimination of risky behavior (sexual promiscuity).

Possible Complications: Damage caused by *N gonorrhoeae* infection causes an increased risk of recurrent pelvic infection, chronic pelvic pain, or infertility resulting from tubal damage or hydrosalpinx formation. The impact of a gonorrheal infection is much greater for women than it is for men. For every three men infected, two women are hospitalized for 1 or more days. For every 18 men infected, one woman undergoes surgery. It is estimated that one episode of gonorrhea is associated with a 15% infertility rate and this rises to 75% for three or more infections. The risk of an ectopic pregnancy is increased 7–10 times in women with a history of salpingitis. Neonatal infections acquired from an infected mother may result in conjunctivitis or pneumonia. Pregnant patients are more likely to experience disseminated gonococcal infection. They account for 7%–40% of all cases.

Expected Outcome: If detected early, successful treatment with minimal sequelae may be expected. Significant permanent damage is common despite treatment because of the indolent course of many infections and the late institution of therapy.

MISCELLANEOUS

Pregnancy Considerations: Pregnant patients should be treated with ceftriaxone 250 mg IM as a single dose. Erythromycin (erythromycin base, 500 mg PO qid for 7 days) may be added if there is a possibility of a coexisting chlamydial infection. Neonatal conjunctivitis and ophthalmia neonatorum may result if the infant does not receive adequate prophylaxis.

ICD-9-CM Codes: 098.0 (Acute, lower genital tract), 098.1 (Acute, upper genital tract) (others based on chronicity and organ involved).

REFERENCES

American College of Obstetricians and Gynecologists. *Gonorrhea and Chlamydial Infections.* Washington, DC: ACOG; 1994. ACOG Technical Bulletin 190.

Centers for Disease Control and Prevention. 1998 guidelines for treatment of sexually transmitted diseases. *MMWR Morb Mortal Wkly Rep* 1998;47(RR-1):60.

Centers for Disease Control and Surveillance. Decreased susceptibility of *Neisseria gonorrhoeae* to fluoroquinolones—Ohio and Hawaii, 1992–1994. *MMWR Morb Mortal Wkly Rep* 1994;43:325.

Phillips RS, Hanff PA, Wertheimer A. Aronson MD. Gonorrhea in women seen for routine gynecologic care: criteria for testing. *Am J Med* 1988;85:177.

Ramus R, Mayfield J, Wendel G. Evaluation of the current CDC recommended treatment guidelines for gonorrhea in pregnancy. *Am J Obstet Gynecol* 1996; 174:409.

SEXUALLY TRANSMITTED INFECTIONS: GRANULOMA INGUINALE

INTRODUCTION

Description: Granuloma inguinale (also called donovanosis) is relatively common in the tropics, New Guinea, and Caribbean areas, but accounts for less than 100 cases per year in the United States. This infection is caused by the bipolar, gram-negative bacterium *Calymmatobacterium granulomatis.*

Prevalence: Uncommon, 100 cases per year in United States, up to 25% of the population in some subtropical areas.

Predominant Age: Younger reproductive.

Genetics: No genetic pattern.

ETIOLOGY AND PATHOGENESIS

Causes: Infection is caused by the bipolar, gram-negative bacterium *C granulomatis.*

Risk Factors: Sexual trauma and exposure to the infective agent.

CLINICAL CHARACTERISTICS

Signs and Symptoms:

- Single or multiple subcutaneous papules that evolve to raised, red, granulomatous lesions that bleed on contact and undergo ulceration and necrosis and heal slowly (lesions are confined to the genitalia in 80% of patients; lesions generally appear within 2 weeks of exposure)
- Painless papules with rolled borders and friable base
- Marked adenopathy not present

DIAGNOSTIC APPROACH

Differential Diagnosis:

- Chancroid
- Lymphogranuloma venereum
- Herpes simplex
- Syphilis

Associated Conditions: Brawny edema of the external genitalia.

Workup and Evaluation

Laboratory: Gram's stain and culture of material from open ulcers. Culture for other sexually transmitted infections should also be considered.

Imaging: No imaging indicated.

Special Tests: Samples for biopsy may be taken from the edge of the ulcer to confirm the diagnosis. A crushed tissue smear may be examined for Donovan bodies.

Diagnostic Procedures: Diagnosis is established clinically or through the identification of intracytoplasmic bacteria (Donovan bodies) in mononuclear cells.

Pathologic Findings

Granulation tissue associated with an extensive chronic inflammatory cell infiltrate and endarteritis. The ulcer is filled with fibrinous exudate and necrosis; plasma cells and mononuclear cells predominate. Donovan bodies (large vacuolated histiocytes with encapsulated bacilli) are diagnostic. Granuloma inguinale extends by local infiltration and by lymphatic permeation in later stages.

MANAGEMENT AND THERAPY

Nonpharmacologic

General Measures: Evaluation, culture or Gram's stain, topical cleansing and care.

Specific Measures: Antibiotic therapy.

Diet: No specific dietary changes indicated.

Activity: No restriction. (Sexual continence required until infection is resolved.)

Patient Education: American College of Obstetricians and Gynecologists Patient Education Pamphlet AP009 (*How to Prevent Sexually Transmitted Diseases*). Patients should be advised to have all sexual partners seen for diagnosis and treatment.

Drug(s) of Choice

Trimethoprin-sulfamethoxazole, one double strength tablet PO bid for a minimum of 3 weeks or

Doxycycline 100 mg PO bid for a minimum of 3 weeks or

Ampicillin 500 mg PO q6h continued until lesions heal (may take up to 3 months).

Contraindications: Known or suspected allergy.

Precautions: Tetracyclines should not be used during pregnancy if at all possible because staining of teeth and inhibition of bone growth are both possible. Sulfonamides should not be used during pregnancy.

Interactions: See individual agents.

Alternative Drugs

Ciprofloxacin 750 mg PO bid for a minimum of 3 weeks.

Erythromycin 500 mg PO qid for a minimum of 3 weeks.

If lesions fail to show improvement after the first week of treatment, chloramphenicol (500 mg PO tid) or gentamicin (1 mg/kg bid) should be considered.

FOLLOW-UP

Patient Monitoring: Because of relapse and late scarring, these patients should be followed carefully for several weeks. Follow-up evaluation for cure with culture or other tests should be carried out, as well as screening for other sexually transmitted diseases. (As with all sexually transmitted diseases, all sexual partners within the preceding 30 days should be screened and treated for probable infections as well.)

Prevention/Avoidance: None.

Possible Complications: Secondary infection or significant scarring may occur in patients with untreated disease.

Expected Outcome: Gradual healing with antibiotic treatment, but scaring and vulvar stenosis are common and may require surgical treatment.

MISCELLANEOUS

Pregnancy Considerations: No direct effect on pregnancy. Women who are pregnant or lactating should be treated with erythromycin plus parenteral aminoglycoside (eg, gentamicin).

ICD-9-CM Codes: 099.2.

REFERENCES

Centers for Disease Control and Prevention. 1998 guidelines for treatment of sexually transmitted diseases. *MMWR Morb Mortal Wkly Rep* 1998:47(RR-1):26.

Dougherty CM, Pastorek JG II. Sexually transmitted diseases and miscellaneous pelvic infections. In: Sciarra JJ, ed. *Gynecology and Obstetrics.* Vol 1. Philadelphia, Pa: JB Lippincott; 1990;41:1.

Kuberski T. Granuloma inguinale (donovanosis). *Sex Transm Dis* 1980;7:29.

Morse SA. *Atlas of Sexually Transmitted Diseases.* Philadelphia, Pa: JB Lippincott; 1990.

Sweet RL, Gibbs RS. *Infectious Diseases of the Female Genital Tract.* Baltimore, Md: Williams & Wilkins; 1995:166.

Wilkinson EJ, Freidrich EF Jr. Disease of the vulva. In: Kurman RJ, ed. *Blaustein's Pathology of the Female Genital Tract.* 4th ed. New York, NY: Springer-Verlag; 1994:46.

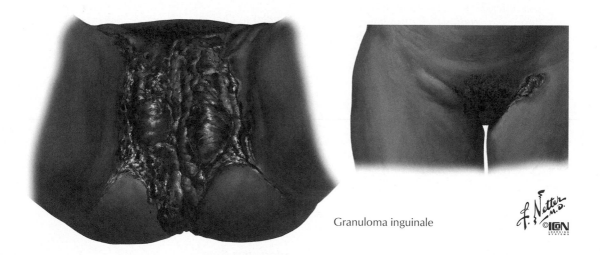

Granuloma inguinale

SEXUALLY TRANSMITTED INFECTIONS: HERPES

INTRODUCTION

Description: Infection by the herpes simplex virus results in recurrent symptoms that range from uncomfortable to disabling and there is a special risk to the neonate when herpes infection occurs during pregnancy.

Prevalence: Twenty million recurrent cases; 300,000–500,000 new cases per year; 1 in 200 asymptomatic women.

Predominant Age: 15–30 (85%).

Genetics: No genetic pattern.

ETIOLOGY AND PATHOGENESIS

Causes: Roughly 80% of genital herpes infections are caused by herpes simplex virus type 2, with the remaining 20% caused by the type 1 virus. Exposure to type 1 virus often happens in childhood and causes oral "cold sores." Previous infection with type 1 virus appears to provide some immunity to type 2 infections. The incubation period from infection to symptoms is generally approximately 6 days (range 3–9), with first episodes lasting from 10–12 days.

Risk Factors: Roughly 75% of sexual partners of infected individuals contract the disease if intercourse occurs during viral shedding. Patients are infectious during the period from first prodrome through crusting of the lesions. Viral shedding may also occur asymptomatically. Nonsexual transmission has not been documented.

CLINICAL CHARACTERISTICS

Signs and Symptoms:
- Prodromal phase—mild paresthesia and burning (beginning approximately 2–5 days after infection)
- Progresses to very painful vesicular and ulcerated lesions, 3–7 days after exposure (may prompt hospitalization in up to 10% of patients)
- Dysuria caused by vulvar lesions, urethral and bladder involvement, or autonomic dysfunction (may lead to urinary retention)
- Malaise, low-grade fever, and inguinal adenopathy (40%)
- Systemic symptoms, including aseptic meningitis, fever, headache, and meningismus can be found in 70% of patients 5–7 days after the appearance of the genital lesions in primary infections

DIAGNOSTIC APPROACH

Differential Diagnosis:
- Chancroid
- Syphilis
- Granuloma inguinale
- Folliculitis

Associated Conditions: Other sexually transmitted diseases, cervicitis.

Workup and Evaluation

Laboratory: Viral cultures of material taken by swab from the lesions (95% sensitivity). Smears of vesicular material may also be stained with Wright's stain to visualize giant multinucleated cells with characteristic eosinophilic intranuclear inclusions.

Imaging: No imaging indicated.

Special Tests: Scrapings from the base of vesicles may be stained using immunofluorescence techniques to detect the presence of viral particles.

Diagnostic Procedures: History, physical examination, viral culture and serologic testing.

Pathologic Findings

The virus replicates in the parabasal and intermediate cells of the skin. It passes from cell to cell until it encounters nerve cell endings, providing access to local ganglia. Typical lesions consist of clear vesicles that lyse, progressing to shallow, painful ulcers with a red border. These may coalesce, becoming secondarily infected and necrotic.

MANAGEMENT AND THERAPY

Nonpharmacologic

General Measures: Topical cleansing, sitz baths followed by drying with a heat lamp or hair dryer, analgesics.

Specific Measures: Topical analgesics (lidocaine [Xylocaine] 2% jelly, nonprescription throat spray with phenol), antiviral agents. If secondary infections occur, therapy with a local antibacterial cream, such as Neosporin, is appropriate.

Diet: No specific dietary changes indicated.

Activity: Pelvic rest until lesions have healed.

Patient Education: American College of Obstetricians and Gynecologists Patient Education Pamphlet AP009 (*How to Prevent Sexually Transmitted Diseases*). Patients should be advised to have all sexual partners seen for diagnosis and treatment.

Drug(s) of Choice

Acute (begun within 48 hours of onset)—acyclovir ointment (Zovirax or generic 5%

applied locally every 3 hours) or acyclovir (400 mg PO tid or 200 mg PO five times a day while lesions are present) or valacyclovir (Valtrex, 1 g PO bid for 5 days) will decrease the duration of symptoms and viral shedding, but this therapy has not been shown to decrease the likelihood of recurrence and the shortening of symptom duration is often minimal.

For frequent recurrences— acyclovir (200 mg PO tid or 400 mg PO bid, increased to five times per day with lesions) or famciclovir (Famvir, 125 mg PO bid for 5 days) is effective in decreasing frequency and severity of flare ups, but use is limited to less than 6 months.

Contraindications: Known or suspected hypersensitivity. Acyclovir is pregnancy category C; famciclovir and valacyclovir are pregnancy category B. Suppressive therapy should not be used for pregnant patients.

Precautions: Thrombotic thrombocytopenic purpura/hemolytic uremic syndrome has been reported in some patients with HIV taking valacyclovir. It has not been encountered in immunocompetent patients. Antiviral agents should be used with caution in patients with compromised renal function.

Interactions: Antiviral agents may interact with or enhance the effects of nephrotoxic agents.

Alternative Drugs

In severe infections, acyclovir 5–10 mg/kg IV q8h for 5–7 days may be required.

FOLLOW-UP

Patient Monitoring: Normal health maintenance. Watch for possible recurrence.

Prevention/Avoidance: Sexual continence during prodrome to full healing, use of condoms to reduce risk, sexual monogamy.

Possible Complications: Between 60% and 90% of patients have recurrences of the herpetic lesions in the first 6 months after initial infection. Although generally shorter and milder, these recurrent attacks are no less virulent.

Expected Outcome: Healing of the lesions is generally complete. Inguinal adenopathy may persist for several weeks after the resolution of the vulvar lesions. Suppuration is uncommon. Complete resolution of all symptoms occurs in 2–4 weeks.

MISCELLANEOUS

Pregnancy Considerations: Significant risk to neonate if acute infection or viral shedding is occurring at the time of delivery or rupture of the membranes. Infection is also associated with an increased risk of early fetal loss. Suppressive therapy should not be used for pregnant patients.

ICD-9-CM Codes: 054.11 (Vulvovaginal).

REFERENCES

American College of Obstetricians and Gynecologists. *Gynecologic Herpes Simplex Virus Infections.* Washington, DC: ACOG; 1988. ACOG Technical Bulletin 119.

Bryson Y, Dillon M, Bernsterin DI, Radolf J, Zakowski P, Garratty E. Risk of acquisition of genital herpes simplex virus type 2 in sex partners of persons with genital herpes: a prospective couple study. *J Infect Dis* 1993;167:942.

Centers for Disease Control and Prevention. 1998 guidelines for treatment of sexually transmitted diseases. *MMWR Morb Mortal Wkly Rep* 1998:47(RR-1):21.

Cone RW, Swenson PD, Hobson AC, Remington M, Corey L. Herpes simplex virus detection from genital lesions: a comparative study using antigen detection (HerpChek) and culture. *J Clin Microbiol* 1993; 31:1774.

deRuiter A, Thin RN. Genital herpes. A guide to pharmacological therapy. *Drugs* 1994;47:297.

Maccato ML, Kaufman RH. Herpes genitalis. *Dermatol Clin* 1992;10:415.

Lesions of Herpes Simplex

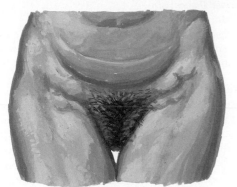

Regional lymphadenopathy, common
in genital herpes

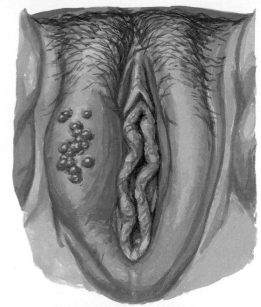

Marked edema and vesicle
formation in primary herpes

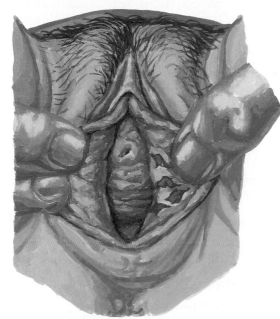

Ulcerative lesions of genitalia

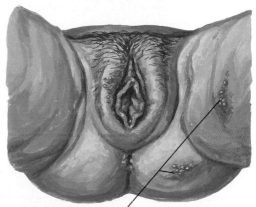

Autoinoculation lesions

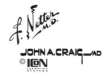

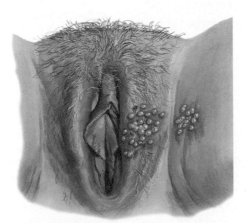

Herpes genitalis

SEXUALLY TRANSMITTED INFECTIONS: HUMAN IMMUNODEFICIENCY VIRUS

INTRODUCTION

Description: Infection by the human immunodeficiency virus (HIV) preferentially involves the immune system and leads to progressive deterioration in immune function. Women make up the fastest growing group of HIV-infected individuals. Many states have specific laws governing HIV screening, reporting, disclosure, and breech of confidence. All care providers should become familiar with the requirements imposed in their area.

Prevalence: Two million Americans or 0.7% of the entire population.

Predominant Age: Median age 35; 84% of cases occur between 15–44.

Genetics: No genetic pattern.

ETIOLOGY AND PATHOGENESIS

Causes: Infection by the HIV, a retrovirus that preferentially infects helper lymphocytes but may infect macrophages, cells of the central nervous system, and possibly the placenta. Incubation from infection to clinical symptoms ranges from 5 days to 3 months, with an average of 2–4 weeks.

Risk Factors: Sexual activity (multiple partners or infected partner—37% of all infections), parenteral exposure to blood (sharing needles, inadvertent needle stick), perinatal exposure of infants. There is no evidence that HIV infection may be transmitted by casual contact, immune globulin preparations, hepatitis B vaccine, or contact with biting insects. HIV infection following donor insemination has been reported.

CLINICAL CHARACTERISTICS

Signs and Symptoms:

- Nonspecific symptoms, often mimicking mononucleosis with aseptic meningitis (90%) (Febrile pharyngitis is the most common, with fever, sweats, lethargy, arthralgia, myalgia, headache, photophobia, and lymphadenopathy lasting up to 2 weeks.)
- Signs of loss of immune function: fever, weight loss, malaise, lymphadenopathy, central nervous system dysfunction, abnormal Pap smear, recurrent cervical intraepithelial neoplasia (CIN), oral or vaginal candidiasis

DIAGNOSTIC APPROACH

Differential Diagnosis:
- Mononucleosis

Associated Conditions: Gynecologic—abnormal Pap smears, CIN and cervical cancer, condyloma acuminata, increased risk of pregnancy loss.

Workup and Evaluation

Laboratory: Enzyme-linked immunosorbent assay (ELISA) with positive results confirmed by Western blot analysis (sensitivity and specificity >99%). (Informed consent is recommended before testing. False-positive Western blot test results are uncommon and are found on the order of less than 1 in 130,000.) Antibodies may not be detectable until 6–12 weeks after infection. Other tests include complete blood count, with differential white count, electrolytes, glucose 6-phosphate dehydrogenase, hepatitis B screen, liver and renal function tests, platelet count, Venereal Disease Research Laboratory (VDRL), or rapid plasma reagent (RPR) test.

Imaging: No imaging indicated.

Special Tests: Tests for tuberculosis (Tuberculin skin test with control [*Candida,* mumps, tetanus]) and other infections should be considered in HIV-infected individuals, Pap smear.

Diagnostic Procedures: ELISA and Western blot analysis.

Pathologic Findings

Reduced CD4 counts and diffuse evidence of immunocompromise.

MANAGEMENT AND THERAPY

Nonpharmacologic

General Measures: Health maintenance, avoidance of stress and infection.

Specific Measures: Management is focused on stabilization of HIV disease, prevention of opportunistic infections, and prevention of perinatal transmission. When CD4 counts are less than 200, antibiotic prophylaxis should be started.

Diet: No specific dietary changes indicated.

Activity: No restriction.

Patient Education: American College of Obstetricians and Gynecologists Patient Education Pamphlet AP009 (*How to Prevent Sexually Transmitted Diseases*). Patient counseling should include the risk of infections associated with sexual behavior, intravenous drug use, the risk of transmission to an infant, the availability of treatment to reduce that risk, and the risk and benefits of treatment for the patient.

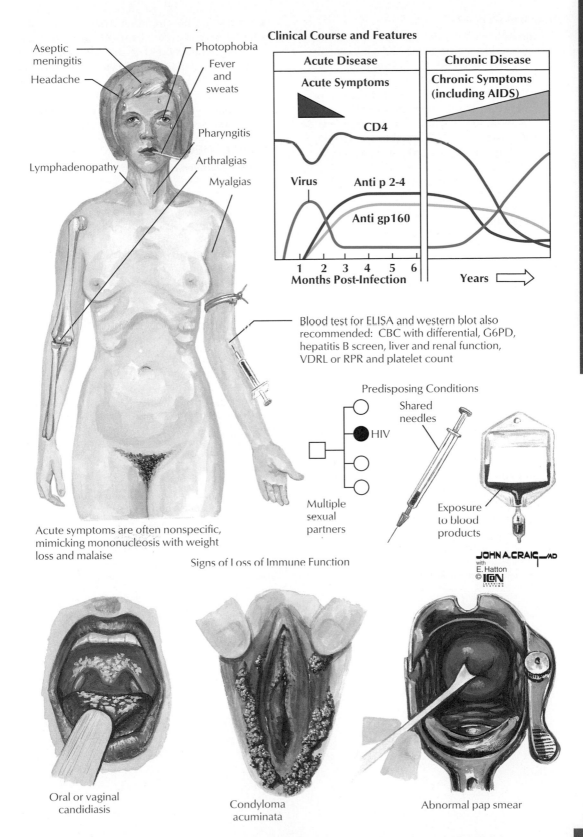

Aseptic meningitis

Photophobia

Headache

Fever and sweats

Pharyngitis

Lymphadenopathy

Arthralgias

Myalgias

Clinical Course and Features

Acute Disease

Acute Symptoms

CD4

Virus

Anti p 2-4

Anti gp160

1 2 3 4 5 6
Months Post-Infection

Chronic Disease

Chronic Symptoms (including AIDS)

Years

Blood test for ELISA and western blot also recommended: CBC with differential, G6PD, hepatitis B screen, liver and renal function, VDRL or RPR and platelet count

Predisposing Conditions

HIV

Shared needles

Multiple sexual partners

Exposure to blood products

Acute symptoms are often nonspecific, mimicking mononucleosis with weight loss and malaise

Signs of Loss of Immune Function

JOHN A. CRAIG __AD
with
E. Hatton
© ICON

Oral or vaginal candidiasis

Condyloma acuminata

Abnormal pap smear

Drug(s) of Choice

Zidovudine (ZVD, 100 mg PO five times daily) is used to reduce vertical transmission during pregnancy. Multiple drug therapy is common for HIV-infected individuals, but the best combination has yet to be determined, and guidelines are rapidly changing. Referral to a specialist is recommended.

Prophylactic drugs—Trimethoprim (160 mg) sulfamethoxazole (800 mg) daily as prophylaxis for those at risk (CD4 <200). (Significant infections must be treated specifically and aggressively.)

FOLLOW-UP

Patient Monitoring: Increased frequency of monitoring, including periodic assessment of blood and CD4 counts.

Prevention/Avoidance: Avoidance of risky behaviors such as intravenous drug use or multiple sexual partners, universal precautions for health care workers, consistent use of condoms, substance abuse prevention and treatment programs, and counseling programs. Prophylaxis after acute exposure (eg, needle stick) with ZVD singly or in combination with other agents has been shown to reduce the risk of infection.

Possible Complications: Opportunistic infections (bacterial, mycotic, and viral), increased risk of malignancy (cervical, Kaposi sarcoma, lymphoma), central nervous system dysfunction.

Expected Outcome: After recovery from the initial infection, the patient enters a carrier state during which symptoms are absent, but viral shedding occurs. Immune dysfunction generally becomes apparent roughly 10 years after the initial infection. The development of immunocompromise is rare before 3 years after infection, and less than 35% develop symptoms of AIDS before 5 years. Despite continuing progress in treatment of HIV infection and AIDS, the outcome is generally poor.

MISCELLANEOUS

Pregnancy Considerations: Significant risk of vertical transmission and worsening of maternal disease.

ICD-9-CM Codes: V08, 042 (With symptoms).

REFERENCES

American Medical Association Advisory Group on HIV Early Intervention. *HIV Early Intervention. Physician Guidelines.* 2nd ed. Chicago, Ill.: American Medical Association, 1994:8.

Bardequez AD. Management of HIV infection for the childbearing age woman. *Clin Obstet Gynecol* 1996; 39:344.

Carpenter CCJ, Fischl MA, Hammer SM, Hirsch MS, Jacobsen DM, Katzenstein DA, et al. Antiretroviral therapy for HIV infection in 1996: recommendations of an international panel. *JAMA* 1996;276:146.

Centers for Disease Control. AIDS in women—United States. *MMWR Morb Mortal Wkly Rep* 1990;39:845.

Centers for Disease Control and Prevention. 1998 guidelines for treatment of sexually transmitted diseases. *MMWR Morb Mortal Wkly Rep* 1998:47(RR-1):11.

Letvin NL. Progress in the development of an HIV-1 Vaccine. *Science* 1998;280:1875.

Waller SC. A meta-analysis of condom effectiveness in reducing sexually transmitted HIV. *Soc Sci Med* 1993;36:1635.

SEXUALLY TRANSMITTED INFECTIONS: LYMPHOGRANULOMA VENEREUM

INTRODUCTION

Description: A potentially destructive infection caused by one of a number of serotypes (L-1, L-2, L-3) of *Chlamydia trachomatis*. Although uncommon in the United States, this infection causes significant morbidity.

Prevalence: Uncommon (600 cases per year in the United States).

Predominant Age: Younger reproductive.

Genetics: Lymphogranuloma venereum (LVG) is 20 times more common in men than in women.

ETIOLOGY AND PATHOGENESIS

Causes: LGV is caused by several serotypes of *Chlamydia trachomatis*.

Risk Factors: Sexual trauma and exposure to the infective agent.

CLINICAL CHARACTERISTICS

Signs and Symptoms:
- Painless vesicle that heals quickly leaving no scar, generally located on posterior aspect of vulva or vestibule
- Proctitis, tenesmus, or bloody rectal discharge in anorectal infections (anal intercourse)
- Progressive adenopathy with bubo formation (groove sign—the "groove sign" is not specific to LGV: it may also be seen in other inflammatory processes such as hidradenitis suppurativa)
- Severe fibrosis and scarring (elephantiasis, "esthiomene") (rectal stenosis may occur)

DIAGNOSTIC APPROACH

Differential Diagnosis:
- Granuloma inguinale
- Chancroid
- Herpes simplex
- Syphilis
- Cancer (vulvar or colon)

Associated Conditions: Other sexually transmissible infections, HIV, dyspareunia, rectal stricture or stenosis.

Workup and Evaluation

Laboratory: Complement fixation test (a titer of greater than 1:64 is highly suspicious for LGV). Approximately 20% of patients with LGV will have false positive VDRL tests.

Imaging: No imaging indicated.

Special Tests: None indicated. (Biopsy of the lesions is not diagnostic because of the nonspecific damage present. Enlarged lymph nodes should not be biopsied or opened: chronic sinuses will result.)

Diagnostic Procedures: Complement fixation testing—80% of patients have a titer of 1:16 or greater.

Pathologic Findings

None (nonspecific inflammatory changes).

MANAGEMENT AND THERAPY

Nonpharmacologic

General Measures: Evaluation, culture or Gram's stain, topical cleansing and care.

Specific Measures: Antibiotic therapy. Treatment should be started even before results of confirmatory tests are received.

Diet: No specific dietary changes indicated.

Activity: No restriction. (Sexual continence required until infection is resolved.)

Patient Education: American College of Obstetricians and Gynecologists Patient Education Pamphlet AP009 (*How to Prevent Sexually Transmitted Diseases*). Patients should be advised to have all sexual partners seen for diagnosis and treatment.

Drug(s) of Choice

Doxycycline 100 PO bid for 3 weeks or tetracycline, 500 mg PO qid, for 3 weeks.

Contraindications: Erythromycin estolate and tetracyclines are contraindicated in pregnancy and should not be used.

Precautions: See individual agents.

Interactions: See individual agents.

Alternative Drugs

Erythromycin (500 mg PO qid for 3 weeks) or sulfadiazine (2 g PO loading dose, 1 g PO qid for 14–21 days) may be substituted.

FOLLOW-UP

Patient Monitoring: Follow-up evaluation for cure with culture or other tests should be carried out, as well as screening for other sexually transmitted diseases. (As with all sexually transmitted diseases, all sexual partners within the preceding 30 days should be screened and treated for probable infections as well.)

Prevention/Avoidance: Use of barrier contraception (condoms, diaphragm), limitation or elimination of risky behavior (sexual promiscuity).

Possible Complications: In one third of patients, abscess formation, rupture, and fistula formation occurs. Chronic progressive lymphangitis with chronic edema and sclerosing fibrosis may occur, causing extensive destruction of the vulva. Rectal stenosis also may occur and may be life threatening.

Expected Outcome: If detected early, successful treatment with minimal sequelae may be expected. Long-term scarring and disfigurement are common.

MISCELLANEOUS

Pregnancy Considerations: No effect on pregnancy, although the possibility of vertical transmission of other associated conditions (such as HIV infection) should be considered.

***ICD-9-CM* Codes:** 099.1.

REFERENCES

Ballard RC, Ye H, Matta A, Dangor Y, Radebe F. Treatment of chancroid with azithromycin. *Int J STD AIDS* 1996;7(suppl 1):9.

Centers for Disease Control and Prevention. 1998 guidelines for treatment of sexually transmitted diseases. *MMWR Morb Mortal Wkly Rep* 1998:47(RR-1):28.

Osewe PL, Peterman TA, Ransom RL, Zaidi AA, Wroten JE. Trends in the acquisition of sexually transmitted diseases among HIV-positive patients at STD clinics, Miami 1988–1992. *Sex Transm Dis* 1996;23:230.

Pearlman MD, McNeeley SG. A review of the microbiology, immunology and clinical implications of *Chlamydia trachomatis* infections. *Obstet Gynecol Surv* 1992;47:448.

Sevinsky LD, Lambierto A, Casco R, Woscoff A. Lymphogranuloma venereum: tertiary stage. *Int J Dermatol* 1997;36:47.

Wilkinson EJ, Stone IK. *Atlas of Vulvar Disease.* Baltimore, Md: Williams & Wilkins; 1995:154.

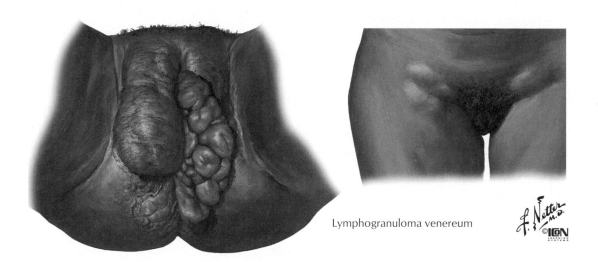

Lymphogranuloma venereum

SEXUALLY TRANSMITTED INFECTIONS: *MOLLUSCUM CONTAGIOSUM*

INTRODUCTION

Description: A papillary lesion caused by viral infection (pox virus) that is spread by skin to skin contact.

Prevalence: Two of 100,000, 1 of 40–60 patients with gonorrhea.

Predominant Age: Early reproductive.

Genetics: No genetic pattern.

ETIOLOGY AND PATHOGENESIS

Causes: *Molluscum contagiosum* is caused by the largest member of the pox virus group. This mildly contagious DNA virus infects epithelial tissues and autoinoculation to other sites is common.

Risk Factors: Sexual activity and exposure to the infective agent.

CLINICAL CHARACTERISTICS

Signs and Symptoms:
- Asymptomatic
- After several weeks of incubation, a round, umbilicated papule, 1–5 mm in size, with a yellow, waxy core of cheesy material (these lesions may grow slowly for months; they may be solitary or occur in clusters)

The lesions of molluscum are highly contagious and appropriate precautions should be used when examining the lesions or material from the lesions to avoid infection or spread.

DIAGNOSTIC APPROACH

Differential Diagnosis:
- Sebaceous cysts
- Folliculitis
- Herpes simplex
- Dermal papilloma
- Nevus

Associated Conditions: Other sexually transmitted infections.

Workup and Evaluation

Laboratory: No evaluation indicated. Because immunosuppressed patients are at higher risk for molluscum, testing for HIV infection should be considered.

Imaging: No imaging indicated.

Special Tests: Material from the lesions is examined microscopically; inclusion bodies is seen in material from the core of the lesion.

Diagnostic Procedures: Clinical picture and examination of material from lesion.

Pathologic Findings

Eosinophilic inclusion bodies (intracytoplasmic) in material from the core of the lesion.

MANAGEMENT AND THERAPY

Nonpharmacologic

General Measures: Local care.

Specific Measures: Treatment is based on obliterating the lesion. This is done by desiccation, cryotherapy, curettage, laser ablation, or chemical cautery ($AgNO_3$) (may cause hyperpigmentation and scarring). Curettage of the base of the lesion (with the tip of an 18-gauge needle or curette) is also curative. Bleeding may be controlled with Monsel's solution (ferric subsulfate solution 20%).

Diet: No specific dietary changes indicated.

Activity: No restriction. (Sexual continence required until infection is resolved.)

Patient Education: American College of Obstetricians and Gynecologists Patient Education Pamphlet AP009 (*How to Prevent Sexually Transmitted Diseases*). Patients should be advised to have all sexual partners seen for diagnosis and treatment.

Drug(s) of Choice

None.

FOLLOW-UP

Patient Monitoring: Follow-up should occur in 1 month to look for new lesions.

Prevention/Avoidance: Limitation or elimination of risky behavior (sexual promiscuity).

Possible Complications: Local secondary infection.

Expected Outcome: Good response to lesion destruction—generally heals with little or no scarring.

MISCELLANEOUS

Pregnancy Considerations: No effect on pregnancy.

ICD-9-CM Codes: 078.0.

REFERENCES

Borwn ST, Nalley JF, Kraus SJ. Molluscum contagiosum. *Sex Transm Dis* 1981;8:227.

Gottlieb SL, Myskowski PL. Molluscum contagiosum. *Int J Dermatol* 1994;33:453.

Morse SA. *Atlas of Sexually Transmitted Diseases.* Philadelphia, Pa: JB Lippincott; 1990.

Reed RJ, Parkinson RP. The histogenesis of molluscum contagiosum. *Am J Surg Pathol* 1977;1:161.

Sweet RL, Gibbs RS. *Infectious Diseases of the Female Genital Tract.* Baltimore, Md: Williams & Wilkins; 1995:170.

Wilkinson EJ, Stone IK. *Atlas of Vulvar Disease.* Baltimore, Md: Williams & Wilkins; 1995:57.

Sexually Transmitted Infections: *Molluscum Contagiosum*

Clinical findings

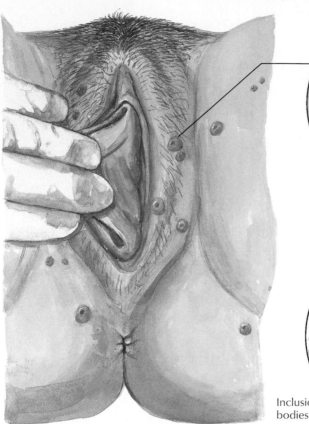

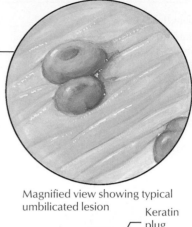

Magnified view showing typical
umbilicated lesion

Keratin
plug

Inclusion
bodies

Scattered distribution of molluscum lesions
over perineum, buttocks and thighs. Lesions
spread by physical contact and autoinnoculation

Histologic section of molluscum
lesions showing pox virus inclusion
bodies and central core of keratin

Evaluation and management

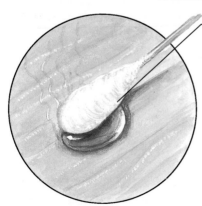

Application of
liquid nitrogen
to lesion
using cotton swab

JOHN A.CRAIG—AD
with
E. Hatton
© ICON
LEARNING SYSTEMS

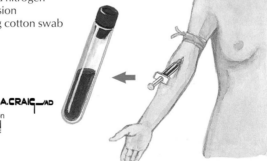

Local eradication of lesions can be obtained
with desiccation, cryotherapy, laser ablation,
chemical cautery or curettage

HIV testing may be warranted because
molluscum is a common complication
in immunosuppressed patients

SEXUALLY TRANSMITTED INFECTIONS: PARASITES

INTRODUCTION

Description: *Phthirus humanus* (pubic or crab lice) and *Sarcoptes scabiei* (scabies or itch mite) are parasitic insects that may be transferred through sexual activity or through contact with contaminated clothing or bedding.

Prevalence: Three million cases per year in the United States.

Predominant Age: Reproductive.

ETIOLOGY AND PATHOGENESIS

Causes: Parasitic insects (*P humanus* [pubic or crab lice] and *S scabiei* [scabies or itch mite]).

Risk Factors: Contact with infected person or fomites.

CLINICAL CHARACTERISTICS

Signs and Symptoms:
- Intense itching (greatest at night), most frequently in the area of the pubic hair

Infestations occur most frequently in the area of the pubic hair. Spread to other hairy areas can and does take place. Scabies infections are not confined to hairy area, but may be found in any area of the body.

DIAGNOSTIC APPROACH

Differential Diagnosis:
- Dermatoses
- Contact dermatitis
- Norwegian (crusted) scabies

Associated Conditions: Other sexually transmitted diseases.

Workup and Evaluation

Laboratory: No evaluation indicated.

Imaging: No imaging indicated.

Special Tests: Close inspection of the affected area generally reveals nits, feces, burrows, or the insects themselves.

Diagnostic Procedures: History and physical examination, microscopic examination of nits.

Pathologic Findings

Inflammatory reaction to the bite, burrow, and feces of the insect.

MANAGEMENT AND THERAPY

Nonpharmacologic

General Measures: Local cleansing, soothing creams, or lotions may be used.

Specific Measures: Topical applications of insecticide. Other family members should be treated and the home disinfected at the same time.

Diet: No specific dietary changes indicated.

Activity: No restriction.

Patient Education: American College of Obstetricians and Gynecologists Patient Education Pamphlet AP009 (*How to Prevent Sexually Transmitted Diseases*). Patients should be advised to have all sexual partners seen for diagnosis and treatment.

Drug(s) of Choice

Permethrin cream (5%) applied to all areas of the body from the neck down and washed off 8–14 hours later. Topical applications of lindane 1% (Kwell) lotion and shampoo applied for 4 minutes then washed off.

Contraindications: Lindane is contraindicated in premature neonates, pregnant or lactating patients, children younger than 2 years of age, or patients with Norwegian (crusted) scabies. Patients with seizure disorders or known or suspected hypersensitivity should not use the product.

Precautions: Care must be taken to avoid the eyes. The dose of lindane should be reduced in elderly patients because of increased skin absorption.

Interactions: Oils and ointments may increase the rate of absorption and should not be used.

Alternative Drugs

Crotamiton (Eurax) (10%) applied to all areas of the body from the neck down for two nights; on the third night, wash off the medication. Repeat the cycle beginning the fourth night.

FOLLOW-UP

Patient Monitoring: Normal health maintenance.

Prevention/Avoidance: Sexual monogamy.

Possible Complications: Secondary skin infection from scratching.

Expected Outcome: Generally good response to insecticide therapy. Reinfection is possible if both partners, family members, and fomites are not all treated simultaneously.

MISCELLANEOUS

Pregnancy Considerations: No direct effect on pregnancy.

ICD-9-CM Codes: 132.2 (*Phthirus pubis*), 131.0 (Scabies).

REFERENCES

Centers for Disease Control and Prevention. 1998 guidelines for treatment of sexually transmitted diseases. *MMWR Morb Mortal Wkly Rep* 1998;47(RR-1):105.

WOMEN'S HEALTH/PRIMARY CARE

Faber BM. The diagnosis and treatment of scabies and pubic lice. *Primary Care Update Ob/Gyn* 1996;3:20.

Landers DV, Sweet RL. Sexually transmitted infection. In: Glass RH, ed. *Office Gynecology.* Baltimore, Md: Williams & Wilkins; 1993:1.

Smith RP. *Gynecology in Primary Care.* Baltimore, Md: Williams & Wilkins; 1997:549.

Sweet RL, Gibbs RS. *Infectious Diseases of the Female Genital Tract.* Baltimore, Md: Williams & Wilkins; 1995:168.

Clinical Findings

Intense itching in pubic area (often nocturnal) is a hallmark of parasitic infection and excoriations are common

Bluish skin discolorations (maculae caerulae) often seen with *Phthirus* pubis infestations

Secondary infection of excoriations or bites may yield eczematoid lesions

Examination of pubic area and pubic hair may reveal ova and parasites

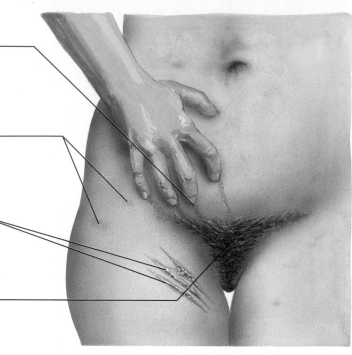

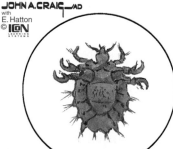

Phthirus pubis

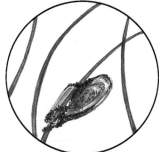

Phthirus pubis egg case (nit) on pubic hair

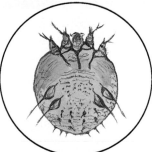

Sarcoptes scabei

Management

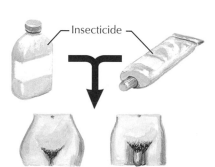

Insecticide

Increased general hygiene and treatment of household members and all sexual partners with insecticide shampoos and creams

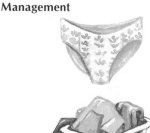

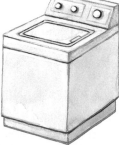

General house cleaning with emphasis on disinfection and laundering of underclothing and bedding

WOMEN'S HEALTH/PRIMARY CARE

SEXUALLY TRANSMITTED INFECTIONS: SYPHILIS

INTRODUCTION

Description: Since antiquity, syphilis has been the prototypic venereal disease. This disease presents with an easily overlooked first stage and, if left untreated, can slowly progress to a disabling disease noted for central nervous system, cardiac, and musculoskeletal involvement.

Prevalence: Increasing; 50,000 new cases were reported in 1990.

Predominant Age: 15–30 (85%).

Genetics: No genetic pattern.

ETIOLOGY AND PATHOGENESIS

Causes: *Treponema pallidum* is one of a very small group of spirochetes that are virulent for humans. This motile anaerobic spirochete can rapidly invade even intact moist mucosa (epithelium).

Risk Factors: It is estimated that roughly one third of patients exposed to early syphilis acquire the disease.

CLINICAL CHARACTERISTICS

Signs and Symptoms (Based on Stage):
- Painless chancres (shallow, firm, punched out, with a smooth base and rolled edges; on the vulva, anus, rectum, pharynx, tongue, lips, fingers, or the skin of almost any part of the body) 10 to 60 days (average, 21 days) after inoculation
- Low-grade fever, headache, malaise, sore throat, anorexia, generalized lymphadenopathy, and a diffuse, symmetric, asymptomatic maculopapular rash over the palm and soles ("money palms"), mucous patches, condyloma lata (second stage).

DIAGNOSTIC APPROACH

Differential Diagnosis:
- Herpes vulvitis
- Condyloma acuminata
- Lymphogranuloma venereum
- Chancroid

Associated Conditions: Tabes dorsalis, aortic aneurysm, and gummas.

Workup and Evaluation

Laboratory: The VDRL and RPR tests are nonspecific tests that are good screening tests because they are rapid and inexpensive. The fluorescent treponemal antibody absorption or microhemagglutination *Treponema pallidum* tests are specific treponemal antibody tests that are confirmatory or diagnostic that are not used for routine screening but are useful to rule out a false-positive screening test. If neurosyphilis is suspected, a lumbar puncture with a VDRL performed on the spinal fluid is required. Screening for HIV infection should also be strongly considered. False-positive screening results may occur in patients with lupus, hepatitis, sarcoidosis, recent immunization, drug abuse, or during pregnancy. These test results may be falsely negative in the second stage of the disease as a result of high levels of anticardiolipin antibody that interferes with the test (prozone phenomenon). Up to 30% of patients with a primary lesion have negative test results.

Imaging: No imaging indicated.

Special Tests: The diagnosis may be made by identifying motile spirochetes on darkfield microscopic examination of material from primary or secondary lesions or lymph node aspirates.

Diagnostic Procedures: Physical examination, suspicion, serologic testing.

Pathologic Findings

Based on stage of disease.

MANAGEMENT AND THERAPY

Nonpharmacologic

General Measures: Evaluation and diagnosis.

Specific Measures: Antibiotic therapy based on stage of disease.

Diet: No specific dietary changes indicated.

Activity: No restriction. (Sexual continence required until infection is resolved.)

Patient Education: American College of Obstetricians and Gynecologists Patient Education Pamphlet AP009 (*How to Prevent Sexually Transmitted Diseases*). Patients should be advised to have all sexual partners seen for diagnosis and treatment.

Drug(s) of Choice

Based on stage of disease. See table.

Contraindications: Known or suspected allergy.

Alternative Drugs

See table. Pregnant patients who are allergic to penicillin should be desensitized and then treated with penicillin.

Superficial Syphilitic Lesions

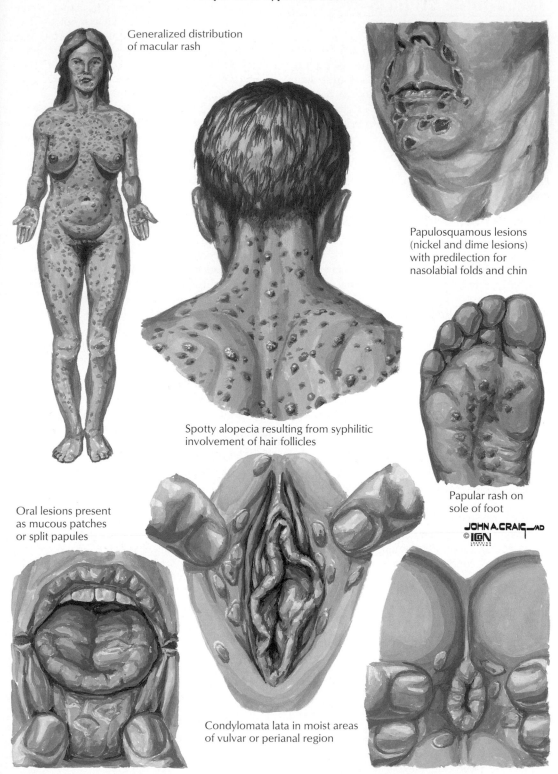

Generalized distribution of macular rash

Papulosquamous lesions (nickel and dime lesions) with predilection for nasolabial folds and chin

Spotty alopecia resulting from syphilitic involvement of hair follicles

Papular rash on sole of foot

Oral lesions present as mucous patches or split papules

Condylomata lata in moist areas of vulvar or perianal region

JOHN A. CRAIG_AD
© ICON

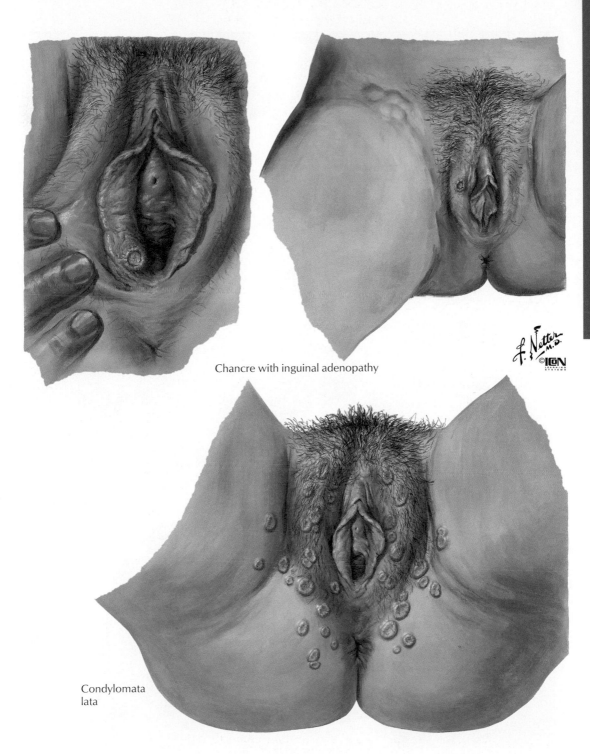

Chancre with inguinal adenopathy

Condylomata
lata

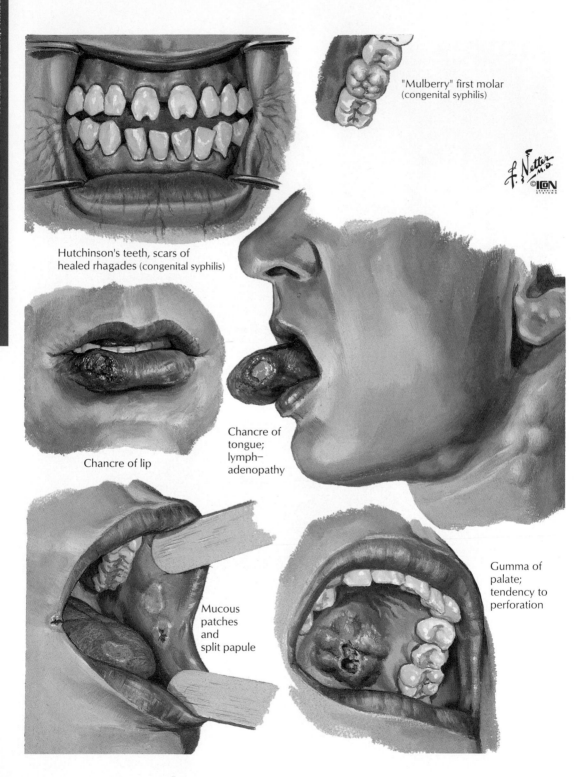

"Mulberry" first molar
(congenital syphilis)

Hutchinson's teeth, scars of
healed rhagades (congenital syphilis)

Chancre of lip

Chancre of
tongue;
lymph–
adenopathy

Mucous
patches
and
split papule

Gumma of
palate;
tendency to
perforation

SYPHILIS THERAPY

	Preferred Treatment	**Alternative Treatment**
Primary or secondary	Benzathine penicillin G, 2.4 mU IM or aqueous procaine penicillin G 600,000 U IM every other day for 8 days	Tetracycline 500 mg PO qid for 15 days (erythromycin 500 mg PO qid for 15 days in pregnant patients)
Cardiovascular/latent	Benzathine penicillin G, 2.4 mU IM weekly for 3 weeks or aqueous procaine penicillin G 600,000 U IM every other day for 15 days	Tetracycline 500 mg PO qid for 30 days (erythromycin 500 mg PO qid for 15 days in pregnant patients)
Neurosyphilis	Crystalline penicillin G 3–4 mU IM q4h for at least 10 days	Penicillin G procaine 2–4 mU IM daily + probenecid 500 mg PO for 10–14 days

FOLLOW-UP

Patient Monitoring: Screening for other sexually transmitted diseases. (As with all sexually transmitted diseases, all sexual partners within the preceding 30 days should be screened and treated for probable infections as well.)

Prevention/Avoidance: Limitation or elimination of risky behavior (sexual promiscuity).

Possible Complications: If untreated, crippling damage to the central nervous or skeletal systems, heart, or great vessels often ensues in the form of destructive, necrotic, granulomatous lesions (gummas), which develop from 1–10 years after the initial infection. Serious cardiovascular or neurologic complications occur in 5%–20% of patients.

Expected Outcome: Early treatment is associated with resolution; permanent damage may occur if disease is treated at a later stage.

MISCELLANEOUS

Pregnancy Considerations: Transplacental spread of syphilis occurs at any time during pregnancy and can result in congenital syphilis. Transplacental infection occurs in roughly 50% of patients with untreated primary or secondary disease. Half of these patients have premature deliveries or stillbirths.

ICD-9-CM **Codes:** 091.0 (Primary, genital chancre), 091.3 (Secondary) (others based on organ system and extent of disease).

REFERENCES

Berry MC, Dajani AS. Resurgence of congenital syphilis. *Infect Dis Clin North Am* 1992;6:19.

Centers for Disease Control and Prevention. 1998 guidelines for treatment of sexually transmitted diseases. *MMWR Morb Mortal Wkly Rep* 1998;47(RR-1):28.

El-Zaatari MM, Martens MG, Anderson GD. Incidence of the prozone phenomenon in syphilis serology. *Obstet Gynecol* 1994;84:609.

Rolfs RT. Treatment of syphilis, 1993. *Clin Infect Dis* 1995;20(suppl 1):S23.

Romanowski B, Sutherland R, Fick GH, Mooney D, Love EJ. Serologic response to treatment of infectious syphilis. *Ann Intern Med* 1991;114:1005.

St Louis ME, Wasserheit JN. Elimination of syphilis in the United States. *Science* 1998;281:353.

Wilkinson EJ, Stone IK. *Atlas of Vulvar Disease.* Baltimore, Md: Williams & Wilkins; 1995:171.

Wong TY, Mihm MC Jr. Primary syphilis. *N Engl J Med* 1994;331:1492.

SEXUALLY TRANSMITTED INFECTIONS: *TRICHOMONAS VAGINALIS*

INTRODUCTION

Description: Infection by the anaerobic flagellate protozoan, *Trichomonas vaginalis* is most often acquired by sexual contact with an infected person.

Prevalence: Roughly 3 million cases per year, 25% of "vaginal infections."

Predominant Age: 15–50 (may occur at any age).

Genetics: No genetic pattern.

ETIOLOGY AND PATHOGENESIS

Causes: *Trichomonas vaginalis*, an anaerobic flagellate protozoan.

Risk Factors: Multiple sexual partners, vaginal pH that is less acidic. (Blood, semen, or bacterial pathogens increase the risk.) Thirty to eighty percent of asymptomatic partners of women with *Trichomonas* infections have a positive culture. The incubation period for *Trichomonas* infections is thought to be between 4 and 28 days.

CLINICAL CHARACTERISTICS

Signs and Symptoms:
- Forty percent may be asymptomatic; a carrier state may exist for many years
- Vulvar itching or burning
- Copious discharge with a rancid odor (generally thin, runny, and yellow-green to gray in color, "frothy" in 25%)
- "Strawberry" punctation of the cervix and upper vagina (15%)
- Dysuria
- Dyspareunia
- Edema or erythema of the vulva

DIAGNOSTIC APPROACH

Differential Diagnosis:
- Bacterial vaginitis
- Bacterial vaginosis
- Chlamydial cervicitis
- Gonococcal cervicitis

Associated Conditions: Other sexually transmitted infections (specifically gonorrhea and chlamydial infection).

Workup and Evaluation

Laboratory: Culture or monoclonal antibody staining may be obtained but are seldom necessary. Evaluation for concomitant sexually transmitted infections should be strongly considered. Detection of *Trichomonas* by Pap smear results in an error rate of 50%.

Imaging: No imaging indicated.

Special Tests: Vaginal pH 6–6.5 or above.

Diagnostic Procedures: Physical examination, microscopic examination of vaginal secretions in normal saline.

Pathologic Findings

T vaginalis is a fusiform protozoan, slightly larger than a white blood cell, with three to five flagella extending from the narrow end, which provide active movement.

MANAGEMENT AND THERAPY

Nonpharmacologic

General Measures: Perineal hygiene, education regarding sexually transmissible infections.

Specific Measures: Medical therapy, vaginal acidification.

Diet: No specific dietary changes indicated. Avoid alcohol during metronidazole treatment.

Activity: Sexual continence until partner(s) are examined and treated.

Patient Education: American College of Obstetricians and Gynecologists Patient Education Pamphlet AP009 (*How to Prevent Sexually Transmitted Diseases*). Patients should be advised to have all sexual partners seen for diagnosis and treatment.

Drug(s) of Choice

Metronidazole 1 g in AM and PM, 1 day or metronidazole 250 mg q8h for 7 days.

Contraindications: Metronidazole is relatively contraindicated in the first trimester of pregnancy.

Precautions: Metronidazole may produce a disulfiramlike reaction resulting in nausea, vomiting, headaches or other symptoms if the patient ingests alcohol. Patients should not use metronidazole if they have taken disulfiram in the preceding 2 weeks. Metronidazole must be used with care or the dose reduced in patients with hepatic disease.

Interactions: Metronidazole may potentiate the effects of warfarin or coumarin and alcohol (as noted above).

Alternative Drugs

Topical clotrimazole, povidone iodine (topical), hypertonic (20%) saline douches.

FOLLOW-UP

Patient Monitoring: Follow-up serologic testing for syphilis and HIV infection as indicated.

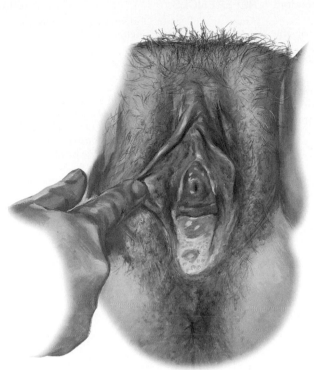

Trichomoniasis

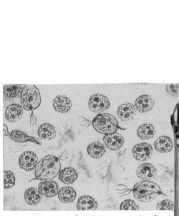

Trichomonas vaginalis

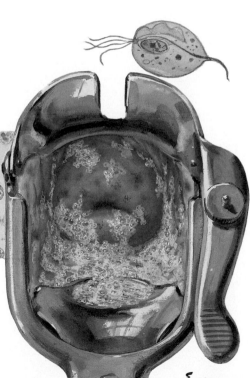

Prevention/Avoidance: Sexual monogamy, condom use for intercourse.

Possible Complications: Cystitis, infections of the Skene's or Bartholin's glands, increased risk of PID, pelvic pain, infertility, and other sequelae of sexually transmitted infections.

Expected Outcome: Resistance to metronidazole is uncommon. Most treatment failures are actually caused by reinfection or failure to comply with treatment.

MISCELLANEOUS

Pregnancy Considerations: Vaginal infections are associated with an increased risk of prematurity and premature rupture of the membranes.

ICD-9-CM **Codes:** 131.0, 131.01 (Vaginal).

REFERENCES

American College of Obstetricians and Gynecologists. *Vulvovaginitis.* Washington, DC: ACOG; 1989. Technical Bulletin 135.

American College of Obstetricians and Gynecologists. *Vaginitis.* Washington, DC: ACOG; 1996. ACOG Technical Bulletin 226.

Centers for Disease Control and Prevention. 1998 guidelines for treatment of sexually transmitted diseases. *MMWR Morb Mortal Wkly Rep* 1998:47(RR-1):74.

Lossick JG. Single-dose metronidazole treatment for vaginal trichomoniasis. *Obstet Gynecol* 1980;56:508.

McLellan R, Spence MR, Brockman M, Raffel L, Smith JL. The clinical diagnosis of trichomoniasis. *Obstet Gynecol* 1982;60:30.

Smith RP. *Gynecology in Primary Care.* Baltimore, Md: Williams & Wilkins; 1997:603.

Summers P. Vaginitis in 1993. *Clin Obstet Gynecol* 1993; 36:105.

Thomason JL, Gelbart SM. *Trichomonas vaginalis. Obstet Gynecol* 1989;74:536.

THROMBOPHLEBITIS

INTRODUCTION

Description: An inflammatory condition of the veins with secondary thrombosis. This may occur in two forms: aseptic or suppurative (septic). The vessels may be either superficial or deep. There may be risk factors present or the onset may be idiopathic. Risk varies with location and cause.

Prevalence: Two million cases per year in United States, 10% of nosocomial infections, intravascular (venous or arterial) catheter-related—88 of 100,000.

Predominant Age: Septic—childhood; aseptic—20–30; superficial— older than 40.

Genetics: Uncommon—antithrombin III, proteins C and S, and factor XII deficiencies (autosomal dominant with variable penetrance).

ETIOLOGY AND PATHOGENESIS

Causes: Sepsis (*Staphylococcus aureus* [65%–75%], multiple organisms [14%]), hypercoagulable states (congenital deficiencies, malignancy, pregnancy, high-dose oral contraceptives, Behçet's syndrome, Buerger's disease, factor V Leiden deficiency), venous stasis (varicose veins), injury to vessel wall. Septic thrombophlebitis may be caused by *Candida albicans* in unusual cases.

Risk Factors: Trauma (general or vascular), prolonged immobility, advanced age, obesity, pregnancy or puerperium, recent surgery, intravascular catheters, steroid or high-dose estrogen therapy (high-dose oral contraceptives), high altitude, hemoglobinopathies, malignancy, nephrotic syndrome, homocystinuria, congenital abnormality.

CLINICAL CHARACTERISTICS

Signs and Symptoms:
- Asymptomatic
- Generalized limb pain or swelling
- Swelling, tenderness, redness along the course of the vein
- Fever (70% of patients)
- Warmth, erythema, tenderness, or lymphangitis (32%)
- Systemic sepsis (84% in suppurative cases)
- Red, tender cord
- Swelling of collateral veins

DIAGNOSTIC APPROACH

Differential Diagnosis:
- Cellulitis
- Erythema nodosa
- Cutaneous polyarteritis nodosa
- Sarcoid
- Kaposi's sarcoma
- Ruptured synovial cyst (Baker's cyst)
- Lymphedema
- Muscle tear, sprain, strain
- Venous obstruction (secondary to tumor, lymph node enlargement)

Associated Conditions: Budd-Chiari syndrome (hepatic vein thrombosis), renal vein thrombosis, homocystinuria, hypercoagulability states (antiphospholipid antibody syndrome), Behçet's syndrome, and varicose veins.

Workup and Evaluation

Laboratory: Complete blood count, blood culture (positive in 80%–90% of superficial cases), D-dimer assay, coagulation profiles (antithrombin III levels are suppressed during the acute event—evaluations for abnormal levels should await completion of therapy), activated partial thromboplastin time (APTT) and prothrombin time (PT) to monitor anticoagulant therapy. For patients with septic thrombosis—periodic white blood cell counts.

Imaging: Contrast venography is the "gold standard" for diagnosis. Doppler studies of vascular flow may be effective for some deep vessels. Chest radiograph if embolism is suspected.

Special Tests: Impedance plethysmography, I^{125}-fibrinogen scans (not widely available and requires 4+ hours), bone or gallium scans for associated periosteal sepsis, ventilation/perfusion scans of the lungs if an embolism is suspected.

Diagnostic Procedures: History, physical examination, imaging or other diagnostic study (impedance plethysmography, [1] I^{125}-fibrinogen scans).

Pathologic Findings

Clot attached to vessel wall with variable degrees of inflammation present in the vessel wall. Enlargement of the vessel with thickening is common. Perivascular suppuration or hemorrhage may be seen.

MANAGEMENT AND THERAPY

Nonpharmacologic

General Measures: For superficial aseptic conditions—heat, elevation, observation. For deep or septic thrombophlebitis—hospitalization, anticoagulation, bed rest for 1–5 days with progressive return to normal activity. Patients with deep vein thrombosis confined to the calf

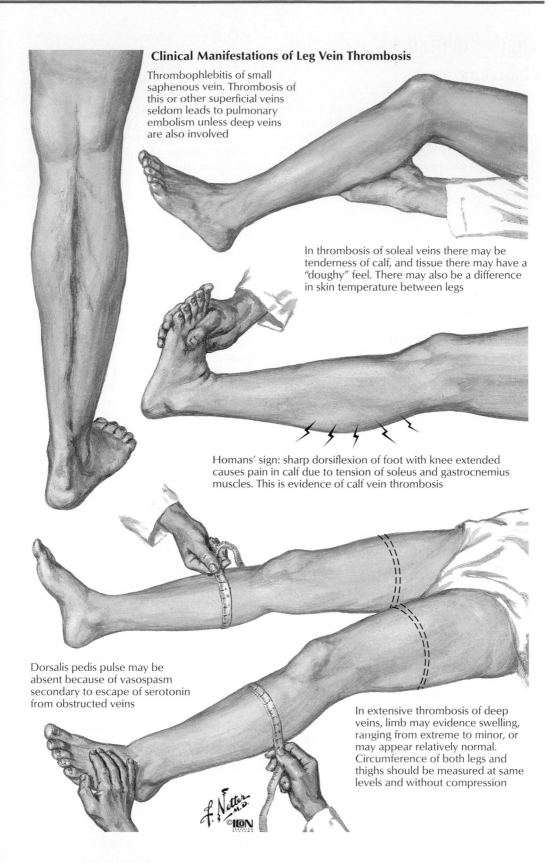

Clinical Manifestations of Leg Vein Thrombosis

Thrombophlebitis of small saphenous vein. Thrombosis of this or other superficial veins seldom leads to pulmonary embolism unless deep veins are also involved

In thrombosis of soleal veins there may be tenderness of calf, and tissue there may have a "doughy" feel. There may also be a difference in skin temperature between legs

Homans' sign: sharp dorsiflexion of foot with knee extended causes pain in calf due to tension of soleus and gastrocnemius muscles. This is evidence of calf vein thrombosis

Dorsalis pedis pulse may be absent because of vasospasm secondary to escape of serotonin from obstructed veins

In extensive thrombosis of deep veins, limb may evidence swelling, ranging from extreme to minor, or may appear relatively normal. Circumference of both legs and thighs should be measured at same levels and without compression

(distal to the popliteal system) may be managed as outpatients.

Specific Measures: Heparin anticoagulation initially followed by oral maintenance therapy (warfarin) for 3–6 months for first episodes or 12 months for recurrent episodes. Filtering devices ("umbrellas") should be considered for those who cannot receive anticoagulation therapy or those with evidence of emboli. Surgical excision of involved superficial veins (and tributaries) may be required.

Diet: No specific dietary changes indicated.

Activity: Initially, bed rest for deep or extensive thrombosis with gradual return to activity in 1–5 days. No restriction once acute episode is resolved.

Patient Education: Patients who have had an episode of thrombosis should be instructed in risk reduction and warning signs that require reevaluation.

Drug(s) of Choice

Heparin 5000–10,000 U IV bolus followed by 1000 U/h IV (may also use bolus of 80 U/kg, followed by 18 U/kg/h). Dosage must be titrated based on APTT: target = 2 times control.

Maintenance with warfarin (Coumadin) starting at 1–5 days. Initial dose 5–10 mg PO qd, adjusted based on PT: target = 1.3–1.5 times control (international normalized ratio [INR] of 2.0–3.0). (Intermittent subcutaneous heparin therapy with 15,000 U bid may also be used.)

Antibiotic therapy should be added for any patient suspected of sepsis (nafcillin 2 g IV q6h + gentamicin 1–1.7 mg/kg IV).

Contraindications: Acute bleeding, recent neurosurgical procedure, known adverse reaction. Warfarin is contraindicated in pregnancy—these patients must continue heparin therapy. Relative contraindications—recent hemorrhage or surgery, peptic ulcer disease (severe), recent nonembolic stroke.

Precautions: Patients should continue to receive heparin until the target PT level is reached. Heparin therapy may cause thrombocytopenia. Intramuscular injections should be avoided while patients are receiving anticoagulant therapy. Warfarin therapy may be associated with necrotic skin lesions in a small number of patients (warfarin necrosis). Desogestrel-containing oral contraceptives are associated with a higher incidence of thromboembolism than other oral contraceptive formulations. This difference is small (20–30 of 100,000 versus 10–15 of100,000 for levonorgestrel and 4 of 100,000 for nonpregnant women).

Interactions: Agents that prolong or intensify the action of anticoagulants—alcohol, allopurinol, amiodarone, steroids, androgens, many antimicrobials, cimetidine, chloral hydrate, disulfiram, all nonsteroidal antiinflammatory agents, sulfinpyrazone, tamoxifen, thyroid hormone, vitamin E, ranitidine, salicylates. Agents such as aminoglutethimide, antacids, barbiturates, carbamazepine, cholestyramine, diuretics, griseofulvin, rifampin, and oral contraceptives reduce the efficacy of oral anticoagulants.

Alternative Drugs

Thrombolytic agents (urokinase, streptokinase, tissue plasminogen activator) are effective in dissolving clots but remain investigational for the treatment of thrombosis. For mild superficial clots, nonsteroidal antiinflammatory agents may be used.

FOLLOW-UP

Patient Monitoring: Patients must be carefully monitored for embolization or further thrombosis. At the start of heparin therapy, the APTT must be monitored several times daily until the dose has been stabilized. The dose of warfarin must be monitored with periodic evaluation of the PT. Monitoring should be done daily until the target has been achieved, weekly for several weeks, and then monthly during maintenance therapy. Periodic checks should be made for hematuria and fecal occult blood.

Prevention/Avoidance: Avoid prolonged immobilization. Active prophylaxis (eg, for patients after surgery) using low-dose subcutaneous heparin, low-molecular-weight heparin (enoxaparin), mechanical leg compression, and early ambulation. Changing intravenous sites every 48 hours reduces the risk of infection and inflammation.

Possible Complications: Pulmonary embolism (fatal in up to 20% of patients), phlegmasia ceruleus dolens (rare). Hematuria or gastrointestinal bleeding may occur while patients are receiving anticoagulants. Any bleeding must be investigated and not presumed to be related to therapy; therapy may unmask an underlying condition such as cancer or ulcer disease. After thrombophlebitis, persistent pain and swelling of the limb may occur. Septic thrombophlebitis is associated with bacteremia (85%), septic emboli (45%), or abscess formation or pneumonia (45%).

Expected Outcome: Superficial thrombophlebitis and distal deep disease generally respond to prompt therapy with eventual resolution of symptoms. Up to 20% of proximal thrombosis may lead to embolization.

MISCELLANEOUS

Pregnancy Considerations: The use of warfarin is contraindicated. Patients who must receive anticoagulant therapy should be given heparin (intermittent subcutaneous therapy). Pregnancy causes a 49-fold increase in the incidence of phlebitis. Risk is increased with increased maternal age, multiparity, multiple pregnancy, hypertension, and preeclampsia.

***ICD-9-CM* Codes:** Based on location and type.

REFERENCES

American College of Obstetricians and Gynecologists. *Thromboembolism in Pregnancy.* Washington, DC: ACOG; 1997. ACOG Technical Bulletin 234.

Hirsh J. Venous thromboembolism. In: Rubenstein E, Federman DD, eds. *Scientific American Medicine.* New York, NY: Scientific American, 1994.

Kontos HA. Vascular diseases of the limbs. In: Wyngaarden JB, Smith LH Jr, Bennett JC, eds. *Cecil Textbook of Medicine.* 19th ed. Philadelphia, Pa: WB Saunders Co, 1992: 671.

Samlaskie CP, James WD. Superficial thrombophlebitis. I. Primary hypercoagulable states. *J Am Acad Dermatol* 1990;22:975.

Samlaskie CP, James WD. Superficial thrombophlebitis. II. Secondary hypercoagulable states. *J Am Acad Dermatol* 1990;23:1.

Weinman EE, Salzman EW. Deep-vein thrombosis. *N Engl J Med* 1994;331:1630.

TOXIC SHOCK SYNDROME

INTRODUCTION

Description: Toxic shock syndrome (TSS) is caused by toxins produced by an often asymptomatic infection with *Staphylococcus aureus*. Although most commonly associated with prolonged tampon use, about 10% of TSS cases are associated with other conditions.

Prevalence: Seen in 0.22–1.23 of 100,000.

Predominant Age: 30–60.

Genetics: No genetic pattern.

ETIOLOGY AND PATHOGENESIS

Causes: *S aureus* exotoxins (toxic shock syndrome toxin-1, enterotoxins A, B and C). For toxic shock to develop three conditions must be met: there must be colonization by the bacteria, it must produce toxin, and there must be a portal of entry for the toxin. The presence of foreign bodies, such as a tampon, is thought to reduce magnesium levels, which promotes the formation of toxin by the bacteria.

Risk Factors: Infection by *S aureus*, use of super absorbency tampons, or prolonged use of regular tampons.

CLINICAL CHARACTERISTICS

Signs and Symptoms:
- Most common—Fever greater than 38.9°C (102°F), hypotension, diffuse rash (the rash caused by toxic shock syndrome is commonly absent in places where clothing presses tightly against the skin)
- Other typical findings—Agitation, arthralgias, confusion, diarrhea, erythema of pharynx, vulva, or vagina, conjunctiva, headache, myalgias, nausea, vomiting

DIAGNOSTIC APPROACH

Differential Diagnosis:
- Other exanthems (acute rheumatic fever, bullous impetigo, drug reaction, erythema multiforme, Kawasaki disease, leptospirosis, meningococcemia, Rocky Mountain spotted fever, rubella, rubeola, scarlet fever, viral disease)
- Gastrointestinal illness (appendicitis, dysentery, gastroenteritis, pancreatitis, staphylococcal food poisoning)
- Acute pyelonephritis
- Hemolytic uremic syndrome
- Legionnaires' disease
- PID
- Reye's syndrome
- Rhabdomyolysis
- Septic shock
- Stevens-Johnson syndrome
- Systemic lupus erythematosus
- Tick typhus

Associated Conditions: Other sources—surgical wounds (including dilation and curettage), nonsurgical focal infections, cellulitis, subcutaneous abscesses, mastitis, infected insect bites, postpartum (including transmission to the neonate), nonmenstrual vaginal conditions, vaginal infection, PID, steroid cream use.

Workup and Evaluation

Laboratory: Cultures for *S aureus*, complete blood count, liver and renal function studies.

Imaging: No imaging indicated.

Special Tests: None indicated.

Diagnostic Procedures: History and physical findings.

Pathologic Findings

Lymphocyte depletion, subepidermic cleavage planes, cervical or vaginal ulcers.

Characteristics That Define Toxic Shock Syndrome

- Fever >38.9°C (102°F)
- Diffuse, macular, erythematous rash
- Desquamation of palms and soles 1–2 weeks after onset
- Hypotension (<90 torr systolic or orthostatic change)
- Negative blood, pharyngeal, and cerebrospinal fluid culture
- Negative serologic tests for measles, leptospirosis, Rocky Mountain spotted fever
- Three or more of the following organ systems:
  - Cardiopulmonary (respiratory distress, pulmonary edema, heart block, myocarditis
  - Central nervous (disorientation or altered sensorium)
  - Gastrointestinal (vomiting, diarrhea)
  - Hematologic (thrombocytopenia of ≤100,000/mm³)
  - Hepatic (>2-fold elevation of total bilirubin or liver enzymes, serum albumin >2 g/dL)
  - Mucous membrane inflammation (vaginal, oropharyngeal, conjunctival)
  - Musculoskeletal (myalgia, >2-fold elevation of creatine phosphokinase)
  - Renal (pyuria, >2-fold elevation of blood urea nitrogen or creatinine)

From Smith RP. *Gynecology in Primary Care.* Baltimore, Md: Williams & Wilkins; 1997:363.

Etiology and Pathogenesis

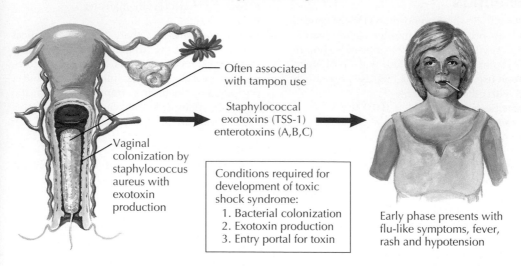

Often associated with tampon use

Staphylococcal exotoxins (TSS-1) enterotoxins (A,B,C)

Vaginal colonization by staphylococcus aureus with exotoxin production

Conditions required for development of toxic shock syndrome:
1. Bacterial colonization
2. Exotoxin production
3. Entry portal for toxin

Early phase presents with flu-like symptoms, fever, rash and hypotension

Clinical Features of Toxic Shock Syndrome

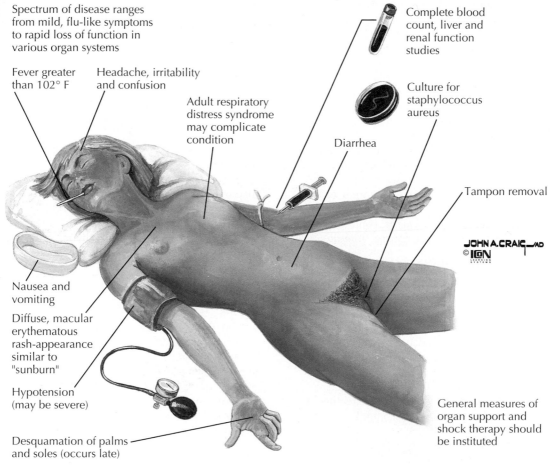

Spectrum of disease ranges from mild, flu-like symptoms to rapid loss of function in various organ systems

Complete blood count, liver and renal function studies

Fever greater than 102° F

Headache, irritability and confusion

Adult respiratory distress syndrome may complicate condition

Culture for staphylococcus aureus

Diarrhea

Tampon removal

Nausea and vomiting

Diffuse, macular erythematous rash-appearance similar to "sunburn"

Hypotension (may be severe)

General measures of organ support and shock therapy should be instituted

Desquamation of palms and soles (occurs late)

JOHN A. CRAIG—AD
© ICON

MANAGEMENT AND THERAPY

Nonpharmacologic

General Measures: Rapid evaluation and supportive intervention. Aggressive support and treatment of the attendant shock is paramount. (Frank shock is common by the time the patient is first seen for care.)

Specific Measures: The site of infection must be identified and drained, most commonly by removing the contaminated tampon. Antibiotic therapy with a β-lactamase-resistant antistaphylococcal agent should be started, but does not alter the initial course of the illness. Other support (eg, mechanical ventilation, pressor agents) as needed.

Diet: As tolerated and dictated by the patient's clinical status during acute disease.

Activity: Bed rest during initial diagnosis and therapy.

Patient Education: American College of Obstetricians and Gynecologists Patient Education Pamphlet AP116 (*Menstrual Hygiene Products*).

Drug(s) of Choice

Oxacillin or nafcillin 100 mg/kg/d given in divided doses q6h.

Contraindications: Known or suspected allergy.

Precautions: The dose of oxacillin must be reduced if renal failure is present.

Interactions: See individual agents.

Alternative Drugs

Clindamycin 25 mg/kg/d given in divided doses q8h. Vancomycin 30 mg/kg/d given in divided doses q6h.

FOLLOW-UP

Patient Monitoring: Intense monitoring is required during the initial phase of treatment. After resolution, normal health maintenance.

Prevention/Avoidance: Frequent changes of tampons. Use of sanitary pads at night. Although the risk of recurrence is low (10%–15%), patients who have had TSS should refrain from the use of tampons in the future.

Possible Complications: Adult respiratory distress syndrome is a common sequela of TSS and patients must be monitored for the development of this complication. Acute renal failure, alopecia, and nail loss may also occur.

Expected Outcome: Although the prognosis for patients with toxic shock syndrome is generally good, mortality rates of 5%–10% are common.

MISCELLANEOUS

Pregnancy Considerations: Uncommon during pregnancy. May occur postpartum as a complication of operative delivery, endometritis, episiotomy infection, or nursing.

***ICD-9-CM* Codes:** 040.89.

REFFRENCES

Broome CV. Epidemiology of toxic shock syndrome in the United States. *Rev Infect Dis* 1989;11:S14.

Chesney PJ, Davis JP, Purdy WK, Wand PJ, Chesney RW. Clinical manifestations of toxic shock syndrome. *JAMA* 1981;246:741.

Davis JP, Vergernot JM, Amsterdam LE, et al. Long-term effects of toxic shock syndrome in women: sequelae, subsequent pregnancy, menstrual history, and long-term trends in catamenial product use. *Rev Infect Dis* 1989;11:S50.

Kain KC, Schulzer M, Chow AW. Clinical spectrum of nonmenstrual toxic shock syndrome (TSS): comparison with menstrual TSS by multivariate discriminant analyses. *Clin Infect Dis* 1993;16:100.

Reingold AL. Toxic shock syndrome: an update. *Am J Obstet Gynecol* 1991;165(suppl):1236.

Reingold AL, Shards KN, Dan BB, Broome CV. Toxic-shock not associated with menstruation. A review of 54 cases. *Lancet* 1982;1:1.

ULCERATIVE COLITIS

INTRODUCTION

Description: An inflammatory bowel disease characterized by an inflammation limited to the mucosa of the large bowel and found primarily in the descending colon and rectum (although the entire colon may be involved). The disease is characterized by intermittent bouts of symptoms interspersed by periods of quiescence.

Prevalence: Seventy to 150 in 100,000.

Predominant Age: 20–50, 20% of patients are younger than 21.

Genetics: Family history present in 8%–2% of cases. More common in some ethnic groups (eg, Jews).

ETIOLOGY AND PATHOGENESIS

Causes: An inflammatory process limited to the mucosa of the large bowel and found primarily in the descending colon and rectum, although the entire colon may be involved. Genetic, infectious, immunologic, and psychologic factors have been postulated to underlay the process.

Risk Factors: Family history. Negatively related to smoking.

CLINICAL CHARACTERISTICS

Signs and Symptoms:
- Abdominal pain (generally mild to moderate) (the pain is frequently relieved by a bowel movement, but many report the sensation of incomplete evacuation)
- Diarrhea (voluminous, watery, with occasional blood)
- Fever and weight loss
- Arthralgias and arthritis (15%–20%)
- Aphthous ulcers of the mouth (5%–10%)

DIAGNOSTIC APPROACH

Differential Diagnosis:
- IBS (ulcerative colitis may be differentiated from IBS by the frequent presence of fever or bloody stools in ulcerative colitis)
- Crohn's disease
- Hemorrhoids
- Colon carcinoma
- Diverticulitis
- Infectious diarrhea (*E coli, Salmonella, Shigella, Entamoeba histolytica*)
- Iatrogenic (antibiotic associated)
- Radiation proctitis/colitis

Associated Conditions: Ocular complications (uveitis, cataracts, keratopathy, corneal ulceration, retin-opathy; 4%–10% of patients), liver and biliary complications (cirrhosis, 1%–5%; sclerosing cholangitis, 1%–4%; bile duct carcinoma), and ankylosing spondylitis.

Workup and Evaluation

Laboratory: No specific evaluation indicated. Complete blood count to evaluate blood loss or inflammation. Albumen and potassium levels may be reduced or liver functions test results may be elevated.

Imaging: Barium enema (air contrast).

Special Tests: Sigmoidoscopy, colonoscopy, or rectal biopsy.

Diagnostic Procedures: History, sigmoidoscopy, barium enema, or rectal biopsy.

Pathologic Findings

Superficial inflammation with ulceration is common. Hyperemia and hemorrhage is also common. The rectum is involved in 95% of cases, but the inflammation extends proximal in a continuous manner, at times even involving the terminal ileum.

MANAGEMENT AND THERAPY

Nonpharmacologic

General Measures: Evaluation and control of inflammation, prevention of complications, maintenance of nutrition (including adequate iron intake).

Specific Measures: Severe exacerbations may require hospitalization. Patients whose disease is refractory to antibiotic therapy may require surgical resection.

Diet: No specific dietary changes indicated except for those based on other indications (such as lactose intolerance).

Activity: No restriction.

Drug(s) of Choice

Sulfasalazine 1–4 g PO qd (useful for both mild flare-ups and chronic suppression; approximately 10% of patients require chronic suppressive therapy).

Steroid enemas or mesalamine (5-aminosalicylic acid [5-ASA]) enemas or suppositories.

Prednisone 40–60 mg PO qd for flare-ups (tapered off over 2 months).

Contraindications: Known or suspected allergy or intolerance.

Precautions: Antidiarrheal agents may precipitate toxic megacolon.

Interactions: See individual agents.

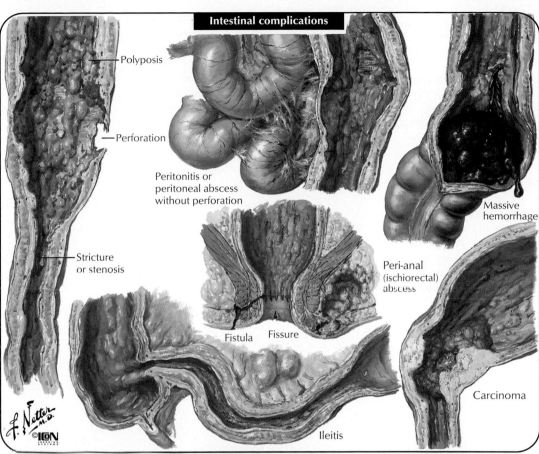

Intestinal complications

Polyposis

Perforation

Peritonitis or peritoneal abscess without perforation

Stricture or stenosis

Massive hemorrhage

Peri-anal (ischiorectal) abscess

Fistula Fissure

Carcinoma

Ileitis

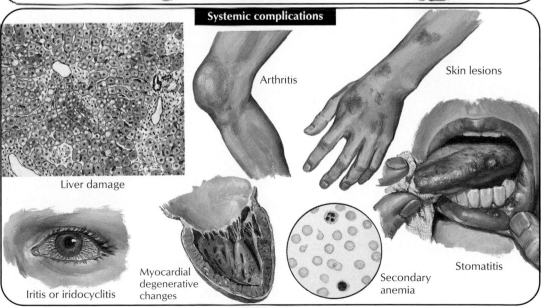

Systemic complications

Liver damage

Arthritis

Skin lesions

Iritis or iridocyclitis

Myocardial degenerative changes

Secondary anemia

Stomatitis

545

Alternative Drugs

Oral 5-ASA derivatives are being studied. Antidiarrheal agents (diphenoxylate-atropine and loperamide) may be used but may precipitate toxic megacolon.

FOLLOW-UP

Patient Monitoring: Normal health maintenance, periodic follow-up to monitor status of disease and possible complications. Colonoscopy to watch for the possible development of cancer should be performed every 1–2 years beginning 7–8 years after the onset of disease. Annual testing of liver function is desirable.

Prevention/Avoidance: None (prevention of complications as above).

Possible Complications: Perforation, toxic megacolon, hepatic disease, bowel stricture and obstruction, colon cancer (30% after 25 years, less for left-sided disease). Mortality for initial attack is approximately 5%.

Expected Outcome: Highly variable; 75%–85% of patients experience relapses, 20% require colectomy. Colon cancer risk is the greatest factor affecting long-term prognosis and management.

MISCELLANEOUS

Pregnancy Considerations: No effect on pregnancy. Thirty percent of patients with inactive disease have relapses during pregnancy, 15% in the first trimester. Treatment with sulfasalazine does not affect the outcome of the pregnancy. It is recommended that pregnancy be delayed until the disease is in remission.

ICD-9-CM **Codes:** 556.9.

REFERENCES

Hannauer SB. Inflammatory bowel disease. *N Engl J Med* 1996;334:841.

Hannauer SB. Inflammatory bowel disease. In: Wyngaarden JB, Smith LH Jr, Bennett JC, eds. *Cecil Textbook of Medicine.* 19th ed. Philadelphia, Pa: WB Saunders Co, 1992: 699.

Rapkin AJ, Mayer EA. Gastroenterologic causes of chronic pelvic pain. *Obstet Gynecol Clin North Am* 1993;20:663.

URINARY INCONTINENCE: BYPASS, OVERFLOW, STRESS, AND URGE

INTRODUCTION

Description: Urinary incontinence is a sign, a symptom, and a disease all at the same time. Bypass incontinence is continuous incontinence occurring when the normal continence mechanism is bypassed, as with fistulae. Symptoms may be intermittent or continuous, making the establishment of a diagnosis difficult in some patients. Overflow incontinence is continuous or intermittent insensible loss of small volumes of urine resulting from an overfilled or atonic bladder. Stress and urge incontinence are limited almost exclusively to women. Stress incontinence is the passive loss of urine in response to increased intraabdominal pressure, such as that caused by coughing, laughing, or sneezing. Urge incontinence is the involuntary loss of urine accompanied by a sense of urgency or impending loss and is associated with increased bladder activity.

Prevalence: Of all women who have hysterectomies, 0.05% develop a fistula and subsequent bypass incontinence. Overflow incontinence is uncommon and generally follows trauma, instrumentation, surgery, or anesthesia. Stress incontinence affects 10%–15% of all women, and 30%–60% of women after menopause. Urge incontinence accounts for 35% of patients with incontinence.

Predominant Age: Mid-reproductive age and onward. Overflow incontinence is more common in later years. Both stress and urge incontinence become more common during the 40s and beyond and are most common after menopause.

Genetics: No genetic pattern.

ETIOLOGY AND PATHOGENESIS

Causes: Bypass incontinence–fistulae may result from surgical or obstetrical trauma, irradiation, or malignancy, although the most common cause by far is unrecognized surgical trauma. Roughly 75% of fistulae occur after abdominal hysterectomy. Signs of a urinary fistula (watery discharge) usually occur from 5–30 days after surgery, although they may be present in the immediate postoperative period.

Overflow incontinence—Trauma (vulvar, perineal, radical pelvic surgery), irritation/infection (chronic cystitis, herpetic vulvitis, herpes zoster), anesthesia (spinal, epidural, caudal), pressure (uterine leiomyomata, pregnancy), anatomic defect (cystocele, retroversion, or prolapse of the uterus), neurologic (multiple sclerosis, diabetes, spinal cord tumors, herniated disc, stroke, amyloid disease, pernicious anemia, Guillain-Barré syndrome, neurosyphilis), systemic disease (hypothyroidism, uremia), medications (antihistamines, appetite suppressants, β-adrenergic agents, parasympathetic blockers, vincristine, carbamazepine), radiation therapy, behavioral (psychogenic, infrequent voiding).

Stress incontinence—Unequal transmission of intraabdominal pressure to the bladder and urethra. Generally associated with an anatomic defect such as a cystocele, urethrocele, or cystourethrocele. The degree of incontinence is often not correlated with the scale of pelvic relaxation.

Urge incontinence—allergy, bladder stone, bladder tumor, caffeinism, central nervous system tumors, detrusor muscle instability, interstitial cystitis, multiple sclerosis, Parkinson's disease, radiation cystitis, radical pelvic surgery, spinal cord injury, urinary tract infections (acute or chronic).

Risk Factors: Bypass incontinence—Surgery or radiation treatment. Most common after uncomplicated hysterectomy, although pelvic adhesive disease, endometriosis, or pelvic tumors increase the individual risk. Overflow incontinence—None known other than causes listed above. Stress incontinence—Multiparity, obesity, chronic cough, or heavy lifting, intrinsic tissue weakness or atrophic changes resulting from estrogen loss. Urge incontinence—Frequent urinary tract infections.

CLINICAL CHARACTERISTICS

Signs and Symptoms:
- Bypass incontinence—Continuous loss of urine (often from the vagina or rectum)
- Fistulae from the vagina to the bladder (vesicovaginal), urethra (urethrovaginal), or ureter (ureterovaginal) (Rarely, communication between the bladder and the uterus [vesicouterine] may also occur through the same mechanisms. Multiple fistulae are present in up to 15% of patients.)
- Overflow incontinence—Frequent loss of small volumes of urine (may or may not be related to increases in intraabdominal pressure)
- Midline lower abdominal mass (with or without tenderness) that disappears with catheterization

Stress Incontinence

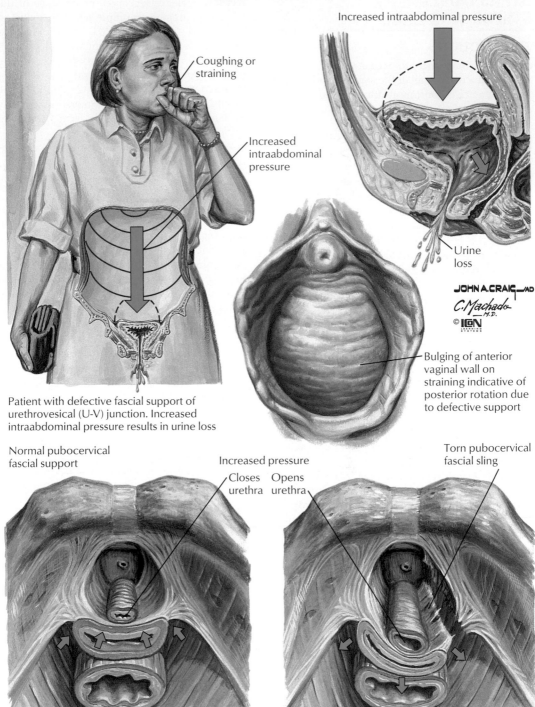

Coughing or straining

Increased intraabdominal pressure

Increased intraabdominal pressure

Urine loss

Patient with defective fascial support of urethrovesical (U-V) junction. Increased intraabdominal pressure results in urine loss

Bulging of anterior vaginal wall on straining indicative of posterior rotation due to defective support

JOHN A. CRAIG—MD

C. Machado M.D.

© ICON

Normal pubocervical fascial support

Increased pressure

Closes urethra   Opens urethra

Torn pubocervical fascial sling

Increased intraabdominal pressure forces urethra against intact pubocervical fascia, closing urethra and maintaining continence

Defective fascial support allows posterior rotation of U-V junction due to increased pressure, opening urethra and causing urine loss

- Ability for spontaneous voiding may or may not be compromised
- Stress incontinence—Loss of small spurts of urine in association with transient increases in intraabdominal pressure
- Associated cystocele, urethrocele, or cystourethrocele
- Urge incontinence—Reduced bladder capacity and early, intense, sensations of bladder fullness
- Spontaneous and uninhibitable contractions of the bladder muscles, resulting in large volume, uncontrolled urine loss
- Loss possibly provoked by activities such as hand washing or a change in position or posture or after (not during) changes in intraabdominal pressure such as a cough or sneeze

DIAGNOSTIC APPROACH

Differential Diagnosis:
- Bypass incontinence—Overflow incontinence
- Urge incontinence
- Ectopic ureter
- Overflow incontinence—Other forms of incontinence (stress, bypass/fistula)
- Chronic urinary tract infections
- Urinary tract obstruction
- Neurologic conditions presenting as an adynamic bladder
- Stress incontinence—Mixed incontinence (stress and urge)
- Urge incontinence (detrusor instability)
- Intrinsic sphincter defect (ISD)
- Low pressure urethra
- Urinary tract fistula
- Urinary tract infection
- Urethral diverticulum
- Overflow incontinence
- Urge incontinence—Mixed incontinence (stress and urge)
- Stress incontinence
- Urinary tract infection
- Urinary tract fistula
- Interstitial cystitis
- Urethritis

Associated Conditions: All forms—vulvitis, vaginitis. Stress incontinence—pelvic relaxation, uterine prolapse, other hernias, vaginitis, vulvitis, recurrent urinary tract infection. Urge incontinence—Nocturia, enuresis (bed wetting).

Workup and Evaluation

Laboratory: No evaluation indicated. Urinalysis is generally recommended, although results are nonspecific. Abrupt onset incontinence in older patients should suggest infection, which may be confirmed through urinalysis or culture.

Imaging: Ureterovaginal fistulae should be evaluated by excretory urography to evaluate possible ureteral dilation or obstruction. Retrograde urography, with the passage of ureteral stents, may also be required. Ultrasonography demonstrates a distended bladder in patients with overflow incontinence.

Special Tests: If a vesicovaginal fistula is found, cystoscopy is required to evaluate the location of the fistula in relation to the ureteral opening and bladder trigone. For most patients, urodynamics testing (including a cystometrogram) should be considered. For patients with stress incontinence a "Q-tip test" should be performed. (A cotton-tipped applicator dipped in 2% lidocaine [Xylocaine] is placed in the urethra and rotation anteriorly with straining is measured. Greater than 30 degrees is abnormal.) A bladder biopsy should be performed if interstitial cystitis is suspected. Neurologic testing should be considered in younger patients with urge incontinence. An evaluation of urinary function is advisable especially if surgical therapy is being considered. In the past, the functional significance of a cystourethrocele was gauged by elevating the bladder neck (using fingers or an instrument) and asking the patient to strain (referred to as a Bonney or Marshall-Marchetti test). This test has fallen out of favor as non-specific and unreliable.

Diagnostic Procedures: When a fistula is suspected, the installation of a dilute solution of methylene blue (or sterile milk) into the bladder while a tampon is in place in the vagina documents a vesicovaginal fistula. A ureterovaginal fistula may be documented in a similar fashion using intravenous indigo carmine. For patients with overflow incontinence, physical examination and catheter drainage of the bladder are diagnostic. Urodynamics testing (cystometrogram) generally confirms the diagnosis. The best way to confirm stress incontinence is by pelvic examination—loss is best demonstrated by having the patient strain or cough while observing the vaginal opening. Urodynamics testing (simple or complex) may be used to evaluate other possible causes of incontinence. History and physical examination, urodynamics testing (simple or complex), and evaluation of sphincter tone and function (as an indication of neurologic function) are the best ways to establish the diagnosis of urge incontinence.

Detrusor Instability and Hyperreflexia

Detrusor instability

Detrusor hyperreflexia

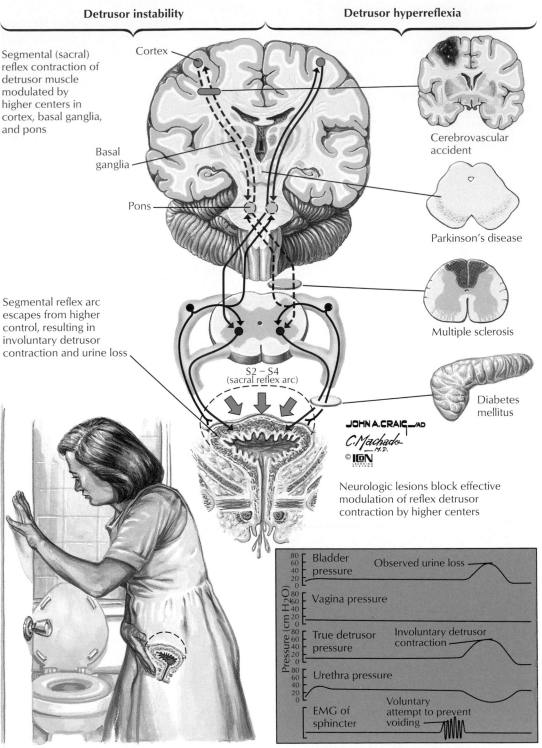

Segmental (sacral) reflex contraction of detrusor muscle modulated by higher centers in cortex, basal ganglia, and pons

Cortex

Basal ganglia

Pons

Cerebrovascular accident

Parkinson's disease

Multiple sclerosis

Diabetes mellitus

Segmental reflex arc escapes from higher control, resulting in involuntary detrusor contraction and urine loss

S2 – S4
(sacral reflex arc)

JOHN A. CRAIG _AD
C. Machado
M.D.
© ICON

Neurologic lesions block effective modulation of reflex detrusor contraction by higher centers

Pressure (cm H₂O)

Bladder pressure — Observed urine loss

Vagina pressure

True detrusor pressure — Involuntary detrusor contraction

Urethra pressure

EMG of sphincter — Voluntary attempt to prevent voiding

Urgency and urge incontinence typical of detrusor instability or hyperreflexia

Cystometry documents involuntary detrusor contraction in bladder filling phase

Pathologic Findings

Based on cause. A distended, often hypotonic bladder is typical of patients with overflow incontinence. Evidence of a loss of support for the urethra and/or bladder is generally apparent on physical examination in patients with stress urinary incontinence. Patients with urge incontinence have a reduced bladder capacity, early first sensation, and uninhibited bladder contractions.

MANAGEMENT AND THERAPY

Nonpharmacologic

General Measures: Bypass incontinence—urinary diversion, protection of the vulva from continuous moisture (zinc oxide, diaper rash preparations). Overflow incontinence—treatment of urinary tract infection (if present). Stress incontinence—weight reduction, treatment of chronic cough (if present), timed voiding, topical or systemic estrogen replacement or therapy as indicated. Urge incontinence—treatment of any urinary tract infection present, timed voiding.

Specific Measures: Bypass incontinence—Vesicovaginal fistulae that occur in the immediate postoperative period should be treated by large caliber transurethral catheter drainage. Spontaneous healing is evident within 2–4 weeks. Similarly, in patients with a ureterovaginal fistula, prompt placement of a ureteral stent, left in place for 2 weeks, allows spontaneous healing for roughly 25% of patients. Surgical repair of genitourinary fistulae is generally delayed 2–4 months, to allow complete healing of the original insult. In all cases, successful surgical repair consists of meticulous dissection of the fistulous tract and careful reapproximation of tissues. Overflow incontinence—prompt and continuous drainage if retention is present, timed voiding to reduce bladder volume, suprapubic pressure or Crede maneuver to reduce residual volume. Stress incontinence—pessary therapy, pelvic muscle exercises (Kegel exercises), collagen injections (ISD), surgical repair; limited role for medical therapy. Urge incontinence—medical therapy; limited role for surgical repair.

Diet: No specific dietary changes indicated. Reduction in caffeine use and other bladder irritants may help some patients with symptoms of urgency incontinence.

Activity: No restriction, although some reduction in heavy lifting may be prudent for women with symptoms of stress incontinence.

Patient Education: Reassurance, American College of Obstetricians and Gynecologists Patient Education Pamphlet AP081 (*Urinary Incontinence*).

Drug(s) of Choice

Bypass incontinence—None.

Overflow incontinence—pharmacologic therapy for these patients is often unsatisfactory and many require long-term catheter drainage or intermittent self-catheterization to manage their problem.

Urinary tract antibiotics if infection is present.

Acetylcholinelike drugs (bethanechol chloride [Urecholine] 10–50 mg three to four times per day, may also be given as 2.5–5 mg SC).

Stress incontinence—phenylpropanolamine (75–150 mg PO daily) may improve mild stress incontinence.

Phenylpropanolamine plus chlorpheniramine (75 mg/12 mg PO q6h) is better tolerated than phenylpropanolamine alone.

Imipramine hydrochloride (Tofranil) 50–150 mg PO daily is good for mixed incontinence and enuresis. Use with care in elderly patients.

Estrogen, either topically or systemically, is often prescribed to improve tissue tone, reduce irritation, and prepare tissues for surgical or pessary therapy.

Urge incontinence—flavoxate hydrochloride (Urispas) 100–200 mg PO tid–qid (fewer side effects, more expensive than some).

Imipramine hydrochloride (Tofranil) 25–50 mg PO bid–tid (good for mixed incontinence and enuresis, 60%–75% effective).

Oxybutynin hydrochloride (Ditropan) 5–10 mg PO tid–qid (side effects common [75%], 60%–80% effective).

Phenylpropanolamine hydrochloride (Propadrine) 50 mg PO bid (α-adrenergic sympathomimetic).

Propantheline bromide (Pro-Banthine) 15–30 mg PO tid–qid (few side effects, variable absorption, 60%–80% effective).

Contraindications: Overflow incontinence—Hyperthyroidism, peptic ulcer, latent or active bronchial asthma, pronounced bradycardia or hypotension, vasomotor instability, coronary artery disease, epilepsy, or Parkinsonism. Stress incontinence—known or suspected sensitivity to medication, undiagnosed vaginal bleeding, breast cancer. Urge incontinence—Most agents are contraindicated in patients with urinary retention, narrow-angle glaucoma, or known or suspected hypersensitivity.

Precautions: Overflow incontinence—it is preferred that bethanechol be given when the stomach is empty (1 hour before or 2 hours after meals). The sterile solution must *not* be given IM or IV.

Other Causes of Incontinence

Secondary detrusor instability

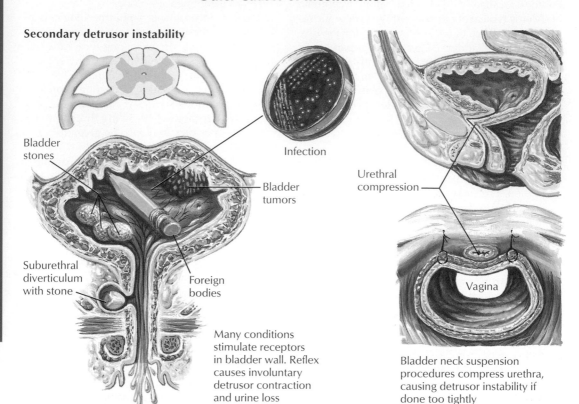

Bladder
stones

Infection

Bladder
tumors

Urethral
compression

Suburethral
diverticulum
with stone

Foreign
bodies

Vagina

Many conditions
stimulate receptors
in bladder wall. Reflex
causes involuntary
detrusor contraction
and urine loss

Bladder neck suspension
procedures compress urethra,
causing detrusor instability if
done too tightly

Other types of incontinence

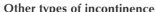
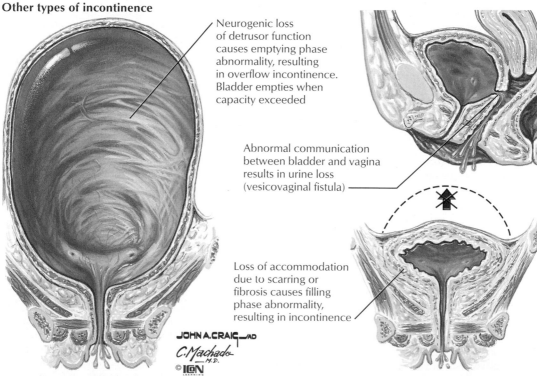

Neurogenic loss
of detrusor function
causes emptying phase
abnormality, resulting
in overflow incontinence.
Bladder empties when
capacity exceeded

Abnormal communication
between bladder and vagina
results in urine loss
(vesicovaginal fistula)

Loss of accommodation
due to scarring or
fibrosis causes filling
phase abnormality,
resulting in incontinence

JOHN A. CRAIG—AD
C. Machado
M.D.
© ICN
LEARNING
SYSTEMS

Bethanechol should not be given if the integrity of either the bladder wall or the gastrointestinal tract is in question or may be mechanically obstructed. Stress incontinence—α-blocking agents used to treat hypertension may reduce urethral tone sufficiently to result in stress incontinence in patients with reduced pelvic support. Patients treated with angiotensin-converting enzyme inhibitors may develop a cough as a side effect of medication, worsening incontinence symptoms and accelerating the appearance or worsening of a cystourethrocele. Urge incontinence—anticholinergic drugs must be used in caution in patients with obstructive gastrointestinal disease or tachycardia. Dry mouth is experienced by 40%–50% of patients.

Interactions: Overflow incontinence—bethanechol should be used with extreme care in patients receiving ganglion blocking compounds. Urge incontinence—patients taking cytochrome P450 3A4 inhibitors (macrolide antibiotics or antifungal agents) must reduce their doses of tolterodine tartrate.

Alternate Therapies: Overflow incontinence—intermittent self-catheterization, electrical stimulation, reduction cystoplasty, urinary diversion. Urge incontinence—tolterodine tartrate (Detrol) 1–2 mg PO bid, dicyclomine hydrochloride (Bentyl) 20 mg IM qid (requires parenteral use), terodiline hydrochloride (Micturin) 12.5–25 mg PO bid (available outside of United States).

FOLLOW-UP

Patient Monitoring: Normal health maintenance. Patients are at increased risk for urinary tract infections, vaginitis, and vulvitis. Patients who have experienced overflow incontinence have an increased risk of recurrence.

Prevention/Avoidance: Careful surgical technique should be used to reduce the risk of fistula formation. Surveillance in situations that predispose to retention (eg, after regional anesthesia, childbirth). Avoidance of and prompt treatment for urinary tract infections is thought to reduce the risk of developing urgency incontinence in the future.

Possible Complications: Social isolation and vulvar and perineal irritation are common complications of any type of urinary incontinence. Ascending urinary tract infection (including pyelonephritis) may occur if a fistula or bladder distension is present.

Expected Outcome: Recurrence after surgical repair of a fistula is common, especially in patients who have undergone radiation therapy for malignancies. For patients with time-limited causes for overflow incontinence a complete resolution with drainage should be expected. For patients with idiopathic retention or retention caused by chronic causation, frequent recurrence, possible dependence on self-catheterization, urinary diversion, and electrical stimulation are possible. Generally favorable results may be obtained for patients with symptoms of stress incontinence through the use of a carefully chosen and fitted pessary. Surgical therapy is associated with 40%–95% success in long-term correction of the anatomic defect and the associated symptoms. (Success rates vary based on the type of procedure performed and duration of follow-up.) Patients with urge incontinence can expect generally good results with medical therapy and timed voiding.

MISCELLANEOUS

Pregnancy Considerations: No effect on pregnancy, although pregnancy (and vaginal delivery) may contribute to a worsening of pelvic support problems. Pregnancy often induces frequency and urgency because of bladder compression by the fetal presenting part near term. Bethanechol is a pregnancy category C drug.

ICD-9-CM Codes: Bypass incontinence: 788.30, 788.37 (Continuous leakage); overflow incontinence—788.39, 788.21 (Incomplete bladder emptying), 788.37 (Continuous leakage of urine), 788.34 (Without sensory awareness); Stress incontinence—625.6; Urge incontinence—788.31.

REFERENCES

Abrams P, Blaivas JG, Stanton SL, Andersen JT. The standardization of terminology of lower urinary tract function produced by the International Continence Society Committee on Standardization of Terminology. *Scand J Urol Nephrol* 1988;114:5.

American College of Obstetricians and Gynecologists. *Pelvic Organ Prolapse.* Washington, DC: ACOG; 1995. ACOG Technical Bulletin 214.

American College of Obstetricians and Gynecologists. *Genitourinary Fistulas.* Washington, DC: ACOG; 1985. ACOG Technical Bulletin 83.

American College of Obstetricians and Gynecologists. *Lower Urinary Tract Operative Injuries.* Washington, DC: ACOG; 1997. ACOG Technical Bulletin 238.

Consensus Conference. Urinary incontinence in adults. *JAMA* 1989;261:2685.

Diaz-Ball FL, Moore CA. A diagnostic aid for vesicovaginal fistula. *J Urol* 1969;102:424.

Federkiw DM, Sand PK, Retzky SS, Johnson DC. The cotton swab test. Receiver-operating characteristic curves. *J Reprod Med* 1995;40:42.

Holley RL, Kilgore LC. Urologic Complications. In: Orr JW Jr, Shingleton HM, eds. *Complications in Gynecologic Surgery: Prevention, Recognition, and Management.* Philadelphia, Pa: JB Lippincott; 1994:149.

Kinn AC, Lindskog M. Estrogens and phenylpropanolamine in combination for stress urinary incontinence in postmenopausal women. *Urology* 1988;32:273.

Norton PA, ed. Urinary incontinence. *Clin Obstet Gynecol* 1990;33:293.

Ostergard DR, Bent AE. *Urogynecology and Urodynamics.* 3rd ed. Baltimore, Md: Williams & Wilkins; 1991:346, 478.

Sims JM. On the treatment of vesico-vaginal fistula. *Am J Med Sci* 1852;23:59.

Smith RP. *Gynecology in Primary Care.* Baltimore, Md: Williams & Wilkins; 1997:577.

Symmonds RE. Incontinence: vesical and urethral fistulas. *Clin Obstet Gynecol* 1984;27:499.

Urinary Incontinence Guideline Panel. *Urinary Incontinence in Adults: Clinical Practice Guidelines.* Rockville, Md: Agency for Health Care Policy and Research, US Dept of Health and Human Services; 1992. AHCPR publication 92-0038.

Videla FLG, Wall LL. Diagnosing stress incontinence without multichannel urodynamic studies. *Obstet Gynecol* 1998;91:965.

Wall LL. Diagnosis and management of urinary incontinence due to detrusor instability. *Obstet Gynecol Surv* 1990;45:1s.

URINARY TRACT INFECTION

INTRODUCTION

Description: An infection of the urinary tract causing urethritis, cystitis (including trigonitis), or pyelonephritis. Urinary tract infections are much more common in women because of their shortened urethral length and exposure of the urinary tract to trauma and pathogens during sexual activity.

Prevalence: Seen in 3%–8%, with roughly 45% aged 15–60 experiencing at least one urinary tract infection.

Predominant Age: Any, increases with older age.

Genetics: No genetic pattern.

ETIOLOGY AND PATHOGENESIS

Causes: Most urinary tract infections in women ascend from contamination of the urethra, acquired via instrumentation, trauma, or sexual intercourse. (A history of intercourse within the preceding 24–48 hours is present in up to 75% of patients with acute urinary tract infection.) Coliform organisms, especially *E coli*, are the most common organisms responsible for asymptomatic bacteriuria, cystitis, and pyelonephritis. Ninety percent of first infections and 80% of recurrent infections are caused by *E coli*, with between 10% and 20% resulting from *Staphylococcus saprophyticus*. Infection with other pathogens such as *Klebsiella* species (5%) and *Proteus* species (2%) account for most of the remaining infections. Anaerobic bacteria, *Trichomonas*, and yeasts are rare sources of infections except in diabetic patients, immunosuppressed patients, or those requiring chronic catheterization. Infection with *Neisseria gonorrhoeae, Chlamydia trachomatis, Mycoplasma,* and *Ureaplasma* should all be considered when urethritis is suspected.

Risk Factors: Sexual activity, instrumentation, more virulent pathogens, altered host defenses, infrequent or incomplete voiding, foreign body or stone, obstruction, or biochemical changes in the urine (diabetes, hemoglobinopathies, pregnancy), estrogen deficiency, diaphragm use, and spermicides.

CLINICAL CHARACTERISTICS

Signs and Symptoms:
- Asymptomatic (5%)
- Frequency, urgency, nocturia, or dysuria
- Pelvic pressure (cystitis)
- Fever and chills (pyelonephritis)
- Pyuria (more than 5 white cells per high power field in a centrifuged specimen)
- Hematuria (infrequent)
- Costovertebral angle tenderness (pyelonephritis)
- Suprapubic tenderness (cystitis)

DIAGNOSTIC APPROACH

Differential Diagnosis:
- Traumatic trigonitis
- Urethral syndrome
- Interstitial cystitis
- Bladder tumors or stones
- Vulvitis and vaginitis (may give rise to external dysuria)
- Urethral diverticulum
- Infection in the Skene's glands
- Detrusor instability

Associated Conditions: Dyspareunia.

Workup and Evaluation

Laboratory: Nonpregnant women with a first episode of classic symptoms suggestive of urinary tract infection do not need laboratory confirmation of the diagnosis, but may be treated empirically. Others should have a urinalysis and culture performed. For uncentrifuged urine samples, the presence of more than 1 white blood cell per high power field gives 90% accuracy in detecting infection. Gram's stain of urine samples or sediments may help establish the diagnosis or suggest a possible pathogen.

Imaging: No imaging indicated.

Special Tests: When urethritis is suspected, a swab inserted into the urethra may be used to obtain material for culture and Gram's stain to establish the diagnosis.

Diagnostic Procedures: History and physical examination, urinalysis.

Pathologic Findings

Pyuria with white blood cell casts common.

MANAGEMENT AND THERAPY

Nonpharmacologic

General Measures: Fluids, frequent voiding, and antipyretics. Urinary acidification (with ascorbic acid, ammonium chloride, or acidic fruit juices) and urinary analgesics (phenazopyridine [Pyridium]) may also be added based on the needs of the individual patient.

Specific Measures: Antibiotic therapy.

Diet: Increased fluids and reduction of caffeine.

Activity: No restriction.

Patient Education: Reassurance, American College of Obstetricians and Gynecologists Patient Education Pamphlet AP050 (*Urinary Tract Infections*).

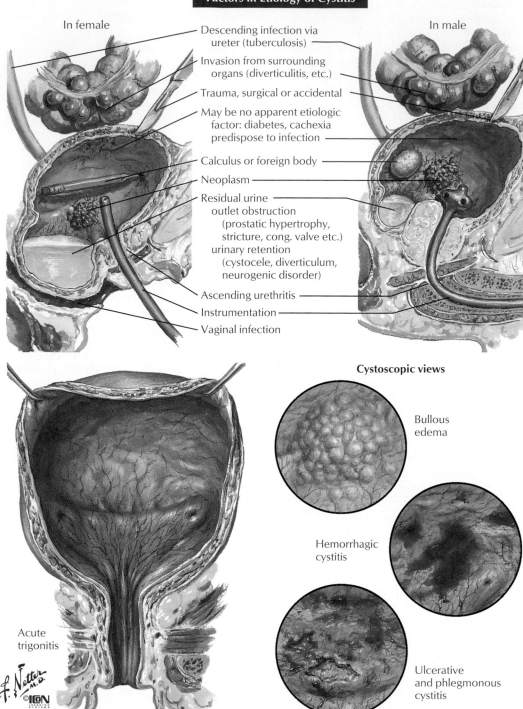

Factors in Etiology of Cystitis

In female

In male

Descending infection via ureter (tuberculosis)

Invasion from surrounding organs (diverticulitis, etc.)

Trauma, surgical or accidental

May be no apparent etiologic factor: diabetes, cachexia predispose to infection

Calculus or foreign body

Neoplasm

Residual urine
outlet obstruction (prostatic hypertrophy, stricture, cong. valve etc.) urinary retention (cystocele, diverticulum, neurogenic disorder)

Ascending urethritis

Instrumentation

Vaginal infection

Cystoscopic views

Bullous edema

Hemorrhagic cystitis

Acute trigonitis

Ulcerative and phlegmonous cystitis

Common Clinical And Laboratory Features Of Acute Pyelonephritis

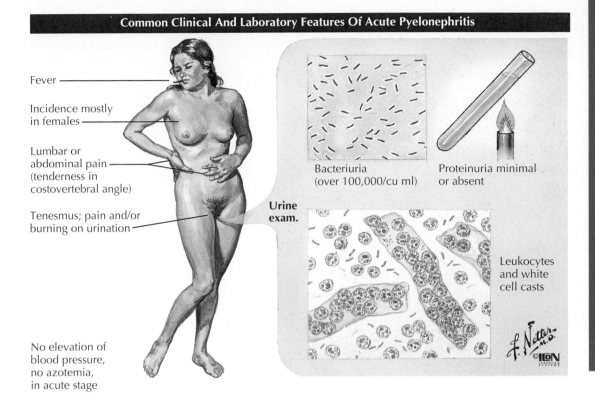

Fever

Incidence mostly in females

Lumbar or abdominal pain (tenderness in costovertebral angle)

Tenesmus; pain and/or burning on urination

Urine exam.

Bacteriuria (over 100,000/cu ml)

Proteinuria minimal or absent

Leukocytes and white cell casts

No elevation of blood pressure, no azotemia, in acute stage

Drug(s) of Choice

Nonpregnant patients: single dose therapy—amoxicillin 3 g, ampicillin 3.5 g, cephalosporin (first generation) 2 g, nitrofurantoin 200 mg, sulfisoxazole 2 g, trimethoprim (TMP) 400 mg, TMP/sulfamethoxazole 300 (1600) mg, fosfomycin tromethamine (Monurol) 3 gm PO.

Three- to seven-day therapy—amoxicillin 500 mg q8h, cephalosporin (first generation) 500 mg q8h, ciprofloxacin 250 mg q12h, nitrofurantoin 100 mg q12h, norfloxacin 400 mg q12h, ofloxacin 200 mg q12h, sulfisoxazole 500 mg q6h, tetracycline 500 mg q6h, TMP/sulfamethoxazole 160/800 mg q12h, TMP 100 (200) mg q12h.

Contraindications: Known or suspected hypersensitivity.

Precautions: Urinary analgesics (phenazopyridine [Pyridium]) should be used for no longer than 48 hours and may stain some types of contact lenses.

Interactions: See individual medications.

Alternative Drugs

Pregnant patients: 7-day therapy—amoxicillin 500 mg q8h, cephalosporin (first generation) 500 mg q6h, nitrofurantoin 100 mg q12h.

FOLLOW-UP

Patient Monitoring: No follow-up is necessary after single dose treatment, or multiday treatment for nonpregnant women who experience resolution of their symptoms. Confirmation of cure for all other patients should be carried out with urinalysis and culture. Those with recurrent infections should be evaluated for possible causes and a program of patient-initiated single-dose therapy should be begun as needed for prophylaxis (after intercourse, daily, or three times weekly based on patient need). Possible causes of recurrent infection include incorrect or incomplete (eg, noncompliant) therapy, mechanical factors (such as obstruction or stone), or compromised host defenses.

Prevention/Avoidance: Frequent voiding, adequate fluid intake, and voiding after intercourse.

Possible Complications: Urethral syndrome and interstitial cystitis. Bacteremia, septic shock, adult respiratory distress syndrome, and other serious sequelae are associated with pyelonephritis. Recurrence rates may be as high as 20% (90% represent reinfection). Up to one third of patients may develop pyelonephritis.

Expected Outcome: For most patients, symptoms should resolve within 2–3 days of the initiation of therapy. Some authors estimate that up to 50% of infections resolve without intervention.

MISCELLANEOUS

Pregnancy Considerations: Asymptomatic bacteriuria is more common during pregnancy (5%). Those at high risk (eg, diabetic patients) should be monitored carefully.

***ICD-9-CM* Codes:** 599.0, 646.6 (Complicating pregnancy).

REFERENCES

American College of Obstetricians and Gynecologists. *Antimicrobial therapy for obstetric patients.* Washington, DC: ACOG; 1988. ACOG Technical Bulletin 117.

Bump RC. Urinary tract infection in women. Current role of single-dose therapy. *J Reprod Med* 1990;35:785.

Greenberg RN, Reilly PM, Luppen KL, Weinandt WJ, Ellington LL, Bollinger MR. Randomized study of single-dose, three-day, and seven-day treatment of cystitis in women. *J Infect Dis* 1986;153:277.

Kunin CM. Urinary tract infections in females. *Clin Infect Dis* 1994;18:1.

Pappas P. Laboratory in the diagnosis and management of urinary tract infections. *Med Clin North Am* 1991; 75:313.

Powers R. New directions in the diagnosis and therapy of urinary tract infections. *Am J Obstet Gynecol* 1991; 164:1387.

Smith RP. *Gynecology in Primary Care.* Baltimore, Md: Williams & Wilkins; 1997:577.

URODYNAMICS TESTING

THE CHALLENGE

An important part of the evaluation of urinary symptoms or incontinence of any type is urodynamic testing of bladder function. This may be performed in the office setting using readily available equipment or may require complex equipment and expertise.

Scope of the Problem: Almost one half of all women have involuntary loss of a few drops of urine at some time in their lifetime, with 10%–15% of women suffering significant, recurrent loss. It has been estimated that more than one quarter of women of reproductive age suffer from some degree of urinary incontinence. This number increases to 30%–40% of women after the age of menopause.

Objectives of Test: To evaluate bladder function and aid in the diagnosis of bladder symptoms such as urgency and incontinence.

TACTICS

Relevant Pathophysiology: The bladder is designed to gradually distend as urine is delivered by the ureters. This distention proceeds with little or no change in bladder pressure (normal compliance). When bladder volume reaches a certain point (generally 150–200 mL) the first sensation of bladder fullness occurs. Additional increases in volume can be accomplished with an increasing sense of urgency but without uninhibited bladder contraction or incontinence. When bladder emptying is allowed, it should happen in an expeditious and efficient manner. While the specific content of urodynamics testing varies, at a minimum it includes cystometrics and provocative tests (such as coughing or straining while the bladder is full). Most centers include sophisticated evaluation of bladder compliance and contractility, cystoscopy, and evaluations of the voiding process itself. Pressure profiles of the bladder and urethra, electromyography, cystoscopy, and fluoroscopic examinations may also be included.

Strategies: The patient should be in a relaxed supine position with her bladder emptied. The patient is catheterized with sterile technique using a straight catheter. Any residual urine is caught, measured for volume, and sent for culture to detect occult infection. The bladder is slowly filled (with sterile saline) by gravity at a rate of less than 3 mL/s. The patient is asked to report her first sensation of bladder fullness and the volume infused at that point is noted.

Filling continues in 25-mL aliquots until the patient is unable to tolerate more, and this volume is recorded as the maximal bladder capacity. Any upward movement of the fluid column, intense sensation of urgency, or leakage around the catheter is abnormal, suggests detrusor instability, and should be noted. The catheter is removed, and the patient asked to cough several times: leakage should be noted. Leakage that occurs immediately after removal, is prolonged, or is of large volume suggests detrusor instability. These maneuvers may be repeated in the standing position.

Patient Education: American College of Obstetricians and Gynecologists Patient Education Pamphlet AP081 (*Urinary Incontinence*), AP050 (*Urinary Tract Infections*), AP012 (*Pelvic Support Problems*).

IMPLEMENTATION

Special Considerations: "Urinary incontinence" may be a sign, a symptom, or a condition. It is defined as a condition in which involuntary loss of urine may be objectively demonstrated, and the loss presents a social or hygienic problem. The volume of the loss is not as important as the impact it has on the patient and her life. More exact measurements of bladder function may be made by assembling intravenous tubing, a spinal manometer (or limb of extra tubing), and a three-way connector. The pressure inside the fluid column may be monitored and the presence of bladder contractions more easily detected and documented. When this greater degree of accuracy is required, many prefer to proceed to formal urodynamics testing. An assessment of voiding may be carried out by filling the bladder with 200 mL of fluid and listening to the patient's voiding from outside a bathroom door or while the patient voids behind a screen. The volume of flow (rate) may be estimated by the sound; the duration of flow may be timed with a stop watch. Sophisticated measures of voiding parameters are typically included in formal urodynamics testing.

REFERENCES

American College of Obstetricians and Gynecologists. *Urinary Incontinence.* Washington, DC: ACOG; 1995. ACOG Technical Bulletin 213.

Bradley WE, Timm GW. Cystometry VI. Interpretation. *Urology* 1976;7:231.

Jarvis GJ, Hall S, Stamp S, Millar DR, Johnson A. An assessment of urodynamic examination in incontinent women. *Br J Obstet Gynaecol* 1980;87:893.

Massey A, Abrams P. Urodynamic of the female lower urinary tract. *Urol Clin North Am* 1985;12:231.

Office Testing Procedures

Standing stress test

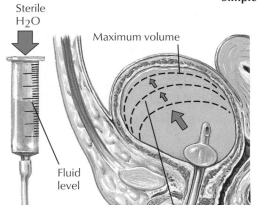

Cough

Towel or sheet

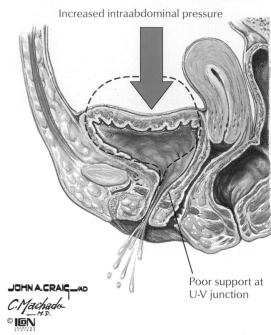

Increased intraabdominal pressure

Poor support at U-V junction

JOHN A. CRAIG_MD
C. Machado
_M.D._
© ICON
LEARNING
SYSTEMS

As physician observes, patient coughs and bears down. Immediate loss of urine suggests stress incontinence

Simple cystometry

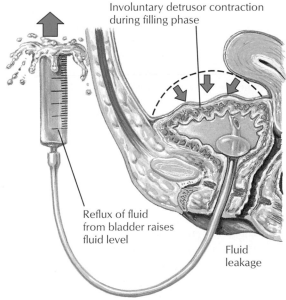

Sterile H$_2$O

Maximum volume

Fluid level

Retrograde filling of bladder with 50 ml sterile H$_2$O

Volume at first urge

Normal

Involuntary detrusor contraction during filling phase

Reflux of fluid from bladder raises fluid level

Fluid leakage

Detrusor instability

Complex Cystometry

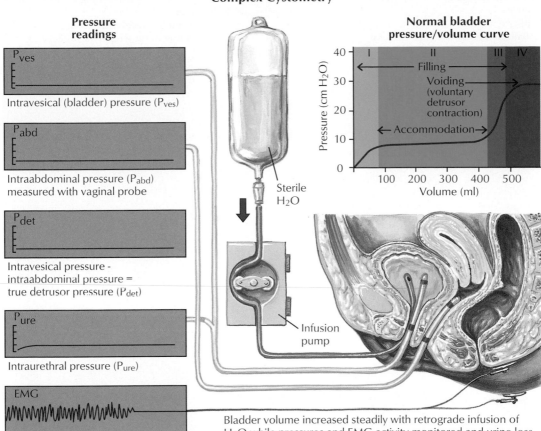

Pressure readings

P_{ves}

Intravesical (bladder) pressure (P_{ves})

P_{abd}

Intraabdominal pressure (P_{abd}) measured with vaginal probe

P_{det}

Intravesical pressure - intraabdominal pressure = true detrusor pressure (P_{det})

P_{ure}

Intraurethral pressure (P_{ure})

EMG

Electromyography (EMG)

Sterile H_2O

Infusion pump

Normal bladder pressure/volume curve

Filling

Voiding (voluntary detrusor contraction)

Accommodation

Bladder volume increased steadily with retrograde infusion of H_2O while pressures and EMG activity monitored and urine loss observed

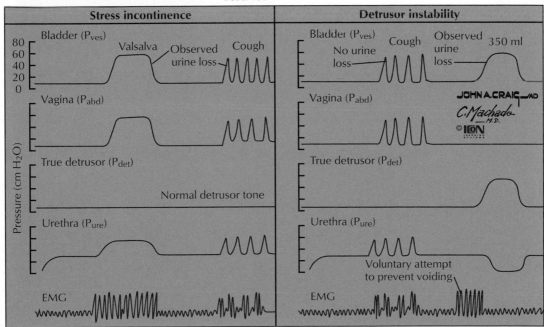

Stress incontinence	Detrusor instability
Bladder (P_{ves}) — Valsalva, Observed urine loss, Cough	Bladder (P_{ves}) — No urine loss, Cough, Observed urine loss, 350 ml
Vagina (P_{abd})	Vagina (P_{abd})
True detrusor (P_{det}) — Normal detrusor tone	True detrusor (P_{det})
Urethra (P_{ure})	Urethra (P_{ure}) — Voluntary attempt to prevent voiding
EMG	EMG

JOHN A.CRAIG—MD

C.Machado—M.D.

© ICON

Ostergard DR, Bent AE, eds. *Urogynecology and Urodynamics*. 4th ed. Baltimore, Md: Williams & Wilkins, 1996.

Smith RP, Ling FW. *Procedures in Woman's Health Care.* Baltimore, Md: Williams & Wilkins; 1997:411, 415.

Sutherst JR, Brown MC. Comparison of single and multichannel cystometry in diagnosing bladder instability. *BMJ* 1984;288:1720.

Walters MD, Realini JP. The evaluation and treatment of urinary incontinence in women: a primary care approach. *J Am Board Fam Pract* 1992;5:289.

VARICOSE VEINS

INTRODUCTION

Description: Dilated, elongated, and tortuous superficial veins with incompetent or congenitally absent valves. Although these may occur anywhere in the body, they are most common in the legs where gravity produces reverse flow. Varicose veins are 5 times more common in women than in men.

Prevalence: Twenty percent of adults.

Predominant Age: Middle age and beyond.

Genetics: Familial as an X-linked dominant condition.

ETIOLOGY AND PATHOGENESIS

Causes: Faulty or absent valves in one or more perforating veins that may result in secondary incompetence at the saphenofemoral junction. Other causes—deep vein thrombophlebitis, increased venous pressure from any source (eg, obstruction by tumor, pregnancy, pelvic mass).

Risk Factors: Pregnancy, family history, prolonged standing.

CLINICAL CHARACTERISTICS

Signs and Symptoms:
- Asymptomatic
- Leg pain or cramps (worse during menstruation)
- Dilated, tortuous superficial veins
- Spider veins (idiopathic telangiectases)
- Limb edema
- Superficial ulceration

DIAGNOSTIC APPROACH

Differential Diagnosis:
- Radiculopathy (nerve root compression)
- Arthritis
- Peripheral neuritis

Associated Conditions: Stasis ulcers and dermatitis.

Workup and Evaluation

Laboratory: No evaluation indicated.

Imaging: Doppler studies may be used to evaluate the possibility of deep vein thrombosis but are generally not required for the diagnosis of varicose veins.

Special Tests: Trendelenburg-Brodie test (elevate leg, compress greater saphenous vein at midthigh, have patient stand: rapid refilling of vein indicates incompetent communicating veins).

Diagnostic Procedures: History and physical examination.

Pathologic Findings

Elongated, tortuous veins with medial fibrosis and absent or atrophic valves.

MANAGEMENT AND THERAPY

Nonpharmacologic

General Measures: Frequent rest, elevation of affected limb, lightweight compression (hosiery), avoidance of proximal compression (girdles).

Specific Measures: Superficial veins may be eliminated with intracapillary injection of hypertonic saline (20%–25%) or 1%–3% solution of sodium tetradecyl sulfate (must be followed by compression for up to 3 weeks). Ligation or stripping of the saphenous veins should be considered in patients with pain, ulcers, recurrent phlebitis, or significant cosmetic problems.

Diet: No specific dietary changes indicated. Weight loss when appropriate.

Activity: Avoid prolonged standing or inactivity, active exercise routines including walking, use of elastic stockings (applied before arising).

Patient Education: Education about risk factors and avoidance, American College of Obstetricians and Gynecologists Patient Education Pamphlet AP119 (*Exercise During Pregnancy*), AP044 (*Working During Your Pregnancy*), AP045 (*Exercise and Fitness: A Guide for Women*).

Drug(s) of Choice

None.

Precautions: Some authors suggest that oral contraceptives not be used within 6 weeks of sclerotherapy.

Alternative Drugs

Antibiotic therapy for infected ulcers.

FOLLOW-UP

Patient Monitoring: Normal health maintenance, evaluation for progression of disease or emergence of complications (skin ulcers).

Prevention/Avoidance: Avoidance of prolonged standing or inactivity, use of compression stockings.

Possible Complications: Petechial hemorrhages, chronic edema, superficial ulceration and infection, chronic pigment change, eczema.

Expected Outcome: Generally a chronic condition with control possible through treatment.

MISCELLANEOUS

Pregnancy Considerations: No effect on pregnancy. Pregnancy often worsens existing disease and

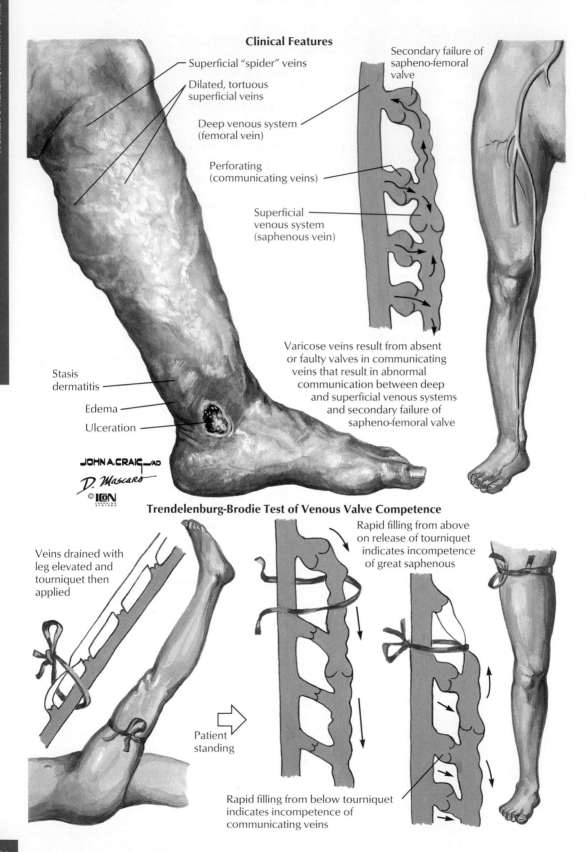

Clinical Features

Superficial "spider" veins

Dilated, tortuous superficial veins

Deep venous system (femoral vein)

Perforating (communicating veins)

Superficial venous system (saphenous vein)

Secondary failure of sapheno-femoral valve

Varicose veins result from absent or faulty valves in communicating veins that result in abnormal communication between deep and superficial venous systems and secondary failure of sapheno-femoral valve

Stasis dermatitis

Edema

Ulceration

JOHN A. CRAIG—MD
D. Mascaro
©ICON
LEARNING
SYSTEMS

Trendelenburg-Brodie Test of Venous Valve Competence

Veins drained with leg elevated and tourniquet then applied

Patient standing

Rapid filling from above on release of tourniquet indicates incompetence of great saphenous

Rapid filling from below tourniquet indicates incompetence of communicating veins

increases the risk of future occurrence. Use of compression stockings should be encouraged for those at increased risk.

***ICD-9-CM* Codes:** 454.1.

REFERENCES

Baccaglini U, Spreafico G, Castoro C, Sorrentino P. Sclerotherapy of varicose veins of the lower limbs. Consensus paper. North American Society of Phlebology. *Dermatol Surg* 1996;22:883.

Green D. Sclerotherapy for the permanent eradication of varicose veins: theoretical and practical considerations. *J Am Acad Dermatol* 1998;38:461.

Helmerhorst FM, Bloemenkamp KW, Rosendaal FR, Vandenbroucke JP. Oral contraceptives and thrombotic disease: risk of venous thromboembolism. *Thromb Haemost* 1997;78:327.

Hobson J. Venous insufficiency at work. *Angiology* 1997; 48:577.

Houghton AD, Panayiotopoulos Y, Taylor PR. Practical management of primary varicose veins. *Br J Clin Pract* 1996;50:103.

Ramelet AA. Complications of ambulatory phlebectomy. *Dermatol Surg* 1997;23:947.

Sapira JD. *The Art and Science of Bedside Diagnosis.* Baltimore, Md: Williams & Wilkins; 1990:368.

Index

dysgerminoma, 240–241, 242f, 254f
  germ cell tumors and, 253
epithelial stromal, 250, 251f, 252
  adenofibroma and, 232
germ cell, 253, 254f, 255
granulosa cell tumors, 256, 257f, 258, 259f
irregular menstrual periods and, 126
menorrhagia and, 128
Overflow incontinence. *See* Urinary incontinence
Overweight problems. *See* Obesity
Ovulation
  anovulation. *See* Anovulation
  assessment of, 368f
  menopause. *See* Menopause
Oxytocin challenge test, 177

P

Paget's disease of the breast, 332, 333f
  lichen sclerosus and, 27
  osteoporosis and, 486
Pap smears
  AGCUS/ASCUS, 80
  atypical squamous or glandular cells of undetermined
    significance, 78, 79f, 80
  carcinoma in situ (cervix), 84
  cervical cancer and, 88
  cervical condyloma, 509
  cervical polyps and, 94
  endometrial cancer, 111, 113
  HGSIL/LGSIL, 81, 83
  high-grade squamous intraepithelial lesion, 81, 82f, 83
  HIV infection and, 520
  low-grade squamous intraepithelial lesion, 81, 82f, 83
  Müllerian sarcomas, 134
  Trichomonas vaginalis, 534
Parasites, sexually transmitted, 527–528, 528f
  pruritus ani and, 498
Pelvic inflammatory disease (PID), 278–280, 279f
  cervicitis and, 98
  Chlamydia trachomatis and, 506
  chronic. *See* Hydrosalpinx
  Crohn's disease and, 422
  dysfunctional uterine bleeding and, 108
  ectopic pregnancy and, 242
  endometritis and, 118
  gonorrhea and, 512
  low back pain and, 474
  toxic shock syndrome and, 541
  Trichomonas vaginalis and, 75, 536
Peptococcus species. *See* Bacterial vaginitis; Bacterial vaginosis
Pessary therapy, 491, 492f
Phthirus humanus, 527–528, 528f
Physical abuse, 396, 397f, 398f, 399
  deep thrust dyspareunia and, 433
  insertional dyspareunia and, 9
  postpartum depression and, 179
  pregnancy trauma, 224, 225f, 226
PID. *See* Pelvic inflammatory disease (PID)
Placental abruption, 207, 208f, 209
  breech birth and, 163
  cholecystitis and, 174
  intrauterine growth restriction and, 198
  placenta previa and, 204
  preeclampsia/eclampsia and, 212
  trauma in pregnancy, 222
  uterine rupture and, 228
Placental implantation, abnormalities of, 146, 147f, 148
  abortion and, 149
  intrauterine growth restriction and, 198
Placenta previa, 204, 205f, 206
  breech birth and, 163
  intrauterine growth restriction and, 198
  placental abruption and, 207
PMS. *See* Premenstrual syndrome (PMS)
Polycystic ovarian disease, 373–374, 374f
Polyhydramnios, 210–211, 211f
Polyps
  cervical. *See* Cervical polyps
  dysmenorrhea and, 430
  endometrial. *See* Endometrial polyps
  hemorrhoids and, 459

pseudosarcoma botryoides, 54
Postcoital bleeding, 493, 494f
  cervical eversion and, 93
  cervical polyps and, 94
  cervicitis and, 98
  endometritis and, 118
Postmenopausal bleeding, 131, 132f, 133
  endometrial cancer and, 111
  endometrial hyperplasia and, 114
  uterine prolapse and, 142
  vaginal prolapse and, 65
Postpartum breast engorgement, 321, 322f
Postpartum depression, 182, 183f, 184f, 185
Postpartum uterine atony, 225, 226f, 227
Precocious pseudopuberty, 256, 257f
Preeclampsia and eclampsia, 212, 213f, 214f, 215
  acute fatty liver and, 155
  cholecystitis and, 174
  gestational trophoblastic disease and, 188
  HELLP syndrome and, 193
  hepatitis in pregnancy and, 195
  placental abruption and, 207
Pregnancy. *See also* Obstetrical conditions
  abortion. *See* Abortion
  acne during, 402
  AGCUS/ASCUS and, 80
  amenorrhea (secondary) and, 342
  amniotic fluid. *See* Amniotic fluid
  anemia during, 406
  anovulation and, 347
  bacterial vaginitis/vaginosis and, 72
  bicornuate, septate, and unicornuate uterus and, 138
  breast cancer and, 295
  carcinoma in situ (cervix) and, 87
  cardiovascular disease in, 168, 169f, 170
    preeclampsia/eclampsia and, 212
  cervical cancer and, 88, 90
  cervical incompetence, 171, 172f, 173
  chancroid and, 505
  Chlamydia trachomatis and, 507–508
  cholecystitis in, 174, 175f, 176
  condyloma acuminata and, 510, 511
  constipation and, 420
  contraception. *See* Contraception
  contraction stress testing, 161, 177, 178f
  cystocele/urethrocele and, 46
  depression after, 179, 180f, 185
  depression during, 426
  dermoid cyst and, 237, 239
  diabetes mellitus in, 182, 183f, 184
    caput succedaneum and, 166
    gingivitis and, 191
    polyhydramnios and, 210
  Down syndrome testing during, 356
  dysfunctional uterine bleeding and, 108, 110
  dysuria and, 438
  ectopic. *See* Ectopic pregnancy
  endometrial cancer and, 111, 113
  endometriosis and, 246
  endometritis and, 119
  female circumcision and, 12
  fibroadenomas and, 304
  fibrocystic breast change and, 309
  galactorrhea and, 325, 327
  gingivitis in, 191, 192f
  gonadal dysgenesis and, 359
  gonorrhea and, 514
  granuloma inguinale and, 516
  hair loss and, 447, 448f, 449
  headaches and, 455
  hemorrhoids and, 459, 461
  hepatitis in, 195, 196f, 197
    acute fatty liver and, 155, 196
  HGSIL abnormality and, 83
  hidradenitis suppurativa treatment and, 15
  HIV infection and, 520, 522
  hydrosalpinx and, 259
  hyperprolactinemia and, 363
  hyperthyroidism and, 462, 464
  infertility. *See* Infertility
  intermenstrual bleeding and, 124